D1608479

THIS PACK HAS BEEN GENEROUSLY DONATED TO MEDICINE AND
HEALTH PROFESSIONALS BY
DOUG STEAD,
DIRECTOR OF CHILD PROTECTION
RAMAS

*Doug Stead has devoted an extraordinary amount of time and resources for the
protection of children. He also provides assistance to law enforcement agencies in
combating the illegal use of technology to facilitate and hide sexual crimes against
children. Over the years, Doug Stead has frequently been on radio and TV as a
guest speaker and as a presenter at numerous international, national and local
conferences on the subject of child pornography and the adults involved in these
types of crimes. Doug Stead has also developed and funded "Reveal", a free
software application which enables a technologically challenged parent to easily
and quickly scan the family computer for indicators (words and images) that may
be of an unhealthy interest by child users.*

Medical, Legal, & Social Science Aspects of

Child Sexual

Exploitation

A Comprehensive Review of Pornography, Prostitution, and Internet Crimes

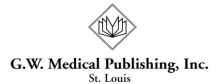

G.W. Medical Publishing, Inc.
St. Louis

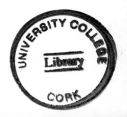

Medical, Legal, & Social Science Aspects of

Child Sexual

Exploitation

A Comprehensive Review of Pornography, Prostitution, and Internet Crimes

Richard J. Estes, DSW, ACSW
Professor
Chair, Concentration in Social and
    Economic Development
Director, International Programs
University of Pennsylvania School of Social
    Work
Philadelphia, Pennsylvania

Victor I. Vieth, JD
Director
APRI's National Child Protection Training
    Center
Winona State University
Winona, Minnesota

Sharon Cooper, MD, FAAP
Adjunct Associate Professor of Pediatrics
University of North Carolina School of
    Medicine
Chapel Hill, North Carolina
Clinical Assistant Professor of Pediatrics
Uniformed Services University of Health
    Sciences
Bethesda, Maryland
Chief , Developmental Pediatric Service
    Womack Army Medical Center
Fort Bragg, North Carolina

Angelo P. Giardino, MD, PhD, FAAP
Associate Chair – Pediatrics
Associate Physician-in Chief/
Vice-President, Clinical Affairs
St. Christopher's Hospital for Children
Associate Professor in Pediatrics
Drexel University College of Medicine
Adjunct Professor of Pediatric Nursing LaSalle
University School of Nursing
Philadelphia, Pennsylvania

Nancy D. Kellogg, MD
Professor of Pediatrics
University of Texas Health Science Center at
    San Antonio
Medical Director
Alamo Children's Advocacy Center

G.W. Medical Publishing, Inc.
St. Louis

Publishers: Glenn E. Whaley and Marianne V. Whaley

Assistant Publisher: Jonathan M. Taylor

Design Director: Glenn E. Whaley

Managing Editors: Karen C. Maurer
Megan E. Ferrell

Associate Editors: Jonathan M. Taylor
Christine Bauer

Book Design/Page Layout: G.W. Graphics
Sudon Choe
Charles J. Seibel, III

Print/Production Coordinator: Charles J. Seibel, III

Cover Design: G.W. Graphics

Color Prepress Specialist: Richard Stockard

Copy Editor: Bonnie F. Spinola

Developmental Editors: Aimee E. Loewe
Laurie Sparks

Proofreader/Indexer: Robert A. Saigh

Printed in Canada.

Publisher:
G.W. Medical Publishing, Inc.
77 Westport Plaza, Suite 366, St. Louis, Missouri, 63146-3124 U.S.A.
Phone: (314) 542-4213 Fax: (314) 542-4239 Toll Free: 1-800-600-0330
http://www.gwmedical.com

Library of Congress Cataloging-in-Publication Data

Cooper, Sharon 1952-
Medical, legal, & social science aspects of child sexual exploitation: a comprehensive review of pornography, prostitution, and internet crimes /
Sharon Cooper . . . [et al.] -- 1st ed.
        p. cm.
Includes bibliographical references and index.
    ISBN 1-878060-70-8 (v. 1, hardcover : alk. paper) -- ISBN 1-878060-71-6 (v. 2, hardcover : alk. paper) -- ISBN 1-878060-37-6 (v. 1 & 2, casebound : alk. paper)
  1. Child sexual abuse -- United States -- Prevention. 2. Children -- Crimes against -- United States. 3. Abused children -- Services for -- United States. 4. Child prostitution -- United States. 5. Children in pornography -- United States. 6. Internet pornography -- United States. I. Title: Medical, legal, and social science aspects of child sexual exploitation. II. Title.
HV6570.2.C65 2005
362.76`0973 -- dc22
                                        2005005612

CONTRIBUTORS

Mary P. Alexander, MA, LPC
MA Counseling-Marriage and Family Therapy
MEd Educational Psychology and Special Education
Certified School Counselor
Eagle Nest, New Mexico

Elena Azaola, PhD
PhD in Social Anthropology
Psychoanalyst
Professor at the Center for Advanced Studies and Research in
    Social Anthropology
Mexico City, Mexico

Joseph S. Bova Conti, BA
Detective Sergeant, Maryland Heights Police Department
Crimes Against Children Specialist
Certified Juvenile Specialist — State of Missouri
Member MPJOA, MJJA, SLCJJA
Lecturer, Author, Consultant
Maryland Heights, Missouri

Duncan T. Brown, Esq
Assistant District Attorney
Sex Crimes/Special Victims Bureau
Richmond County District Attorney's Office
Staten Island, New York

Cormac Callanan, BA, MSc
Secretary General
Association of Internet Hotline Providers in Europe (INHOPE)

Lt. William D. Carson, MA, SPSC
Commander, Bureau of Investigation
Maryland Heights Police Department
Maryland Heights, Missouri

Michelle K. Collins, MA
Director, Exploited Child Unit
National Center for Missing & Exploited Children (NCMEC)
Alexandria, Virginia

Peter I. Collins, MCA, MD, FRCP(C)
Manager, Forensic Psychiatry Unit
Behavioural Sciences Section
Ontario Provincial Police
Associate Professor, Department of Psychiatry
University of Toronto
Toronto, Canada

Jeffrey A. Dort, JD
Deputy District Attorney
Team Leader Family Protection Division
Lead Prosecutor — ICAC: Internet Crimes Against Children
San Diego District Attorney's Office
San Diego, California

V. Denise Everett, MD, FAAP
Director, Child Sexual Abuse Team
WakeMed
Raleigh, North Carolina
Clinical Associate Professor, Department of Pediatrics
University of North Carolina at Chapel Hill School of Medicine
Chapel Hill, North Carolina

Fadi Barakat Fadel
Director of Programmes of the International Centre to Combat
    Exploitation of Children
Founder of Sexually Exploited Youth Speak Out Network
    (SEYSO)

James A. H. Farrow, MD, FSAM
Professor, Medicine & Pediatrics
Director, Student Health Services
Tulane University
New Orleans, Louisiana

David Finkelhor, PhD
Director, Crimes Against Children Research Center
Family Research Laboratory
Professor, Department of Sociology
University of New Hampshire
Durham, New Hampshire

Katherine A. Free, MA
Program Manager
Exploited Child Unit
National Center for Missing & Exploited Children (NCMEC)
Alexandria, Virginia

Nadine Grant
Director of Programs
Save the Children Canada
Toronto, Canada

Ernestine S. Gray, JD
Judge
Orleans Parish Juvenile Court
Section "A"
New Orleans, Louisiana

Donald B. Henley
Senior Special Agent
US Department of Homeland Security
Immigration and Customs Enforcement (ICE)

Marcia E. Herman-Giddens, PA, DrPH
Child Maltreatment Consulting
Senior Fellow, North Carolina Child Advocacy Institute
Adjunct Professor, University of North Carolina School of
    Public Health
Pittsboro, North Carolina

Nicole G. Ives, MSW
Doctoral Candidate
University of Pennsylvania, School of Social Work
Philadelphia, Pennsylvania

Eileen R. Jacob
Supervisor Special Agent
Crimes Against Children Unit
Federal Bureau of Investigation
Washington, DC

Terry Jones, BA (Hons), PGCE
Consultant: Internet Paedophilia Training Awareness
Consultancy (IPTAC)
Former Head Greater Manchester Police Abusive Images Unit
United Kingdom

Aaron Kipnis, PhD
Professor — Clinical Psychology
Pacifica Graduate Institute
Carpenteria, California
Psychologist
Santa Barbara, California

Susan S. Kreston, JD, LLM
Consultant
New Orleans, Louisiana

Kenneth V. Lanning, MS
(Retired FBI)
CAC Consultants
Fredericksburg, Virginia

Mary Anne Layden, PhD
Codirector
Sexual Trauma and Psychopathology Program
Director of Education
Center for Cognitive Therapy
Department of Psychiatry
University of Pennsylvania
Philadelphia, Pennsylvania

Shyla R. Lefever, PhD
Assistant Professor of Communication
Hampton University
Hampton, Virginia

Ingrid Leth
Former Senior Adviser
UNICEF HQ, USA
Associate Professor — Clinical Child Psychology
Department of Psychology
University of Copenhagen
Copenhagen, Denmark

Elizabeth J. Letourneau, PhD
Assistant Professor
Department of Psychiatry and Behavioral Sciences
Medical University of South Carolina
Charleston, South Carolina

L. Alvin Malesky, Jr, PhD
Assistant Professor, Department of Psychology
Western Carolina University
Cullowhee, North Carolina

Bernadette McMenamin, AO
National Director of CHILD WISE
ECPAT in Australia
Director, NetAlert (Internet safety advisory board)
Director, KidsAP (Internet safety advisory board)
Advisor to the Federal Government for the National Plan of
Action on CSEC (Commercial Sexual Exploitation of Children)
South Melbourne, Australia

Kimberly Mitchell, PhD
Research Associate — Crimes Against Children Research Center
Assistant Research Professor of Psychology
University of New Hampshire
Durham, New Hampshire

Thomas P. O'Connor, BA, MA
Chief of Police, Maryland Heights Police Department
Law Enforcement Instructor, Specialty Crimes Against Persons,
    Criminal Investigation Procedures
Maryland Heights, Missouri

John Patzakis, Esq
Vice Chairman and Chief Legal Officer
Guidance Software, Inc.

David S. Prescott, LICSW
Treatment Assessment Director,
    Sand Ridge Secure Treatment Center
Mauston, Wisconsin

Ethel Quayle, BA, MSc, PsychD
Lecturer
Researcher with the COPINE Project
Department of Applied Psychology
University College Cork
Cork, Ireland

Erika Rivera Ragland, JD
Staff Attorney
National Center for Prosecution of Child Abuse
American Prosecutors Research Institute (APRI)
Alexandria, Virginia

Thomas Rickert
Attorney at Law
President, Association of Internet Hotline Providers in
    Europe (INHOPE)
Chair, Internet Content Task Force eco
Cologne, Germany

Migael Scherer
Director, Dart Award for Excellence in Reporting on Victims of
    Violence
Dart Center for Journalism and Trauma
Department of Communication
University of Washington
Seattle, Washington

Daniel J. Sheridan, PhD, RN, FAAN
Assistant Professor
Johns Hopkins University School of Nursing
President, International Association of Forensic Nurses
Baltimore, Maryland

Linnea W. Smith, MD
Psychiatrist
Chapel Hill, North Carolina

Raymond C. Smith
Assistant Inspector in Charge
Fraud, Prohibited Mailings and Asset Forfeiture
US Postal Inspection Service
Washington, DC

Max Taylor, PhD, C. Forensic Psychology
Professor and Head of Department
    of Applied Psychology
University College Cork
Director, COPINE Project
Cork, Ireland

Govind Prasad Thapa, MA, BL, MPA, PhD
Additional Inspector General, Nepal Police
Chief — Crime Investigation Department
Police Headquarters
Kathmandu, Nepal

Phyllis L. Thompson, LCSW
OUR KIDS Center
Nashville General Hospital
Instructor in the Department of Pediatrics
Vanderbilt University Medical Center
Nashville, Tennessee

Christopher D. Trifiletti
Special Agent
Federal Bureau of Investigation
Baltimore, Maryland
Chair, Interpol Specialists Group on Crimes Against Children,
Child Pornography, and Internet Investigations Theme Groups
Lyon, France

Dawn Van Pelt, BSN, RN
Graduate Student
Johns Hopkins University School of Nursing
Baltimore, Maryland

Bharathi A. Venkatraman, Esq
United States Department of Justice
Civil Rights Division
Washington, DC

F. Bruce Watkins, MD
Assistant Clinical Professor of Ob/Gyn
University of Illinois College of Medicine
Medical Director, Women's Health Service
Crusader Clinic
Rockford, Illinois

Bruce Watson, LLB, CA
Past President, Enough Is Enough
Fairfax, Virginia

Neil Alan Weiner, PhD
Senior Research Investigator
Center for Research on Youth and Social Policy
School of Social Work
University of Pennsylvania
Philadelphia, Pennsylvania

Cathy Spatz Widom, PhD
Professor of Psychiatry and University Professor
UMDNJ — New Jersey Medical School
Department of Psychiatry
Newark, New Jersey

Janis Wolak, JD
Research Assistant Professor
Crimes Against Children Research Center
University of New Hampshire
Durham, New Hampshire

G.W. Medical Publishing, Inc.
St. Louis

OUR MISSION

To become the world leader in publishing and

information services on child abuse, maltreatment

and diseases, and domestic violence. We seek to

heighten awareness of these issues and provide

relevant information to professionals and consumers.

A portion of our profits is contributed to nonprofit organizations
dedicated to the prevention of child abuse and the care of victims of abuse
and other children and family charities.

FOREWORD

In my career as a prosecutor, and now a Congressman, I have seen tremendous improvements in our nation's response to cases of child maltreatment. In most communities today, multidisciplinary teams work together for the benefit of children. Many elected district attorneys, sheriffs, and police chiefs have developed specialized units to respond to cases of child abuse.

Through the work of the American Prosecutors Research Institute's National Center for Prosecution of Child Abuse, the National Child Protection Training Center at Winona State University, Fox Valley Technical College, the National Center for Missing & Exploited Children, and other federally funded programs, thousands of frontline professionals are trained annually in the art and science of handling child protection cases.

Perhaps the most important development is the Children's Advocacy Center program. Children's Advocacy Centers (CACs) are child-friendly facilities where children can be interviewed sensitively and receive medical and psychological services. As a district attorney, I had the privilege of starting the nation's first Children's Advocacy Center. As a member of Congress, I championed support for the National Children's Advocacy Center in Huntsville, Alabama, and the National Children's Alliance, a coalition of CACs from across the nation that is headquartered in Washington, DC. Today there are hundreds of CACs in every part of our country.

We can not, however, rest on our laurels. As detailed in the pages of this book, modern technology poses a new threat to our children. It is increasingly easy for perpetrators to exploit children through the Internet, to create and disseminate child pornography, and to solicit children for illicit purposes.

The commercial exploitation of children is a global problem that impacts every community in the United States. Through the pioneering work of Dr. Richard Estes and other researchers, we know that hundreds of thousands of children are at risk of commercial exploitation. Although more research needs to be done, there is some evidence to suggest these children are just as likely to come from rural and suburban communities as urban centers.

I commend GW Medical Publishing as well as the editors and contributors to this book for producing a treatise that addresses child sexual exploitation from every angle. I am particularly grateful to the survivors of child pornography, commercial exploitation, and online solicitation for sharing their pain with those of us who will read this book. I hope the courage of these survivors spurs all of us to do more to protect children.

Finally, I want to commend the frontline investigators, prosecutors, medical and mental health professionals, and other child advocates who are in the trenches daily trying to spare children from every form of exploitation. You labor long hours for little pay or honor on behalf of someone else's children. Please know that your selfless dedication is not unnoticed. Indeed, your heroism is an inspiration to us all.

Congressman Robert E. "Bud" Cramer, Jr.
Member of the US House of Representatives (1991-present)
Founder of the Children's Advocacy Center movement

FOREWORD

It is common to hear pronouncements from public figures that children are society's most important and treasured assets. To an overwhelming majority, this concept is fundamentally true. To a marginal and deviant minority, however, children are viewed as commodities to be traded, imported, and exported like any other merchandise. Parents and professionals need help combating the alarming growth of child exploitation and this book is a valuable tool in the fight to protect our children from predators who would use them for financial gain or prurient reasons.

Global in scope, these 2 volumes are written by individuals who represent a wide array of backgrounds, disciplines, and perspectives. Some authors are the authentic voices of those who were victimized and forced to navigate a system that was intended to help but found to be less than helpful. Some speak from distant lands that are growing ever closer with the ease of air travel and where the youth are being sold to travelers seeking to indulge their perverse needs with someone else's children. Some voices are actually electronic particles from cyberspace delivering images of unspeakable abuse to our home and office computers.

Some of the highlights of this book that I found interesting include:

— A chapter discussing exploitation in advertising and the need for healthcare providers to be aware of the "slippery slope" that can occur when girls and teens are used in sexualized marketing

— A chapter about the resources of the National Center for Missing & Exploited Children with a focus on their Exploited Child Unit

— A chapter from UNICEF on the global commodification of children for sexual work and exploitation

— A chapter from the University of Washington School of Journalism discussing the importance of addressing child victims of sexual exploitation in an empathetic and nonvictimizing manner in the newspapers; the chapter includes excerpts and photographs from a focused series in the *Atlanta Journal Constitution* called "The Selling of Atlanta's Children," which played an important role in convincing the Georgia State Legislature to change its laws to make the selling of children a felony, as compared to its history of misdemeanor status for over a century

— A chapter from the Association for the Treatment of Sexual Abusers (ATSA) regarding the ethical issues in child sex offender assessments and the benchmarks for parole and probation determinations

— Chapters relating to the medical and surgical complications of prostitution

— A chapter discussing the demographics of girls who are brought into the criminal justice system and recommendations for communities to avoid the incarceration of prostituted children and youths

— A chapter that explains the nuts and bolts of "cloning a computer" when an investigation is conducted in a child pornography case

— A chapter describing other aspects of federal laws that are involved when children and youths are trafficked into the United States for sexual exploitation purposes, including civil rights violations and labor law violations

— A chapter on the AMBER Alert legislation and the several children whose lives contributed to its inception

— A chapter detailing the frequently overlooked concept of child sexual exploitation in rural communities

This book represents the culmination of the efforts of an impressive collection of premier investigators, judicial participants, child protection agency personnel, and clinicians to gather and organize information about child exploitation. It is the most comprehensive text on this subject and it is a welcome addition to the literature on child maltreatment.

Robert M. Reece, MD
Clinical Professor of Pediatrics
Tufts University School of Medicine
Visiting Professor of Pediatrics
Dartmouth Medical School
Editor, *The Quarterly Update*

FOREWORD

In 1981, my worst nightmare became a reality when my 6-year-old son, Adam, was abducted and murdered. The prime suspect in Adam's case was never charged. He died in prison while serving a life sentence for other crimes. With determination to spare other families from enduring a similar tragedy, my wife Revé and I worked to help enact the Missing Children Act of 1982 and the Missing Children's Assistance Act of 1984. We founded the National Center for Missing & Exploited Children (NCMEC) in 1984. In the past 20 years, the rate of recovery of missing children has increased from 62% to 95%.

While the NCMEC is best known for its work in tracking down missing children, the Exploited Child Unit, established in 1997, has also been a primary resource for law enforcement and families in the investigation and prosecution of the sexual exploitation of children. Child sexual exploitation is a worldwide problem, encompassing child pornography, molestation, and prostitution. In recent years, computers and the Internet have become favorite tools of child molesters as they collect and trade pornographic images and solicit new victims online.

Medical, Legal, & Social Science Aspects of Child Sexual Exploitation: A Comprehensive Review of Pornography, Prostitution, and Internet Crimes is a 2-volume text that addresses this pervasive problem. Written by physicians, nurses, attorneys, social workers, and law enforcement officials who are leading experts in the field, the text takes a multidisciplinary approach to the medical and legal issues faced by victims of sexual exploitation. The contributions of authors from countries outside the United States help to highlight the international nature of this problem. First-person accounts by adults who were exploited as children and teenagers help to put a human face on the issue. The role of the media is addressed, both as contributors to the problem and as partners in creating and implementing solutions. Other chapters discuss the role of the United States Postal Inspection Service, the investigation of Internet exploitation cases, prosecutorial and judicial issues, the role of the medical expert, and the establishment of criminal liability for groups promoting child sexual exploitation.

It is my sincere belief that this book will be a significant contribution to the literature in this field, and by doing so, will help to combat this worldwide problem.

John Walsh
Cofounder, National Center for Missing & Exploited Children
Host, Fox Television's *America's Most Wanted*

PREFACE

The idea for this work originated from the need to establish a repository of information for multidisciplinary team members who are learning about Internet crimes against children. When the concept of mass communication began with Gutenberg's printing press in the 14th century, the purpose was to disperse information and promote new ideas. Seven centuries later, the Internet has expanded upon the original purpose of the printing press and now includes the deception and entrapment of our most vulnerable resource: children. As methods of victimization have become more innovative, sophisticated, and elusive, professionals are challenged in their efforts to prevent, detect, intervene, and treat children that fall prey to online predators.

Knowledge regarding Internet crimes against children has been primarily limited to media coverage of the topic. This text serves to separate fact from fiction and to dispel several myths and misconceptions, including the belief that prostituted youths typically market themselves by choice and can easily escape from this form of abuse. To the uninformed, it is inconceivable that children and youth are often sold from within their own homes, that the Internet is used in numerous capacities to make such arrangements, and that Internet cafés present a nearly untraceable means of making the deal. Online solicitation has become an increasing threat to children. Many naïve children and youths unwittingly receive unwanted sexual solicitations, and may be enticed to leave their homes and families to meet online predators; such encounters may end tragically in sexual assault, physical assault, abduction, or murder. What was slavery and bondage in the past has now become human trafficking for forced labor and sexual exploitation. These crimes continue to escalate worldwide.

The text begins with the history of child exploitation and proceeds to explain the contemporary and global nature of this form of child victimization. A careful analysis of the acquaintance molester leads the reader to complex types of sexual exploitation, illustrated with online, local, national, and international examples of the scope of these crimes against children. A collage of perspectives is presented, including exploitation in advertising, the role of the journalistic media response to these types of victims of crime, medical evaluation and treatment of victims, offender psychology and victim mental health impact, and social science research in the area of commercial sexual exploitation of children. The reader will experience a judicial and criminal justice view, the perspective of the sexually exploited male, an education regarding the Internet community with respect to offender dynamics, and important aspects of the offender evaluation when potential parole, probation, and public safety is being considered.

From the investigative and prosecuting platform, numerous important issues are discussed: the role of the first responder in an Internet crime against a child; the details of "cloning software" and the best way to present this complex information to a judge or jury; the technology of victim identification from an Internet Web site; the importance of strategy in prostitution cases when the common bias is that the victim is an offender; the recognition of the organized crime aspects of girls domestically trafficked across a country for sexual slavery and prostitution; the international requirements of police agencies in abduction and exploitation cases; and the realization that child pornography production and collection is a highly recidivistic crime. Investigations of high profile cases of sexual exploitation have resulted in an organized response to the sex tourist who travels to exploit young children for sexual purposes. The worst-case scenario of child abduction, sexual assault, and homicide are described, as well as community responses such as the AMBER Alert program, designed to facilitate a rapid and safe recovery of a missing child or youth.

From a child maltreatment perspective, this groundbreaking work provides comprehensive and diverse information for this contemporary, yet misunderstood and daunting, form of child exploitation. It has been an immense honor to work with truly professional contributors, all of whom have been eager and cooperative in providing an international and expert treatise on a subject that all parents and professionals must acknowledge and understand. As the Internet, the "printing press" of the 21st century, has opened new doors for the worldwide exchange of information and ideas, so too has it opened a Pandora's box of opportunities for criminals that victimize children and youths. At present, the knowledge regarding Internet crimes against children is fragmented, scant, and discipline-specific. This text is the first step toward comprehension, effective intervention, and the multidisciplinary coordination of investigations of crimes involving these exploited children. It will open your eyes and your mind to a new dark side of child abuse that we can no longer afford to ignore.

Sharon W. Cooper, MD, FAAP
Richard J. Estes, DSW, ACSW
Angelo P. Giardino, MD, PhD, FAAP
Nancy D. Kellogg, MD
Victor I. Vieth, JD

REVIEWS

As a former Police Chief I know that important policy decisions regarding the establishment of comprehensive child protection strategies are often based upon a tragic case or anecdotal evidence that often ignores the scope and scale of the overall problem. The research conducted by these nationally recognized experts provides important insight into emerging threats to children and serves as a guide for developing an effective national response.

Brad Russ
ICAC Training & Technical Assistance
Program Director
University of New Hampshire
Internet Crimes Against Children
Research Center
Durham, NH

The factual information, practical methodologies, and expertise in this book can be as a practical tool in combating the horror of the commercial sexual exploitation of children. The fact that this text is guided by internationally recognized child rights principles and documents gives one hope that change is possible in a world where exploitation of children is so prevalent. As a survivor and now activist, I encourage the government, professionals, and the public to care about this issue and be practical and humane in their approach to combating exploitation. This book provides us with that template.

Cherry Kingsley
Special Advisor
International Centre to Combat
Exploitation of Children
Vancouver, Canada

With the emergence of the Internet and its worldwide expansion as a favored mode of communication, there is an ever-increasing avenue for the sexual exploitation of children. This informative publication, authored by acknowledged leaders in the field of forensic science, provides professionals working with child abuse victims, their families, and the suspected perpetrators with a wide range of forensic techniques and knowledge that will serve as an essential forensic reference.

Faye Battiste-Otto, RN, SANE
Founder/President of American
Forensic Nurses
Cofounder, International Association
of Forensic Nurses
Palm Springs, CA

In giving a broad scope of understanding about the sexual exploitation of children, this book delineates familial child sexual abuse and commercial sexual exploitation. Its international perspective suggests that the causes are broader than defined by western countries and therefore prevention foci need to be tailored accordingly. While giving information on offender motives and treatment, it emphasizes the victim as blameless, a view that continues to need reinforcement. The detailed nature of the book and the number of worthy contributors reiterate its use as a text for all manner of helping professionals.

Jane Rudd, PhD
Associate Professor
Saint Joseph College
West Hartford, CT

The subject matter is disturbing, but this is a must-read resource book for professionals working in the field of child maltreatment in the 21st century. The contents provide a comprehensive review of research, current programs, and concepts that address intervention, investigation, and prevention.

Jeanie Ming, CPNP
Forensic Pediatric Nurse Practitioner
Child Abuse Services Team
Orange, CA

Medical, Legal, & Social Science Aspects of Child Sexual Exploitation is a rare and welcome departure from the "same old, same old" of recent years and is truly new and innovative. This book is the first to provide in-depth coverage of an emerging and serious global issue. The authors and editors are well qualified to address the complex social, psychological, and legal issues presented by child sexual exploitation.

John E.B. Myers
Distinguished Professor and Scholar
University of the Pacific
McGeorge School of Law
Sacramento, CA

This text brings to light the necessary role of interagency collaboration in child exploitation cases while providing direct guidance through case study and lessons of necessary considerations, benefits and limitations of emerging tools, and strategies for the investigation, proper assessment, and ongoing management of perpetrators.

Margaret Bullens
Forensic Psychophysiologist and Sex
Offender Management Consultant
Grapevine, TX

Very worthwhile and a must-read for law enforcement and other professionals involved in identifying, rescuing, and treating child victims of sexual abuse. This book allows the reader to better understand how and why individuals use the computer to facilitate the sexual exploitation of children.

Det Sgt Paul Gillespie
Officer In Charge
Child Exploitation Section
Toronto Police Service
Toronto, Canada

Whether it is child prostitution, trafficking, cyber-enticement, child pornography, or sex tourism, tens of thousands of children suffer irreparable physical and psychological harm from producers and customers of this form of abuse. As a leader in the education of forensic nurses, the International Association of Forensic Nurses supports all efforts to educate healthcare providers, criminal justice and social service professionals about the crimes of child exploitation. Since there is presently a lack of evidence-based information, we look forward to this new professional resource.

International Association of Forensic
Nurses (IAFN)
Board of Directors, 2005-2006

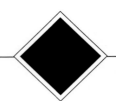

Contents In Brief

VOLUME TWO

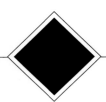

CONTENTS IN DETAIL

VOLUME ONE

CHAPTER 16: PSYCHOSOCIAL CONTEXT LEADING JUVENILES TO PROSTITUTION AND SEXUAL EXPLOITATION

CHAPTER 17: MEDICAL CARE OF THE CHILDREN OF THE NIGHT

CHAPTER 18: THE MEDICAL IMPLICATIONS OF ANOGENITAL TRAUMA IN CHILD SEXUAL EXPLOITATION

CHAPTER 24: THE WORK OF THE UNITED STATES POSTAL INSPECTION SERVICE: COMBATING CHILD SEXUAL EXPLOITATION

CHAPTER 25: THE ROLE OF THE FIRST RESPONDER IN THE CRIMINAL INVESTIGATIVE PROCESS

CHAPTER 26: INVESTIGATING INTERNET CHILD EXPLOITATION CASES

CHAPTER 27: PROSECUTORIAL ISSUES IN THE CHILD
PORNOGRAPHY ARENA

CHAPTER 33: INTERNET PEDOPHILIA

CHAPTER 34: THE MEDICAL EXPERT AND CHILD SEXUAL EXPLOITATION

CHAPTER 35: COMPUTER FORENSIC SOFTWARE AND ITS LEGAL VALIDATION

CHAPTER 37: ESTABLISHING CRIMINAL CONSPIRACY AND AIDER AND ABETTOR LIABILITY FOR GROUPS THAT PROMOTE SEXUAL EXPLOITATION OF CHILDREN

CHAPTER 38: THE HIDDEN TRUTH OF INVOLUNTARY SERVITUDE AND SLAVERY

CHAPTER 45: SHADOW CHILDREN: ADDRESSING THE COMMERCIAL
EXPLOITATION OF CHILDREN IN RURAL AMERICA

CHAPTER 46: RECOMMENDATIONS FOR ACTION FOR DEALING
EFFECTIVELY WITH CHILD SEXUAL EXPLOITATION

Medical, Legal, & Social Science Aspects of

Child Sexual

Exploitation

A Comprehensive Review of Pornography, Prostitution, and Internet Crimes

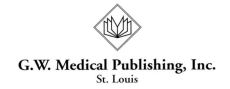

G.W. Medical Publishing, Inc.
St. Louis

ACQUAINTANCE CHILD MOLESTERS: A BEHAVIORAL ANALYSIS*

Kenneth V. Lanning, MS, Former Supervisory Special Agent, Federal Bureau of Investigation

INTRODUCTION

CAUTION

The sexual victimization of children involves varied and diverse dynamics. It can range from one-on-one intrafamilial abuse to multioffender/multivictim extrafamilial sex rings and from stranger abduction of toddlers to prostitution of teenagers. This chapter will focus *primarily* on sexual exploitation of children perpetrated by "acquaintance molesters." This term and related terms will be defined, and insight will be provided into the behavioral patterns of offenders and victims in such cases. The term **compliant** will sometimes be used to describe those children who cooperate in or "consent" to their sexual victimization. Because children can not legally consent to having sex with adults, this compliance does not in any way alter the fact that they are victims of serious crimes. The reasons for and the complexity and investigative significance of this compliance will be discussed.

The goal of this chapter is to describe, in plain language, the behavioral dynamics of these cases. Because of the complexity of human behavior, these dynamics will often be described on a continuum rather than as either/or categories. It is not intended to be a detailed, step-by-step investigative manual, nor does it offer rigid standards for forensic intervention. The material presented here may not be applicable to every case or circumstance. Although the intervention techniques discussed may be used in other cases of sexual victimization of children, they are intended to be applied primarily to cases involving the sexual molestation of children by adult acquaintances. Many real-world constraints, including lack of time and personnel, make following all the techniques discussed here impossible.

In the interest of readability, children alleging sexual abuse or who are suspected of being sexually exploited will sometimes be referred to as "victims," even though their victimization may not have been proven in a court of law. This shorthand should not blur the fact that forensic interveners are expected to keep an open mind and maintain objectivity. Although females can and do molest children, offenders will generally be referred to by the pronoun "he."

The information in this chapter and its application are based on my education, training, and more than 30 years of experience studying the criminal aspects of deviant sexual behavior and interacting with investigators, prosecutors, and other forensic interveners. Although I understand that *data* are not the plural of *anecdote*, the information and opinions in this chapter are based primarily on the totality of my

---

* Adapted from the National Center for Missing & Exploited Children. Lanning KV. Child Molesters: A Behavioral Analysis. 4th ed. Alexandria, Va: NCMEC: 2001.

acquired knowledge and expertise. My database is the thousands of cases on which I have consulted or studied. Its validity is the fact that its application has worked for all these many years. I have great confidence in its behavioral accuracy and reliability. Much of this chapter will set forth its application to criminal investigation. I believe that it can be adapted to varying degrees to forensic fact-finding by many disciplines. Forensic interveners based on departmental policy, rules of evidence, and current case law, however, must carefully evaluate its legal acceptance and application. This chapter is intended to be a practical behavioral analysis with application primarily to the objective, neutral fact-finding process. It is not intended to be a precise legal analysis with technical legal definitions. In addition, the use of terms also used in mental health (eg, impulsive, compulsive, pedophilia) is not meant to imply a psychiatric diagnosis or lack of legal responsibility.

OVERVIEW

In order to understand and intervene in allegations of what constitutes "acquaintance" molestation, it is important to have an historical perspective of society's general attitudes about sexual victimization of children. A brief synopsis of these attitudes in the United States is provided here in order to give a context to this discussion. That context, hopefully, will help investigators better understand some of the problems and investigative difficulties encountered in these cases.

In the United States, society's historical attitude about sexual victimization of children can generally be summed up in one word: *denial.* Most people do not want to hear about it and would prefer to pretend that such victimization just does not occur. Today, however, it is difficult to pretend that it does not happen. Stories and reports about child sexual abuse and exploitation are daily occurrences. Investigators dealing with sexual victimization of children must recognize and learn to address this denial. They must try to overcome it and encourage society to address, report, and prevent the sexual victimization of children.

A complex problem such as the sexual victimization of children can be viewed from 3 major perspectives: personal, political, and professional. The *personal* perspective encompasses the emotional: how the issues affect individual needs and wants. The *political* perspective encompasses the practical: how the issues affect getting elected, obtaining funding or pay, and attaining status and power. The *professional* perspective encompasses the rational and objective: how the issues affect sexually victimized children and what is in their best interest. Often these perspectives overlap or are applied in combination. Because most of us use all 3, sometimes which perspective is in control may not be clear.

The personal and political perspectives tend to dominate emotional issues such as the sexual victimization of children. The personal and political perspectives are real and will never go away. In fact, many positive things can and have been achieved through them, eg, attention, adequate funding, equipment, manpower. In general, however, sexually victimized children need more people addressing their needs from the professional perspective and fewer from the personal and political perspectives.

In their zeal to overcome denial or influence opinion, some individuals allow the personal or political perspectives to dominate by exaggerating or misrepresenting the problem. Presentations and literature with poorly documented or misleading claims about 1 in 3 children being sexually molested, the multibillion-dollar child pornography industry, organized child slavery rings, and 50 000 stranger-abducted children are still common. The documented facts in the United States are bad enough and need no embellishment. True professionals, when communicating about the problem, should clearly define their terms and then *consistently* use those definitions unless indicating otherwise. Professionals should understand and cite reputable and scientific studies, and note the sources of information. Operational definitions for terms (eg, child, pedophile, sexual exploitation) used in cited research should be clearly expressed and not mixed to distort the findings. Once someone is caught using distorted or misleading information and labeled an extremist, people may not listen to what he or she says, no matter how brilliant or profound he or she may be. When the exaggerations and distortions are discovered, the credibility of those people and the issue are diminished.

"Stranger Danger"

During the 1950s and 1960s, the primary focus in the limited literature and discussions on sexual victimization of children was on "stranger danger"—the dirty old man in the wrinkled raincoat approaching an innocent child at play. If one could not totally deny the existence of child sexual victimization, one could describe the victimization in simplistic terms of good and evil. The investigation and prevention of this "stranger danger" are more clear-cut. We immediately know who the good and bad guys are, what they look like, and that the danger is external.

During this time, the Federal Bureau of Investigation (FBI) distributed a poster that epitomized this attitude. It showed a man with his hat pulled down, lurking behind a tree with a bag of candy in his hands. He was waiting for a sweet little girl walking home from school alone. At the top it read, "Boys and Girls, color the page, memorize the rules." At the bottom it read, "For your protection, remember to turn down gifts from strangers, and refuse rides offered by strangers." The poster clearly contrasts the evil of the offender with the goodness of the child victim. When confronted with such an offender, the advice to the child is simple and clear—say no, yell, and tell.

The myth of the typical child molester as the dirty old man in the wrinkled raincoat has been reevaluated based on what we have learned about the kinds of people who sexually victimize children. We are increasingly recognizing that child molesters can look like anyone else and even be someone we know and like.

The other part of this myth, however, is still with us, and it is far less likely to be discussed. It is the myth of the typical child victim as a completely innocent young girl playing in front of her house, going to school, or walking down the street minding her own business. It may be more important to confront this part of the myth than the part about the evil offender, especially when addressing the sexual exploitation of children and acquaintance child molesters. Child victims can be boys as well as girls and can be older as well as younger. Not all child victims are "little angels." They are, however, all human beings.

Society seems to have a problem dealing with any sexual-victimization case in which the adult offender is not completely "bad" or the child victim is not completely "good." The idea that child victims could simply behave like human beings and respond to the attention and affection of offenders by voluntarily and repeatedly returning to an offender's home is a troubling one. It confuses us to see the victims in child pornography giggling or laughing. At professional conferences on child sexual abuse, child prostitution is rarely discussed. It is the form of sexual victimization of children most unlike the stereotype of the innocent victim. Child prostitutes, by definition, participate in and sometimes initiate their victimization. Child prostitutes and the participants in exploitation cases involving multiple victims are frequently boys. A therapist once told me that a researcher's data on child molestation were "misleading" because many of the child victims in question were child prostitutes. This seems to imply that child prostitutes are not "real" child victims. Whether or not it seems fair, when adults and children have sex, the child is *always* the victim.

Although no longer the primary focus of sexual-victimization-of-children literature and training, stranger danger still maintains a disproportionate concern for society.

Intrafamilial Child Sexual Abuse

During the 1970s and 1980s, society began to learn more about the sexual victimization of children. In my opinion, this was primarily as a result of the women's movement. We began to realize that someone a child knows who is often a relative—

a father, stepfather, uncle, grandfather, older brother, or even a female family member—sexually molests most children. Some mitigate the difficulty of accepting this by adopting the view that only family members of socioeconomic, racial, or cultural groups other than their own commonly engage in such behavior.

It quickly became apparent that warnings about not taking gifts or rides from strangers were not good enough to realistically try to prevent most child sexual abuse. Consequently, we began to develop prevention programs based on more complex concepts such as "good touching" and "bad touching," the "yucky" feeling, and the child's right to say no. These are not the kinds of things that can be easily and effectively communicated in 50 minutes to hundreds of kids of varying ages packed into a school auditorium. These are difficult issues, and prevention programs must be carefully developed and evaluated.

By the 1980s, child sexual abuse had become almost synonymous with incest for many professionals, and incest meant father-daughter sexual relations; therefore, much of the focus of child-sexual-abuse intervention and investigation turned to one-on-one, father-daughter incest. Even today a large portion of training materials, articles, and books on this topic refer to child sexual abuse only in terms of intrafamilial, father-daughter incest.

Incest is, in fact, sexual relations between individuals of any age too closely related to marry. It need not, however, necessarily involve an adult and a child, and it goes beyond child sexual abuse. But more important, child sexual abuse goes beyond father-daughter incest. Intrafamilial incest between an adult and child may be the most common form of child sexual victimization, but it is not the only form.

The progress of the 1970s and 1980s in recognizing that child sexual victimization was not simply a result of stranger danger was an important breakthrough in dealing with society's denial. The battle, however, is not over. The persistent voice of society luring us back to the simpler concept of stranger danger never seems to go away.

Acquaintance Child Molestation

Today, for many child advocates and professionals in the field (eg, police, prosecutors, social workers, physicians, therapists), the sexual victimization of children still means one-on-one intrafamilial sexual abuse. Although they are certainly aware of other forms of sexual victimization of children, when discussing the problem in general, their "default setting" (eg, that which is assumed without an active change) always seems to go back to children molested by family members. For the public, however, the "default setting" seems to be stranger abduction. To them, child molesters are sick perverts who physically overpower children and violently force them into sexual activity.

The often forgotten piece in the puzzle of the sexual victimization of children is acquaintance molestation. This seems to be the most difficult manifestation of the problem for society and professionals to face. People seem more willing to accept a sinister stranger from a different location or father/stepfather from a different socioeconomic background as a child molester than a clergy member, next door neighbor, law enforcement officer, pediatrician, teacher, or volunteer with direct access to children. The acquaintance molester, by definition, is one of us. He is not just an external threat. We can not easily distinguish him from us or identify him by physical traits. These kinds of molesters have always existed but society, organizations, and the criminal justice system have been reluctant to accept the reality of these cases. When such an offender is discovered, a common response has been to just move him out of our midst, perform damage control, and then try to forget about it. Sadly, one of the main reasons that the criminal justice system and the public were forced to confront the problem of acquaintance molestation was the preponderance of lawsuits arising from the negligence of many prominent organizations.

One of the unfortunate outcomes of society's preference for the stranger danger concept has a direct impact on intervention into many acquaintance-exploitation cases. It is what I call "say no, yell, and tell" guilt. This is the result of societal attitudes and prevention programs that focus only on "unwanted" sexual activity and tell potential child victims to avoid sexual abuse by saying no, yelling, and telling. This technique might work with the stranger lurking behind a tree. Children who are seduced and actively participate in their victimization, however, often feel guilty and blame themselves because they did not do what they were "supposed" to do. These seduced and, therefore, compliant victims may feel a need to sometimes describe their victimization in more socially acceptable but inaccurate ways that relieve them of this guilt. Except for child prostitution, most acquaintance sexual-exploitation-of-children cases in the United States involve molesters who rarely use physical force on their victims.

Advice to prevent sexual exploitation of children by adult acquaintances is very complex and more difficult to implement. How do you warn children about pedophiles who may be their teachers, coaches, clergy members, or neighbors and whose only distinguishing characteristics are that they will treat the children better than most adults, listen to their problems and concerns, and fulfill their emotional, physical, and sexual needs? Will parents, society, and professionals understand when the victimization is discovered or disclosed? Much prevention advice simply does not distinguish types of sexual victimization. The right to say "no" would be applied differently to a stranger, parent, or teacher.

Although stranger, intrafamilial, and acquaintance child molesters have been described here as seemingly separate and distinct offenders, reality is not so simple. Strangers, family members, or acquaintances should all be viewed on a continuum. The concept of who exactly is a "stranger" is not always clear-cut and obvious. It can range from someone never seen before and unknown to someone seen but nameless to someone named but unknown to someone named and slightly known to someone known from the Internet but never seen and anyone in between. Every acquaintance offender was a "stranger" the first time he met any potential child victim. In addition, an offender molesting children to whom he is an acquaintance can also molest children to whom he is a stranger. He might use the services of a child prostitute who may or may not know him. The "intrafamilial" molester can range from the biological father to the stepfather to mom's live-in boyfriend to mom's rent-paying roommate. An intrafamilial offender can molest children other than his own. He may be either a stranger or an acquaintance to these additional victims. Most acquaintance child molesters use their occupations, hobbies, neighborhoods, or online computers to gain access to child victims; however, in addition to or in lieu of these methods, some romance or marry women who already have children. Such molesters may technically be intrafamilial offenders, but dynamically they are not. An acquaintance molester can be a neighbor the child sees every day or friend the child regularly communicates with on the Internet but sees for the first time when they finally meet in person.

Therefore, in this chapter, the determination of an "acquaintance" child molester will be based more on the process and dynamics of the child victimization and less on the technical relationship between the offender and child victim. Stranger offenders can use trickery to initially lure their child victims but tend to control them more through confrontation, threats of force, and physical force. Intrafamilial offenders tend to control their victims more through their private access and family authority. Acquaintance child molesters, although sometimes violent, tend to control their victims through the grooming or seduction process. This process not only gains the victim's initial cooperation but also decreases the likelihood of disclosure and increases the likelihood of ongoing, repeated access. Acquaintance offenders with a preference for younger victims (younger than 12) are also more likely to have to spend time seducing the potential victim's parents or caretakers to gain their trust and confidence. An acquaintance molester who uses violence is likely to be reported quickly to law enforcement. An acquaintance molester who seduces his victims without violence can sometimes go unreported for 30 years or more.

The acquaintance child molester might get involved in "abduction," usually by not allowing a child he knows and has seduced to return home. He may wind up abducting or not returning this child easily linked to him because he wants or needs the child all to himself away from a judgmental society. Such missing children often voluntarily go with the offender. Abducting or running away with a child with whom you can be linked is high-risk criminal behavior. Investigators can more easily identify this abductor and, therefore, more easily find the missing child. Some acquaintance molesters get violent because they misevaluated their victim or wanted to prevent discovery of the sexual activity.

Peers who are acquaintances also sexually victimize many adolescents. For sexual activity between peers to be a prosecutable crime, it would usually have to involve lack of consent in some form. This is a significant and often overlooked problem. The focus of this chapter, however, will *not* include adolescents sexually victimized by acquaintances who are peers.

The sexual victimization of children by family members and "strangers" is a serious and significant problem. This chapter, however, will focus on the problem of sexual exploitation of children by *adult* acquaintances. It will provide insight into 3 aspects of this relatively common but poorly understood type of child sexual victimization.

The first aspect involves understanding the predatory, serial, and usually extrafamilial acquaintance offenders who sexually exploit children through seduction and/or the collection, creation, or distribution of child pornography. With increasing frequency, such offenders are also using online computers and traveling to underdeveloped countries (ie, sex tourism) to facilitate their sexual activity with children.

The second aspect involves understanding the child victims as human beings with needs, wants, and desires. Child victims can not be held to idealistic and superhuman standards of behavior. Their frequent cooperation in their victimization must be viewed as an understandable human characteristic that should have no criminal-justice significance. In theory, the law recognizes their developmental limitations and affords them with special protection. The repeated use, however, of terms such as "rape," "sexual violence," "assault," "attack," "sexually violent predator," and "unwanted sexual activity" when discussing or inquiring about the sexual exploitation of children assumes or implies in the minds of many that all child victims resist sexual advances by adults and are then overpowered by coercion, trickery, threats, weapons, or physical force. Although cases with these elements certainly exist, when adults and children have sex, lack of "consent" can exist simply because the child is legally incapable of giving consent. Whether or not the child resisted, said no, and was overpowered are, therefore, not necessarily elements in determining if a crime has occurred. Understanding this is especially problematic for the public (eg, potential jurors) and professionals (eg, physicians, therapists) who lack specialized training in criminal law and may not rely on strict legal analysis.

The third aspect involves understanding the scope of behavior that can constitute sexual activity. Sexual victimization of children can run the gamut of "normal" sexual acts from fondling to intercourse but can also include deviant sexual acts. Some acts can be sexual acts if you can prove the intent or motivation of the individual. Seemingly "nonsexual" behavior can be in the service of sexual needs. Law enforcement obviously must look to the law to determine what constitutes a sex offense. Other interveners can take a broader perspective. When evaluating the significance and relevance of offender behavior and children's allegations, interveners should always consider *both* the activity and its motivation.

All 3 aspects of this form of sexual exploitation of children by acquaintance molesters must be recognized, understood, and addressed if these cases are going to be effectively identified, investigated, prosecuted, and prevented. The sad reality is, however, that such behavior does have significance in the perception of society and the "real world" of the courtroom.

Society's lack of understanding and acceptance of the reality of acquaintance molestation and exploitation of children often results in:

— Victims denying and failing to disclose their victimization.

— Incomplete, inaccurate, and distorted victim disclosures when they do happen.

— A lifetime of shame, embarrassment, and guilt for the victims.

— Offenders being able to abuse numerous victims over an extended period of time.

— Ineffective prevention programs that also make the first 4 problems even worse.

This chapter hopes to address and improve this situation for the benefit of the victims and investigators. While society has become increasingly more aware of the problem of the acquaintance molester and related problems such as child pornography and computer use, the voice calling the public to focus only on "stranger danger" and calling many child abuse professionals to focus only on intrafamilial sexual abuse still persists. Sexual exploitation cases involving acquaintance molesters present many investigative challenges, but they also present the opportunity to obtain a great deal of corroborative evidence and help victims.

Definitions

Need

In the previous section, a variety of terms were used and deliberately left undefined in order to make a point. Many of these terms are thought to be basic and are, therefore, frequently not defined. Nonprofessionals and professionals use them regularly.

Disagreements and differences of opinion are often the result of confusion over definitions. Some say that pedophiles can be treated; others claim that they can not. Some say a connection between missing children and child pornography exists; others disagree. Some people say that communities should be notified when sex offenders move into a neighborhood; others say it is an unproductive violation of privacy. This is most often not simply a matter of a difference of opinion.

Referring to the same thing by different names and different things by the same name frequently creates confusion. For example, the same 15-year-old individual can be referred to as a(n) "baby," "child," "youth," "juvenile," "minor," "adolescent," "adult," or (as in one forensic psychological evaluation) "underage adult." A father who coerces, a violent abductor, an acquaintance who seduces, a child-pornography collector, or an older boyfriend can all be referred to as a "child molester" or "pedophile."

In written and spoken communication definitions are crucial to understanding. The problem is that when we use basic or common terms, we rarely define them. What is the difference between the sexual abuse of children and sexual exploitation of children? What is the difference between child molestation and child rape? What does it mean to someone who reads in the newspaper that a child was the victim of "indecent assault," a child was "sodomized," or an offender was convicted of "indecent liberties" or "lewd and lascivious conduct" with a child or "contributing to the delinquency of a minor"? Should statistics on violence against women include cases involving the "rape" of female children?

Terms such as "sexual exploitation of children and youth" or "sexual exploitation of children and adolescents" imply that a youth or an adolescent is not a child. At what age does a child become a youth or adolescent? If such a person is sexually victimized, is that considered youth molestation or sexual abuse of adolescents?

Although many recognize the importance of definitions, a major problem is the fact that many terms do not have one universally accepted definition. They have different meanings on different levels to different disciplines. For example, the dictionary or lay person's definition of a "pedophile" is not the same as the psychiatric definition in the *Diagnostic and Statistical Manual of Mental Disorders*, 4th edition, Text Revision (DSM-IV-TR) (American Psychiatric Association [APA], 2000). Legal definitions may not be the same as societal attitudes. The definition problem is most acute when professionals from different disciplines come together to work or communicate about the sexual victimization of children. Definitions are less important when investigating and prosecuting cases and more important when discussing, researching, and writing about the nature and scope of a problem. This chapter and this book are examples of the latter.

The important point, then, is not that these terms have or should have only one definition but that people using the terms should communicate their definitions, whatever they might be, and then use those definitions consistently. To alert forensic interveners to potential confusion and clarify the intended meaning, a discussion of some key terms as used in this chapter follows.

DEFINING THE TERMS USED
"Sexual Victimization of Children"
The term ***sexual victimization of children*** is used as the broadest term to encompass all the ways in which a child can be sexually victimized. Under this umbrella term are the wide variety of forms of sexual victimization such as *sexual abuse of children, sexual exploitation of children, sexual assault of children,* and *sexual abduction of children.* Many professionals do not deal with or do not realize the wide diversity of ways that children can be sexually victimized. More importantly, they may not recognize how these forms of victimization are alike and different.

"Sexual Exploitation of Children"
The term *sexual exploitation of children* is difficult to precisely define. This difficulty is usually addressed by giving examples instead of a definition. It means different things to different people. For some, it implies a commercial or monetary element in the sexual victimization. For many, including the US federal government, it often implies sexual victimization of a child perpetrated by someone other than a family member or legal guardian. It is contrasted with the term "sexual abuse" of children, which is used most often to refer to one-on-one intrafamilial abuse.

As used in this chapter, ***sexual exploitation of children*** refers to forms of victimization involving significant and complex dynamics that go beyond an offender, a victim, and a sexual act. It includes victimization involving sex rings, child pornography, sex tourism, child prostitution, and computer use. Other than child prostitution, this sexual exploitation does not necessarily involve commercial or monetary gain. In fact, in the United States, child pornography and sex-ring activity most often result in a net financial loss for offenders. Cases of sexual exploitation of children may involve intrafamilial offenders and victims although this is not typical. Depending on definitions, it could be argued that all sexually abused children are exploited but that not all sexually exploited children are abused. For example, a child who has been surreptitiously photographed in the nude has been sexually exploited but not necessarily sexually abused.

Child prostitution is a significant and often ignored aspect of sexual exploitation. Due to its complexity and the narrow focus of this chapter, this prostitution will not be discussed here in any detail. This should in no way be interpreted as meaning that child prostitution is not a serious problem or form of sexual victimization and exploitation of children.

"Investigator"

As used in this chapter, the term *investigator* will refer to any forensic intervener into the sexual victimization of children who is engaging in neutral, objective fact-finding. This would obviously include law enforcement officers and prosecutors, but it could in certain situations also include probation and parole officers, social and child protective service workers, physicians and nurses, and therapists and mental health professionals. Law enforcement officers and prosecutors almost always function from the perspective of objective fact-finding with the criminal justice system and society as their clients. The other disciplines just mentioned, however, may have multiple perspectives with varying "clients" depending on their specific roles in different situations or cases. This sometimes makes their jobs more difficult and complicated. The information in this chapter is obviously written from my law enforcement perspective but for use as much as possible by any "investigators" when functioning from a neutral, objective, fact-finding perspective. In this chapter, "investigation" is, therefore, defined as the work any of these investigators perform from this perspective.

"Sexual Activity"

Defining *sexual activity* is not as easy as many people think. Is a sex crime determined by specific acts performed or by the motivation for the acts? Sexual victimization of children can run the gamut of "normal" sexual acts from fondling to intercourse; however, looking solely at the nature of the acts performed does not necessarily solve the problem. Seemingly "sexual" behaviors (eg, vaginal or anal intercourse) can be in the service of nonsexual needs and may, in fact, be more motivated by power and/or anger. This is why it is often said that rape, a crime involving obvious sexual activity, is not a sex crime but a crime of violence. Obviously such acts may still be considered sexual assaults by the law even if they were motivated by nonsexual needs.

Sex can also include deviant sexual acts involving behavior such as sadomasochism, bondage, urination, and defecation. A sexual act for one person might not be a sexual act for another, or it might not be illegal. Some would argue, therefore, that a sex crime is one motivated by sexual gratification.

Some acts can be sexual acts if you can prove the intent or motivation of the individual. Are kissing, hugging, or appearing naked in front of a child sexual acts? Are giving a child an enema, taking a child's rectal temperature, having a child spit in a cup, or cutting a child's hair sexual acts? Are a physical examination by a doctor, hands-on wrestling instructions by a coach, or photographing a child playing dead sexual acts? Child molesters when interviewed commonly admit their acts but deny the intent (eg, "I was demonstrating a wrestling hold with the child;" "I was taking measurements for a study on adolescent growth;" "It was part of an initiation ceremony"). These acts could be sexual acts if you could prove the intent was for sexual gratification. Seemingly "nonsexual" behavior can be in the service of sexual needs.

It is important to realize that some acts may not be crimes even if proven that they were done for sexual gratification. Photographing children on the playground, tape recording the belching of boys, or listening to children urinate in a public bathroom can be sexual acts for some individuals, but they are most likely not crimes.

Other acts involve societal and cultural judgments. Does allowing children to watch adults have sex or gain access to pornography constitute child sexual abuse or child neglect? Should artists, photographers, and therapists have special privileges under child-pornography statutes? Can a high-quality artistic photograph taken with an expensive camera and printed on expensive paper still be child pornography? Is it child abuse to ask a child to reenact sexual abuse the child has described? Is it a crime to photograph the reenactment? Is burning a child's genitals with a lit cigarette physical abuse, sexual abuse, or both? Does it ever matter? The specific motivation might have important investigative or prosecutive significance in some cases.

Law enforcement officers obviously must look to the law to determine what a sex offense is and the elements of the offense. Some states allow wider latitude in looking at motivation to determine what is a sex crime. In any case, when evaluating the significance and relevance of offender behavior and children's allegations, investigators should always consider both the activity and its motivation.

"Child"

There clearly is a conflict between the law and society when it comes to defining a *child*. Sympathy for victims is inversely proportional to their age and sexual development. Many people using the term sexual abuse of *children* have a mental image of children 12 or younger. The main problem, therefore, is with the definition of the 13- to 17-year-old age group. Those are the child victims who most likely look, act, and have sex drives like adults, but who may or may not be considered children under some laws and by society. Pubescent teenagers can be viable sexual targets of a much larger population of sex offenders. Unlike one-on-one intrafamilial sexual abuse in which the victim is most often a young female, the victim in many sexual-exploitation cases is a boy between the ages of 10 and 16.

Under federal law, a sexually explicit photograph of a mature-looking 16-year-old girl or boy is legally child pornography. Such photographs are not, however, what most people think of when they think of child pornography. This again reflects the problem of definitions. Arguments about child pornography, such as whether it is openly sold or of interest only to pedophiles, may be primarily the result of confusion over its definitions.

Adolescents are frequently considered and counted by child advocates as children in order to emphasize the large scope of the child-victimization problem. But then little or nothing said or done about addressing the problem seems to apply to the reality of adolescent victims. If adolescents are considered child victims of sexual exploitation, then their needs, interests, and desires must be realistically recognized and understood when addressing the problem.

Legal definitions of who is considered a child or minor vary from state to state and even statute to statute when dealing with adolescent victims. During a prosecution, the definition can even vary from count to count in the same indictment. The age of the child may determine whether certain sexual activity is a misdemeanor or felony and what degree of felony. Issues such as whether the victim consented or whether the offender was a guardian or caretaker can have important legal significance. Sixteen-year-olds may be able to consent to have sex with the man down the street but not with their father or schoolteacher. It is unclear to me how the law evaluates consent when dealing with a 14-year-old boy seduced by a 55-year-old adult. The easiest way for an adult to have sex with a child and come under no legal scrutiny is to marry the child. The age and circumstances under which a child can marry an adult also vary from state to state.

To determine who is a child legally, investigators must turn to the law. The penal code will legally define who is a child or minor. But they must still deal with their own perceptions as well as those of the jury and society as a whole. In general, a ***child*** will be defined here as someone who has not yet reached his or her 18th birthday. One of the problems in using this broad, but sentimentally appealing, definition of a child is that it lumps together individuals who may be more unalike than alike. In fact, 16-year-olds may be socially and physically more like 26-year-old young adults than like 6-year-old children.

"Paraphilia"

Paraphilias are psychosexual disorders defined for clinical and research purposes in the DSM-IV-TR (APA, 2000). They are defined as recurrent, intense, and sexually arousing fantasies, urges, or behaviors that generally involve nonhuman objects, the suffering or humiliation of oneself or one's partner, or children or other nonconsenting persons, and that occur over a period of at least 6 months. Better known and more common paraphilias include exhibitionism (exposure), fetishism (objects), frotteurism (rubbing), pedophilia (child), sexual masochism (self-pain), sexual sadism (partner pain), and voyeurism (looking). Less known and less common paraphilias include scatologia (talk), necrophilia (corpses), partialism (body parts), zoophilia (animals), coprophilia (feces), klismaphilia (enemas), urophilia (urine), infantilism (baby), hebephilia (female youth), ephebophilia (male youth), and theoretically many others.

In the real world, each of the paraphilias typically has a slang name (eg, "big baby," "golden showers," "S&M"), an industry that sells related paraphernalia and props (eg, restraining devices, dolls, adult-size baby clothing), a support network (eg, North American Man/Boy Love Association [NAMBLA], Diaper Pail Fraternity, Internet newsgroups and chat rooms), and a body of literature (eg, pornography, newsletters). In fact, the paraphilias are the organizational framework or the "Dewey Decimal System" of pornography, obscenity, adult bookstores, and Internet sex chat rooms.

Paraphilias are psychosexual disorders and not types of sex crimes. They may or may not involve criminal activity. Individuals can and frequently do have more than one of these paraphilias. Individuals suffering from one or more of these paraphilias can just engage in fantasy and masturbate, or they can act out their fantasies legally (eg, with consenting adult partners or objects) or illegally (eg, with nonconsenting partners or underage partners). It is their choice. In addition, not everyone committing a sex offense has a paraphilia. Their behavior patterns may be criminal but might not fit the specific diagnostic criteria of a paraphilia.

"MO" and "Ritual"

On an investigative level, the presence of paraphilias often means highly repetitive and predictable behavior patterns focused on specific sexual interests that go well beyond a *method of operation* (MO). The concept of **MO**—something done by an offender because it works and will help him get away with the crime—is well known to most investigators. MO usually involves patterns of behavior intended to ensure success, protect identity, and facilitate escape. MO is fueled by thought and deliberation. Most offenders change and improve their MO over time and with experience.

The repetitive behavior patterns of some sex offenders can and do involve some MO, but are more likely to also involve the less-known concept of sexual *ritual*. Sexual *ritual* is the repeated engaging in an act or series of acts in a certain manner because of a sexual need; that is, in order to become fully aroused and/or gratified, a person must engage in the act in a certain way. If repeated often enough during sexual activity, some aspects of the MO of sex offenders can, through behavioral conditioning, become part of the sexual ritual. Other types of ritual behavior can be motivated by psychological, cultural, or spiritual needs or some combination. Unlike an MO, ritual is necessary to the offender but not to the successful commission of the crime. In fact, instead of facilitating the crime, ritual often increases the odds of identification, apprehension, and conviction because it causes the offender to make need-driven mistakes.

Sexual ritual and its resultant behavior are determined by erotic imagery, are fueled by fantasy, and can often be bizarre in nature. Most important to investigators, offenders find it difficult to change and modify their psychological, cultural, spiritual, or sexual ritual, even when their experience tells them they should or they suspect law-enforcement scrutiny. The ritual patterns of sex offenders have far more significance as prior and subsequent like acts than the MO of other types of offenders. Understanding sexual ritual is the key to investigating certain sex offenders. The courts in this country have, however, been slow to recognize and understand the difference between MO and ritual.

From a forensic point of view, it is not always easy to distinguish between MO and ritual. Putting on your shoes and socks every morning is a noncriminal/nonsexual example of MO. It serves a practical, functional purpose. Every morning putting on your right sock, then your right shoe, hopping once, then putting on your left sock, then your left shoe is a noncriminal/nonsexual example of ritual. It serves only a psychological need. Depending on the offender's intention, blindfolding or tying up a victim could be either MO or ritual. Tying up someone so he or she can not resist or escape is MO. Tying up someone for sexual gratification is called bondage and is a ritual. The ability to interpret this distinction is in the detailed analysis of the behavior. Investigators must, therefore, keep an open mind and continually accumulate and evaluate even the small details of offender *physical, sexual,* and *verbal* behavior.

"Child Molester"

The term *child molester* is fairly common and used by professionals and nonprofessionals alike, including law-enforcement officers. Although Random House Webster's College Dictionary (1991) defines molest as "to bother, interfere with, or annoy," it has generally come to convey sexual activity of some type with children.

In spite of its common usage, the term child molester conveys many different images and variations of meanings to different individuals. For many, it brings to mind the image of the dirty old man in a wrinkled raincoat hanging around a school playground with a bag of candy waiting to lure little children. For some, the child molester is a stranger to his victim and not a father having sex with his daughter. For others, the child molester is one who exposes himself to or fondles children without engaging in vaginal or anal intercourse. Still others believe the child molester is a nonviolent offender. Some differentiate between nonviolent child "molesters" who coax or pressure the child into sexual activity and violent child "rapists" who overpower or threaten to harm their victims. Most would probably not apply the term child molester to a man who uses the services of an adolescent prostitute. For law enforcement officers and prosecutors, the term child molester is more likely to conform to various legal definitions of sexual molestation set forth in the penal code.

For the purposes of this chapter, a **child molester** will be defined as a significantly older individual who engages in any type of sexual activity with individuals legally defined as children. When using only the term "child molester," no distinctions will be made between male and female, single and repeat offenders, or violent and nonviolent offenders. No distinctions will be made as to whether the child victims are prepubescent or pubescent, known or unknown, or related or unrelated to the offender. Finally, no distinctions will be made based on the type of sexual activity engaged in by the offender. Although such distinctions may have important legal and evaluation significance, they have no bearing on whether or not an individual is labeled a child molester.

How much older is "significantly older"? Clearly, in many cases, the dynamics of the case may be more important than simply the chronological age of the individuals. There are, however, some working guidelines. The rule of thumb that psychiatrists and others use is that there must be an age difference of at least 5 years. There are, however, cases in which the age difference is less than 5 years and yet the sexual behavior seems to fit the power-abuse dynamics of child sexual exploitation (CSE). The younger the child, the more significant the age difference. There are also cases in which the age difference is greater than 5 years, but the behavior does not seem to fit the dynamics. One of the most difficult cases to evaluate is that involving a younger and an older adolescent—for example, a 13-year-old girl and a 19-year-old boy. It is more than 5 years' difference, but is it CSE? What does the law say? What does society say? As previously stated, the focus of this chapter will not include adolescents sexually victimized by acquaintances who are clearly peers.

A central theme of this chapter is to emphasize the "big picture" approach to intervention. In short, a reported case of a 12-year-old child molester requires an investigation of more than just the reported crime. Many people have the idea that the cycle of abuse only means that child victims grow up and become adult offenders. It can also mean that the same individual is simultaneously a victim and offender. For example, say that a man sexually molests a 13-year-old boy. The 13-year-old boy goes home and molests his 7-year-old brother. The 7-year-old brother then molests the baby his mother is babysitting. The intervention into the last activity should lead back to the first crime.

"Pedophile"

Although the use of the term child molester is commonplace, publicity and awareness concerning sexual victimization of children has resulted in increasing use of the term *pedophile*. In the DSM-IV-TR, pedophilia is classified as a paraphilia, one of the psychosexual disorders. It is important for investigators to understand that the DSM-IV-TR diagnostic criteria for pedophilia require that there be recurrent, intense, *and* sexually arousing fantasies, urges, *or* behaviors involving *prepubescent* children, generally *aged 13* or younger. The absence of *any* of the key criteria could technically eliminate the diagnosis. For example, an individual who has a strong preference for and repeatedly engages in sex with large numbers of 14-year-olds could correctly be evaluated by a mental-health professional as *not* a pedophile. In spite of this, some mental-health professionals continue to apply the term to those with a sexual preference for pubescent teenagers. In addition, reaching puberty is a complex phenomenon that does not occur overnight or during everyone's 13th year.

The terms *hebephilia* and *ephebophilia* (ie, sexual preference for pubescent children) are not specifically mentioned in the DSM-IV-TR and are used far less often, even by mental-health professionals. They are, however, being increasingly used in forensic evaluations submitted to the court by defendants attempting to minimize their sexual behavior with teenagers. If you can be a hebephile, then you can have a mental disorder but not be a pedophile, and you may be able to confuse the court. Although sexual attraction to pubescent children by adults has the obvious potential for criminal activity, it does not necessarily constitute a sexual perversion as defined by psychiatry.

Technically, pedophilia is a psychiatric diagnosis that can be made only by qualified psychologists or psychiatrists. For many, therefore, the word is a diagnostic term, not a legal one. At one time, the term pedophile was used almost exclusively by mental-health professionals. Today many people, including those in the media, routinely refer to those who sexually abuse children as pedophiles. The term pedophile is also being used more and more by law enforcement and prosecutors. It has even entered their slang usage—with some talking about investigating a "pedo case" or being assigned to a "pedo squad." Although people in the United States most often pronounce the "ped" in "pedophilia" with a short "e" as the "ped" in "pedestrian" (from the Latin for foot), the correct pronunciation is "ped" with a long "e" as in "pediatrician" (from the Greek for child).

This increasing use has to some degree brought this term outside the exclusive purview of psychiatric diagnosis. Just as someone can refer to another as being "paranoid" without implying a psychiatric diagnosis or assuming psychiatric expertise, a social worker, physician, prosecutor, or law enforcement officer can refer to an individual who has sexually victimized a child as a pedophile. Random House Webster's New College Dictionary (1991) contains a good layperson's definition for pedophilia: "sexual desire in an adult for a child."

For the purposes of this chapter, the term "*pedophile*," when used, will be defined as a significantly older individual who *prefers* to have sex with individuals legally considered children. Pedophiles are individuals whose erotic imagery and sexual fantasies focus on children. They do not settle for child victims, but, in fact, clearly prefer to have sex with children. The law, not puberty, will determine who is a child.

To refer to someone as a pedophile is to say only that the individual has a sexual preference for children. It says little or nothing about the other aspects of his character and personality. To assume that someone is not a pedophile simply because he is nice, goes to church, works hard, is kind to animals, helps abused children, reports finding child pornography on the Internet to law enforcement, and/or searches for missing children is absurd. Pedophiles span the full spectrum from saints to monsters. In spite of this fact, over and over again pedophiles are not recognized, investigated, charged, convicted, or sent to prison simply because they are "nice guys." One of the best indicators of the continuing lack of understanding of pedophilia is that the media and society still view as a contradiction that someone could be a caring, dedicated teacher (eg, clergy member, coach, therapist, doctor, children's volunteer) and sexually victimize a child in his care. The vast majority of dedicated schoolteachers are not pedophiles, but many pedophiles who become schoolteachers are dedicated teachers.

Though pedophiles *prefer* to have sex with children, they can and do have sex with adults. Adult sexual relationships are more difficult for some pedophiles than for others. Some pedophiles have sex with adults as part of their effort to gain or continue their access to preferred children. For example, one might have occasional sex with a single mother to ensure continued access to her children.

OFFENDER TYPOLOGY
CHILD MOLESTER VERSUS PEDOPHILE
Even professionals are confused with regard to the terms child molester and pedophile. For many the terms have become synonymous. For them the word pedophile is just a fancy term for a child molester. The public, the media, and many child abuse professionals frequently use the terms interchangeably and simplistically refer to all those who sexually victimize children as pedophiles. No single or uniform definition for the word "pedophile" exists. As previously stated, for mental health professionals, it is a psychiatric diagnosis with specific criteria. Labeling all child molesters as pedophiles is, however, potentially confusing. Clear differences can be found between the types of individuals who sexually abuse children, and investigators handling these cases need to understand that and make such distinctions when appropriate.

Not all pedophiles are child molesters. A child molester is an individual who sexually molests children. A pedophile might have a sexual preference for children and fantasize about having sex with them, but if he does not act on that preference or those fantasies, he is not a child molester. Whether or not a person acts on deviant sexual fantasies and urges may be influenced by other factors such as personality traits, the severity of psychosocial stressors, personal inhibitions, substance abuse, or opportunities. Inhibiting factors such as guilt, moral beliefs, or fear of discovery may limit or reduce the sexual activity with children.

Some pedophiles might act out their fantasies in legal ways by simply talking to or watching children and later masturbating. Some might have sex with dolls and mannequins that resemble children. Some pedophiles might act out their fantasies in legal ways by engaging in sexual activity with adults who *look* (small stature, flat-chested, no body hair), *dress* (children's underwear, school uniform), or *act* (immature, baby talk) like young children. Others may act out child fantasy games with adult prostitutes. A difficult problem to detect and address is that of individuals who act out their sexual fantasies by socially interacting with children (ie, in-person or via an online computer), or by interjecting themselves into the child-sexual-abuse or exploitation "problem" as overzealous child advocates (ie, cyber vigilantes). It is almost impossible to estimate how many pedophiles exist who have never molested a child. What society can or should do with such individuals is an interesting area for discussion but beyond the role of investigators or prosecutors. People can not be arrested and prosecuted just for their fantasies.

Not all child molesters are pedophiles. A pedophile is an individual who prefers to have sex with children. A person who prefers to have sex with an adult partner may, for any number of reasons, decide to have sex with a child. Such reasons might include simple availability, opportunity, curiosity, or a desire to hurt a loved one of the molested child. The erotic imagery and sexual fantasies of such individuals are not necessarily recurrent, intense, and focused on children; therefore, these people are not pedophiles.

Are child molesters with adolescent victims pedophiles? Is an individual who collects both child and adult pornography a pedophile? Is everyone who uses a computer to facilitate having sex with children a pedophile? Is everyone who traffics in child pornography a pedophile? Many child molesters are, in fact, pedophiles, and many pedophiles are child molesters. But they are not necessarily one and the same. Often it may be unclear whether the term is being applied with its diagnostic meaning or some other definition. Most investigators are not qualified to apply the term with its diagnostic meaning. Distinctions between the types of child molesters, however, can have important and valuable implications for the investigation of sexual exploitation of children.

Most classification systems for child molesters were developed for and are used primarily by psychiatrists and psychologists evaluating and treating them. These systems and the DSM-IV-TR diagnostic system usually require that the offender be identified and available for evaluation. This chapter will set forth a model for investigators that places sex offenders along a motivational continuum and into several patterns of behavior. These categories are *not* intended for use by mental-health professionals doing *clinical* work. They are intended for use by forensic investigators and other professionals in evaluating cases and developing the evidence needed to assess, evaluate, identify, arrest, or convict child molesters. If the investigator already has enough evidence to convict a child molester, then whether or not the molester is a pedophile or any other category of offender may be of little importance. But if the investigator is still attempting to evaluate the case and develop incriminating evidence, such distinctions can be invaluable. Even if there is enough evidence to convict a child molester, the fact that a molester is a certain type of sex offender could still be important in evaluating the potential for additional child victims and other types of criminal behavior.

There is one answer to the questions investigators most commonly ask about child molesters, such as, "What is the best way to interview them?" "Do they collect child pornography?" "How many victims do they have?" "How did they get away with it for so long?" "Can I use an expert search warrant?" "Can they be reliably polygraphed?" "Can they be treated?" "Should the community be notified if one lives in the area?" The answer to all of these questions is—"It depends." It depends on what kind of child molester you have. Understanding and documenting offender patterns of behavior is one of the most important and overlooked steps in the assessment and corroboration of cases. If investigators accept the fact that there are different kinds of child molesters and that those differences can have criminal-justice significance, then they need a classification system or typology to label and distinguish among them.

Obtaining the kind of comprehensive, accurate, and reliable information necessary to apply a typology effectively, however, is far more difficult than developing a typology.

TYPOLOGY OF SEX OFFENDERS

When distinctions among types of offenders need to be made by investigators, I recommend the use of a descriptive typology developed for criminal justice purposes. After consulting on hundreds of cases in my work at the FBI Academy and not finding a typology that fit investigative needs, I decided to develop my own typology of child molesters for criminal-justice professionals. I deliberately avoided all use of diagnostic terminology (eg, pedophile, antisocial-personality disorder) and used instead descriptive terms. After developing the basic categories, I consulted with Dr. Park Dietz, a forensic psychiatrist. Dr. Dietz advised that in his work he sometimes divided sex offenders into the 2 broad categories: *situational* and *preferential* (Dietz, 1983). His concept was totally consistent with my new typology. With his permission, I then incorporated the use of these descriptive terms into my typology and expanded on his ideas.

My original typology of child molesters was developed in the mid-1980s and published and widely disseminated by the National Center for Missing & Exploited Children (NCMEC) (Lanning, 1986). It was revised in April 1987 (Lanning, 1987) and again in December 1992 (Lanning 1992a). It divided child molesters into 2 categories (Situational or Preferential) and into 7 patterns of behavior, as shown in **Table 23-1**. In the years that followed, I presented this typology at training conferences all over the world, and I applied it to and continued to learn from thousands of cases on which I consulted.

Although still useful, several limitations in this old typology gradually became evident to me. I realized that complex human behavior did not easily fit into neat little boxes. I, therefore, slowly began to revise it, and it has been replaced by the typology presented in **Table 23-2**. This newer typology places all sex offenders, not just child molesters, along a motivational continuum (Situational to Preferential) instead of into 1 of 2 discrete categories. The patterns are not necessarily mutually exclusive. The fact that an offender is motivated predominately by deviant sexual needs does not mean he can not also be motivated by some nonsexual needs. Offenders can demonstrate both situational and preferential motives and behavior patterns, but one is usually more dominant. It is a motivational continuum, but motivation can be difficult to determine. Offenders must be placed along the continuum based on the totality of known facts. Motivation is most often evaluated and determined by behavior patterns as well as other indicators and evidence. A more detailed discussion of this newer typology was published by the NCMEC in September 2001 (Lanning 2001).

At one end of the continuum are the more "situational" sex offenders (**Table 23-2**). Although they can be smart and rich, they tend to be less intelligent and more likely to be from lower socioeconomic groups. Their criminal sexual behavior tends to be in

---

Table 23-1. Child Molesters: A Behavioral Analysis (1985-1992)

SITUATIONAL CHILD MOLESTER	PREFERENTIAL CHILD MOLESTER
— Regressed	— Seduction
— Morally indiscriminate	— Introverted
— Sexually indiscriminate	— Inadequate
	— Sadistic

the service of basic sexual needs (eg, "horniness" and lust) or nonsexual needs (eg, power and anger). Their sexual behavior is often opportunistic and impulsive but primarily thought-driven. They are more likely to consider the risks involved in their behavior but often make stupid or sloppy mistakes. If they collect pornography, it is often violent in nature, reflecting their power and anger needs. Their thought-driven criminal sexual behavior tends to focus on general victim characteristics (eg, age, race, gender) and their perception of themselves as entitled to the sex. Much of their criminal behavior is intended simply to obtain and control their victims. Their verbal skills are usually low, and they are more likely to use physical violence to control victims. They are more likely to have a history of varied crimes against both person and property. Their sex crimes are usually either spontaneous or planned. Their victims tend to be targeted based primarily on availability and opportunity. They are

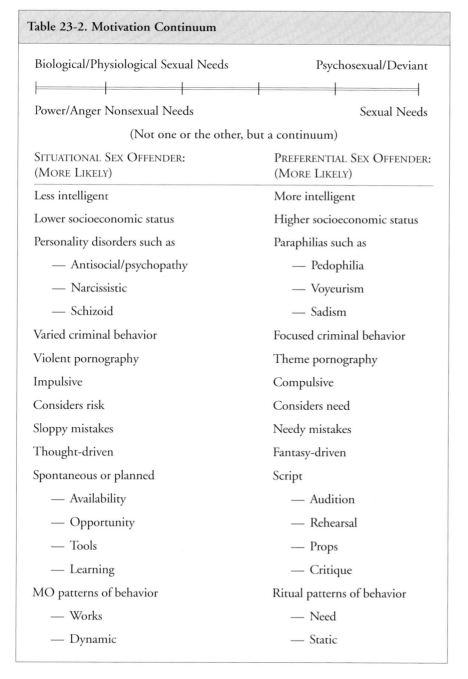

Table 23-2. Motivation Continuum

Biological/Physiological Sexual Needs   Psychosexual/Deviant

Power/Anger Nonsexual Needs   Sexual Needs

(Not one or the other, but a continuum)

Situational Sex Offender: (More Likely)	Preferential Sex Offender: (More Likely)
Less intelligent	More intelligent
Lower socioeconomic status	Higher socioeconomic status
Personality disorders such as	Paraphilias such as
— Antisocial/psychopathy	— Pedophilia
— Narcissistic	— Voyeurism
— Schizoid	— Sadism
Varied criminal behavior	Focused criminal behavior
Violent pornography	Theme pornography
Impulsive	Compulsive
Considers risk	Considers need
Sloppy mistakes	Needy mistakes
Thought-driven	Fantasy-driven
Spontaneous or planned	Script
— Availability	— Audition
— Opportunity	— Rehearsal
— Tools	— Props
— Learning	— Critique
MO patterns of behavior	Ritual patterns of behavior
— Works	— Need
— Dynamic	— Static

more likely to use practical tools (eg, weapons, lock picks, gloves, masks) and learn from and then modify their criminal sexual behavior. Their patterns of criminal sexual behavior are more likely to involve the previously discussed concept of method of operation.

Situational-type offenders sexually victimizing children do not have a true sexual preference for children. They may molest them, however, for a wide variety of situational reasons. They are more likely to view and be aroused by adult pornography but engage in sex with children in certain situations. Situational sex offenders frequently molest children to which they have easy access, such as their own children or those they may live with or have control over. Pubescent teenagers are high-risk, viable sexual targets. Younger children may also be targeted because they are weak, vulnerable, or available. Morally indiscriminate situational offenders may select children, especially adolescents, simply because they have the opportunity and think they can get away with it. Social misfits may situationally select child victims out of insecurity and curiosity. Others may have low self-esteem and use children as substitutes for preferred adults.

At the other end of the motivation continuum are the more "preferential" sex offenders (**Table 23-2**). Although they can be unintelligent and poor, they tend to be more intelligent and are likely to be from higher socioeconomic groups. Their criminal sexual behavior tends to be in the service of *deviant* sexual needs known as paraphilias. This behavior is often persistent and compulsive and is primarily fantasy-driven. Their erotic imagery creates the needs, which are then fueled over time by repeated fantasy. They are more likely to consider these needs rather than the risks involved and therefore make "needy" mistakes that often seem almost stupid. When they collect pornography and related paraphernalia, it usually focuses the themes of their paraphilic preferences. Their fantasy-driven behavior tends to focus not only on general victim characteristics and their entitlement to sex but also on their paraphilic preferences including specific victim preferences, their relationship to the victim (eg, teacher, rescuer, mentor), and their detailed scenario (eg, education, rescue, journey) (Hazelwood & Warren, 2001). Their criminal sexual behavior is rooted in their sexual fantasies and their need to turn fantasy into reality. Their verbal skills are usually high, and they are less likely to use physical violence to control victims. They are more likely to have a history of primarily sex offenses. Their sex crimes usually stem from a fantasy-fueled and elaborate script that is far more detailed and elaborate (eg, dialogue, exact sequence, clothing) than the "plan" of a situational-type sex offender or common criminal. They tend to "audition" their potential victims, selecting them primarily based on their similarity to and consistency with that script. There can be a lengthy "rehearsal" or grooming process leading up to the victimization. They are more likely to use fantasy "props" (eg, fetish items, costumes, toys) and critique the activity but not necessarily learn from or then modify their criminal sexual behavior. Their patterns of behavior are more likely to involve the previously discussed concept of ritual.

As this descriptive term implies, preferential-type sex offenders have specific sexual preferences or paraphilias. For instance, those with a preference for children could be called "pedophiles." Those with a preference for peeping could be called voyeurs, and those with a preference for suffering could be called sadists. But one of the purposes of this typology is to limit the use of these diagnostic terms for investigators and prosecutors. Preferential-type sex offenders are more likely to view, be aroused by, and collect theme pornography. A pedophile would be just one example or subcategory of a preferential sex offender. A preferential sex offender whose sexual preferences do not include children, and is therefore not a pedophile, can still sexually victimize children.

As previously stated, this new typology is a continuum. A preferential sex offender can have some of the motives and behavior patterns of a situational sex offender and vice versa. It is a matter of degree. In one case, an offender who was a schoolteacher had a child-pornography videotape mailed to him at the school where he worked. The "smart" thing to do would have been to take it home and view it in private; however, the teacher took it to a videocassette recorder (VCR) at the school for immediate viewing. This was a fantasy-driven, "needy" mistake typical of preferential sex offenders. To make it worse, he forgot to move a switch, and the tape was shown on numerous monitors around the school, which led to his identification. This was a "sloppy" mistake.

Although this typology continuum will be applied here primarily to child molesters, it can be applied to any sex offender. Nuisance sex offenders (eg, window peepers, fetish burglars, obscene telephone callers, flashers) are the sex offenders most likely to exhibit predominately preferential motives and patterns. Child molesters are more evenly distributed between offenders exhibiting predominately preferential and situational motives and patterns. Offenders who rape adults are the sex offenders most likely to exhibit predominately situational motives and patterns. In my opinion, this is why one hears it said so often that "rape is not about sex" and is not really a sex crime. In spite of this common and "politically correct" view, some rapists are preferential-type sex offenders, and for them, rape *is* primarily about sex. One rarely hears it said, however, that child molesting is not about sex or is not a sex crime. This is most likely due to the fact that more child molesters exhibit preferential patterns of sexual behavior and do not use physical force or violence to control their victims.

Situational-Type Child Molesters

The situational-type child molester does *not* usually have compulsive-paraphilic sexual preferences, including a preference for children. He may, however, engage in sex with children for varied and sometimes complex reasons. For such a child molester, sex with children may range from a "once-in-a-lifetime" act to a long-term pattern of behavior. The more long-term the pattern, the further down the continuum he may move. He will exhibit more and more of the behavior patterns of the preferential-type offender. The situational-type molester usually has fewer child victims. Other vulnerable individuals, such as the elderly, sick, or disabled, may also be at risk for sexual victimization by him. For example, the situational-type child molester who sexually abuses children in a day care center might leave that job and begin to sexually abuse elderly people in a nursing home. Situational offenders are not "better" than or not as "bad" as preferential offenders; they are just different. Within this category at least 3 major patterns of behavior emerge: *regressed, morally indiscriminate,* and *inadequate* (Lanning 2001).

Preferential-Type Child Molesters

Preferential-type child molesters have definite sexual inclinations. For many, that preference includes children, and they are the ones it would be most appropriate to refer to as "pedophiles." Some preferential-type sex offenders *without* a preference for children do, however, molest children. They might do so in order to carry out their bizarre sexual fantasies and preferences with young, less threatening, less judgmental, and highly vulnerable victims. Some of these offenders' sexual activity with children may involve deviant acts they are embarrassed or ashamed to request or do with a more experienced adult partner they actually prefer. Such offenders, even if they do not have a sexual preference for children, would still be preferential sex offenders and, therefore, engage in similar patterns of behavior.

Those with a definite preference for children (ie, pedophiles) have sexual fantasies and erotic imagery that focus on children. They have sex with children not because of some situational stress or insecurity but because they are sexually attracted to and prefer children. They have the potential to molest large numbers of child victims. For many of them, their problem is not only the nature of the sex drive (attraction to children) but also the quantity (need for frequent and repeated sex with children). They usually have age and gender preferences for their victims. Their sexual preference for children may also be accompanied by other paraphilic preferences. Preferential-type child molesters seem to prefer more boy than girl victims. Within this category, at least 4 major patterns of behavior emerge: *seduction, introverted, sadistic,* and *diverse* (Lanning 2001).

Who Cares?

The purpose of this descriptive typology is not to gain insight or understanding about *why* child molesters have sex with children in order to help or treat them but to recognize and evaluate *how* child molesters have sex with children in order to identify, arrest, and convict them. Things such as what evidence to look for, whether there are additional victims, how to identify those victims, and how to interview a victim or suspect depend on the type of child molester involved.

As this descriptive term implies, preferential-type sex offenders have specific sexual preferences or paraphilias. Those with a preference for children could be called "pedophiles." Those with a preference for peeping could be called voyeurs, with a preference for suffering could be called sadists, etc. But one of the purposes of this typology is to avoid these diagnostic terms. Preferential-type sex offenders are more likely to view, be aroused by, and collect theme pornography. Some preferential sex offenders *without* a preference for children do molest children in order to carry out their bizarre sexual fantasies and preferences with young, less threatening, less judgmental, and highly vulnerable victims. Some of these offenders' sexual activity with children may involve acts they are embarrassed or ashamed to request or do with a preferred adult partner. Such offenders, even if they do not have a sexual preference for children, would still be preferential sex offenders and, therefore, engage in similar patterns of behavior.

This criminal-justice descriptive typology has many advantages. If there is a need to distinguish a certain type of sex offender, this typology provides a name or label instead of just calling them "these guys." The label is professional in contrast to calling them "pervert," "sicko," or worse. Because the terms are descriptive (not diagnostic) and probative (not prejudicial), they may be more acceptable in reports, search warrants, and testimony by criminal justice professionals. For example, the currently popular term "predator" might be considered too prejudicial for some court testimony. The continuum concept also better addresses the complexity of and changes in human behavior. Using the term "preferential sex offender" instead of "preferential child molester" addresses the issue of applying it to offenders who collect child pornography without physically molesting children. The term preferential sex offender eliminates the need for investigators to distinguish between child pornography collectors and child molesters, between pedophiles and hebephiles, and among numerous other paraphilias. How to recognize and identify such offenders will be discussed shortly.

Investigators might argue that it is their job to investigate individuals who violate the law, and whether or not that offender is a pedophile or preferential sex offender is not important to them. There is no legal requirement to determine that a subject or suspect in a case is a pedophile or preferential-type sex offender. Often it is irrelevant to the investigation or prosecution. There are, however, clear differences between the types of individuals who sexually victimize children, and investigators handling these cases sometimes need to make such distinctions. The terms situational and preferential sex offender are merely descriptive labels to be used only to identify, for investigative and prosecutive purposes, a certain type of offender. The terms do *not* appear in the DSM-IV-TR, and they are *not* intended to imply or be used for a clinical diagnosis.

Although there is not *a* "profile" that will determine if someone is a child molester, preferential sex offenders tend to engage in highly predictable and recognizable behavior patterns. The potential evidence available as a result of the long-term, persistent, and ritualized behavior patterns of many sexual exploiters of children makes these cases almost "investigators' heaven."

Need-driven behavior often leads to bewildering mistakes. For example, why would a reasonably intelligent individual do such things as use his computer at work to download child pornography, deliver his computer filled with child pornography for repair, send his film with child pornography on it to a store to be developed, appear in child-pornography images he is making, discuss engaging in serious criminal activity with a "stranger" he met on the Internet, transmit identifiable photographs of himself to such an individual, maintain incriminating evidence knowing investigators might soon search his home or computer, give investigators permission to search his home or computer knowing it contains incriminating evidence, give investigators the names of victims or former victims as character references, and agree to be interviewed without his lawyer?

Although a variety of individuals sexually abuse children, preferential-type sex offenders, and especially pedophiles, are the *primary* acquaintance sexual exploiters of children. A preferential-acquaintance child molester might molest 10, 50, hundreds, or even thousands of children in a lifetime depending on the offender and how broadly or narrowly child molestation is defined. Although pedophiles vary greatly, their sexual behavior is repetitive and highly predictable. Knowledge of these sexual-behavioral patterns or characteristics is extremely valuable to the law enforcement investigator.

These highly predictable and repetitive behavior patterns make cases involving preferential-type offenders far easier to investigate than those involving situational-type offenders. An important step in investigating cases of sexual exploitation of children by adult acquaintances is to recognize and identify, if present, the highly predictable sexual-behavior patterns of preferential sex offenders or pedophiles. To do this, it is important that investigators continually attempt to place a suspected acquaintance child molester along the motivational continuum.

A classification system or typology to determine the type of offender with whom one is dealing can not be applied unless the most complete, detailed, and accurate information possible is obtained in order. To properly evaluate the significance of any offender or victim behavior, investigators must have and be able to professionally process the *details* of that behavior. The fact that a suspect was previously convicted of "sodomizing" or engaging in "indecent liberties" with a child is almost meaningless if the *details* (ie, verbal, physical, and sexual behavior) of the crime are not available and known. Reports that sanitize or describe, in politically correct terms, an offender's language and sexual behavior are almost worthless in evaluating sex offenses. This is one reason why investigators who can not easily and objectively communicate about regular and deviant sex have problems dealing with sex crimes.

The investigator must understand that doing a background investigation on a suspect means more than obtaining the date and place of birth and credit and criminal checks. School, juvenile, military, medical, driving, employment, bank, sex-offender and child-abuse registry, sex offender assessment, computer, and prior investigative records can all be valuable sources of information about an offender. Relatives, friends, associates, and current and former sex partners can be identified and interviewed. Other investigative techniques (eg, mail cover, pen register, trash run, surveillance) can also be used. Indicators and counter-indicators must be identified and evaluated.

Many investigators like to jokingly refer to such behavior as examples of "criminal stupidity." Defense attorneys might even argue that such behavior indicates that their clients are innocent, lack criminal intent, or are not criminally responsible. Why else would an intelligent individual do something so obviously "stupid?" Such behavior does not necessarily mean the offender is stupid, insane, or not criminally responsible. Another explanation is much more probable—it is need-driven. The fantasy- or need-driven behavior of preferential sex offenders has little to do with thinking. As a father cautioned his son in the movie *A Bronx Tale*, it is more a matter of the "little head" telling the "big head" what to do. It is what makes preferential sex offenders so vulnerable to proactive investigations even though the techniques used have been well publicized. If necessary, an expert could be used to educate the court concerning certain patterns of behavior. The use of such an expert was upheld in *United States v Romero*, 189 F3d 576 (7th Cir 1999).

Investigators should be aware of a "Cautionary Statement" that appears on page xxxvii of the DSM-IV-TR and reads in part that:

It is to be understood that inclusion here, for clinical and research purposes, of a diagnostic category such as *Pathological Gambling or Pedophilia* does not imply that the condition meets legal or other nonmedical criteria for what constitutes mental disease, mental disorder, or mental disability. The clinical and scientific considerations involved in categorization of these conditions as mental disorders may not be wholly relevant to legal judgments, for example, that take into account such issues as individual responsibility, disability determination, and competency [emphasis added](APA, 2000).

Profiling?

It should be noted that the above-described applications of this typology have little, if anything, to do with "profiling." As used by the FBI's Behavioral Science Unit and National Center for the Analysis of Violent Crime (NCAVC), the term "profiling" refers to analyzing the criminal behavior of an *unknown* subject and determining likely personality and behavioral characteristics of that offender. It has nothing to do with cases in which a particular suspect is identified.

In addition, this typology is not intended to be used in a court of law to *prove* that someone is guilty of child molestation because he or she fits a certain "profile." It would be inappropriate and improper to claim that because someone has certain traits and characteristics, we know with certainty that he or she is a child molester and he or she should therefore be convicted. The level of proof necessary to take action on information is dependent on the consequences of that action. The level of proof necessary to convict someone in a court of law and incarcerate him is very high: proof beyond a reasonable doubt.

Applying this typology, however, in the ways discussed here (eg, assess allegations, identify potential victims, evaluate intent, develop interview strategies, address staleness of probable cause, assess prior and subsequent like acts, educate juries, compare consistency) has less direct and immediate severe consequences for a suspected offender. Any additional evidence obtained from applying this typology can hopefully be used in court. Even if an expert educates a jury about certain patterns of behavior, the jury still decides how it applies, if it applies, and if the evidence constitutes proof beyond a reasonable doubt. The expert is not giving an opinion about the guilt of the accused. (See *United States v Romero*, 1999.)

In essence, the criminal investigative analysis involved in applying this typology to the investigation of acquaintance molestation cases often consists of determining and assessing the *details* (ie, verbal, physical, and sexual behavior) of "what" happened, evaluating and deciding "why" something did or did not happen (ie, motivation continuum), and then comparing that for consistency to the known behavioral patterns and characteristics of "who" is identified or suspected. This, of course, can only be done if you have accurate, detailed information about "what" allegedly happened and comprehensive, reliable information about "who" allegedly did it. As previously stated, no one "profile" will determine if someone is a child molester. But there are some child molesters who tend to engage in highly predictable and recognizable behavior patterns. The potential evidence available as a result of the long-term, persistent, and ritualized behavior patterns of many preferential sex offenders makes the understanding and recognition of these patterns important and useful to investigators and prosecutors in legally appropriate ways.

SUMMARY OF TYPOLOGIES

Although there are few absolutes in human behavior, situational-type sex offenders tend to be less predictable, more "criminally" intelligent, less likely to retain corroborative evidence intentionally, more vulnerable to appeals to their need to have their egos flattered and, when confronted with the facts of the case, more willing to make a thought-driven deal with the criminal justice system to limit the legal consequences of their behavior. Preferential-type sex offenders tend to be more predictable, less "criminally" intelligent, more likely to retain corroborative evidence intentionally, more vulnerable to appeals to their need to have their activities validated and, when confronted with the facts of the case, more willing to make a need-driven deal with the criminal justice system to avoid public disclosure of the details of their behavior.

POTENTIAL PROBLEM AREAS

In applying any offender typology, the investigator must recognize the difficulty of attempting to put complex human behavior into neat categories. There are few absolutes in human behavior. The words "always" and "never" rarely apply, except to say there will always be exceptions and difficulties. One of the biggest problems with any diagnostic or classification system is taking the time to apply it carefully and properly. Because of heavy work loads or lack of training, law enforcement officers, social workers, prosecutors, and other forensic interveners frequently do not take the time to evaluate offender patterns of behavior adequately. Split-second decisions and stereotypes often determine how an alleged perpetrator is classified and investigated.

COMBINATION OFFENDERS

A pedophile might have other psychosexual disorders, personality disorders, or psychoses or may be involved in other types of criminal activity. A pedophile's sexual interest in children might be combined with other sexual deviations (paraphilias), which include indecent exposure (exhibitionism), peeping (voyeurism), obscene telephone calls (scatologia), exploitation of animals (zoophilia), urination (urophilia), defecation (coprophilia), binding (bondage), baby role playing (infantilism), infliction of pain (sadism, masochism), and real or simulated death (necrophilia). The pedophile is interested in sex with children that might, in some cases, involve other sexual deviations. The morally indiscriminate or diverse-type child molester is interested in a variety of sexual deviations that might, in some cases, involve children. There are cases in which pedophiles are also psychopathic con artists, paranoid survivalists, or even serial killers. One particularly difficult offender to deal with is the morally indiscriminate pedophile. If an offender has a sexual preference for children and at the same time has no conscience, there is no limit to how he might sexually victimize children. He does not have to spend a lot of time validating his behavior. Such an offender is more likely to abduct or murder children. While his preferential sexual interest in children affects his victim selection, however, most of his behavior is determined by a stunning lack of conscience. He is best viewed as a morally indiscriminate offender and should be investigated and interviewed as such. When an offender seems to fit into more than one pattern of behavior, it is best to choose the broadest or most comprehensive one.

NUISANCE SEX OFFENDERS

The word "nuisance" is an unfortunate but descriptive term commonly applied to sex offenses that occur frequently and are viewed as causing little or no harm (eg, financial loss or physical injury). Examples with which most law enforcement officers are familiar include window peepers (voyeurism), flashers (exhibitionism), and obscene callers (scatologia). Nuisance sex offenders are often linked to the sexual paraphilias. As previously stated, nuisance sex offenders are the sex offenders most likely to exhibit predominately preferential motives and patterns. These cases, therefore, are highly solvable if the cases can be captured and linked and the patterns and rituals can be identified. However, they are usually given a low priority and not solved because:

— Most incidents are not reported to law enforcement.

— When incidents are reported they are either not recorded or recorded in a way that makes retrieval difficult.

— Little, if any, manpower and resources are committed to the investigation.

— Law-enforcement agencies frequently do not communicate and cooperate with each other concerning these cases.

— The crimes often involve minor violations of the law.

Importance

Investigators dealing with the sexual exploitation of children need to be interested in and concerned about nuisance sex offenses because of (1) progression, (2) substitution, (3) assessment and evaluation, and (4) corroboration.

Progression

Sex offenders can progress in the following ways: types of victims; types of acts; frequency, intensity, skill of crimes; and physical and emotional harm to a victim. Many sex offenders progress in gaining confidence and in acting out their deviant sexual fantasies by moving from inanimate objects to paid adult partners (prostitutes) to compliant adult partners and then to crime victims who are family members, acquaintances, or strangers. Although prostitution is a crime, this acting-out behavior is usually criminal only when the victims are children or nonconsenting adults. The violence used by sex offenders can also progress. They can progress to violence and in violence. Their sexual violence can be part of general aggression or true sexual sadism. It can be incidental to the sex crime or an integral part of it. Almost any sex offender can become violent to avoid discovery or identification. If the sex offender's preference includes children (ie, pedophilia), this progression can obviously lead to child victims.

Nuisance sex offenses with child victims can be part of the evolving process of a pedophile developing his criminal skills and overcoming inhibitions. The nuisance offenses with the child victims can also be because the pedophile has other paraphilias and has a sexual interest in these particular behaviors (eg, indecent exposure, obscene calls, peeping) with children.

Substitution

Many preferential sex offenders who commit these nuisance sex offenses do not have a sexual preference for children but often select child victims because they are ashamed and embarrassed of their deviant sexual preferences or because the children are more vulnerable and less intimidating. Some of them select children as victims when the true target or victim is a relative of the child or someone linked to the child in some way. This indirect victimization is even more likely if the child victim is especially young and incapable of understanding and providing the anticipated reaction to the "nuisance" sexual behavior (eg, obscene notes and photographs, indecent exposure).

Assessment and Evaluation

Understanding the paraphilias and considering both the activity and its motivation are an important part of assessing and evaluating the significance and relevance of offender behavior and children's allegations. This can be useful when child victims describe what sounds like bizarre activity involving such things as urine, feces, enemas, bondage, and playing dead. It is often said at child-abuse conferences that when young children talk about "pee pee" coming out of an offender's penis, they are actually referring to semen. If the offender is into urophilia, however, the child may in fact be referring to urine, and it is still sexual activity. A few "child-sexual-abuse experts" decided that the only explanation for allegations of this type was that the offenders were "satanists." The only paraphilia that many professionals dealing with child sexual abuse have heard of is pedophilia. Knowledge of this kind of behavior can also assist in evaluating narrative material found in the possession or on the computer of child molesters. Even noncriminal behavior related to sexual preferences can and should be used to assess and evaluate allegations of child sexual victimization. Even when children are the victims of this unusual, bizarre sexual activity, it is still sometimes considered to be a "nuisance" sex offense.

Corroboration

Understanding the paraphilias and nuisance sex offenses can sometimes help investigators to prove intent, identify prior and subsequent like acts, and recognize collateral evidence in sexual-exploitation-of-children cases. Because a high percentage of nuisance sex offenders are preferential sex offenders, they engage in similar patterns of predictable and persistent sexual behavior and are vulnerable to the same investigative techniques discussed in this chapter. These techniques can be used to help prove the sexual motivation of some of these poorly understood nuisance sex offenses as well as evaluating their possible connection to sexual-exploitation-of-children cases.

Evaluation

Some "nuisance" sex offenses against children are more common than others. Some of the more bizarre behaviors include stealing soiled diapers being worn by a baby; photographing children wearing diapers; squirting children with a water pistol filled with semen; listening to children urinate in a school bathroom; video-taping cheerleaders at a high school football game; having parents send photographs of their children getting an enema; playing the master/servant game by having children rest their feet on his prone body; tape-recording boys belching; window peeping at his own children; urinating on prostitutes, girlfriends, and his own child; masturbating to videotapes of children's autopsies; having children spit in cups; buying soiled underwear from adolescent boys; and soliciting body fluids from boys on the Internet. The investigative priority of these types of crimes can change rapidly when it is discovered that the offender carries the human immunodeficiency virus (HIV) or is entering homes in the middle of the night. In many of these cases, proving the sexual motivation is difficult unless one understands preferential sex offenders. Some are still not considered sex crimes or crimes at all, even if one can prove the sexual motivation.

A big investigative question in nuisance sex offenses is always the progression to more serious offenses. Some nuisance sex offenders progress little over the years in their criminal sexual behavior. Some progress to more serious sex crimes, and some move back and forth. Many investigators consider the possibility that a nuisance sex offender might progress to more serious crimes in the future, but they ignore the possibility that he *already* has.

When evaluating nuisance sex offenders, investigators should consider: (1) *focus,* (2) *escalation,* (3) *theme,* and (4) *response to identification.* The fact that a nuisance sex offender moves from victims meeting general criteria to specific victims is an example of focus and a potential danger sign. Escalation over time is also a danger sign. Escalation can be evaluated only when multiple offenses occur. Because of the low priority of the cases enumerated above, this can be difficult to do. The cases that the investigator believes are the first, second, and third may actually be the 10th, 16th, and 22nd. Investigators should also consider the theme of the nuisance sex offenses. Not all obscene calls or indecent exposures are the same. As discussed, specific details, not general labels, are needed. Lastly, in evaluating dangerousness, investigators should consider the nuisance sex offender's reaction to identification. Did he become violent and aggressive? Is he indifferent to or aroused by the response of his victims? Is he cooperative? Whatever their personal feelings, investigators will almost always get more information, details, and admissions from these offenders when they treat them with respect, dignity, and empathy.

MULTIPLE OFFENDERS

When investigations involve multiple offenders, the investigator must recognize that the subjects involved could include different kinds of molester patterns. The staff at a day care center where children are being molested might include inadequate, seduction, morally indiscriminate, or any other combination of the traits of the previously discussed situational and preferential sex offenders. A religious group involved in sexually abusing children might include morally indiscriminate, diverse, inadequate, and sadistic patterns of behavior. The behavior of the individuals involved must be carefully evaluated in order to develop appropriate investigative and interview strategies.

An important application of this typology is the simple recognition that not all child molesters are the same. Not all child molesters are pedophiles. Not all child molesters are passive, nonaggressive people. Child molesters can look like everyone else and are motivated by a wide variety of influences. No single investigative or interview technique deals with all of them.

INCEST CASES

It is commonly accepted that incestuous fathers are typically "regressed" child molesters who molest only their own children, do not collect child pornography, and are best dealt with in noncriminal treatment programs. This is not true all of the time. There are cases in which the incestuous father is a seduction or introverted preferential-type child molester (ie, pedophile) who "married" simply to gain access to children. In many cases, he has molested children outside the marriage or children in previous "marriages."

Such individuals frequently look for women who already have children who meet their age and gender preferences. Their marriages or relationships usually last only as long as there are children in the victim preference range. In today's more liberal society, such an offender frequently no longer marries the woman but simply moves in with her and her children. On some occasions, they merely befriend the mother and do not even pretend romantic interest in her but only express a desire to be a "father figure" for her children and help with expenses. Another technique is to marry a woman and adopt children or take in foster children. The last and least desirable stratagem they use is to have their own children. This is the least desirable method because it requires offenders to have frequent sex with their wives, and then there are few guarantees that the baby will be of the preferred sex.

In order to engage in sexual relations with his wife, the true pedophile must create a fantasy. To aid in this fantasy, some pedophiles have their wives dress, talk, or behave like children. After the birth of a baby of the preferred sex, such pedophiles may terminate or greatly reduce sexual relations with their wives. Of course, these facts are difficult for the law enforcement investigator to learn. Most wives or even ex-wives would be embarrassed to admit these sexual problems. Some ex-wives or ex-girl-friends might even exaggerate or embellish such information. Although such of-fenders are technically intrafamilial molesters, they are more properly and effectively investigated and prosecuted as acquaintance molesters.

Many incestuous fathers and live-in boyfriends, however, are morally indiscriminate individuals whose sexual abuse of children is only a small part of their problems. They have no real sexual preference for children but sexually abuse the available children because they can. They sometimes victimize and abuse the children in the home because they are competition for mom's attention and time. They can be cun-ning, manipulative individuals who can convincingly deny the allegations against them or, if the evidence is overwhelming, claim they need "help with their problem." Their personality disorder is more serious than even pedophilia and probably more difficult to treat.

The possibility that an incestuous father might molest children outside the home or commit other sex offenses seems to be beyond the comprehension of many child-abuse professionals. Even when they intellectually admit the possibility, their pro-fessional actions indicate otherwise.

FEMALE OFFENDERS
Where do female child molesters fit into this typology? The answer is unknown at this time. I have not consulted on a sufficient number of cases involving female of-fenders to properly include them in this typology. Although they certainly comprise a minority of cases, I believe that the sexual victimization of children by females is far more prevalent than most people believe.

Many people view sex between an older woman and acquaintance adolescent boy not as molestation but a "rite of passage." Furthermore, sexual activity between women and young children is difficult to identify. Females are the primary care-takers in our society and can dress, bathe, change, examine, and touch children with little suspicion.

Many of the cases involving alleged sexual abuse in day care centers involve female offenders. The apparent sexual activity in some of these cases may in fact be physical abuse directed at sexually significant body parts (eg, genitals, nipples). There are many cases in which females actively participate in the sexual abuse of children with an adult male accomplice. Sometimes the female assumes the role of "teaching" the child victim about sexual activity. In other cases, the female appears to be motivated by more serious emotional and psychological problems. It is rare to find a case, how-ever, in which a female offender fits the dynamics of the preferential-type child molester. This may be due to the fact that preferential molesting (eg, multiple vic-tims, paraphilias, theme pornography) has been defined from a male-sexual-behav-ior perspective.

This area still needs additional research and study. For additional information on female sex offenders, see "Female sex offenders: a typological and etiological overview" (Warren & Hislop, 2001).

ADOLESCENT OFFENDERS
Another area that has received increased attention involves adolescent offenders. In past years, adolescent child molesters were usually dismissed with "boys will be boys" or "he's just going through a stage." Adolescent child molesters can fit anywhere along the continuum and into any of the patterns of behavior described in this book. Frighteningly, though, many cases involving adolescent child molesters seem to fit the morally indiscriminate pattern of behavior. These adolescent offenders must be carefully evaluated for proper intervention and treatment when-ever possible.

In addition, adolescent (and even younger) sex offenders should *always* be viewed as past or current victims of sexual victimization in the broadest sense. This might also include psychological sexual abuse, inappropriate exposure to sexually explicit material, and the repeated or inappropriate witnessing of adult sexual activity. Recognizing and then investigating this victimization can lead to the identification of additional offenders and victims. The sexual abuse of younger children by an older child should always be viewed as a *possible* indication that the older child was also sexually victimized.

As previously stated, this chapter will not address the issue of children, especially adolescents, sexually victimized by peers. For additional information on adolescent sex offenders, see "The sex crimes of juveniles" (Hunter, 2001).

ACQUAINTANCE-EXPLOITATION CASES

OVERVIEW

This section discusses cases in which multiple children are sexually exploited by acquaintances. The majority of offenders who simultaneously sexually victimize multiple children are acquaintance child molesters, and most acquaintance child molesters who victimize multiple children are preferential sex offenders. Recognizing, understanding, and managing these dynamics are crucial to the proper forensic intervention into these cases. Cases involving multiple child victims are sometimes referred to as *child sex rings*. Many people, however, have extreme and stereotypical ideas of what a child sex ring is. They believe it must involve organized groups buying and selling children and shipping them around the country or the world for sexual purposes. In this chapter, the term **child sex ring** is simply defined as one or more offenders simultaneously involved sexually with several child victims. Because of the stereotypical images conjured up by the term, however, its use will be kept to a minimum.

Acquaintance-exploitation cases with multiple victims need not have a commercial component or involve group sex. Although that has happened in some cases, it is more likely that the offender is sexually interacting with the children one at a time. The offender more than likely has sex with other children before terminating the sexual relationship with prior victims. The activity can involve any of the wide range of "sexual" behaviors discussed in this chapter. The various child victims being molested during a certain period of time usually know each other but may or may not know that the offender is having sex with the other children. Some victims may believe they are the only ones having a "special" relationship with the offender. Other victims may actually witness the sexual activity of the offender with other children. Offenders may have favorite victims that they treat differently than the other victims.

Acquaintance-exploitation cases with multiple victims need not involve highly structured or organized groups such as organized crime, satanic cults, or pedophile organizations. Burgess (1984) identified 3 types of child sex rings: *solo, transition,* and *syndicated.* In the solo ring, the offender keeps the activity and photographs completely secret. Each ring involves one offender and multiple victims. In the transition ring, offenders begin to share their experiences, pornography, or victims. Photographs and letters are traded, and victims may be tested by other offenders and eventually traded for their sexual services. In the syndicated ring, a more structured organization recruits children, produces pornography, delivers direct sexual services, and establishes an extensive network of customers. In the United States, even the syndicated-type rings rarely have a hierarchical structure with a clear chain of command. They are more likely to be informal networks of individuals who share a common sexual interest and who will betray each other in a minute if it helps their criminal case.

DYNAMICS OF CASES

Cases in which children are exploited by acquaintances have many dynamics different from "typical" intrafamilial-abuse cases.

"Experts"

Many of the nation's experts on the "sexual abuse of children" have little or no experience dealing with acquaintance-exploitation cases, especially those involving multiple victims. Most of their experience is with one-on-one, intrafamilial-incest cases. The investigation of acquaintance-exploitation cases requires specialized knowledge and techniques. The intervention model for dealing with one-on-one, intrafamilial-child sexual abuse has only limited application when dealing with multiple-victim, extrafamilial, CSE cases.

Risk to Other Children

Preferential sex offenders are more likely to have multiple victims. Those who focus on intrafamilial abuse rarely think of the danger to other children in the community because, in their minds, intrafamilial offenders molest only their own children. In one case that I was asked to evaluate, a military officer had sexually molested his own daughter from shortly after birth to shortly before her seventh birthday. He was convicted and sent to prison. After several years, he was released and returned to live with his wife and daughter. When hearing about this case, most people operating only from the intrafamilial perspective of child sexual abuse react with disgust or outrage at the notion that the offender is back in the home with the victim. Although that is of some concern to me, it is minor compared with my concern for other young female children in the community where the offender now lives. Having reviewed and analyzed the offender's behavior patterns and extensive collection of child pornography and erotica, I know a great deal about the sexual fantasies and desires of this clearly preferential sex offender. His daughter is now too old to be a preferred sexual partner, and any young female child in the neighborhood fitting his preferences is at significant risk of victimization. If neighborhood children were molested, he would be both an intrafamilial and acquaintance offender.

How and when to notify the community of this possible risk to other children is a very difficult and important judgment call by investigators. The need to protect society must be weighed against the rights of the accused and the opportunity to obtain reliable evidence. Investigators must carefully consider what and how much information can be disseminated to the public. Do you notify everyone in the neighborhood, only parents of high-risk victims, only parents who had contact with the suspected offender, or only parents of children allegedly molested? Alerting parents too soon or improperly can result in destroying the life of an innocent individual, vigilante "justice," and contamination of a valid case.

Role of Parents

The role of the child victim's parents is a third major difference between acquaintance exploitation cases and intrafamilial-child sexual abuse. In intrafamilial cases, there is usually an abusing and a nonabusing parent. In such cases, a nonabusing mother may protect the child, pressure the child not to talk about the abuse, or persuade the child to recant the story so that the father does not go to jail. Dealing with these dynamics is important and it can be difficult.

Since parents are usually not the abusers in these acquaintance cases, their role is different. However, to underestimate the importance of that role is a potentially serious mistake. Their interaction with their victimized child can be crucial to the case. If the parents pressure or interrogate their children or conduct their own investigation, the results can be damaging to the proper investigation of the case. It is also possible that a child sexually exploited by an acquaintance was or is possibly being sexually, physically, or psychologically abused at home.

Disclosure Continuum Status

When investigators interview children in intrafamilial cases, the victim has usually already disclosed the abuse to someone. In cases involving sexual exploitation by acquaintances, the children interviewed often have not previously disclosed their victimization. They are likely being interviewed only because the victimization was discovered or is suspected because an alleged or known sex offender had access to them. These types of interviews are extremely difficult and sensitive. The disclosure/reporting continuum is discussed in detail later in this chapter.

Multiple Victims

There is frequently interaction among the multiple victims in acquaintance-exploitation cases. In intrafamilial cases, the sexual activity is usually a secret that the victim has discussed with no one until disclosure takes place. In a child sex ring, there are multiple victims whose interactions *before* and *after* discovery must be examined and evaluated.

Multiple Offenders

Interaction among multiple offenders is another major difference. Offenders sometimes communicate with each other and trade information and material. Offender interaction is an important element in the investigation of these cases. The existence of multiple offenders can be an investigative difficulty, but it can also be an advantage. The more offenderEs involved, the greater the odds that there is a "weak link" who can be used to corroborate the alleged abuse.

Gender of the Victim

The gender of the victim is another major difference between intrafamilial and extrafamilial-sex cases. Unlike intrafamilial sexual abuse, in which the most common reported victim is a young female, in acquaintance-exploitation cases an adolescent boy victim is more common.

SEXUAL EXPLOITATION VERSUS SEXUAL ABUSE CASES

Because so many investigators and prosecutors have more training and experience dealing with intrafamilial, child-sex-abuse cases, a synopsis of this comparison with acquaintance-exploitation cases can be useful (**Table 23-3**). These contrasts are only typical tendencies. There are always exceptions and many variations.

Almost by definition, child-sexual-abuse cases tend to be "intrafamilial." They are more likely to involve situational sex offenders who often coerce a small number of usually younger, female victims into sexual activity. The offenders are less likely to collect child pornography or erotica. They tend to rationalize their sexual activity with children as not being harmful. When most investigators interview victims in these cases, the children have usually first disclosed or reported the abuse to someone else. Family members frequently pressure the child to keep the family "secret" and not report it or recant it once reported. In general, there is usually less corroborative evidence.

Almost by definition, acquaintance-exploitation cases tend to be "extrafamilial." As previously mentioned, however, some true "acquaintance" molesters gain access to their victims through "marriage." Such cases might be superficially classified as intrafamilial. Acquaintance-exploitation cases are more likely to involve preferential sex offenders who seduce a large number of victims, often older, male victims, into sexual activity. The offenders are more likely to collect child pornography or erotica. They tend to validate their sexual activity with children as good or beneficial to the victims. When investigators in these cases interview victims, the children have usually not disclosed the exploitation, and victimization is discovered or only suspected. Family members frequently "interrogate" the child about the exploitation, pressuring the child in a variety of ways to describe the victimization in a more socially "acceptable" way. In general, there is usually more corroborative evidence.

TYPES OF MULTIPLE-VICTIM CASES

CSE cases involving multiple victims fall into 2 major patterns or types: *historical* and *multidimensional*. These terms give a descriptive and generic name to each type of case yet avoid such loaded labels as "traditional," "ritualistic," or "satanic" child sexual

---

Table 23-3. Comparison of Abuse and Exploitation Cases

CHILD SEXUAL ABUSE	CHILD SEXUAL EXPLOITATION
— "Intrafamilial"	— "Extrafamilial"
— Situational offenders	— Preferential offenders
— Female victims	— Male victims
— Younger victims	— Older victims
— Greater number of victims	— Fewer number of victims
— Coercion	— Seduction
— "Disclosure"/ report interviews	— Suspicion interviews
— Family secrecy	— Family "interrogation"
— Rationalization	— Validation
— Child pornography less likely	— Child pornography more likely
— Child erotica less likely	— Child erotica more likely
— Less evidence	— More evidence

---

abuse and exploitation. The dynamics and characteristics of the far more common "historical" multiple-victim cases are described below. The highly controversial dynamics and characteristics of multidimensional cases will not be discussed in this chapter. Those seeking such information should obtain a copy of the monograph titled *Investigator's Guide to Allegations of "Ritual" Child Abuse* from the FBI's NCAVC at the FBI Academy, Quantico, Va (Lanning, 1992c). Investigative techniques specific to these "historical" multiple-victim cases are described in more detail later in this chapter.

"Historical" Multiple-Victim Cases

"Historical" multiple-victim cases can involve a day care center, a school, a scout troop, a little league team, or neighborhood children. Although viewed predominately as acquaintance-exploitation cases, they can also involve marriage as a method of access to children, intrafamilial molestation of children, and the use of family children to attract other victims.

We know much about this kind of case. The information is well documented by law-enforcement investigation and based on my involvement in many hundreds of corroborated cases for more than 25 years. The investigation of these cases can be challenging and time-consuming. Once agencies understand the dynamics and are willing to commit the manpower and resources, however, obtaining corroboration and convictions in these cases can be easier than in one-on-one intrafamilial cases.

Acquaintance-exploitation cases with multiple child victims have the general characteristics described below.

Male Offenders

In a very high percentage of these cases, the offenders are male. Even in those few cases where there is a female offender, she will often have one or more male accomplices who are the ringleaders.

Preferential Sex Offenders

Most of the offenders in these cases are true pedophiles or other preferential sex offenders. Most of the preferential molesters will use the seduction pattern of behavior. The main characteristics of preferential-type child molesters are multiple victims, access to children, and collection of child pornography and/or erotica. These offenders will almost always be acquaintances of the victims.

Male Victims
In my experience, many of the victims in these cases are male, and many are boys between the ages of 10 and 16.

Sexual Motivation
Although pedophiles frequently claim that sex is only a small part of their "love" for children, the fact is that when the sexual attraction is gone, the relationship is essentially over. If it were not for the time spent having sex, they would not be spending the other time with the child. Their primary reason for interacting with the children is to have sex. This is not to say, however, that sex is their only motivation. Some pedophiles do care about children and enjoy spending time with them.

Child Pornography and Child Erotica
Pedophiles almost always collect child pornography and/or erotica. Child pornography can be defined as the sexually explicit visual depiction of a minor and includes sexually explicit photographs, negatives, slides, magazines, movies, videotapes, or computer disks. Child erotica (pedophile paraphernalia) can be defined as any material relating to children that serves a sexual purpose for a given individual. Some of the more common types of child erotica include toys, games, computers, drawings, fantasy writings, diaries, souvenirs, sexual aids, manuals, letters, books about children, psychological books on pedophilia, and ordinary photographs of children.

Control Through Seduction
Child molesters control their victims in a variety of ways. In acquaintance-exploitation cases with multiple victims, they control them primarily through the seduction or "grooming" process. They seduce their victims with attention, affection, kindness, gifts, and money until they have lowered the victims' inhibitions and gained their cooperation and "consent." The nature of this seduction is partially dependent on the developmental stages, needs, and vulnerabilities of the targeted child victims. Offenders who prefer younger child victims are more likely to "seduce" their parents first and then rely more on techniques involving fun, games, and play to manipulate the children into sex. Those who prefer older child victims are more likely to take advantage of normal time away from their family and then rely more on techniques involving ease of sexual arousal, rebelliousness, and curiosity to manipulate the children into sex. These seduced and compliant victims are less likely to disclose their victimization and are more likely to return to be victimized voluntarily again and again.

AGE OF CONSENT
In an infamous case in the early 1980s, a judge sentenced a convicted child molester to a minimal sentence because the judge felt the 5-year-old victim was "sexually promiscuous." Society and professionals were outraged and demanded that the judge be removed from the bench. The sad reality is that most people were outraged for the wrong reason—because they thought it was impossible for a 5-year-old child to be sexually promiscuous. Although not typical or probable, it is possible for such a child to be "sexually promiscuous." Of course this is the result of abuse, not the cause. It should, however, make no difference whether the 5-year-old child was sexually promiscuous. It in no way lessens the offender's crime or responsibility. If you change the case slightly and make the victim 9 years old, does that make a difference? Most people would probably say no. If you change it again and make the victim 12 years old, many people would still say it makes no difference, but they might want to see a

picture of the victim. If you change it again and make the victim 13, 14, 15, or 16 years old, the response of society and the law would vary greatly.

In sex crimes, the fundamental legal difference between victimization of an adult and a child is the issue of consent. With sexual activity between adults, with a few rare exceptions, there must be a lack of consent in order for there to be a crime. With sexual activity between children and adults, there can be a crime even if the child cooperates or "consents." But the reality of age of consent is not so simple.

Age of consent can vary depending on the type of sexual activity and individual involved. At what age can a child consent to get married, engage in sexual activity, appear in sexually explicit visual images, or leave home to have sex with an unrelated adult without parental permission? Federal case law seems to suggest that the consent of a 14-year-old who crosses state lines after running off and having sex with a 40-year-old man she met on the Internet is a valid defense for a kidnapping charge but not for a sexual assault charge. At what age can an adolescent consent to have sex with a relative, a teacher, a coach, an employer, or a 21-year-old boyfriend?

In the United States, society and criminal investigators seem to have a preference for sexual victimization cases where the victim, adult or child, clearly does not consent. Among lack of consent cases, the *least* preferred are cases where the victim could not consent because of self-induced use of drugs or alcohol. Cases where the victim was just verbally threatened are next, followed by cases where a weapon was displayed. For purposes of ease of proof, the *most* preferred lack-of-consent cases are those where the victim has visible physical injuries or is, sad to say, dead. Many seduced child victims may inaccurately claim they were asleep, drunk, drugged, or abducted in part to meet these lack of consent criteria and in part to avoid embarrassment.

Sexual-victimization cases where the child victim is not forced or threatened and co-operates or "consents" are more troubling and harder for society and investigators to deal with. Although "consent" is supposed to be irrelevant in child-sexual-victimization cases, there are "unspoken" preferences in these cases as well. The *most* preferred are "consent" cases where the victim can explain that the cooperation was due to some general fear or ignorance about the activity. The child was afraid to tell or did not understand what was happening. Fear seems to work more effectively as a control tactic with younger victims. The next most preferred are cases where the child was tricked, "duped," or "indoctrinated." If the offender was an authority figure, this "brainwashing" concept is even more appealing. Next on this preference scale are the cases where the victim was willing to trade sex for attention and affection. Many older children welcome perceived "romance" and believe they are in love with the offender. Much less acceptable are cases where the child willingly traded sex for material rewards (eg, clothes, shoes, trips) or money (ie, prostitution). Almost un-acceptable are cases where the child engaged in the sexual activity with an adult because the child enjoyed the sex. In fact, it is almost a sacrilege to even mention such a possibility. These societal and criminal-justice preferences prevail in spite of the fact that almost all human beings trade sex for attention, affection, privileges, gifts, or money. Although any of these reasons for compliance are possible, many seduced child victims inaccurately claim that they were afraid, ignorant, or indoc-trinated in part to meet these societal preferences for cooperation and in part to avoid embarrassment.

Any of the above scenarios in various combinations are certainly possible. A child might cooperate in some sexual acts and be clearly threatened or forced into others. All are crimes. Investigators should always attempt to determine what actually happened and not attempt to confirm their preconceived beliefs about sexual vic-timization of children.

Most acquaintance-exploitation cases involve these seduced or compliant victims. Although applicable statutes and investigative or prosecutorial priorities may vary, individuals investigating sexual exploitation cases must generally start from the premise that the sexual activity is *not* the fault of the victim even if the child:

— Did not say no.

— Did not fight.

— Actively cooperated.

— Initiated the contact.

— Did not tell.

— Accepted gifts or money.

— Enjoyed the sexual activity.

Investigators must also remember that many children, especially those victimized through the seduction process, often:

— Trade sex for attention, affection, or gifts.

— Are confused over their sexuality and feelings.

— Are embarrassed and guilt-ridden over their activity.

— Describe victimization in socially acceptable ways.

— Minimize their responsibility and maximize the offender's.

— Deny or exaggerate their victimization.

All of these things do not mean the child is not a victim. What they do mean is that children are human beings with human needs. Society seems to prefer to believe that children are pure and innocent. The FBI's national initiative on computer exploitation of children is named "Innocent Images." Many children are seduced and manipulated by clever offenders and usually do not fully understand or recognize what they were getting into. Even if they do seem to understand, the law is still supposed to protect them from adult sexual partners. Consent should *not* be an issue with child victims. Sympathy for victims is, however, inversely proportional to their age. As with poorly understood offender patterns of behavior, the dynamics of these "consenting" victim patterns of behavior can be explained to the court by an education expert witness as in *United States v Romero* (1999). The ability to make these explanations, however, is being undermined by the fact that children at an age when they can not legally choose to have sex with an adult partner can choose to have an abortion without their parents' permission or be charged as adults when they commit certain crimes. Can the same 15-year-old be both a "child" and an "adult" in the criminal-justice system?

OFFENDER STRATEGIES

Control

Maintaining control is important in the operation of a case with multiple child victims. A significant amount of ability, cunning, and interpersonal skill is needed to maintain a simultaneous sexual relationship with multiple partners. It is especially difficult if you have the added pressure of concealing illegal behavior. In order to operate a child sex ring, an offender must know how to control and manipulate children.

As stated above, control is maintained primarily through attention, affection, and gifts—all part of the seduction process. Preferential child molesters seduce children much the same way that adults seduce one another. This technique is no great mystery. Between 2 adults or 2 teenagers, it is simply called dating. The major difference, however, is the disparity between the adult authority of the child molester and vulnerability of the child victim. It is especially unfair if the child molester is a prestigious authority figure (eg, teacher, law enforcement officer, clergy member, youth volunteer) and if the child is an easily sexually aroused, curious, rebellious adolescent or an easily confused, naïve, trusting young child. As previously stated, these techniques must also be adjusted for the varying developmental stages, needs, and vulnerabilities of children of different ages.

The Seduction Process

The seduction process begins when the preferential child molester sees a potential victim who fits his age, gender, and other preferences. It may be a dark-eyed, shy, 6-year-old girl or a blond-haired, extroverted, 14-year-old boy. Child molesters, however, can and do have sex with children and sometimes adults who do not fit their exact preferences. A child molester may be experimenting or unable to find a child who fits his preference. Child molesters who prefer adolescent boys sometimes become involved with adolescent girls as a method of arousing or attracting the boys. In addition, child molesters may not molest some children to whom they have access and opportunity because the children do not meet their preferences or are not vulnerable to their advances or seduction techniques.

The offender's next step in the seduction process is to gather information about the potential victim. This may involve nothing more than a 10-minute spot evaluation of the child's demeanor, personality, dress, and financial status. Through practice, many child molesters have developed a real knack for spotting the vulnerability in each victim. Other preferential child molesters may have access to school, medical, mental health, or court records. These records could be valuable in determining a child's interests or vulnerabilities.

The seduction process takes place over time. It may take a few minutes or a few years. The offender who is operating a sex ring has many other victims. He is willing to put in the time it takes to seduce a child. Some molesters may even start grooming a potential victim long before the child has reached their age preference.

In addition to seducing his child victims, the sex-ring operator often "seduces" the victim's parents, gaining their trust and confidence, so that they will allow him free access to their children. A favorite target victim is a child living with a single mother. He may offer to babysit or watch her children after school. The offender will sometimes feign romantic interest in the mother or express a desire to be a father figure or mentor for her child. He may even marry her or move in with her. The relationship with the mother can be used as a cover for his interest in children, and her child can be used as bait to lure or gain access to other children. For example, most parents would not be reluctant to allow their child to go on an overnight trip with the "father" of one of their child's friends. In this case, however, the man in question is not the child's father or even the stepfather. He is just a man who lives with the mother. Some offenders legally adopt or become the legal guardian of potential victims. Once a molester has put in the time and effort to seduce a child, he will be reluctant to give up access to the child until he is finished with the child.

The true pedophile often possesses an important talent in the seduction process: his ability to identify with children. He knows the "in" video games, toys, television shows, movies, music, computers, and Internet sites. He is skilled at recognizing and then temporarily filling the emotional and physical needs of children. This is why such offenders can be the Big Brother of the Year, the most popular teacher, or the most successful soccer coach. They are sometimes described as "pied pipers" who simply attract children. This is not to say that in some cases children will not sense that some adult is "weird" or has a "problem" before other adults or parents recognize it. Parents who desperately want their children to get good grades, become star athletes, get into modeling or show business, have an adult male role model, or have a good babysitter may actually push their children to these offenders.

The essence of the seduction process is the offender providing attention, affection, and gifts to the potential victim. Gifts and financial incentives are important, especially for kids from lower socioeconomic backgrounds, but attention and affection is the real key. How do you tell a child to not respond to attention and affection? All children crave it, but it is craved especially by children who are not getting it at home. Thus, while almost any child can be seduced, the most vulnerable children tend to be those who come from dysfunctional homes or who are victims of emotional neglect. Moreover, because the offender is interested only in short-term gain, he may allow his victims to "break the rules"—play basketball or football in the house, make a mess, swim without a bathing suit, view pornography, drink alcohol, use drugs, drive a car, or go to bars or restaurants known to have physically well-endowed female staff. The homes of many preferential child molesters are miniature amusement parks filled with games, toys, computers, and athletic equipment appealing to children of their age preference.

The typical adolescent, especially a boy, is *easily sexually aroused, sexually curious, sexually inexperienced,* and *somewhat rebellious.* All these traits combine to make the adolescent boy the easiest victim of this seduction. It takes almost nothing to get an adolescent boy sexually aroused. An adolescent boy with emotional and sexual needs is simply no match for an experienced 50-year-old man with an organized plan. Yet adult offenders who seduce them, and the society that judges them, continue to claim that these victims "consented." The result is a victim who feels responsible for what happened and embarrassed about his actions. Once a victim is seduced, each successive sexual incident becomes easier and quicker. Eventually, the child victim may even take the initiative in the seduction.

The next step in the seduction process is the lowering of inhibitions. Being judgmental is easy toward victims when you look at only the end product of their seduction. At the beginning of the relationship, the child is looking for friendship, emotional support, a job, or just some fun. The lowering of sexual inhibitions is usually done so gradually and skillfully that the victim does not realize he or she is a victim until too late. It may begin with simple affection such as a pat, hug, or kiss on the cheek. Sexual activity can begin with conversation about sex. The activity can progress to fondling while wrestling, playing hide-and-seek in the dark, playing strip poker, swimming nude in the pool, drying the child with a towel, massaging an injury, giving a back rub, tickling, playing a physical game, or cuddling in bed. The introduction of photography or video cameras during this process is common. Innocent pictures progress to pictures of the "fun and games" or playing movie star/model that then progress to pictures of the nude or partially nude child that then escalate into more sexually explicit pictures.

Adult pornography is frequently left out for the children to "discover." A collection of adult pornography will sexually arouse and lower the inhibitions of adolescent boys. This is the primary reason why preferential child molesters collect adult pornography. Some of them may, however, attempt to use this collection as proof that they do not have a sexual preference for children. Alcohol and drugs are also used, especially with adolescent boys, to lower inhibitions. By the time the victims realize what is going on, they are in the middle of it and ashamed of their complicity. They did not "say no, yell, and tell." Much of this process can even take place online with a computer without even meeting in person.

Most preferential child molesters usually work toward a situation in which the child has to change clothing, spend the night, or both. If the child molester achieves either of these 2 objectives, the success of the seduction is almost assured. The objectives of changing clothes can be accomplished by such ploys as squirting with the garden hose, turning up the heat in the house, exercising, taking a bath or shower, physically examining the child, or swimming in a pool. Spending the night (eg, field trips, camping, babysitting) with the child is the best way for the sexual activity to progress.

Some victims come to realize that the offender has a greater need for this sex than they do, and this gives them great leverage against the offender. The victims can use sex to manipulate the offender or temporarily withhold sex until they get things they want. A few victims even blackmail the offender, especially if he is married or is a pillar of the community. Though all of this is unpleasant and inconsistent with our idealistic views about children, when adults and children have "consensual" sex, the adult is always the offender, and the child is always the victim. Consent is an issue only for adults.

Operation of Cases Involving Multiple Child Victims

The ongoing sexual victimization of multiple children is dynamic and ever changing. It is like a pipeline. At any given moment, victims are being recruited, seduced, molested, and let go or "dumped." For most acquaintance offenders it is easy to recruit, seduce, and molest the victims, but it is difficult to let the victims go without their turning against the offender and disclosing the abuse.

The offenders control the victims once they are in the pipeline through a combination of bonding, competition, and peer pressure. Most children, especially adolescent children, want to be a part of some peer group. Any offender operating a sex ring has to find a way to bind the victims together. Some offenders use an existing structure such as a scout troop, sports team, or school club. Other offenders create their own group such as a magic club, computer club, or religious group. Some offenders just make up a name and establish their own rules and regulations. They may call themselves the "88 Club" or the "Winged Serpents." Some offenders have used religion, satanism, and the occult as a bonding and controlling mechanism.

Competition, sometimes focusing on sexual acts, is also an effective control technique. Victims may compete over who can do an act first or longest. A series of sexual acts may result in some special reward or recognition. The offender may use peer pressure to control his victims, and the children will enforce the rules on each other. No victim wants to be the one to ruin it for anyone else or embarrass others, and each victim may think he or she is the offender's "favorite." All of these techniques simply capitalize on the developmental needs of children of different ages.

Violence, threats of violence, and blackmail are most likely used by the offender when pushing a victim out or attempting to hold onto a still-desirable victim who wants to leave. Sexually explicit notes, audiotapes, videotapes, and photographs are effective insurance for a victim's silence. Victims worried about disclosure of illegal acts such as substance abuse, joyriding, petty thefts, and vandalism are also subject to blackmail. Victims and their families from higher socioeconomic backgrounds may be more concerned about the public embarrassment of any disclosure. Many victims, however, are most concerned over disclosure and, therefore, more likely to deny *engaging in sex for money, bizarre sex acts, homosexual acts in which they were the active participant*, and *sex with other child victims*. In child sex rings, not only does the offender have sex with the child but also in some cases, the children have sex with each other. While children may report that they were forced by the offender to perform certain acts with him, they find it hard to explain sexual experiences with other children; therefore, they frequently deny such activity. One offender told me that if you select your victims and seduce them "properly," the secret takes care of itself.

When trying to push a victim out the end of the pipeline, the offender may pass the child to another pedophile who prefers older children. The victim now enters a new pipeline as a "pre-seduced" victim. "Dumping" the child can also be made easier and safer if the child is promoted to another grade or school, moves onto another level of scouting or sports, or moves out of the neighborhood.

Offender-Victim Bond

Because victims of acquaintance-exploitation usually have been carefully seduced and often do not realize they are victims, they repeatedly and voluntarily return to the offender. Society and the criminal-justice system have a difficult time understanding this. If a boy is molested by his neighbor, teacher, or clergy members, why does he "allow" it to continue? Most likely he may not initially realize or believe he is a victim. Some victims are simply willing to trade sex for attention, affection, and gifts and do not believe they are victims. The sex itself might even be enjoyable. The offender may be treating them better than anyone has ever treated them. They may come to realize they are victims when the offender pushes them out. Then they recognize that all the attention, affection, and gifts were just part of the master plan to use and exploit them. This may be the final blow for a troubled child who has had a difficult life.

Most of these victims never disclose their victimization. Younger children may believe they did something "wrong" or "bad" and are afraid of getting into trouble. Older children may be more ashamed and embarrassed. Many victims not only do not disclose but also, when confronted, strongly deny it happened. Some will vehemently and publicly defend the offender. In one case, several boys took the stand and testified to the high moral character of the accused molester. When the accused molester changed his plea to guilty, he admitted that the boys who testified for him were also victims. In another case, a 16-year-old victim tried to murder the man who had sexually exploited him but still denied he was sexually victimized. He pled guilty rather than use the abuse as a mitigating circumstance and publicly admit he had engaged in sexual activity with a man. He privately admitted his victimization to a prosecutor but said he would always publicly deny it.

The most common reasons that victims do not disclose are *stigma of homosexuality, lack of societal understanding, presence of positive feelings for the offender, embarrassment or fear over their victimization,* or *the belief that they are not really victims.* Since most of the offenders are male, the stigma of homosexuality is a serious problem for male victims. Although being seduced by a male child molester does not necessarily make a boy a homosexual, the victims do not understand this. If a victim does disclose, he risks significant ridicule by his peers and lack of acceptance by his family.

These seduced or compliant child victims obviously do sometimes disclose. Such victims often disclose because the sexual activity is discovered (eg, abduction by offender, recovered child pornography, overheard conversations) or suspected (eg, statements of other victims, association with a known sex offender, proactive investigation), and they are then confronted. Others disclose because the offender misjudged them, became too aggressive with them, or is seducing a younger sibling or close friend of theirs. Victims sometimes come forward and report because they are angry with the offender for "dumping" them. They might be jealous that the offender found a younger victim. They disclose because the abuse has ended, not to end the abuse.

A particular aspect of this offender-victim bond is especially troubling for the criminal justice system. Some older child victims, when being pushed out, or while still in the pipeline, may assist the offender in obtaining new victims. They still want to trade sex for attention, affection, gifts, or money, but their sexual worth has diminished in value. They have to come up with something else of value. They then become the bait to lure other victims. Such recruiters or "graduate" victims can and should be considered subjects of investigation. Their offenses, however, should be viewed in the context of their victimization and the child sex ring.

High-Risk Situations

Certain high-risk situations that arise in investigating acquaintance-exploitation cases. Unfortunately, certain youth organizations inadvertently provide the child molester with almost everything necessary to operate a child sex ring. A scouting organization, for example, fulfills the offender's needs for *access to children of a specific age or gender, a bonding mechanism to ensure the cooperation and secrecy of victims,* and *opportunities to spend the night with a victim or have a victim change clothing.* The bonding mechanism of the scouts is especially useful to the offender. Loyalty to the leader and group, competition among boys, a system of rewards and recognition, and indoctrination through oaths and rituals can all be used to control, manipulate, and motivate victims. Leaders in such organizations, especially those who are not the parents of children involved, should be carefully screened and then closely monitored.

Another high-risk situation involves high-status authority figures. As stated above, child molesters sometimes use their adult authority to give them an edge in the seduction process. Adults with added authority (eg, teachers, camp counselors, coaches, religious leaders, law-enforcement officers, doctors, judges) present even greater problems in the investigation of these cases. Such offenders are in a better position to seduce and manipulate victims and escape responsibility. They are usually believed when they deny any allegations. In such cases, investigators must always incorporate understanding of the seduction process into interviews, take the "big picture" approach and try to find multiple victims or recover child pornography or erotica in order to get a conviction.

The most difficult case of all involves a subject who has an ideal occupation for any child molester: a therapist who specializes in treating troubled children. This offender need only sit in his office while society preselects the most vulnerable victims and brings them to him. The victims are by definition "troubled" and unlikely to be believed if they do make an allegation. In addition, such therapists, especially if they are psychiatrists or physician's assistants, can claim that certain acts of physical touching were a legitimate part of their examination or treatment. They may also claim to be conducting research on child development or sexual victimization. Again, such a case could probably be proven only through the identification of patterns of behavior, multiple victims, and the recovery of child pornography or erotica. Fortunately for investigators in the United States, but unfortunately for children in the United States, such offenders almost always have highly predictable behavior patterns, multiple victims, and child-pornography and erotica collections.

Summary

In order to effectively evaluate most cases involving sexual exploitation of children by acquaintance molesters, 3 aspects of this relatively common, but poorly understood, type of child sexual victimization must be understood.

The *first* aspect involves understanding the "nice guy" offender who seems to love and is often loved by children. These acquaintance offenders frequently are and are almost always described as "nice guys" and "pillars of the community." It is not uncommon for these offenders to be viewed as "child magnets" or "pied pipers" who have an extraordinary ability to relate to children. They groom and seduce their child victims with the most effective combination of attention, affection, kindness, privileges, gifts, alcohol, drugs, or money. How long such offenders get away with this type of victimization is usually determined by how well they select their victims, how good they are at identifying and filling their victims' needs, how much time they have, and how proficient they are at seducing their victims.

Such offenders usually have strong needs to rationalize and validate their sexual behavior. Most of them seem to have an overwhelming need to convince primarily themselves that: (1) the behavior they engaged in is not really sex, (2) the child does not understand or remember and is therefore not harmed, (3) this is an expression of love and caring, or (4) I am entitled to this because of all the good I do. Their need to rationalize their sexual interests and behavior often leads them to be involved in "good works" that help troubled, needy children. Such activity conveniently also gives them obvious access to vulnerable children and also justification for their contact. These types of offenders will generally try to conceal their sexual behavior from anyone they believe will not accept their rationalizations and disclose at least part of their sexual behavior to those they believe might accept their rationalizations.

The *second* aspect involves understanding the compliant child victim. As human beings, many children are willing to trade "sex" for the affection and attention of a trusted adult. Their frequent cooperation in their victimization must be viewed as an understandable human characteristic that should have no significance for the criminal justice system or society. Compliant child victims and adult survivors usually either deny their victimization or disclose it in inaccurate but socially acceptable ways because they often suffer from shame, guilt, and embarrassment. Society tells them in so many ways that they are not "real" victims. When an adult and a child have sex, unless the adult does not consent, the adult is always the offender, and the child is always the victim.

The *third* aspect involves understanding the scope of behavior that can constitute sexual activity. Sexual victimization of children can run the gamut of "normal" sexual acts from fondling to intercourse. Sex can also include deviant sexual acts involving behavior such as sadomasochism, bondage, urination, and defecation. Seemingly "nonsexual" behavior can be in the service of sexual needs. When evaluating the significance and relevance of offender behavior and children's allegations, interveners should always consider both the activity and its motivation. In properly evaluated cases, there is rarely any doubt as to whether an act was innocent "fun" or sexually motivated behavior. These cases can not be evaluated or investigated by "peeping through the keyhole" in an effort to prove one molestation, by one offender, on one day, many years ago. Instead, someone must open the door, look at the "big picture" and recognize patterns of behavior.

As stated, all 3 of these aspects of the sexual exploitation of children by acquaintance molesters must be recognized, understood, and addressed if these cases are going to be effectively identified, investigated, prosecuted, and prevented.

CONCLUSION

The professional "investigator's" job is to listen to all victims nonjudgmentally, objectively assess and evaluate the relevant information, and conduct an appropriate, proficient investigation. Corroborative evidence exists more often than many investigators realize, especially in acquaintance molestation cases. Investigators should remember that not all childhood trauma is abuse and that not all child abuse is a crime. There can be great frustration when, after a thorough investigation, an investigator is convinced that something traumatic happened to the child victim but does not know with any degree of certainty exactly what happened, when it happened, or who did it. That is sometimes the price we pay for a criminal justice system in which people are considered innocent until proven guilty beyond a reasonable doubt. Investigators must also recognize that their preconceived, stereotypical ideas about the nature of the sexual exploitation of children by acquaintances can interfere with the disclosure, evaluation, and corroboration of many valid cases.

INVESTIGATING ACQUAINTANCE SEXUAL EXPLOITATION

This section is intended to offer general guidelines on how to apply the previously discussed behavioral dynamics to the investigation and evaluation of cases of sexual exploitation of children perpetrated by acquaintance molesters.

Intrafamilial, child-sexual abuse cases can be difficult to prove in a court of law. Frequently, there is only the word of one child against that of an adult. Convicting a prominent, well-respected member of the community will be extremely difficult based only on the testimony of one troubled, delinquent adolescent or one confused, naïve young child. This is, however, rarely the case in child-sexual-exploitation cases, especially those involving preferential acquaintance sex offenders. With multiple victims, no one victim should have to bear the total burden of proof, and cases should rarely, if ever, be selected for prosecution. The best victims and these cases should be selected for prosecution.

It is commonly accepted that child sexual victimization is a complex problem requiring the efforts and coordination of many agencies and disciplines. No one agency or discipline possesses the personnel, resources, training, skills, or legal mandate to deal effectively with every aspect of child maltreatment. In this context, law enforcement interacts with a variety of professions and agencies during the investigation process. For example, some offenders cross jurisdictional boundaries, and many violate a variety of state and federal laws when exploiting children. This often will mean working with other local, state, and federal law-enforcement agencies in multi-jurisdictional investigative teams and with prosecutors, social services, and victim assistance in multidisciplinary teams. This can be done as part of informal networking or a formal task force.

The multidisciplinary approach not only is advantageous in avoiding duplication and making cases but is also in the best interests of the child victim. It may minimize the number of interviews and court appearances and provide the victim with needed support. The team approach can also help investigators deal with the stress and isolation of this work by providing peer support. The multidisciplinary approach is mandated statutorily or authorized in the majority of states and under federal law (US Department of Justice, 1993).

Working together as part of a multidisciplinary team means coordination, not abdication. Each discipline performs a function for which it has specific resources, training, and experience. Although each discipline must understand how its role contributes to the team approach, it is equally important that each discipline understand the respective responsibilities and limitations of that role. For example, child-protection agencies often can not get involved in cases in which the alleged perpetrator is not a parent or caretaker (eg, acquaintance molester). The team approach is a two-way street. Just as medical and psychological professionals are charged with evaluating and treating the abused or neglected child, law-enforcement investigators are responsible for conducting criminal investigations. Just as law-enforcement officers need to be concerned that their investigation might further traumatize a child victim, therapists and physicians need to be concerned that their treatment techniques might hinder the investigation.

Children may furnish information about their victimization to a wide variety of nonprofessional (parents and friends) and professional (clergy, therapists, medical, social workers, and law enforcement) individuals. Coordinating, disseminating, and evaluating the details of all of this information can be complex and difficult due to laws, policies, and privacy issues. In addition, information about the background and behavior patterns of alleged offenders may exist in a variety of places. Multidisciplinary cooperation can obviously aid in addressing these problems.

THE INVESTIGATIVE PERSPECTIVE

The criminal investigative perspective deals with criminal activity and legally defensible, objective fact-finding. The process must, therefore, focus more on admissible evidence of *what* happened than on emotional belief that *something* happened, more on the *accuracy* than on the *existence* of repressed memory, more on objective than on subjective reality, and more on *neutral investigation* than on *child advocacy.*

In their desire to convince society that child sexual victimization exists and children do not lie about it, some professionals interpret efforts to seek corroboration for alleged sexual victimization as a sign of denial or disbelief. Corroboration, however, is essential. Investigators can not just accept that something sexual happened to a child and ignore the necessary context details if it is to be proven in a court of law. When the only evidence offered is the word of a child against the word of an adult, child sexual victimization can be difficult to prove in a court of law. It is not the job of investigators to believe a child or any other victim or witness. The child victim should be carefully interviewed. The information obtained should be assessed and evaluated, and appropriate investigation should be conducted to corroborate any and all aspects of a victim's statement. The investigator should always be an objective fact-finder who considers all possibilities and attempts to determine what happened with an open mind. As previously stated, in a valid case, the best and easiest way to avoid child-victim testimony in court is to build a case so strong that the offender pleads guilty. Most children, however, can testify in court if necessary.

EMOTION VERSUS REASON

Regardless of intelligence and education, and often despite common sense and evidence to the contrary, adults tend to believe what they want or need to believe. The greater the need, the greater the tendency. The extremely sensitive and emotional nature of CSE makes this phenomenon a potential problem in these cases. For some, no amount of training and education can overcome this zealotry. Some people seem to be incapable of becoming objective fact-finders in some sexual-victimization-of-children cases. Investigators must evaluate this tendency in others and minimize it in themselves by trying to do their job in a rational, professional manner.

To be effective interviewers, investigators must be both aware of and in control of their own feelings and beliefs about victims and offenders in child-sexual-exploitation cases. People in the United States tend to have stereotypical concepts of the innocence of children and malevolence of those who sexually victimize them. Most investigators now know that a child molester can look like anyone else and may even be someone we know and like. As previously discussed, the stereotype of the child victim as a completely innocent little girl is still with us and is less likely to be addressed by lay people and even professionals. In reality, child victims of sexual abuse and exploitation can be boys as well as girls, and not all victims are "angels" or even "little." The idea that some children might enjoy certain sexual activity or behave like human beings and engage in sexual acts as a way of receiving attention, affection, gifts, and money is troubling for society and many investigators.

Depending on the nature of the abuse and techniques of the offender, investigators must understand that the victim may have many positive feelings for the offender and even resent law-enforcement intervention. The investigator must be able to discuss a wide variety of sexual activities, understand the victim's terminology, and avoid being judgmental. Not being judgmental is much more difficult with a delinquent adolescent engaged in homosexual activity with a prominent clergyman than with a sweet 5-year-old girl abused by a "lowlife" stranger. Investigators often nonverbally communicate their judgmental attitude through gestures, facial expressions, and body language. Many investigators do not interview children well because deep down inside they really do not want to hear the detailed answers.

Another emotion-related problem that occurs frequently during subject and suspect interviews is the inability of some investigators to control or conceal their anger and outrage at the offender's behavior. They often want to spend as little time as possible with the offender. Occasionally, investigators have the opposite problem and are confused that they have sympathetic feelings for the offender. Many investigators also find it difficult to discuss deviant sexual behavior calmly, objectively, nonjudgmentally, and in detail with anyone, much less an alleged child molester or a child.

An investigator who gets too emotionally involved in a case is more likely to make mistakes and errors in judgment. He or she might wind up losing a case and allowing a child molester to go free because the defendant's rights were violated in some way. The emotionally involved officer is also less likely to interview and assess a child victim properly and objectively. Investigators must learn to recognize and control these feelings. If they can not, they should not be assigned to child-sexual-victimization cases or at least not to the interview phase.

THE "BIG PICTURE" APPROACH

Although this section can not cover in detail the investigation of all types of cases, it can serve to alert investigators to the "big picture" approach to the sexual victimization of children. Investigators must stop looking at CSE through a keyhole—focusing only on one act by one offender against one victim on one day. Investigators must "kick the door open" and take the "big picture" approach—focusing on offender typologies, patterns of behavior, multiple acts, multiple victims, child pornography, and proactive techniques.

The "big picture" approach starts with recognizing 4 basic but often ignored statements about child molesters:

— Child molesters sometimes molest multiple victims.

— Intrafamilial child molesters sometimes molest children outside their families.

— Sex offenders against adults sometimes molest children.

— Other criminals sometimes molest children.

These elements are not always or usually present; nevertheless, their possibility should be incorporated into the investigative strategy. Offenders, unfortunately, often ignore neat categories of offenders and crime. A window peeper, an exhibitionist, or a rapist also can be a child molester. "Regular" criminals can also be child molesters. A child molester put on the FBI's "Ten Most Wanted Fugitives" list was later arrested for burglarizing a service station. Although most professionals now recognize that an intrafamilial child molester might victimize children outside his or her family and that identifying other victims can be an effective way to corroborate an allegation by one victim, few seem to incorporate a search for additional victims into their investigative approaches. An acquaintance molester may also use marriage as a method of access to children.

In numerous cases, offenders have not been effectively prosecuted or have continued to operate for many years after first being identified because no one took the "big picture" approach. Convicting an acquaintance child molester who is a "pillar of the community" is almost impossible based only on the testimony of one confused 5-year-old girl or one delinquent adolescent boy. Investigation, especially of preferential sex offenders, should never be "he said, he or she said," but "he said, they said." To stop the offender, investigators must get details, be willing to evaluate the allegations, conduct background investigation, document patterns of behavior, review records, identify other acts and victims, and, as soon as possible, develop probable cause for a search warrant. Simply interviewing the child or obtaining the results of someone else's interview, asking the offender if he did it, polygraphing him, and then closing the case does not constitute a thorough investigation and is certainly not consistent with the "big picture" approach.

The "big picture" investigative process consists of 3 phases. They are *interview, assess and evaluate,* and *corroborate.* These 3 phases do not always happen in this sequence and may occur simultaneously or intermittently.

INTERVIEW

This section will not include a detailed discussion of the latest research and specific techniques for forensic interviewing of children (see Saywitz et al, 2002). Only the investigative perspective of child-victim interviewing and some general guidelines will be briefly discussed here.

Law-Enforcement Role

For some, the criminal investigation of child sexual victimization has evolved into using newly acquired interviewing skills to get children to communicate and then believing whatever they say. For others, it has become letting someone else do the interview and then blindly accepting the interviewer's opinions and assessments. Law-enforcement officers should take advantage of the skills and expertise of other disciplines in the interviewing process. If the primary purpose of an interview of a child is to gain investigative information, however, law enforcement must be actively involved. This involvement can range from actually doing the interview to carefully monitoring the process. Although nothing is wrong with admitting short-comings and seeking help, law enforcement should *never* abdicate its control over the *investigative* interview.

The solution to the problem of poorly trained investigators is better training, not therapists and physicians independently conducting investigative interviews. Even if, for good reasons, an investigative interview is conducted by or with a forensic interviewer, social worker, or therapist, law enforcement should be in control. In cases where child protection rather than investigation is more the focus of the interview, a more collaborative approach with child protective services may be in order. The key is for each discipline to attempt to coordinate its response without abdicating its responsibilities.

The Disclosure/Reporting Continuum

Before applying interviewing research, training, and skills, investigators first must attempt to determine where the child is on the disclosure/reporting continuum. This determination is essential to developing a proper interview approach that maximizes the amount of legally defensible information and minimizes allegations of leading and suggestive questioning. The disclosure process is set forth as a continuum because there can be many variations, combinations, and changes in situations involving the disclosure status of child victims. Training material and presentations often fail to consider and emphasize the determination of this disclosure/reporting status prior to conducting a child-victim interview.

At one end of the continuum are children who already have made voluntary and full disclosures to one or more people. These are generally the easiest children to interview. The child has made the decision to disclose, and the child has done so at least once. Determining the length of time between the abuse and disclosure is of course important.

At another point along the continuum are children who have voluntarily decided to disclose but appear to have made only incomplete or partial reports. For understandable reasons, some children fail to disclose, minimize, or even deny all or part of their victimization; however, not every child who discloses sexual victimization has more horrible details yet to be revealed.

Further down the continuum are children whose sexual victimization was discovered rather than disclosed (eg, recovered child pornography, medical evidence). This can often be the situation in cases in which child pornography or computer records are found. These interviews can be more difficult because these children have not decided to disclose and may not be ready to do so. They also can be easier, however, because the investigator knows with some degree of certainty that the child was victimized. The interview can now focus more on determining additional details.

At the far end of the continuum are children whose sexual victimization is only suspected. These may be the most difficult, complex, and sensitive interviews. The investigator must weigh a child's understandable reluctance to talk about sexual victimization against the possibility that the child was not victimized. The need to protect the child must be balanced with concern about leading or suggestive questioning. This is often the situation in acquaintance-exploitation cases.

Establishing Rapport and Clarifying Terms

The interviewer's first task, with a child at any age, is to establish rapport. Investigators should ask primarily open-ended questions that encourage narrative responses. It is hoped that this will set the stage for more reliable responses to investigative questions that follow.

Part of developing rapport with victims of acquaintance molestation is to subtly communicate the message that the child is not at fault. If they think they are going to be judged, many children will deny their victimization and some may exaggerate it by alleging threats, force, and even abduction that did not occur to make the crime more socially acceptable. Although many of the same interview principles apply to the interview of adolescent victims, it can be far more difficult to develop rapport with an older child than with a younger child.

Another critical task early in the interview is to clarify the suspected victim's terminology for various body parts and sexual activities. If this clarification is not achieved early on, much misunderstanding can occur. Similarly, it is just as important to find out exactly what the adolescent victim means by the terms he or she uses for sexual activity. Terms such as "head job" and "rim job" are not so readily acceptable as the 5-year-old's "pee-pee" and "weiner." The interview of an adolescent boy victim of sexual exploitation is extremely difficult at best. The stigma of homosexuality and embarrassment over victimization greatly increases the likelihood that the victim may deny or misrepresent the sexual activity. The investigator must accept the fact that even if a victim discloses, the information is likely to be incomplete, minimizing his involvement and responsibility and, in some cases, exaggerating the offender's.

Videotaping

The taping of victim interviews was once thought to be the ultimate solution to many of the problems involving child victim interviews and testimony. Many legislatures rushed to pass special laws allowing it. Aside from the constitutional issues, *there are advantages and disadvantages to videotaping or audiotaping child victims' statements.* The *advantages* include the following:

— Knowing exactly what was asked and answered

— The potential ability to reduce the number of interviews

— The visual impact of a videotaped statement

— The ability to deal with recanting or changing statements

— Potential to induce a confession when played for an offender who truly cares for the child victim

The *disadvantages* include the following:

— The artificial setting created when people "play" to the camera instead of concentrating on communicating

— Determining which interviews to record and explaining variations between them

— Accounting for the tapes after the investigation; copies are sometimes furnished with little to control defense attorneys and expert witnesses; many are played at training conferences without concealing the identity of victims

— Interpretation and criticism of each tape by "experts" because there are conflicting criteria on how to conduct such an interview

Many experts now feel that child-victim interviews must be videotaped in order to be assessed and evaluated properly. Some judges and courts now require videotaping of child-victim interviews. Many people in favor of videotaping argue, "If you are doing it right, what do you have to hide?" When videotaping a victim interview, however, a piece of evidence is created that did not previously exist, and that evidence can become the target of a great deal of highly subjective scrutiny. Words, inflections, gestures, and movements become the focus of attention rather than whether or not the child was molested. Unreliable information and false victim denials can be obtained from "perfect" interviews, and reliable information and valid disclosures can be obtained even from highly imperfect interviews. This fact can be lost when there is an excessive focus on how the interview was conducted. This in no way denies the fact that repetitive, suggestive, or leading interviews are real problems and can produce false or inaccurate information.

Many videotaping advocates do not seem to recognize the wide diversity of circumstances and dynamics comprising sexual-victimization-of-children cases. Interviewing a 12-year-old boy who is suspected of having been molested by his coach is far different from interviewing a 9-year-old girl who has disclosed having been sexually abused by her father. Interviewing a runaway 15-year-old inner-city street prostitute is far different from interviewing a middle-class 5-year-old kidnapped from her backyard by a child molester. Interviewing a Native American child in a hogan without electricity on a remote reservation is far different from interviewing a white child in a specially designed interview room at a child advocacy center in a wealthy suburb. In addition, videotape equipment can be expensive, and it can malfunction.

Although some of the disadvantages can be reduced if the tapes are made during the medical evaluation, it is still my opinion that the disadvantages of taping generally outweigh the advantages. This is especially true of the interviews of adolescents who are only suspected of having been sexually exploited because of their known contact with an acquaintance child molester and who have not previously disclosed.

Many experienced child-sexual-victimization prosecutors oppose taping child-victim statements although special circumstances may alter this opinion on a case-by-case basis. One such special situation might be the interview of a child who is younger than the age of 7. Departments should be careful of written policies concerning taping. It is potentially embarrassing and damaging to have to admit in court that such interviews are usually not in this case. It is better to be able to say that such interviews usually are not taped but were in a certain case because of some special circumstances that can be clearly articulated. In this controversy over videotaping, investigators should be guided by their prosecutors' expertise and preferences, legal or judicial requirements, and their own common sense.

General Rules and Cautions

Investigative interviews should always be conducted with an open mind and the assumption that there are multiple hypotheses or explanations for what is being described, alleged, or suspected. Investigative interviews should emphasize open ended, age-appropriate questions that are designed to elicit narrative accounts of events. All investigative interaction with victims must be documented carefully and thoroughly.

The interview of an alleged or potential child victim as part of a criminal investigation should always be conducted as quickly as possible. It is important to interview as many potential victims as is legally and ethically possible. This is especially important in cases involving adolescent boy victims, most of whom will deny their victimization no matter what the investigator does. Unfortunately for victims, but fortunately for the investigative corroboration, men who victimize adolescent boys are, in my experience, the most persistent and prolific of all child molesters. The small percentage of their victims who disclose still may constitute a significant number.

The investigation of allegations of recent activity from multiple young children should begin quickly with interviews of all potential victims being completed as soon as possible. The investigation of adult survivors' allegations of activity 10 or more years earlier presents other problems and, unless victims are at immediate risk, should proceed more deliberately with gradually increasing resources as corroborated facts warrant.

Children rarely get the undivided attention of adults, even their parents, for long periods. Investigators must be cautious about subtly rewarding a child by allowing this attention to continue only in return for furnishing additional details. The investigator should make sure this necessary attention is unconditional.

Interviews of children younger than 7 years of age are potentially problematic and should be done by investigators trained and experienced in such interviews. Because suggestibility is potentially a bigger problem in younger children, the assessment and evaluation phase is especially important in cases involving these young victims, and videotaping is more justified.

ASSESS AND EVALUATE

This part of the investigative process in child-sexual-victimization cases seems to have gotten lost. Is the victim describing events and activities that are consistent with criminal behavior and prior cases documented in law enforcement, or are they more consistent with distorted media accounts and erroneous public perceptions of criminal behavior? Investigators should apply the "template of probability." Accounts of child sexual victimization that are more like books, television, and movies (eg, big conspiracies, snuff films, child sex slaves, highly organized sex rings) and less like documented cases should be viewed with skepticism but still be *thoroughly investigated.* It is the investigator's job to consider and investigate all possible explanations of events. In addition, the information learned will be invaluable in counteracting the defense attorneys when they raise alternative explanations.

The so-called "backlash" has had both a positive and negative impact on the investigation and prosecution of child sexual victimization cases. In a positive way, it has reminded criminal-justice investigators of the need to do their jobs in a more professional, objective, and fact-finding manner. Most of the damage caused by the backlash is actually self-inflicted by well-intentioned child advocates. In a negative way, it has cast a shadow over the validity and reality of child sexual victimization and has influenced some to avoid properly pursuing cases (Lanning, 1996).

For many years, the statement, "Children never lie about sexual abuse. If they have the details, it must have happened," was almost never questioned or debated at training conferences. During the 1970s, there was a successful crusade to eliminate laws requiring corroboration of child-victim statements in child-sexual-victimization cases. It was believed that the way to convict child molesters was to have the child victims testify in court. If we believe them, the jury will believe them. Any challenge to this basic premise was viewed as a threat to the progress made and denial that the problem existed. Both parts of this statement—"Children never lie about sexual abuse" and "If they have the details, it must have happened"—are receiving much-needed reexamination, a process that is critical to the investigator's task of assessing and evaluating the alleged victim's statements.

"Children Never Lie"

The available evidence suggests that children rarely lie about sexual victimization if a lie is defined as a statement deliberately and maliciously intended to deceive. If children in exploitation cases do lie, it may be because factors such as shame or embarrassment over the nature of the victimization increase the likelihood they will misrepresent the sexual activity. Seduced victims sometimes lie to make their victimization more socially acceptable or to please an adult. Occasionally children lie because they are angry and want to get revenge. Some children, sadly, lie about sexual victimization to get attention and forgiveness. A few children may even lie to get money or as part of a lawsuit. This can sometimes be influenced by pressure from their parents. Objective investigators must consider and evaluate all of these possibilities. It is extremely important to recognize, however, that just because children might lie about part of their victimization does not mean that the entire allegation is necessarily a lie and that they are not victims. As previously discussed, acquaintance-exploitation cases often involve complex dynamics and numerous incidents that often make it difficult to say "it" is all true or false.

In addition, just because a child is not lying, does not mean that he or she is making an accurate statement. Children might be telling you what they have come to believe happened to them even though it might not be literally true. Other than lying, there are many possible alternative explanations for why victims might allege things that do not seem accurate:

— The child might be exhibiting distortions in traumatic memory.

— The child's account might reflect normal childhood fears and fantasy.

— The child's account might reflect misperception and confusion caused by deliberate trickery or drugs used by perpetrators.

— The child's account might be affected by suggestions, assumptions, and misinterpretations of overzealous interveners.

— The child's account might reflect urban legends and shared cultural mythology.

Such factors, alone or in combination, can influence a child's account to be inaccurate without necessarily making it a "lie." Children are not adults in little bodies. Children go through developmental stages that must be evaluated and understood. In many ways, however, children are no better or worse than other victims or witnesses of a crime. They should not be automatically believed or dismissed. Of what victims allege, some statements may be true and accurate, some may be misperceived or distorted, some may be screened or symbolic, and some may be "contaminated" or false. The problem and challenge, especially for law enforcement, is to determine which is which. This can be done only through evaluation and active investigation.

The investigator must remember, however, that almost anything is possible. Though an allegation sounds farfetched or bizarre, it may still have happened. The debate over the literal accuracy of grotesque allegations of ritual abuse has obscured the well-documented fact that child sex rings, bizarre paraphilias, and cruel sexual sadists do exist. Even if only a portion of what these victims allege is factual, it still may constitute significant criminal activity.

"If They Have the Details, It Must Have Happened"

The second part of the basic statement also must be evaluated carefully. The details in question in some cases have little to do with sexual activity. Investigators must do more than attempt to determine how a child could have known about sex acts. Some cases involve determining how a child could have known about a wide variety of bizarre activities. Young, nonabused children usually might know little about sex, but they might "know" more than you realize about monsters, torture, kidnapping, and even murder.

When considering a child's statement, investigators should remember that lack of sexual detail does not mean abuse did not happen. Some children are reluctant to discuss the details of what happened. In evaluating reported details, it is also important to consider that victims might supply details of sexual or other acts using information from sources other than their own direct victimization. Such sources must be evaluated carefully and may include the items noted below.

— *Personal Knowledge.* The victim might have personal knowledge of the activity but not as a result of the alleged victimization. The knowledge could have come from participating in cultural practices; viewing pornography, sex education, or other pertinent material; witnessing sexual activity in the home; or witnessing the sexual victimization of others. It also could have come from having been sexually or physically abused by someone other than the alleged offender(s) and in ways other than the alleged offense.

— *Other Children or Victims.* Young children today interact socially more often and at a younger age than ever before. Many parents are unable to provide simple explanations for their children's stories or allegations because they were not with the children when the explaining events occurred. They do not know what video-tapes their children might have seen, games they might have played, and stories they might have been told or overheard. Some children are placed in day care centers for 8, 10, or 12 hours a day, starting at as young as 6 weeks of age. The children share experiences by playing house, school, or doctor. Bodily functions such as urination and defecation are a focus of attention for these young children. To a certain extent, each child shares the experiences of all the other children. Children of varying ages are also sharing information and experiences on the Internet. The possible effects of the interaction of such children prior to the disclosure of the alleged abuse must be evaluated.

— *Media.* The amount of sexually explicit, bizarre, or violence-oriented material available to children in the modern world is overwhelming. This includes movies, videotapes, music, books, games, and CD-ROMs. Cable television, computers, the Internet, and the home VCR make all this material readily available to even young children. Numerous popular toys and video games are on the market with bizarre or violent themes.

— *Suggestions and Leading Questions.* This problem is particularly important in cases involving children who are younger than the age of 7 and especially those stem-ming from custody/visitation disputes. This is not to suggest that custody/visitation disputes usually involve sex-abuse allegations, but when they do and when the child in question is young, such cases can be difficult to evaluate. It is my opinion that most suggestive, leading questioning of children by interveners is done inadvertently as part of a good-faith effort to learn the truth.

Not all interveners are in equal positions to influence allegations by children. Parents and relatives are in the best position to subtly cause their children to describe their victimization in a certain way. They sometimes question children in a suggestive and accusatory style that casts doubt on the child's statements. In most cases, parents and relatives mean well and do not realize their style of questioning might influence their child to make inaccurate or false statements. Family members sometimes misinterpret innocuous or ambiguous statements as evidence of sexual abuse. Children might overhear their parents discussing the details of the case. They might be trying to pro-long the rarely given undivided attention of an adult.

Children often tell their parents what they believe their parents want or need to hear. For example, a parent may be able to accept oral sex but not anal sex. Some parents may need to believe that their child would engage in sex with an adult of the same gender only if confronted with overwhelming physical force. In one case, a father gave law enforcement a tape recording to "prove" that his child's statements were spontaneous disclosures and not the result of leading, suggestive questions. The tape recording indicated just the opposite. The father voluntarily gave it to law enforcement probably because he truly believed he was not influ-encing his child's statement—but he was.

Usually well-meaning interveners have subtly as well as overtly rewarded some victims for furnishing certain details. Interveners who excessively or emotionally refer to the child's sexual victimization as "rape" may, for example, influence the child's version of events to conform to that view. Some "details" of a child's allegation even might have originated as a result of interveners making assumptions about or misinterpreting what the victim actually said. The interveners then repeat and possibly embellish these assumptions and misinterpretations, and eventually the victims come to agree with or accept this "official" version of what happened.

— Therapists also can be in a good position to influence the allegations of children and adult survivors. Types and styles of verbal interaction, useful in therapy, might create significant problems in a criminal investigation. Some therapists may have beliefs about sexual abuse or may be overzealous in their efforts to help children in difficult circumstances. It should be noted, however, that when a therapist does a poor investigative interview as part of a criminal investigation, it is the fault of the criminal justice system that allowed it and not of the therapist who did it.

— *Misperception and Confusion by the Victim.* Sometimes what seems unbelievable has a reasonable explanation. In one case, a child's description of the impossible act of walking through a wall turned out to be walking between the studs of an unfinished wall in a room under construction. In another case, pennies in the anus turned out to be copper, foil-covered suppositories. The children might describe what they believe happened. It is not a lie, but it is also not an accurate account. It might be due to confusion deliberately caused by the offender or misperception inadvertently caused by youthful inexperience.

Many young and some older children have little experience or frame of reference for accurately describing sexual activity. They might not understand the difference between "in" and "on" or the concept of "penetration." Drugs and alcohol also might be used deliberately to confuse the victims and distort their perceptions.

— *Education and Awareness Programs.* Some well-intentioned awareness and sex education programs designed to prevent child sex abuse and child abduction or provide children with information about human sexuality may, in fact, unrealistically increase fears and provide some of the details that children are telling interveners. Children may describe the often-discussed stranger abduction rather than admit they made an error in judgment and went voluntarily with an offender. The answer to this potential problem, however, is to evaluate the possibility, not to stop education and prevention programs.

Areas of Evaluation

As part of the assessment and evaluation of victim statements, it is important to determine how much time has elapsed between when the victim first made disclosure and when that disclosure was reported to law enforcement or social services. The longer the delay, the greater the potential for problems. The next step is to determine the number and purpose of all prior interviews of the victim concerning the allegations. The more interviews conducted before the investigative interview, the greater the potential difficulties. Problems can also be created by interviews conducted by various interveners after the investigative interview(s).

The investigator must closely and carefully evaluate events in the victim's life before, during, and after the alleged victimization. Events occurring before the alleged exploitation to be evaluated might include the following:

— Background of the victim

— Abuse or drugs in the home

— Pornography in the home

— Play, television, VCR, computer, and Internet habits

— Attitudes about sexuality in the home

— Religious beliefs and training

— Extent of sex education in the home

— Cultural and subcultural attitudes and practices

— Activities of siblings

— Need or craving for attention

— Childhood fears

— Custody/visitation disputes

— Victimization of or by family members

— Interaction between victims

— Family disputes or discipline problems

Events occurring during the alleged exploitation to be evaluated include the following:

— Use of fear or scare tactics

— Degree of trauma

— Use of magic, deception, or trickery

— Use of rituals

— Use of drugs and alcohol

— Use of pornography

— Use of grooming and seduction

Events occurring after the alleged exploitation to be evaluated include the following:

— Disclosure sequence

— Other interviews

— Background of prior interviewers

— Background of parents

— Comingling of victims

— Type of therapy received

— Contact by offender

— Shame and guilt

— Lawsuits

The investigator must understand that doing a background investigation on a suspect means more than obtaining the date and place of birth and credit and criminal checks. School, juvenile, military, medical, driving, employment, bank, sex-offender and child-abuse registry, sex-offender assessment, computer, and prior investigative records can all be valuable sources of information about an offender. Relatives, friends, associates, and current and former sex partners can be identified and interviewed. Other investigative techniques (eg, mail cover, pen register, trash run, surveillance) can also be used. Indicators and counter indicators must be identified and evaluated.

Contagion

Investigators must also evaluate possible contagion. Consistent statements obtained from different interviews and multiple victims are powerful pieces of corroborative evidence—as long as those statements are not "contaminated." Investigation must evaluate both predisclosure and postdisclosure contagion and both victim and intervener contagion carefully. Are the different victim statements consistent because they describe common experiences/events or because they reflect contamination or shared cultural mythology?

The sources of potential contagion are widespread. Victims can communicate with each other both prior to and after their disclosures. Interveners can communicate with each other and the victims. The team or cell concepts are attempts to deal with potential investigator contagion in multivictim cases. The same individuals do not interview all the victims, and interviewers do not necessarily share information directly with each other (Lanning, 1992b).

Documenting existing contagion and eliminating additional contagion is crucial to the successful investigation of many cases. There is no way, however, to erase or undo contagion. The best you can hope for is to identify and evaluate it and attempt to explain it. Mental health professionals requested to evaluate suspected victims must be carefully selected and evaluated.

Once a case is contaminated and out of control, little can be done to salvage what might have been a prosecutable criminal violation. A few cases have even been lost on appeal after conviction because of contamination problems.

To evaluate the contagion element, investigators must investigate these cases meticulously and aggressively. Whenever possible, personal visits should be made to all locations of alleged exploitation and to the victims' homes. Events that took place before the alleged exploitation must be evaluated carefully. Investigators might have to view television programs, movies, video games, computer games, and videotapes seen by the victims. In some cases, it might be necessary to conduct a background investigation and evaluation of everyone who, officially or unofficially, interviewed the victims about the allegations prior to and after the investigative interview(s).

Investigators must be familiar with the information about sexual victimization of children being disseminated in magazines, books, television programs, conferences, and the Internet. Every alternative way that a victim could have learned about the details of the activity must be explored, if for no other reason than to eliminate them and counter defense arguments. There may, however, be validity to these contagion factors. They might explain some of the "unbelievable" aspects of the case and result in the successful prosecution of the substance of the case. Consistency of statements becomes more significant if contagion is identified or disproved by independent investigation.

Munchausen syndrome and Munchausen syndrome by proxy are complex and sometimes controversial issues in child-victimization cases. No attempt will be made to discuss them in detail (see Feldman & Ford, 1994 and Parnell, 2002), but they are well-documented facts. Unfortunately, most of the published literature about them focuses only on their manifestation in the medical setting as false or fabricated illness or injury. For example, Munchausen syndrome by proxy is repeatedly and erroneously *defined* as "a form of child abuse" in which "mothers" deliberately physically harm their children and then under false pretenses seek medical attention. This may be a common manifestation of the condition, but it is neither the definition of the condition nor the only manifestation of the condition.

Munchausen syndrome is a psychological disorder (factitious disorder) in which an individual seeks secondary gain (ie, attention and forgiveness) by falsely claiming to have done something (eg, heroic rescue, awards, furnish information to solve a crime) or have had something happen to them (eg, illness, vandalism, hate crime, assault, rape). **Munchausen syndrome by proxy** is a variation of this psychological disorder in which one individual seeks this same secondary gain but through something done by or to another individual associated with them (eg, child, parent, friend). This syndrome can be caused or influenced by a wide variety of psychological conditions and disorders, but by definition the individual making the claim knows it is a lie. Adults can be the victims and non-parents and children can be perpetrators. Munchausen syndrome and Munchausen syndrome by proxy can and often are manifested in the criminal- justice setting as false or fabricated crime victimization. A child might falsely allege sexual victimization to get attention or forgiveness. If parents would poison their children to prove an illness, they might abuse their children in other ways to provide "proof" that a crime occurred and, therefore, get attention.

Investigators are often baffled by Munchausen syndrome and Munchausen syndrome by proxy cases because they can not imagine why the individual would be lying about these events. Investigators are usually looking for traditional motives such as money, anger, jealousy, and revenge. The key to identifying these syndromes is understanding that people sometimes lie to get attention and forgiveness and then are alert for such motives and needs. These are the unpopular but documented realities of the world. Recognizing the existence of these syndromes does not mean that child sexual victimization is any less real and serious.

Summary of Evaluation and Assessment

As much as investigators might wish, there may be no simple way to determine the accuracy of a victim's allegation. Investigators can not rely on therapists, evaluation experts, or the polygraph as shortcuts to determining the facts. Many mental health professionals might be good at determining that something traumatic happened to a child, but determining exactly *what* happened is another matter. Mental health professionals are now more willing to admit they are unable to determine, with certainty, the accuracy of victim statements in these cases. There is no test or statement-analysis formula that will determine with absolute certainty how or whether a child was sexually abused. Although resources such as expert opinion, statement-validity analysis, phallometric devices (sexual-arousal evaluation), voice-stress analysis, and the polygraph might be useful as part of the evaluation process, none of them should *ever* be the sole criterion for pursuing or not pursuing an allegation of child sexual victimization. Investigators must proceed with the investigation and rely primarily on the corroboration process.

The criminal-justice system must identify or develop and use fair and objective criteria for evaluating the accuracy of allegations of child sexual victimization and filing charges against the accused. Because something is possible does not mean it actually happened. The lack of corroborative evidence *is* significant when there should be corroborative evidence. With preferential sex offenders, there is almost always corroborative evidence. Blindly believing everything in spite of a lack of logical evidence or simply ignoring the impossible or improbable and accepting the possible is *not* good enough. If some of what the victim describes is accurate, some misperceived, distorted, and contaminated, what is the court supposed to believe? Until we come up with better answers, the court should be asked to believe what a thorough investigation can corroborate, understanding that physical evidence is *only one form of corroboration*. In those cases in which there simply is no corroborative evidence, the court may have to make its decision based on carefully assessed and evaluated victim testimony and the elimination of alternative explanations.

Corroborate

As a general principle, valid cases tend to get "better" and false cases tend to get "worse" with investigation. The techniques noted below are offered as ways to corroborate allegations of CSE and avoid child-victim testimony in court. If child-victim testimony can not be avoided, at least the victim will not bear the total burden of proof if these techniques are used. These techniques can, to varying degrees, be used in any child-sexual-victimization case, but my main focus here is on acquaintance molesters. The amount of corroborative evidence available might depend on the type of case, sexual activity, and offender(s) involved. Corroboration might be more difficult in an isolated one-on-one case perpetrated by a situational sex offender and easier in a sex-ring case perpetrated by an acquaintance-preferential sex offender.

Document Behavioral Symptoms of Sexual Victimization

Because the behavioral and environmental indicators of child sexual victimization are set forth in so many publications elsewhere (see Myers & Stern, 2002), they will not be discussed in detail here. Developmentally unusual sexual knowledge and behavior, however, seem to be the strongest symptoms. The documentation of these symptoms can be of assistance in corroborating child-victim statements. It must be emphasized, however, that these are only symptoms, and objective experts must carefully evaluate their significance in context. Many behavioral symptoms of child sexual victimization are actually symptoms of trauma, stress, and anxiety that could be caused by other events in the child's life. Almost every behavioral indicator of sexual victimization can be seen in nonabused children. Because of variables such as the type and length of abuse, the resiliency of the child victim, and society's response to the abuse, not all children react to being abused in the same way; therefore, just as the presence of behavioral symptoms does not prove that a child was sexually victimized, the absence of them does not prove that a child was not.

The use of expert witnesses to introduce this evidence into a court of law is a complex legal issue that will also not be discussed here in detail (see Myers & Stern, 2002). Mental health professionals, social workers, child protective service workers, and law-enforcement investigators can be the source of such expert testimony regarding sexual victimization symptoms. Experts might not be allowed to testify about the guilt and innocence of the accused but might be able to testify about the apparent validity of a case by explaining or offering opinions about the nature of the offense and its consistency with documented cases and offender-victim patterns of behavior. One commonly accepted use of such expert testimony is to impeach defense experts and rehabilitate prosecution witnesses after their credibility has been attacked by the defense. An expert might be able to testify concerning such symptoms to rebut defense allegations that the prosecution has no evidence other than the testimony of a child victim or that the child's disclosure is totally the result of leading and improper questioning.

These and other possible uses of expert testimony should be discussed with the prosecutor of each case. Even if not admissible in court, the symptoms of sexual victimization still can be useful as part of investigative corroboration, particularly when symptoms *predate* any disclosure. Ongoing research reveals that sexually abused girls also may experience physiological changes and symptoms (DeBellis et al, 1994). The investigative and prosecutorial significance of these findings is unknown at this time.

Document Patterns of Behavior

Two patterns of behavior should be documented. They are victim patterns and offender patterns.

By far the most important *victim pattern* of behavior to identify and document is the disclosure process. Investigators must verify, through active investigation, the exact nature and content of each disclosure, outcry, or statement made by the victim. Secondhand information about disclosure is not good enough. To whatever extent humanly possible, the investigator should determine exactly when, where, to whom, with precisely what words, and why the victim disclosed.

It can be important to determine why the child did not disclose sooner and why the child did disclose now. A well-documented, convincing disclosure, especially a spontaneous one with no secondary gain, can be corroborative evidence. The fact that a victim does not disclose the abuse for years or recants previous disclosures might be part of a pattern of behavior that in fact helps to corroborate sexual victimization. The documentation of the secrecy, the sequence of disclosures, the recantation of statements, and the distortion of events can all be part of the corroboration process.

Documenting *offender patterns* of behavior is one of the most important and overlooked steps in the corroboration process. Investigators must make every reasonable effort to document offender patterns of behavior and determine the type of offender involved. Because their molestation of children is part of a long-term pattern of behavior, preferential sex offenders are like human evidence machines. During their lifetime they leave behind a string of victims and collections of child pornography and erotica. In these cases, a wealth of evidence is available to investigators and prosecutors. All they need to uncover it is an understanding of how to recognize these offenders and how these offenders operate and the full commitment of agency/department time and resources.

Knowing the kind of offender being investigated can help determine investigative strategy. For example, it might be useful in:

— Anticipating and understanding need-driven mistakes.

— Comparing consistency of victim statements with offender characteristics.

— Developing offender and victim interview strategies.

— Determining the existence, age, and number of victims.

— Recognizing where and what kind of corroborative evidence might be found.

— Evaluating the likelihood of possessing child pornography or using a computer.

— Utilizing an expert search warrant.

— Addressing staleness.

— Evaluating and proving intent.

— Determining appropriate charging and sentencing.

— Evaluating dangerousness at a bond hearing.

— Assessing the admissibility of prior and subsequent like acts.

— Explaining behavior patterns to a jury.

— Determining suitability for treatment options.

— Notifying the community.

As previously mentioned, comparing the consistency between "what" is alleged to have happened and "who" is suspected of doing it is an important application of the offender typology. If a victim describes his or her victimization as involving what sounds like the behavior patterns of a preferential sex offender, then the fact that the alleged offender fits that pattern is corroborative. If he does not, an inconsistency needs to be resolved. The inconsistency could be because the alleged "what" is inaccurate (eg, distorted account from victim, insufficient details), the suspected "who" has been misevaluated (eg, incomplete background, erroneous assessment), or the alleged "who" is innocent (eg, suspect did not commit alleged crime). In my experience, distorted accounts from victims are frequently caused or influenced by various interveners (eg, therapists, physicians, parents, law enforcement) who are unwilling to accept the reality of the nature of acquaintance molestation of children nonjudgmentally.

It is obviously better to convict a child molester based on his or her past behavior. If all else fails, however, preferential child molesters usually can be convicted in the future based on their continuing molestation of children.

In an *exaggerated example,* an investigation determines that a suspect is a 50-year-old single male who does volunteer work with troubled boys, has 2 prior convictions for sexually molesting young boys in 1974 and 1986, has an expensive state-of-the-art home computer, has an online screen name of "Boy lover," and has at least one online profile that describes himself as a 14-year-old. He has for the last 5 years daily spent many hours online in chat rooms and the alt.sex.preteen newsgroup justifying and graphically describing his sexual preference for and involvement with young boys, and brags about his extensive pornography collection while uploading hundreds of child-pornography files, all focusing on preteen boys in bondage, to dozens of individuals all over the world. If such a determination were relevant to the case, these facts would constitute more than enough probable cause to prove that this suspect is a preferential sex offender.

Identify Adult Witnesses and Suspects

Not all sexual victimization of children is one-on-one, as in cases with multiple offenders and accomplices. One benefit of a multioffender case is that it increases the likelihood of a weak link in the group. Do not assume that accomplices will not cooperate with the investigation. The conspiracy model of building a case against one suspect and then using that suspect's testimony against others can be useful. Because of the need to protect potential child victims, however, the conspiracy model of investigation has limitations in child-sexual-victimization cases. Investigators and prosecutors can not knowingly allow children to be molested as the case is built by "turning" suspects. Corroboration of a child victim's statement with adult-witness testimony, however, is an important and valuable technique.

Medical Evidence

Whenever possible, all children suspected of having been sexually victimized should be afforded a medical examination by a trained and competent physician (Jenny, 2002). The primary purpose of this examination is to assess potential injury, assess the need for treatment, and reassure the patient. A secondary purpose is to determine the presence of any corroborating evidence of acute or chronic trauma. The ability and willingness of medical doctors to corroborate child sexual victimization has improved greatly in recent years, primarily due to better training and the use of protocols, rape kits, the colposcope, toluidine blue dye, ultraviolet light photography, and other such techniques.

When used with a camera, the colposcope can document the trauma without additional examinations of the child victim. Positive laboratory tests for sexually transmitted diseases can be valuable evidence especially in cases involving young children. Statements made to doctors by the child victim as part of the medical examination might be admissible in court without the child testifying.

Investigators should be cautious of doctors who have been identified as child-abuse crusaders or always find—or never find—medical evidence of sexual victimization. In a forensic examination, medical doctors or nurses should be objective scientists. The exact cause of any anal or vaginal trauma needs to be evaluated carefully and scientifically. Many acts of child sexual victimization do not leave any physical injuries that can be identified by a medical examination. In addition, children's injuries can heal rapidly. Thus, lack of medical corroboration does not mean that a child was not sexually victimized or that it can not be proven in court.

Other Victims

The simple understanding and recognition that a child molester might have other victims is one of the most important steps in corroborating an allegation of child sexual victimization. There is strength in numbers. If an investigation uncovers one or two victims, each will probably have to testify in court. If an investigation uncovers multiple victims, the odds are that none of them will testify because a trial will not occur. With multiple victims, the only defense is to allege a flawed, leading investigation.

Because of the volume of crime, limited resources, and lack of knowledge about the nature of crime, many law-enforcement agencies are unable or unwilling to continue an investigation to find more than a couple of victims. If that is the case, they must try to identify as many victims as possible. Other victims are sometimes identified through publicity about the case. Consistency of statements obtained from multiple victims, independently interviewed, can be powerful corroboration.

With preferential acquaintance molesters, especially those who prefer boys, the potential for multiple victims can be overwhelming. If there are a dozen disclosing victims, with a mountain of corroborative evidence, and an offender who is going to jail for many years, does the investigator have to continue to investigate until "all" the victims are found? The US Attorney General's Guidelines for Victim and Witness Assistance indicates that US Department of Justice investigators and prosecutors are responsible for identifying and contacting all the victims of a crime (US Department of Justice, 2000). The exact meaning of this statement is subject to interpretation, but common sense says a decision must be made based on a totality of the facts.

Some unidentified victims may be in need of therapy and counseling. Some, however, may be doing fine, and dredging up the victimization may cause more problems. Some victims may not know or realize that they are victims until informed by investigators. Can victims suffer the psychological consequences of being victimized if they do not know that they are victims? These difficult issues have no easy answers. Investigators must think about these issues and make the best-informed decision.

Search Warrants

The major law-enforcement problem with the use of search warrants in child sexual-victimization cases is that they are not obtained soon enough. In many cases, investigators have probable cause for a search warrant but do not know it. Because evidence can be moved, hidden, or destroyed quickly, search warrants should be obtained as soon as legally possible. Waiting too long and developing, in essence, too much probable cause also might subject investigative agencies to criticism or even lawsuits charging this delay allowed additional victims to be molested. This is a potentially significant problem in sexual exploitation cases. "What did you know and when did you know it" can become a big issue in defending an investigative response as correct and reasonable. Investigators often do not recognize the value and significance of child erotica, pedophile paraphernalia, and other collateral evidence.

The expertise of an experienced investigator and well-documented behavior patterns of preferential sex offenders can be used sometimes to add to the probable cause, expand the scope of the search, or address the legal staleness problem of old information. Such "expert" search warrants should be used when necessary and when there is probable cause to believe the alleged offender fits the preferential pattern of behavior.

Physical Evidence

Physical evidence can be defined as objects that corroborate anything a child victim did, said, saw, heard, tasted, smelled, drew, or had done to him or her. It can be used to prove offender identity and type and location of activity. It could be items such as sheets, articles of clothing, sexual aids, lubricants, fingerprints, and documents. It also could be an object or sign on the wall described by a victim. If the victim says the offender ejaculated on a doorknob, ejaculate on the doorknob becomes physical evidence if found. If the victim says the offender kept condoms in the nightstand by his bed, they become physical evidence if found. An adult pornography magazine with a page missing as described by the victim is physical evidence. Satanic occult paraphernalia is evidence if it corroborates criminal activity described by the victim. Positive identification of a subject through deoxyribonucleic acid (DNA) analysis of trace amounts of biological evidence left on a child or at a crime scene might result in a child victim not having to testify because the perpetrator pleads guilty.

Child Pornography and Child Erotica

Child pornography, especially that produced by the offender, is one of the most valuable pieces of corroborative evidence of child sexual victimization that any investigator can have. Many collectors of child pornography do not molest children, and many child molesters do not possess or collect child pornography. Investigators should, however, always be alert for it. Child erotica can be defined as any material, relating to children, that serves a sexual purpose for a given individual. That purpose is often to validate their sexual interest in children. Some of the more common types of child erotica include drawings, fantasy writings, diaries, souvenirs, letters, books about children, psychological books on pedophilia, and ordinary photographs of children. It must be evaluated in the context in which it is found using good judgment and common sense. Child erotica is not as significant as child pornography, but it can be of value.

Computers

Investigators must be alert to the rapidly increasing possibility that a child molester with the intelligence, economic means, or employment access might use a computer in a variety of ways as part of his sexual victimization of children. As computers have become less expensive, more sophisticated, and easier to operate, the potential for this abuse is growing rapidly. Computer use is discussed in detail in chapter 22, The Use of the Internet for Child Sexual Exploitation.

Consensual Monitoring

Consensual monitoring is a valuable but often underused investigative technique. It includes the use of body recorders and pretext telephone calls. Because of the legal issues involved and variations in state laws, use of this technique should always be discussed with prosecutors and law-enforcement legal advisers.

It is important to remember that children are not small adults and must never be endangered by investigators. The use of this technique with child victims presents ethical issues as well as legal considerations. Its use with victims who have emotional problems or are in therapy, for example, should be carefully evaluated. Pretext telephone calls are more suitable than body recorders with child victims but are not always appropriate. They might not be suitable for use with very young victims or victims who have developed a strong bond with the offender and do not believe they are victims. Because victims who are seduced or compliant may feel pressured by parents or investigators to furnish a more socially acceptable, stereotypical version of their victimization, they may falsely pretend no such a bond with the offender exists and/or may feign a desire to have the offender arrested and prosecuted. If the child victim states one thing but feels differently, "participating" in the investigation in this way could lead to the child "tipping off" the alleged offender or more serious consequences for the child ranging from further victimization to suicide.

The use of this technique should be discussed with the parents of a victim who is a minor. The parent, however, might not be trusted to be discreet about the use of this technique or might even be a suspect in the investigation. Although further emotional trauma can occur, many victims afterward describe an almost therapeutic sense of empowerment or return of control through their participation in pretext telephone calls.

Investigators using the pretext telephone call should ensure that they have a telephone number that can not be traced to law enforcement and method to verify the date and time of the calls. In addition to victims, investigators can also make such calls themselves by impersonating a wide variety of potentially involved or concerned individuals. Sometimes victims or their relatives or friends do the monitoring and recording on their own. Investigators need to check appropriate laws concerning the legality of such taping and admissibility of the material obtained.

Consensual monitoring with body recorders is probably best reserved for use with undercover investigators and adult informants. Under no circumstance should an investigative agency produce or wind up with a videotape or audiotape of the actual or simulated molestation of a child as part of an investigative technique; however, the child victim might be used to introduce the undercover investigator to the subject.

Inappropriate responses obtained through consensual monitoring can be almost as damaging as outright admissions. When told by a victim over the telephone that law enforcement or a therapist wants to discuss the sexual relationship, "Let's talk about it later tonight" is an incriminating response by a suspect.

Subject Confessions

Getting a subject to confess obviously can be an effective way to corroborate child sexual victimization and avoid child-victim testimony in court. Unfortunately, many investigators put minimal effort into subject interviews. Simply asking an alleged perpetrator if he molested a child does not constitute a proper interview. Any criminal investigator needs effective interviewing skills. In view of the stakes involved, child-sexual-victimization investigators must do everything reasonably possible to improve their skills in this area. Entire books and chapters have been written about interview techniques and strategies. In this limited space, I will offer a brief review of some basic interviewing issues.

Investigators need to collect background information and develop an interview strategy before conducting a potentially important discussion with the alleged offender. Many sexual offenders against children really want to discuss their behavior or at least their rationalization for it. If treated with professionalism, empathy, and understanding, many of these offenders will make significant admissions. If the offender is allowed to rationalize or project some of the blame for his behavior onto someone or something else, he is more likely to confess. Most sex offenders will admit only what they can rationalize and that which has been discovered. Revealing *some* irrefutable "facts," therefore, can be an effective strategy. In a computer case, this might involve showing him some of the chat logs of his online conversations. If investigators do not confront the subject with all available evidence, the suspect might be more likely to minimize his acts rather than totally deny them. Many child molesters admit their acts but deny the intent. A tougher approach can always be tried if the soft approach does not work. Investigators should consider noncustodial (ie, no arrest), nonconfrontational interviews of the subject at home or work. Interviews during the execution of a search warrant also should be considered. Investigators should not overlook admissions made by the offender to wives, girlfriends, neighbors, friends, and even the media.

The polygraph and other lie-detection devices can be valuable tools when used as part of the interview strategy by skilled interviewers. Their greatest value is in the subject's belief that they will determine the truth of any statement he makes. Once used, their value is limited by their lack of legal admissibility. The polygraph, or any lie-detection device, should never be the sole criterion for discontinuing the investigation of child-sexual-victimization allegations.

Surveillance

Surveillance can be a time consuming and expensive investigative technique. In some cases, it also can be effective. Time and expense can be reduced if the surveillance is not open-ended but is based on inside information about the subject's activity. One obvious problem, however, is what to do when the surveillance team comes to believe that a child is being victimized. How much reasonable suspicion or probable cause does an investigator on physical or electronic surveillance need to take action? If a suspected child molester simply goes into a residence with a child, does law enforcement have the right to intervene? What if the offender is simply paying the newspaper boy or watching television with a neighborhood child? Consider these important legal and ethical issues when using this surveillance technique. Sometimes the surveillance may discover that the offender is making contact with children in violation of his parole. In spite of potential problems, surveillance is a valuable technique, especially in the investigation of multiple-victim-exploitation cases.

INVESTIGATING MULTIPLE-VICTIM CASES

The general investigative techniques discussed can be applicable in varying degrees to the acquaintance-exploitation cases involving multiple victims. The "big picture" approach is the key to the successful investigation and prosecution of these cases. Multiple victims corroborated by child pornography, erotica, and other physical evidence make a powerful case likely to result in a guilty plea, no trial, and no child-victim testimony. The techniques noted below apply *primarily* to the investigation of acquaintance-exploitation cases involving multiple victims.

Understanding the Seduction Process

Most child victims in multiple-victim-exploitation cases were seduced or groomed over time. The seduction process was discussed earlier in this chapter. True understanding of this process must be incorporated into the investigation of these cases. For example, pediatricians or therapists who discuss forced or unwanted sexual activity with their patients are potentially missing a significant area of sexual victimization of children. Because a child wanted to have sex with an adult does not mean it is not abuse and a crime. After understanding the seduction process, the investigator must be able to communicate this understanding to the victim. This is the difficult part. An investigator once contacted me and described what sounded like a classic case involving an acquaintance-seduction preferential offender. The investigator stated, however, that his first disclosing victim, a 12-year-old boy, described being gagged and tied up by the offender. While this is certainly possible, it is not typical of such offenders. When asked when and how the victim furnished this information, the investigator admitted that it was after he had asked the boy why he did not scream or fight when the offender abused him sexually.

By asking such questions in this way, the investigator is communicating to the boy that the investigator has no insight into the nature of this crime nor an understanding or acceptance of the subtle seduction of the boy. Obviously, the investigator is back in the world of dirty old men in wrinkled raincoats jumping out from behind trees. The investigator did not understand that the molester was probably the boy's best friend who seduced him with attention and affection. The victim realized that the investigator would not understand what happened, so the boy "adjusted" the story and tried to explain with an excuse that the investigator would accept and understand. The boy was suffering from the "say no, yell, and tell" guilt.

I have given many presentations describing the dynamics of multiple-victim cases and seduction techniques of preferential child molesters (pedophiles). After many of these presentations, adult members of the audience, especially males, have approached me in private and admitted that they were victimized as children. Most stated they had never before told anyone of their victimization but were able now to tell because they realized that I understood the problem and that they were not the only ones victimized in this way. The key, then, to getting child victims who were compliant to disclose their victimization is to communicate subtly to them your understanding of the seduction process without engaging in repetitive, leading, or suggestive interviewing that might damage the reliability and credibility of the information obtained. After the first few victims disclose, the others usually come forward more readily. Some individuals, however, may come forward and falsely claim to be victims in order to get attention, forgiveness, or part of a financial settlement in a civil lawsuit. All allegations must be thoroughly and objectively evaluated and investigated.

Investigators must understand and learn to deal with the incomplete and contradictory statements of seduced victims of acquaintance molesters. The dynamics of their victimization must be considered. They are embarrassed and ashamed of their behavior and correctly believe that society will not understand their victimization. Many younger child victims are most concerned about the response of their parents and often describe their victimization in ways they believe will please their parents. Adolescent victims are also typically concerned about the response of their peers. Victims and their families from higher socioeconomic backgrounds may be more concerned about the public embarrassment of any disclosure. Investigators who have a stereotyped concept of child-sexual-abuse victims or who are accustomed to interviewing younger children molested within their family will have a difficult time interviewing adolescents molested in a sex ring. Many of these victims will be streetwise, troubled, or even delinquent children from dysfunctional homes. Such victims should not blindly be believed but should not be dismissed because the accused is a pillar of the community and the victims are delinquent or troubled. Such allegations should be objectively investigated.

When attempting to identify potential victims in a multiple-victim-exploitation case, I recommend trying to start with victims who are about to or have just left the offender's "pipeline." The victim most likely to disclose would be one who has just left the ring and has a sibling or close friend about to enter the ring. The desire to protect younger victims from what they have endured is the strongest motivation for overcoming their shame and embarrassment. The next best choice would be a victim who has just entered the "pipeline."

Before beginning the interview, the investigator must understand that the victim may have many positive feelings for the offender and even resent any intervention. Because of the bond with the offender, victims may even warn the offender. Even the occasional victim who comes forward and discloses may feel guilty and then warn the offender. They may even return to law enforcement with a hidden tape recorder to try to catch the investigator making inappropriate comments or utilizing improper interview techniques. Reluctance to disclose may be more due to affection for rather than fear of the offender.

Time must be spent attempting to develop a working relationship with the victim. The investigator must be able to discuss a wide variety of sexual activities, understand the victim's terminology, and not be judgmental. Being nonjudgmental, as with developing rapport, may be much more difficult with a delinquent adolescent who actively participated in his victimization. Investigators often nonverbally communicate their judgmental attitude unknowingly through gestures, facial expressions, and body language.

In interviewing victims of acquaintance sexual exploitation, investigators should consider—in their own minds—pretending that the victim is actually more like a subject or suspect, and expect the victim to deny or minimize his or her acts. Some victims will continue to deny their victimization no matter what the interviewer says or does. Some children even deny victimization that the offender has admitted or other evidence discloses. Some will make admissions but minimize the quality and quantity of the acts. They may minimize their compliance and maximize the offender's involvement by claiming he drugged them, threatened them, had a weapon, or had even abducted them. Of course, some of these allegations may be accurate and should be investigated. They are, however, atypical of acquaintance-exploitation cases. Violence is most likely used to prevent disclosure. Sadistic preferential offenders may also use violence during sex, but this is relatively rare in cases involving seduction. As previously discussed, these potential inaccuracies in the details of the allegations of seduced victims may explain some of the inconsistencies between the alleged "what" and the suspected "who."

The investigator must communicate to the victim that he or she is not at fault even though the victim did not say no, did not fight, did not tell, initiated the sex, or even enjoyed it. When the victim comes to believe that the investigator understands what he experienced, he or she is more likely to talk. Victims often reveal the details little by little, testing the investigator's response. The investigator must recognize and sometimes allow the victim to use face-saving scenarios when disclosing victimization. For example, such victims might claim they were confused, tricked, asleep, drugged, drunk, or tied up when they were not. Adolescents, who pose special challenges for the interviewer, use these face-saving devices most often. Even if a victim discloses, the investigator must accept that the information is likely to be incomplete, minimizing the victim's involvement and acts. Some of these victims simply do not believe they were victims.

In the absence of some compelling special circumstance, the interview of a child possibly seduced by an acquaintance molester should *never* be conducted in the presence of parents. The presence of the parent increases the likelihood that the child will just deny or give the socially or parentally acceptable version of the victimization. This is especially true of younger victims. Investigators also should consider unannounced interviews of victims of acquaintance molesters.

If all else fails, the investigator can try the no-nonsense approach. No matter what the investigator does, most compliant adolescent boy victims will deny they were victims. It is important, therefore, that as many potential victims as legally and ethically possible must be interviewed. It is also possible that some troubled teenagers may exaggerate their victimization or even falsely accuse individuals. Allegations must be objectively investigated considering all possibilities. After disclosing, some victims will later recant or change their stories.

The offender also may continue to manipulate the victims after investigation and disclosure. The offender may appeal to the victim's sympathy. He may make a feeble attempt at suicide to make the victims feel guilty or disloyal. Some offenders may threaten the victims with physical harm or disclosure of the blackmail material. Some offenders may bribe the victim and his family. Even after they disclose and testify in court, some victims then recant and claim they perjured themselves. Although in some cases the recantation may be valid, it is most likely the result of blackmail, feelings of guilt about the offender being in prison, or shame over their behavior.

Some victims in acquaintance-child-exploitation cases disclose incomplete and minimized information about the sexual activity. This creates significant problems for the investigation and prosecution of such cases. For instance, when the investigator finally gets a victim to disclose the exploitation and abuse, the victim furnishes a version of his victimization that he or she swears is true. Subsequent investigation then uncovers additional victims, child pornography, or computer chat logs and other records—directly conflicting with the first victim's story. A common example is that the victim admits the offender sucked his penis but denies that he sucked the offender's penis. The execution of a search warrant then leads to the seizure of photographs of the victim sucking the offender's penis. Additional victims may also confirm this but then lie when they vehemently deny that they did the same thing.

The allegations of multiple victims often conflict with each other. Victims tend to minimize their behavior and maximize the behavior of other victims or the offender. Some victims continue to deny the activity even when confronted with the pictures. Today, investigators must be especially careful in computer cases where easily recovered chat logs, records of communication, and visual images may directly contradict the socially acceptable version of events the victim is now giving.

Understanding the Preferential Molester

Preferential sex offenders may be "pillars of the community" and are often described as "nice guys." They almost always have a means of access to children (eg, marriage, neighborhood, occupation). Determining their means of access helps identify potential victims. Investigations should always verify the credentials of those who attempt to justify their acts as part of some "professional" activity. It must be understood, however, that just because an offender is a doctor, clergy member, or therapist, for example, he could still be a child molester.

As previously stated, because the molestation of children is part of a long-term persistent pattern of behavior, preferential child molesters are like human evidence machines. During their lifetime they leave behind a string of victims and a collection of child pornography and erotica. The preferential child molester, therefore, can be thoroughly investigated and corroborative evidence easily found if investigators understand how to recognize him, how he operates—*and if their agencies give them the time and resources.*

Men sexually attracted to young adolescent boys are the most persistent and prolific child molesters known to the criminal-justice system. Depending on how one defines molestation, they can easily have dozens if not hundreds of victims in a lifetime. They usually begin their activity when they are teenagers themselves and continue throughout their lives as long as they are physically able.

Many pedophiles spend their entire lives attempting to convince themselves and others that they are not evil sexual perverts but good guys who love and nurture children. This is a major reason why they do such things as join organizations where they can help troubled children and volunteer to search for missing children. Because so many of them have successfully hidden their activities for so long, when identified and prosecuted they try to convince themselves that they will somehow continue to escape responsibility. This is why they often vehemently proclaim their innocence right up to the time of their trial. If, however, the criminal investigator and prosecutor have properly developed the case, preferential offenders almost always change their plea to guilty.

Investigators also should be aware of offenders too eager to plead guilty. They may be hiding much more extensive or serious behavior that they hope will not be discovered by additional investigation.

Proactive Approach

Because this chapter is available to the public, specific details of proactive investigative techniques will not be discussed. These techniques are, for the most part, only appropriate for use by law enforcement investigators. In general, however, proactive investigation involves the use of surveillance, mail covers, undercover correspondence, "sting" operations, reverse "sting" operations, and online computer operations. For example, when an offender who has been communicating with other offenders is arrested, law enforcement investigators can assume his identity and continue the correspondence.

It is not necessary for each law-enforcement agency to "reinvent the wheel." Federal law-enforcement agencies such as the US Postal Inspection Service, the US Customs Service, the FBI, and some state and local departments have been using these techniques for years. Because child prostitution and the production and distribution of child pornography frequently involve federal violations, the US Postal Inspection Service, the US Customs Service, and the FBI all have intelligence information about such activity. It is recommended that any law-enforcement agency about to begin the use of these proactive techniques, especially those involving online Internet activity, should contact nearby federal, state, and local law-enforcement agencies to determine what is already being done and what protocols and policies have been developed. Many areas of the country have organized task forces on sexual abuse, exploitation, and computer exploitation of children. Law enforcement agencies must learn to work together in these proactive techniques, or else they may wind up "investigating" each other. Some child molesters are actively trying to identify and learn about these proactive techniques.

Investigators must give careful thought and consideration before utilizing a child in any way in proactive investigation. Child safety and protection come first. As previously stated, investigators should *never* put child pornography on the Internet or in the mail because of the harm of such uncontrolled circulation. The end does not justify the means. Investigators also must ensure their undercover activity does not cross the line into entrapment or outrageous government conduct. This is even more important if the investigator forwards his or her investigative "findings" to another law enforcement agency for appropriate action.

The proactive approach also includes the analysis of records and documents obtained or seized from offenders during an investigation. In addition to being used to convict these offenders, such material can contain valuable intelligence information about other offenders and victims. This material must be evaluated carefully in order not to overestimate or underestimate its significance.

Establish Communication With Parents

The importance and difficulty of this technique in extrafamilial cases can not be overemphasized. Because the parents are not the alleged perpetrators, their investigative significance is different, not less than in intrafamilial cases. Parents should be advised of the general nature of the investigation. Investigators should seek their cooperation and maintain ongoing communication with them. Not all parents react the same way to the alleged sexual victimization of their children. Some are supportive and cooperative. Others overreact, and some even deny the victimization. Sometimes, there is animosity and mistrust among parents with differing reactions. Some parents even support the accused perpetrator. Others want him immediately put in jail.

Parents must be told that in the absence of some extraordinary circumstance, investigators need to interview their children outside their presence. In some cases, departmental policy or the law may give parents the right to be present during the interview of their minor children. If that is the situation, every effort should be made to get parental and/or departmental permission to waive that right. If parents are present during the interviews, any information so obtained must be carefully assessed and evaluated with the understanding of the parents' potentially significant influence on their children's statements. Compromises involving one-way mirrors, video cameras, and out-of-eye-contact sitting positions may be possible. Eventually, parents will have to be told something about what *their* children disclose. It is best if this happens after the information is obtained in a way that increases the likelihood of its accuracy and reliability. Parents should not be given the details of the disclosures of any other victims. Parents should be told of the importance of keeping the details of their child's disclosures confidential, especially from the media and other parents.

Parents should be interviewed regarding any behavioral indicators of possible abuse they have observed and the history of their child's contact with the alleged offender. They must be reminded, however, that their child's credibility will be jeopardized when and if the information was obtained through repetitive or leading questioning and/or turns out to be exaggerated, unsubstantiated, or false. To minimize these problems, within the limits of the law and without jeopardizing investigative techniques, parents must be told on a regular basis how the case is progressing. Parents can also be assigned constructive things to do (eg, lobbying for new legislation, working on awareness and prevention programs) to channel their energy, concern, and guilt.

If the parents lose faith in professionals and begin to interrogate their children and conduct their own investigation, the proper evaluation of the case may be lost forever. Parents from one case communicate the results of their "investigation" with each other, and some have even contacted the parents in other cases. Such parental activity, while understandable, is an obvious source of potential contamination.

In addition, it must be remembered that children sexually exploited outside the home can also be sexually victimized inside the home.

REFERENCES

American Psychiatric Association (APA). *Diagnostic and Statistical Manual of Mental Disorders.* 4th ed. Text revision. Washington, DC: American Psychiatric Association; 2000.

Burgess AW, ed. *Child Pornography and Sex Rings.* Lexington, Mass: Lexington Books; 1984.

DeBellis M, Lefter L, Trickett P, Putnam F. Urinary catecholamine excretion in sexually abused girls. *J Am Acad Child Adolesc Psychiatry.* 1994;33:320-327.

Dietz PE. Sex offenses: behavioral aspects. In: Kadish SH et al. *Encyclopedia of Crime and Justice.* New York, NY: Free Press; 1983.

Feldman MD, Ford CV. *Patient or Pretender.* New York, NY: John Wiley & Sons; 1994.

Hazelwood RR, Warren JI. The sexually violent offender: impulsive or ritualistic? In: Hazelwood RR, Burgess AW. *Practical Aspects of Rape Investigation.* 3rd ed. Boca Raton, Fla: CRC Press; 2001:97-113

Hunter JA. The sexual crimes of juveniles. In: Hazelwood RR, Burgess AW. *Practical Aspects of Rape Investigation.* 3rd ed. Boca Raton, Fla: CRC Press; 2001: 401-419

Jenny C. Medical issues in child sexual abuse. In: Myers JEB, Berliner L, Briere J, Hendrix CT, Jenny C, Reid TA. *APSAC Handbook on Child Maltreatment.* 2nd ed. Thousand Oaks, Calif: Sage Publications; 2002:235-248.

Lanning KV. *Child Molesters: A Behavioral Analysis.* Alexandria, Va: National Center for Missing & Exploited Children; 1986.

Lanning KV. *Child Molesters: A Behavioral Analysis.* 2nd ed. Alexandria, Va: National Center for Missing & Exploited Children; 1987.

Lanning, KV. *Child Molesters: A Behavioral Analysis* 3rd ed. Alexandria, Va: National Center for Missing & Exploited Children; 1992a.

Lanning KV. *Child Molesters: A Behavioral Analysis.* 4th ed. Alexandria, Va: National Center for Missing & Exploited Children; 2001.

Lanning KV. *Child Sex Rings: A Behavioral Analysis.* 2nd ed. Alexandria, Va: National Center for Missing & Exploited Children; 1992b.

Lanning KV. *Investigator's Guide to Allegations of "Ritual" Child Abuse.* Quantico, Va: US Dept of Justice; 1992c.

Lanning KV. The "witch hunt," the "backlash," and professionalism. *The APSAC Advisor.* 1996;9(4):8-11

Myers JEB, Stern P. Expert testimony. In: Myers JEB, Berliner L, Briere J, Hendrix CT, Jenny C, Reid TA, eds. *APSAC Handbook on Child Maltreatment.* 2nd ed. Thousand Oaks, Calif: Sage Publications; 2002:379-402.

Parnell TF. Munchausen by proxy syndrome. In: Myers JEB, Berliner L, Briere J, Hendrix CT, Jenny C, Reid TA, eds. *APSAC Handbook on Child Maltreatment.* 2nd ed. Thousand Oaks, Calif: Sage Publications; 2002:131-138.

Random House Webster's College Dictionary. New York, NY: Random House; 1991.

Saywitz KJ, Goodman GS, Lyon TD. Interviewing children in and out of court: current research and practice implications. In: Myers JEB, Berliner L, Briere J, Hendrix CT, Jenny C, Reid TA, eds. *APSAC Handbook on Child Maltreatment* 2nd ed. Thousand Oaks, Calif: Sage Publications; 2002:349-378.

United States v Romero, 189 F3d 576 (7th Cir 1999), *cert denied.*

US Department of Justice (USDOJ). *Attorney General Guidelines for Victim and Witness Assistance.* Washington, DC: US Dept of Justice; 2000.

US Department of Justice (USDOJ). *Joint Investigations of Child Abuse: Report of a Symposium.* Washington, DC; 1993.

Warren JI, Hislop J. Female sex offenders: a typological and etiological overview. In: Hazelwood RR, Burgess AW, eds. *Practical Aspects of Rape Investigation.* 3rd ed. Boca Raton, Fla: CRC Press; 2001:421-434

The Work of the United States Postal Inspection Service: Combating Child Sexual Exploitation

Raymond C. Smith

The sexual exploitation of children spans all social and economic classes, and the perpetrators have no regard for the enduring grief and trauma they bring to their victims. Every child is a potential victim. The dangers of child sexual exploitation should never be minimized. This most despicable of crimes—a crime against a child—results in physical and emotional suffering, ruined lives, and shattered dreams. Through public awareness, vigorous investigation, certain prosecution, and just sentencing, the incidence of this horrible crime can be reduced. Members of society have an obligation to help protect children and their families.

The United States Postal Inspection Service

As one of America's oldest federal law enforcement agencies, the US Postal Inspection Service (USPIS), founded by Benjamin Franklin, has a long, proud, and successful history of fighting criminals who attack the nation's postal system and misuse it to defraud, endanger, or otherwise threaten the American public. As the primary law enforcement arm of the US Postal Service, the USPIS is a specialized, professional organization performing investigative and security functions essential to a stable and sound postal system.

As fact-finding and investigative agents, Postal Inspectors are federal law enforcement officers who carry firearms, make arrests, execute federal search warrants, and serve subpoenas. Inspectors work closely with US attorneys, other law enforcement agencies, and local prosecutors to investigate cases and prepare them for court. Approximately 2000 Postal Inspectors are stationed throughout the United States and enforce more than 200 federal laws regarding crimes that involve the US mail and postal system.

Early Enforcement Efforts: Obscenity Investigations

For more than a century, the USPIS has had specific responsibility for investigating the mailing of obscene matter. In the 1860s and 1870s, Special Agents (as Postal Inspectors were called then) had to deal with European smut peddlers who were invading American shores with obscene material. Special Agent Anthony Comstock, or "Mad Anthony," as he was known, waged a relentless battle against anyone who used the US mail in an attempt to corrupt the morals of young people. In 1873, Congress passed the Comstock Act, a forerunner to the existing postal obscenity statute (18 USC § 1461). In a letter dated June 11, 1875, now in the Inspection Service Archives, Comstock wrote to his superior reporting on an investigation:

I have the honor to report that yesterday in the city of New York I caused the arrest of one Zephir M. Caille, of 261 West 27th St., and doing business opposite 602 Broadway. He is charged with selling obscene pictures, and today waived examination at Tombs Police Court and was committed in default of $1,000—for trial in Special Sessions court. I seized about 175 pictures in his possession. I have found I had a good case in State court and therefore I took him there instead of waiting to work up a case in United States Court. He is a Frenchman, and I am informed owned a set of 37 different negatives for printing obscene photographs and supplied the trade throughout the country, although ostensibly keeping a stand on Broadway.

I have the honor to be
Very Respectfully Sir:
Your Obedient Servant

Anthony Comstock

P.S. This fellow had a clasp knife sharpened as a dirk, but he did not get a chance to use it as I ironed him.

PROTECTING CHILDREN FROM SEXUAL EXPLOITATION: A NATIONAL PRIORITY

Through the years, child pornography has been investigated along with obscenity matters; however, it was not until the late 1970s that Congress took action to create federal legislation protecting children from sexual exploitation.

Prior to the late 1970s, most Americans were unaware of the proliferation and commercial distribution of magazines, films, photographs, and videotapes depicting children in explicit sexual acts. Fortunately, we have come to realize that child pornography is not an "art form" but a manifestation of aberrant behavior resulting in the sexual molestation and abuse of children.

Individuals with a preferred sexual interest in children, sometimes referred to as preferential offenders or **pedophiles**, are the primary producers and users of this insidious material. The primary reasons why these individuals produce, use, and collect child pornography are:

— For their own sexual arousal and gratification.

— To lower the inhibitions of their child victim.

— As "blackmail" to ensure that the child does not tell the "secret" of the activity that he or she is being forced to endure.

— To preserve the child's "youth" by maintaining a pictorial record of the child's appearance at the "desirable" age even after he or she has grown older and matured.

— As a medium of exchange with other like-minded individuals to enlarge their child pornography collections.

— For commercial gain.

Who are the victims? The popular notion that runaways and children from broken homes are the main targets of child molesters and pornographers is inaccurate. Often, the victim is the "child down the street" who has been seduced into a relationship by a trusted adult. Children may fail to disclose the abuse because of guilt, shame, blackmail, or, in some instances, because for the first time in their life they have received the attention all children crave in what is interpreted to be affection from an adult.

In 1977, the Protection of Children Against Sexual Exploitation Act became law (18 USC § 2251-2253). This was the first federal law specifically designed to protect children from commercialized sexual exploitation. It was the culmination of years of effort by Congress, the US Department of Justice (USDOJ), concerned members of the public, and the law enforcement community to take action against the pernicious effects of pornography and the sexual exploitation of children. Under this law, a child, or minor, was defined as a person younger than age 16.

America had finally awakened to the devastating effects of child pornography in this country. In the landmark 1982 US Supreme Court case, *New York v Ferber* (1982), the Court found that child pornography is "intrinsically related to the sexual abuse of children. ... First, the materials produced are a permanent record of circulation. Second, the distribution network for child pornography must be closed if the production of material which requires the sexual exploitation of children is to be effectively controlled." The Court ruled that the standards used to determine obscenity in adult pornography cases are not applicable to child pornography, and child pornography is not protected under the First Amendment.

On May 21, 1984, 7 years after the first federal child pornography statutes were enacted, President Ronald Reagan signed into law the Child Protection Act of 1984. This act amended the original act and created some new statutes, making the federal laws against child pornography more substantial. Some of the more noteworthy changes included the following:

— Raising the age of a minor to younger than age 18

— Eliminating the requirement that child pornography be transported "for sale or distribution for sale"

— Amending the federal wiretap statute to include the Child Protection Act

— Raising the maximum fines from $10 000 to $100 000 for violation by an individual and $250 000 for violation by an organization

— Allowing certain property, including profits and proceeds from the pornographic activity of the violator, to be civilly or criminally forfeited—a change of great importance in the attempt to put child pornographers out of business

For the first time, legal authority to take the profit out of child pornography existed. Congress recognized that to combat sexual exploitation of children, the economic benefits had to be removed, so, in addition to being prosecuted, child pornographers could now be deprived of their property and profits obtained as a result of their criminal acts.

In 1985, President Reagan called upon Attorney General Edwin Meese to create a panel to examine the effects of pornography, in particular, child pornography, on American society. The Commission on Pornography, as it was known, was comprised of a chairman and 10 members. The Commission had several full-time staff investigators, including Postal Inspector Daniel Mihalko.

One of the witnesses who appeared before the Commission and testified was a victim by the name of "Mary."

I was sexually abused as a child in my own home. My abuse started at the age of 3. My father kept suitcases full of pornographic pictures and magazines. From the earliest years, he would have me perform oral sex on him. He would hang me upside down in a closet and push objects like screwdrivers or table knives into me. Sometimes he would heat them first. He would look at his porno pictures almost every day, using them to get ideas of what to do to me or my siblings. I have had my hands tied and my feet tied. He would tell me I was very fortunate to have a father that would teach me the facts of life (Attorney General's Commission on Pornography, 1986).

This is not fantasy or exaggeration. These are the words of a person who was victimized by sexual abuse and pornography as a child and continues to be haunted. Over half of the 92 recommendations made by the Commission specifically addressed the problem of child sexual exploitation. Some of the more significant recommendations were the following:

— State legislatures should amend laws, where necessary, to make knowing possession of child pornography a felony.

— State legislatures should enact legislation that requires photofinishing laboratories to report suspected child sexual abuse and pornography.

— Judges should use, when appropriate, a sentence of lifetime probation for convicted child pornographers after they are released from prison.

— Congress should enact legislation to prohibit the exchange of information concerning child pornography or children to be used in child pornography through computer networks.

— Legislation should recognize and accommodate the limitations involved with the child victim as a witness.

— Social service agencies should be actively involved in treating the victimization that results from the production and distribution of child pornography.

Today, most of the recommendations made by the Attorney General's Commission on Pornography in 1986 have been put into place. Since the Commission concluded its work, Congress has continually passed new legislation to protect our children better and close all possible "loopholes" in existing laws. Some of the more significant legislation created by Congress are listed in **Table 24-1**.

CHILD EXPLOITATION PROGRAM OVERVIEW

The USPIS was the first federal law enforcement agency to begin aggressively identifying, targeting, and arresting commercial child pornography distributors. Recognizing that child molesters and pornographers often seek to communicate with one another through what they perceive as the security and anonymity provided by US mail, Postal Inspectors have been extensively involved in child sexual exploitation and pornography investigations since 1978. They are specially trained to conduct child exploitation investigations and are assigned to each of the USPIS's field divisions nationwide. Use of "undercover operations" designed to flush out mail-order child pornography dealers proved to be most effective, and hundreds of offenders have been

Table 24-1. Legislation Related to Child Pornography	
YEAR	LEGISLATION
1986	Unlawful to place any kind of advertisement offering to provide or seeking to obtain child pornography
1988	Unlawful to use a computer to transmit or knowingly receive child pornography
1990	Unlawful to possess child pornography
1996	Unlawful to use any kind of communication facility, including the mail, to induce, coerce, or entice a minor to engage in sexual conduct, if such conduct would constitute a criminal offense
2002	(a) Unlawful to transport an individual under the age of 18 in interstate or foreign commerce or in any commonwealth, territory, or possession of the United States with intent that the individual engage in prostitution or any other sexual activity
	(b) Unlawful for any person (US citizen or alien admitted into the United States for permanent residency) to travel to a foreign country, or to conspire to do so, for the purpose of engaging in any sexual act with a person under the age of 18

arrested and convicted under the new federal laws. More than 4500 child molesters and pornographers have been arrested since the enactment of the Federal Child Protection Act of 1984.

Due to public outcry and a series of well-publicized incidents involving child exploitation and abuse, state and local law enforcement efforts have eliminated the over-the-counter sale and/or viewing of child pornography in the United States. Unfortunately, the clandestine purchasing and trafficking of this illegal material flourishes and has readily adapted itself to alternative methods and routes of reproduction and dissemination.

Since the advent of publicly available Internet service, the opportunity for exchange and barter involving sexually explicit materials has dramatically increased the amount of child pornography available online. Child molesters and pornographers frequently communicate in select online newsgroups and facilitate through technology videographic and still images of child sexual abuse, both from existing collections as well as in response to requests for new materials. The increase in the victim pool as manifested by newer child pornographic images and bold production techniques has necessitated an equally innovative investigative response. The USPIS has risen to this challenge and continues to prevent the trafficking of videotapes and computer disks through the mail. Approximately 70% of the child sexual exploitation investigations conducted by Postal Inspectors have a common nexus with the Internet and the US mail.

OPERATION AVALANCHE

There has been no investigation in the history of child sexual exploitation cases comparable to Operation Avalanche. This landmark investigation was conducted under the direction of the USPIS and illustrates the success that can be achieved through the cooperation of multiple national and international law enforcement agencies.

In 1999, an alert Postal Inspector in St. Paul, Minnesota, discovered a company called Landslide Productions, Inc, advertising child pornography on the Internet. Further investigation determined Landslide Productions was operating from Ft. Worth, Texas, and appeared to be selling subscriptions to child pornography Web sites. The investigation was passed on to Postal Inspector Robert Adams, assigned to the Ft. Worth USPIS office. Inspector Adams teamed up with Detective Steven Nelson of the Dallas Police Department's Internet Crimes Against Children (ICAC) Task Force, and they launched an undercover investigation into the activities of Landslide Productions. Their work was the beginning of an investigation of unprecedented magnitude since they had a "lion by the tail."

Owned by Thomas and Janice Reedy, Landslide Productions was determined to be a multimillion-dollar child pornography enterprise. Using the screen names of "Houdini" and "Money," the Reedys used their business to advertise and sell prepaid subscriptions to adult and child pornography Web sites to customers from around the world. Landslide Productions was, in fact, a gatekeeper for a number of international Web masters, advertising and marketing child pornography from countries such as Indonesia and Russia as well as the United States.

Initially, the Reedys were bold in their online marketing, using banners such as "Child Porn—Click Here" and "CH!LD R@PE." They eventually changed their advertisements to more covert suggestions of the content of the Web site. For $29.95, an individual could purchase a 1-month subscription to any number of graphic child pornography Web sites. Most customers used credit cards for their purchase; some customers mailed checks, cash, or money orders to Landslide's post office box address in Ft. Worth. The cash flow for Landslide Productions was significant at times, amounting to as much as $1.4 million per month. Not surprisingly, the Reedys enjoyed the fruits of their labors, living in an upscale community in Fort Worth and driving top-end Mercedes Benz automobiles, all of which proved the personal gain motives of their business. The Reedys were living a grand lifestyle at the expense of sexually abused and exploited children.

In September 1999, Adam's investigation, being conducted in concert with the US Attorney's Office for the Northern District of Texas and the Child Exploitation and Obscenity Section (CEOS) of the Department of Justice, gathered sufficient probable cause to obtain multiple federal search warrants for evidence related to the advertisement and distribution of child pornography. On September 8, 6 federal and state agencies executed a series of federal search warrants on the primary business location of Landslide Productions, a secondary Landslide office in Dallas, Texas, and the Reedys' personal residence. The simultaneous raids, led by the USPIS, took more than 18 hours to complete. Under the direction of the USPIS's Forensic and Technical Services Division, Digital Evidence Section, careful efforts were taken to seize, secure, and protect the numerous computer systems located within the properties searched. The data extracted from the computer servers would later be known as the "Holy Grail." Among the evidence seized under the scope of the warrants were financial records revealing that one Web master from Indonesia alone received more than $98 000 in 1 month for his contribution to the criminal enterprise, providing some of the child pornography Web sites for the paying customers.

Through Landslide Productions' network of computer systems and the World Wide Web, the Reedys provided child pornography to thousands of paying customers throughout the world. The success of their endeavor was based on supply and demand. This reinforced the understanding that reproduction and sale of child pornography promoted further production as well as a need for additional and new materials. The tragedy of this form of trade is the fact that real children are sexually abused and photographed or videotaped for the continued enjoyment of a specific clientele.

In April 2000, the Reedys were charged with their crimes in Fort Worth US District Court. A federal grand jury returned an 89-count indictment against them, charging conspiracy to advertise and distribute child pornography and possession of child pornography. Subsequent plea offers by the prosecutors were declined and the case went to trial. During the trial, defense attorneys offered that the Reedys had a lack of content knowledge and intent with respect to the various Web sites that they marketed; however, evidence obtained from the examination of Landslide's computers refuted this. The evidence showed that the Reedys did have knowledge of the child pornography Web sites and payments made by them to the Web masters for the child pornography content.

Testimony was provided by excellent government witnesses, including a detective from the United Kingdom's National Crime Squad, who summarized the problem of child pornography on the Internet through a discussion of the discovery of 2 children who are well known in the child pornography world, Helen and Gavin. Helen and Gavin are British children who were sexually abused and exploited by their stepfather. The detective testified to the extent of abuse and exploitation of the children and how the children have been revictimized, in case after case, by those who reproduce and disseminate their images.

At the conclusion of the case, the jury found the defendants guilty as charged on all counts of the indictment. On August 6, 2001, Thomas Reedy was sentenced to 15 years in federal prison on each of the 89 counts charged. The judge ordered that each 15-year term run consecutive to the previous term for a total of 1335 years. Janice Reedy was sentenced to a 14-year term. The sentences were appealed to the US Court of Appeals for the Fifth Circuit. On appeal, Thomas Reedy's sentence was reduced to 180 years—in essence, a life sentence—and Janice's remained the same.

Through Operation Avalanche, Postal Inspectors conducted undercover investigations and worked with the federally funded ICAC Task Forces across the country, resulting in the arrests of hundreds of offenders. Internationally, the USPIS worked closely with the international police organization, Interpol, and other law enforcement agencies around the world. As a direct result of these international partnerships and the intelligence gained through the Landslide investigation, more than 5000 searches have been carried out in other countries, making this the largest global operation ever undertaken. To this day, subscribers to the child pornography Web sites offered through Landslide Productions, Inc, continue to be investigated in countries around the world.

No offender profile could be created for those individuals who purchased child pornography from Landslide's criminal business. Occupations of the offenders included, but were not limited to, attorneys, physicians, firemen, professional counselors for children, teachers, clergy, and law enforcement officers.

Through Operation Avalanche, vast quantities of child pornography have been seized, scores of individuals have been arrested, and many children have been rescued from further sexual abuse and exploitation.

On October 23, 2002, President George W. Bush was personally briefed by representatives of the USPIS on the Landslide investigation and Operation Avalanche. Following the briefing, the President addressed a group of law enforcement personnel and child protection advocates gathered at the White House. In his statement, the President made a commitment to the American people: "Anyone who targets a child for harm will be a primary target of law enforcement. That's our commitment. Anyone who takes the life or innocence of a child will be punished to the full extent of the law" (Bush, 2002). The President used Operation Avalanche as an example of the government's aggressive efforts to combat the sexual exploitation of children.

OPERATION LOST INNOCENCE

On April 15, 2004, the USPIS and the USDOJ announced the results of a 2-year undercover sting operation that dismantled a large international child pornography ring. Operation Lost Innocence netted 45 child pornographers and molesters in 35 states, Puerto Rico, Cuba, and Ecuador, and shut down a major international child pornography production and distribution network. Over the 2-year period, 103 searches were conducted throughout the country, resulting in the 45 arrests. Most importantly, 150 children were rescued from further sexual abuse.

The announcement of the results of Operation Lost Innocence was made after 45-year-old Angel Mariscal, an Ecuadorian national, was convicted in Miami, Florida, Federal District Court on April 13, 2004, of multiple federal child exploitation crimes. Postal Inspectors began looking into Mariscal's activities in April 2002 after a videotape, suspected of being produced and mailed by Mariscal, was found among other evidence seized from another child pornographer's home in the Detroit, Michigan area. Mariscal was arrested in September 2002 by Postal Inspectors and charged with distributing child pornography by mail. That December, Mariscal was indicted by a federal grand jury in Miami, Florida, on charges of conspiracy to advertise, produce, and ship child pornography.

The Mariscal investigation revealed a horrifying case of sexual abuse, rape, and commercial exploitation of more than 150 children, unraveling an international child pornography ring of staggering proportions. In 1998, Mariscal began conducting a mail-order child pornography business from Miami Beach, Florida. He produced the child pornography outside of the United States, smuggled it into the United States, and then mailed it to customers who had previously placed orders in response to advertisements or catalogs.

The majority of the victims were Cuban and Ecuadorian children between the ages of 6 and 14. The pornography was personally produced by Mariscal and his accomplices, and displayed Mariscal sexually abusing the young children. A 30-minute video or DVD, produced using the customer's own script, sold for as much as $975. At the time of his arrest, Mariscal stated that he was HIV positive. A number of the child victims who were identified and located were tested for the HIV virus but tested negative.

Based on information provided by Postal Inspectors, law enforcement authorities in Cuba and Ecuador arrested 5 coconspirators and identified a number of the child victims. During the international phase of the investigation, invaluable assistance was provided by the Department of State, Bureau of Diplomatic Security, and the Bureau of Immigration and Customs Enforcement.

Nationally, Postal Inspectors worked in conjunction with the USDOJ, CEOS, and the US Attorney's Office, Southern District of Florida. Following Mariscal's arrest, Postal Inspectors, armed with the seized customer list, conducted an undercover operation that led to more than 100 searches in the United States. More than 40 US citizens have been arrested at the time of this writing and more arrests are anticipated. Individuals arrested included police officers, school teachers, a school custodian, a college professor, and a school bus driver.

As found with Operation Avalanche, these offenders come from all walks of life and are difficult to profile but oftentimes are in a "position of trust" and surrounded by children. Tragically, many of these offenders were child pornographers and child molesters.

CONCLUSION

It is a hope that a time will come when textbooks like this will no longer be necessary and our children will be able to grow up in a world free of danger. We have come a long way over the last several decades, but we have much further to go. Only through our continual efforts, individually and collectively, will we help ensure that victimized children and their families receive the attention and services they need and deserve and that their offenders will receive the swift and righteous justice that we as a global society demand.

REFERENCES

Attorney General's Commission on Pornography. *Attorney General's Commission on Pornography final report*. Washington, DC: US Government Printing Office; 1986.

Bush GW. Increasing online safety for America's children. Remarks from: Presidential Action, Dwight D. Eisenhower Executive Office Building; October 23, 2002; Washington, DC.

New York v Ferber, 458 US 747 (1982).

Chapter 25

THE ROLE OF THE FIRST RESPONDER IN THE CRIMINAL INVESTIGATIVE PROCESS

Det Sgt Joseph S. Bova Conti, BA
Col Thomas P. O'Connor, BA, MA

The exploitation of children has been a problem for countless years. Curiosity and trust—innate qualities of children—are normally considered positive character traits, but they can make children particularly vulnerable to sexual predators. Today, under the veil of secrecy provided by electronic technology, the number of exploited children is growing at an alarming rate. The Internet introduces unique and sometimes difficult challenges to the law enforcement community. Jurisdictional boundaries previously recognized by child protection services and police have become blurred. Child exploitation is a worldwide phenomenon. It takes communication and cooperation by those who protect children to bring the criminals to justice.

This chapter reviews the investigative process and the role of the first responder, the uniformed officer, and the investigators and detectives assigned to a case. In most jurisdictions, the first responder is the uniformed officer receiving a call for police. Many times the call coming in is vague, with little information. Therefore, the first officer on the scene is responsible for evaluating the situation and taking the first steps in the investigation. Specialized training and a great deal of experience are required to handle exploitation crimes. The information in this chapter is a culmination of more than 70 combined years of law enforcement experience in the field—experience that includes in-depth interviews with perpetrators. The suggestions contained in this chapter are the result of numerous cases handled personally by the authors and offer a unique perspective into the behavior of the sexual predator. The hope is that this information can help a first responder identify the traits and qualities of sexual predators, effectively elicit confessions, and successfully prosecute the perpetrators.

PRELIMINARY INVESTIGATION BY FIRST RESPONDERS

The criminal investigative process begins with and is based on a well-documented account of all observations, actions, parties present, and evidence relevant to the initial scene. This compilation of facts and ideas helps determine whether a crime has been committed. It is the responsibility of the law enforcement community to make the critical link between mere suspicion and a formal accusation.

Patrol officers responding to a child exploitation call should consider the following factors as an integral part of the preliminary investigative process:

— The investigation starts immediately on arrival at the scene. Visual observations and details about what is being said are important. In particular, anything said spontaneously that is relevant to the issue at hand should be noted and incorporated into the initial report. The first responder's responsibility is to ascertain whether a crime has been committed and if it has, who is responsible.

— The officer should immediately determine whether the victim needs medical assistance and initiate the necessary procedures to provide the appropriate care.

— All witnesses should be identified and interviewed. Their relative involvement in the incident should be noted.

— If applicable, a timeline should be established detailing as much as possible of the who, what, where, when, how, and why of the situation. This timeline becomes a work sheet for the investigation.

— Find and appropriately seize any physical evidence that could help determine what occurred. It may be necessary to obtain a suspect's consent before searching for evidence. Recognize potential evidence, and take the steps necessary to preserve it. Keep in mind the complexities involving electronic imaging and the associated technological equipment. Experience in the field of sexual exploitation of children has revealed that perpetrators often keep a cache of souvenir images. If located, these images become the permanent record of a crime in progress. They can help identify additional victims, witnesses, and suspects.

— A first responder must address the motives involved in the case. If relevant, review the victim's or the witness's motivation for reporting the incident. These should be used in conjunction with observed behavior to show a connection, or lack thereof, with the potential suspects.

— Interview and obtain statements from all parties involved, including but not limited to individuals from other jurisdictions and child protection intervention workers. Include the victim's statements (if appropriate, considering the victim's age and relationship to the potential suspect). Medical records should also be obtained.

— Determine exactly what occurred by specifying the nature of the criminal event and the overt acts associated with the incident.

— If the suspect is at the scene, the on-site officers' responsibility is to identify the individual and establish probable cause. Additionally, an investigator or a first responder may decide to have the suspect voluntarily go to the designated interview area (police department) and then talk with the suspect before making an arrest. Often, circumstances unique to each case influence the timing of an interview strategy and arrest. Numerous factors can be involved, one of which includes establishment of rapport with the suspect. The first responder should evaluate whether it is appropriate to handcuff a suspect in the presence of the victim or the suspect's family, friends, or co-workers. In some situations, it may be better to delay the physical arrest in an attempt to gain the trust and acceptance of the suspect. Consideration should be given to any circumstances that may adversely affect the likelihood of obtaining a confession.

— Police officers should draw on their overall police experience to determine immediately whether they should initiate the interview of the suspect or defer to a more experienced investigator who may be better trained for this intricate communication process.

— If an officer has sufficient training and experience, a confession from the suspect should be obtained that meets all of the criteria associated with current laws (eg, the Miranda decision). A written statement and, if possible, a videotaped statement are crucial for the successful prosecution of the perpetrator.

The initial phase of a child exploitation case involves a complicated sequence of events that involves various activities. Officers should consider their experience and capabilities when assessing the complexity of a case. In addition, only officers who have the appropriate combination of experience and training should use additional resources such as cameras, videos, anatomical dolls, and evidence collection kits.

The responsibility of first responders (police officers) is to establish the initial scope of the investigative process. The second phase of the criminal investigative process is historically the job of investigators (detectives). In traditional police organizations, the detectives are responsible for follow-up investigations. Detectives have the ability, time, and resources to make an in-depth investigation. This is why first responders must be detailed in their findings. Depending on jurisdictions, these roles can be interchangeable or concurrent.

THE INVESTIGATOR

The investigator or detective's role is to obtain the pertinent information that will allow the case to be successfully adjudicated in court. Communication with the witnesses, suspects, victims, and complainants depends on the communication skill level of the investigator.

Information is the essential catalyst of criminal investigations. The predominant body of information is collected by investigators through verbal communication. It is the unique ability of the investigators that elicits appropriate, useful, and accurate information to allow the case to proceed successfully. Cases are made or lost by the effectiveness of the investigators.

A successful investigator of crimes against children has particular character traits, which include but are not limited to the following:

— *An authoritative presence.* Authority should be paired with calmness; overall, a confident demeanor is important.

— *An extroverted personality.* Extroversion is a readily identifiable trait reflected by the investigator's ability to communicate and to show a basic fondness for people.

— *A professional appearance and sense of being capable.* Professionalism helps the suspect perceive the investigator as trustworthy and as a competent problem solver.

— *An accepting and sociable personality.* Acceptance and sociability make the investigator seem more trustworthy to the suspect. For example, what is the investigator's attitude toward the offender? What are the verbal, analytical, and problem-solving skills of the investigator? Is the investigator composed? Does the investigator exhibit empathy and know the difference between empathy and sympathy? Does the investigator display accepted skills of persuasion and influence, justification and rationalization? Are the investigator's behavior and personality reflective of one another? Does the investigator's speech convey a feeling of consistency? Is the interviewer able to address the suspect's fear with a balance of empathetic kindness and concern? Is the interviewer able to control "emotional leakage," which could unintentionally give the offender a glimpse of the investigator's true feelings?

— *An understanding of the difference between guilt and shame (identify with the suspect).* The concepts of guilt and shame are simple but often overlooked. If a suspect feels more ashamed than guilty, the likelihood of obtaining a confession decreases. Shame is an externally based feeling. An ashamed suspect is worried "everybody knows," and the crime will become public knowledge. In contrast, guilt is an internally based feeling involving the suspect's conscience. An investigator should attempt to minimize the suspect's feelings of shame and accentuate the feelings of guilt to elicit a confession.

— *An ability to recognize and address the rationalization process.* Rationalization is nothing more than a justification of behavior by faulty logic. Rationalization involves "poor me" thoughts, feelings of hopelessness and anger, isolationism, inappropriate spontaneous decision making, use of recent life events and previous child abuse as explanations, and use of religious background and confessions to a higher power. Suspects may try everything possible to avoid taking responsibility for their actions.

The methodology of resolving child exploitation cases is partly based on the following investigative goals:

— Identification of the full scope of the crime, remembering that cases involving child exploitation through the Internet, child pornography, and child sexual abuse often encompass more than one crime scene and more than one victim

— Collection and proper recording of all information associated with the investigation

— Evaluation of all of the collected data for evidentiary value; identification of the connection between the evidence and the suspect

— Preparation of an investigative approach to resolve the issue by considering all appropriate psychological strategies needed to obtain a confession or secure evidence; establishment of rapport, which is a key element in the preparation to resolve the case

— Resolution of the case using all resources and skills legally available to the police

The primary goals should be the identification of the perpetrator and determination of the most effective way to obtain a confession. A perfect investigative case would consist of the following 3 elements, known collectively as the *investigative trifecta*:

1. *Physical evidence* showing a relationship between the victim and the perpetrator

2. *Witnesses* with firsthand information

3. A *confession* from the perpetrator

Although not the primary component of most cases, the collection and preservation of physical evidence is critical. Evidence collection is a task best performed by a proficient member of the investigative team. Physical evidence is nonrefutable, provides an association between the suspect and the victim, and can become an advantage for the prosecution in courtroom testimony (**Table 25-1**).

The Interview Process

The development of a theme is a critical part of the interview process, especially with perpetrators of sexual crimes against children. A theme is a scenario or rationalization used to help the suspect make an admission. Ideally, the theme serves to minimize the action of the perpetrator in favor of gaining a confession to the alleged act. To develop a theme, the investigator has to be keenly aware of the suspect's frame of mind. The profile of a sexual offender varies and is complex yet is remarkably linked to victimology, motive, and behavior (see Chapter 30, An Investigation of Victim and Offender Dynamics in Prostitutes and Incarcerated Pedophiles). Sexual offenders are more likely to answer key questions if the questions are presented in a way that allows for rationalization. For example, allowing suspects to take responsibility for their action but on their own terms. Many times, people who molest children believe they are "helping" the child, and in their own mind, never feel as though they have hurt the child. To this end, the investigator may find it helpful to evaluate the following through careful questioning and listening:

— Previous arrest record

— Work experience (especially computer expertise if the case involves the Internet)

— Family background

— History of childhood sexual abuse

Table 25-1. Examples of Evidence

— Souvenirs, including photographs, videos, electronic images, clothing, catalogs, magazines, and all images depicting children, even if not sexual in nature

— Sex toys

— Bindings and sadomasochistic paraphernalia

— Suspect's unwashed clothing and bed linens

— Suspect's DNA

— Suspect's fingerprints

— Cell phone and home phone records

— Computer hard drives, floppy disks, CDs, and DVDs

— Items obtained from search of suspect's employment site (including items from lockers, vehicles, desks, and computers)

— Address books, general and credit card receipts, and cash withdraw and bank records

— History of process addictive behavior, substance addictive behavior, or both

— Current and past residences

— Education

— Social affiliations

— Experience with pornography, voyeurism, and other paraphilia

— Victim preference

— Victim selection and approach

— Grooming techniques

— Whether professional help has ever been sought

— Opinions regarding issues of sexual contact with children and teenagers

Additional interviewing tips are contained in **Table 25-2**. The investigator should also keep the following in mind when interviewing:

— *Victimology.* Victimology involves a detailed assessment of what caused the person to become a victim and the manner in which the person was victimized.

— *Motivation and behavior of the perpetrator (and possibly the victim).* The perpetrator's personality and behavior reflect one another.

— *Power of the police in the interview process.* The suspect and the police should be keenly aware that the interview process may have numerous ramifications for the suspect: a loss of freedom, a loss of substantial finances, separation from mainstream society, and possibly legal execution.

To overcome a suspect's denials and bring closure to a case, you must understand why a perpetrator may try to deceive an investigator. Reasons generally fit into 1 of 2 categories. The first category involves *fear*, including fear of prosecution, termination from a job, embarrassment, restitution, physical safety, punishment, and loss of loving relationships.

Table 25-2. Interviewing Tips

— Learn as much as possible about the suspects before the interview.

— As completely as possible, attempt to detail suspects' recent activities, including their whereabouts at the time of the crime as well as any significant triggers, events, or stressors they have recently experienced.

— Obtain background information by interviewing the suspects' associates, family, and friends, and then develop an interview strategy. The best interview strategies are created when the history is known. Use a standard set of questions to ensure uniformity.

— Schedule uninterrupted time for an interview or interrogation session. These sessions take a lot of time, so plan on it.

— Always interview suspects in a police office or a neutral site. Never interview suspects in their environment.

— Begin the interview process by establishing rapport through conversation and nonthreatening, open-ended questions. Observe (and if possible have someone else watch) and record in detail suspects' nonverbal behavior during the rapport-building process.

— When a particular suspect is determined responsible for a crime, confront the suspect with the conclusion and present themes to elicit an admission, a confession, or both. These themes vary and are created from the information obtained during the interview and preinterview background work. During this direct confrontation, the interviewer must not become condescending or judgmental and must remain empathetic to maintain rapport.

Table 25-3. Occam's Razor
Ancient philosopher William of Occam is credited with the following translated quote: "Of two competing theories or explanations, all other things being equal, the simpler one is to be preferred."

The second category involves *profits* and is especially relevant when the lucrative business of child pornography is involved. Factors include personal gain, greed, and acceptance or losing face. In the pornography business, acceptance by others in the field is critical. By extension, not gaining that acceptance by getting caught or confessing causes one to lose face. Acceptance equals money and losing face cuts profits considerably. By understanding a suspect's reasons for being deceitful, the investigator can tailor the interview questions and evaluate the suspect's psychological responses to structured questions. When formulating questions, use a deductive reasoning approach, in which questions and conclusions are created based on existing information. In contrast, inductive reasoning involves past similarities but no factual data and can cause the investigative process to fail. All statements are relevant even if no statement is made. All cases are different and need to be treated individually even if similarities exist among situations. Finally, remember that when multiple theories exist, the most straightforward is the most likely to be true (**Table 25-3**).

WHEN INVESTIGATIONS FAIL
A rarely talked about topic in criminal investigation is failure, more specifically, the reason an investigation fails. Failure involving any part of the investigative team happens partly because humans are creatures of habit. Some habits inhibit the ability to think clearly and rationally, thus hindering an investigator's ability to effectively solve a case.

As stated previously, inductive reasoning can result in an unsuccessful investigation. More commonly, though, a culmination of factors causes the process to fail. The most common reasons for a failed criminal investigation include the following:

— Tunnel vision or failure to see the big picture

— Excessive reliance on past experiences

— Personal interpretation rather than factual analysis of the evidence

— False identification of and false confessions from a suspect

— Failure to recognize false witnesses

— Preconceived prejudices based on personal value systems and past conditioning

— Excessive reliance on intuition, a powerful and emotional force rarely based in fact and, thus, prone to error

— Inability to use logical reasoning and overcome emotions, often because the physical and psychological trauma of a young victim can be unnerving, making it difficult to suppress emotions

— Failure to accept an external review of the case by disinterested parties

CONCLUSION
The success of the entire investigative process depends on the knowledge, dedication, and tenacity of investigators and their passion to speak up for the victims of these life-changing crimes. Being calm and unemotional, evaluating all components of a case, documenting all pertinent information, carefully interviewing all parties involved, and realizing personal limitations allows an investigator to successfully pursue a case and convict the perpetrators.

Chapter 26

INVESTIGATING INTERNET CHILD EXPLOITATION CASES

Sp Agt Christopher D. Trifiletti

One of the primary reasons many offenders use the Internet to exploit children sexually is because of the expectation of anonymity on the Internet; however, this feeling of anonymity is often false. A good investigator, even an investigator with limited Internet knowledge, can penetrate cyberspace to identify and arrest a suspect.

This chapter provides investigators with the basic knowledge to be a competent first responder to an Internet child sexual exploitation complaint and begin the investigation process. Since this chapter uses many technology-specific terms, **Appendix 26-1** provides a glossary.

An effective response to the growing problem of Internet-based crimes, especially those committed against children, must be a mission rooted in 3 components—enforcement, training, and education. The cooperation of all levels of law enforcement working with civilian groups that have an interest in protecting children has led to a large, and sometimes ambiguous, matrix of law enforcement coordination. However, that children and their families have various resources to protect them from online dangers makes it worth the effort. Enforcement is the most logical and important task for all investigators; however, since the Internet continues to grow and evolve, this medium demands more than enforcement. Proper training of fellow investigators and other members of the criminal justice system, including judges and prosecutors, is necessary. Lastly, members of the education, child advocacy, and healthcare communities, as well as (and most important) parents and guardians must be educated about the risks their children face when using the Internet. Such education should allow them to find the proper balance between allowing their children to use the Internet as an important resource and protecting their children from the dangers that can be found on the Internet. (See **Table 26-1** for a representation of the complex matrix that makes up the discovery and investigation of child exploitation on the Internet.)

Though this educational mission may seem daunting, providing simple brochures and other printed materials through existing community and law enforcement programs is an important first step (**Table 26-2**). These printed guides provide important information for parents who are not as knowledgeable about the Internet as their children and who may not obtain this information by other means. The development of a comprehensive public awareness mission, which includes aggressive media coverage of cases, an Internet Service Provider (ISP) liaison, guidance for computer and other private sector companies, and an educational campaign for parents, teachers, and children, is equally important.

Table 26-1. Investigators and Complainants
ONLINE INVESTIGATORS
— Federal Bureau of Investigation (FBI)
— Immigration and Customs Enforcement (ICE)
— US Postal Inspection Service (USPIS)
— Internet Crimes Against Children (ICAC) Task Forces
LAW ENFORCEMENT COMPLAINANTS
— FBI Offices and Legats
— ICE Field Offices and Attaches
— USPIS Field Offices
— Police Departments
CIVILIAN COMPLAINANTS
— National Center for Missing & Exploited Children (NCMEC)
— Internet Service Providers (ISPs)
— Child Advocates
— Physicians and Other Healthcare
CHILDREN AND FAMILIES

Table 26-2. What Can You Do to Minimize the Chances of an Online Exploiter Victimizing Your Child?

— Communicate with your child about sexual victimization and potential online danger.

— Spend time with your children online. Have them teach you about their favorite online destinations.

— Keep the computer in a common room in the house, not in your child's bedroom. It is much more difficult for a sex offender to communicate with a child when the computer screen is visible to a parent or another member of the household.

— Use parental controls provided by your ISP and/or blocking software but do not totally rely on them. Though an electronic chat room can be a great place for children to make new friends and discuss various topics of interest, it is also prowled by computer sex offenders. Use of chat rooms, in particular, should be heavily monitored.

— Always maintain access to your child's online account and randomly check his/her e-mail. Be aware that your child could be contacted through the US mail. Be upfront with your child about your access and reasons why.

— Teach your child the responsible use of online resources. There is more to the online experience than chat rooms.

— Find out what computer safeguards are used by your child's school, the public library, and at the homes of your child's friends. These are all places, outside of your normal supervision, where your child could encounter an online predator.

— Understand, even if your child was a willing participant in any form of sexual exploitation, that he/she is not at fault and is the victim. The offender always bears the complete responsibility for his or her actions.

— Instruct your children never to do the following:

    — Arrange a face-to-face meeting with someone they met online

    — Upload (post) pictures of themselves onto the Internet or online service to people they do not personally know

    — Give out identifying information such as their name, home address, school name, or telephone number

    — Download pictures from an unknown source as there could be sexually explicit images

    — Respond to messages or bulletin board postings that are suggestive, obscene, belligerent, or harassing

    — Not to believe that whatever they are told online; it may or may not be true

Adapted from Federal Bureau of Investigation (FBI). A parent's guide to Internet safety. FBI Publications Web site. Available at: http://www.fbi.gov/publications/pguide/pguidee.htm. Accessed August 23, 2004.

Stimulating public interest and involvement is important, but investigators should be familiar with organizations formed by private citizens to help fight child exploitation on the Internet. Though the mission of such groups is admirable, investigators in some countries, including the United States, have encountered difficulties (eg, insufficient information, the improper handling of potential evidence) when working with these groups. Most alarming is the activity of some unauthorized members who go against the principles of the group to conduct their own Internet investigations, thereby opening themselves to potential criminal liability. Sadly, some agencies have seen members of these organizations use their affiliation as a cover or alibi when being prosecuted for violations of the law. Since background investigations or references are not required of their members, a person with a criminal history or poor morals will usually not be discovered until it is too late. Investigators are reminded to consider this when receiving complaints from the Internet community.

A New Area to Patrol

Identifying Suspects and Potential Crime Areas on the Internet

Law enforcement personnel should think of the Internet as a new type of community that should be patrolled for crime. This is especially true when comparing an Internet investigation to a more well-known type of criminal investigation (eg, a drug investigation). For example, a drug investigator's typical day is comprised of looking for "bad" people or patrolling "bad" areas. (In this chapter, a "bad" person or area is considered a person or place "predicated" or predisposed to commit a crime.) In most countries, predications about who or what area is bad allow investigators to begin the process of identifying, investigating, and arresting suspects who have become known to law enforcement officials by citizen complaint, forensic evidence, or through undercover techniques, where legally acceptable (**Table 26-3**).

Table 26-3. Examples of Predication

Predicated Location	Predicated Person

— Chat room name:
    — littlegirlsexchat
    — underage_boy_pics
— File names:
    — lolita
    — 8yo
    — Twinks
    — illegal teen
	— Citizen complaint:
	    — "He is saying sexual things to my son."
	    — "He tried to meet my daughter online."
	— Criminal history:
	    — Registered sex offender and known
	      suspicious Internet use

Law enforcement officials patrol bad areas to gather intelligence information for future investigations. In Internet investigations, investigators obtain this information by reading material posted on the Internet by potential abusers and by monitoring known, predicated areas that draw potential abusers. The resulting intelligence helps identify the bad people who posted the recovered information. In addition, investigators may predicate suspects from citizen and/or parent complaints. As a result of the sheer volume of information and areas on the Internet, information received from technical and professional sources helps focus the investigators' limited resources as they search for suspects regardless of the way in which these suspects were initially predicated. Since most countries lack laws requiring ISPs to provide information useful to law enforcement officials, such assistance from outside sources helps. As a result of working together, positive, friendly relationships are encouraged between law enforcement officials and information technology employees.

Prosecution of Suspects

Regardless of the way a suspect was identified, whenever possible, investigators are urged to prosecute the suspect in the jurisdiction in which he or she resides in order to facilitate the potential identification of other victims. Prosecution in the suspect's place of residence generates the greatest amount of community impact through media and neighborhood attention. Such attention helps increase public awareness about this crime problem and potentially reaches families so that future victimization of this kind may be prevented.

Since the Internet community is global, if a suspect is believed to live in another country, investigators are encouraged to refer these suspects to the appropriate law enforcement agencies. A suspect who commits an offense in North America one moment could easily commit the same type of crime in Europe moments later without changing his or her physical location. Working on international cases or multistate investigations is challenging because of differing laws and investigative procedures; however, the virtual mobility of the Internet offender and the various information and resources necessary to conduct Internet investigations require investigators to work together.

INVESTIGATION TASK FORCES

Even when working with a local investigation, investigators must pool their investigative skill and resources, which has led to expansive use of the task force concept. Task forces, which include members of multiple agencies and jurisdictions, ensure the best chance of identifying and arresting offenders and the proper sharing of expensive computer and labor resources as well as the resultant criminal intelligence that develops from the work performed. An effective task force has key resources and members available though sometimes one person may have to perform many of these roles simultaneously, as is the case with a smaller task force (**Figure 26-1**). Task force members should include the following:

— Coordinators who serve as liaisons between other task force members and law enforcement agencies

— Computer forensics examiners who review the deluge of equipment and media seized from suspects and victims

— Intelligence analysts who interpret the case evidence, digital or otherwise

— Attorneys who are knowledgeable in this area and can readily interpret the rapidly developing area of computer and Internet law

— Child interviewers who are skilled in working with child victims

— Victim and witness specialists who help protect the welfare of child victims and maintain the integrity of the case

Some investigators may feel helpless to create such a task force; however, the same virtual mobility the offenders seek on the Internet can be used to create a local or regional task force or work group in which the members do not necessarily need to occupy the same office space. Though sensitive case or victim information should *never* be transmitted via the Internet without appropriate security precautions, the use of e-mail and other Internet services for less sensitive information can reduce the need for face-to-face contact, thereby helping to make such virtual work groups effective.

Whether a task force is large or small, local or regional, or real or virtual, most realize that a single group can not handle all of the local complaints received from the public, let alone the national and international Internet child exploitation complaints received. In an effort to meet these obligations on a national basis, many countries have established centers to serve as national collection points for Internet complaint information.

In the United States, the joint publicly and privately funded National Center for Missing & Exploited Children (NCMEC) serves this function. All NCMEC functions are specific to crimes against children, including the NCMEC's CyberTipline for Internet child exploitation complaints.

Figure 26-1. *Various roles in a sample task-force.*

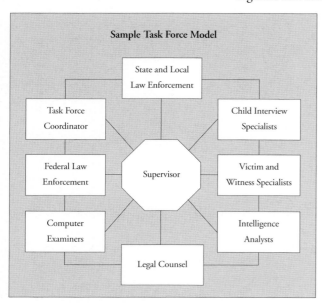

In other countries, these centers may handle other Internet crimes as well as child exploitation crimes. In some countries, a government agency runs the hotline, and other countries have a private interest group, which cooperates with government officials, monitoring and maintaining the hotline (as is the case with the NCMEC). Whether run by a government agency or a private interest group, information centers can be a useful resource to all investigators. Regardless of the information center's size, the investigators, and especially the first responders, must make the case to save the victimized children.

ROLE OF THE INVESTIGATOR

Understanding the basic concepts presented in this chapter will enable investigators to work effectively and efficiently with other cybercrime investigators but will not qualify investigators to work proactively online to seek suspects or perform the computer forensic work necessary for case prosecution. These areas are specific disciplines that require extensive training; an unprepared investigator would do more harm than good. Rather, investigators should use the information provided in this chapter to ask the right questions of suspects, victims, and witnesses and to learn where to find the right information and evidence to begin an investigation.

INTERNET BASICS

TRADER AND TRAVELER CASES

Internet child sexual exploitation complaints typically comprise 2 violations:

1. Complaints about child pornography

2. Complaints about people attempting to meet children via the Internet for sexual exploitation purposes

These crimes are sometimes referred to as **trader** and **traveler** cases, respectively. These terms are admittedly too kind when compared to the ghastly crimes they represent. In fact, many investigators worldwide no longer use the term *child pornography* and instead use the term **child abuse images** since it more accurately describes this crime, which perpetuates the abuse of the child victim long after the images are taken.

While most countries have recognized this and have adopted laws prohibiting the production, transmission, and possession of child pornography (**Table 26-4**), the use of the Internet to meet children for sex may not, by itself, be a violation in many countries. Even in such countries, however, if the suspect is successful in his or her attempt to meet a child and engages in sexual activity, he or she will be prosecutable under relevant sex offense laws and the potential for Internet evidence can not be overlooked.

LOCATING EVIDENCE

If investigators are called to identify a trader or traveler, they must know where to look and how to find the necessary evidence. If the Internet is patrolled as another crime area, as previously suggested, investigators must understand what this Internet "neighborhood" looks like. This can be a bit confusing because no single entity owns or runs the Internet.

The Internet Corporation for Assigned Names and Numbers (ICANN), a multinational organization, performs many of the Internet's managerial functions, such as the assignment of Internet protocol address block assignments and the design and adoption of Internet naming standards, as their name implies. The ICANN took over these functions from the United States-led Internet Assigned Name Authority (IANA). Despite this change, many people believe the Internet remains unduly dominated by the United States. While the ICANN and other Internet managerial bodies typically control key parts of this infrastructure, most widely used services on

Table 26-4. Countries That Submitted Information on Exploitation Laws to Interpol

A	B	C	D	E
— Albania	— Bahamas	— Cambodia	— Denmark	— Ecuador
— Andorra	— Bahrain	— Canada	— Djibouti	— Egypt
— Argentina	— Barbados	— Chile	— Dominican Republic	— El Salvador
— Armenia	— Belarus	— China (Hong Kong)	— Dominica	— Estonia
— Australia	— Belgium	— Colombia		
— Austria	— Bolivia	— Costa Rica		
— Azerbaijan	— Bosnia Herzegovina	— Côte d'Ivoire		
	— Botswana	— Croatia		
	— Brazil	— Cuba		
	— Brunei	— Cyprus		
	— Burundi	— Czech Republic		

F	G	H	I	J
— Fiji	— Georgia	— Honduras	— Iceland	— Jamaica
— Finland	— Germany	— Hungary	— India	— Japan
— France	— Gibraltar		— Indonesia	
	— Greece		— Ireland	
	— Guatemala		— Israel	
	— Guinea		— Italy	
	— Guyana			

K	L	M	M	O
— Kazakhstan	— Latvia	— Macao	— Namibia	— Oman
— Kenya	— Lebanon	— Malta	— Nepal	
	— Lesotho	— Mauritania	— Netherlands	
	— Liechtenstein	— Mauritius	— New Zealand	
	— Lithuania	— Mexico	— Norway	
	— Luxembourg	— Moldova		
		— Monaco		
		— Mongolia		
		— Myanmar		

P	R	S	T	U
— Pakistan	— Romania	— St. Kitts & Nevis	— Tanzania	— Ukraine
— Panama	— Russia	— Senegal	— Thailand	— United Kingdom
— Peru		— Singapore	— Trinidad & Tobago	— United States
— Philippines		— Slovakia	— Tunisia	— Uruguay
— Poland		— Slovenia	— Turkey	— Uzbekistan
— Puerto Rico		— South Africa		
— Portugal		— Spain		
		— Sri Lanka		
		— Swaziland		
		— Sweden		
		— Switzerland		
		— Syria		

V
— Venezuela

Specific legislation can be viewed at and table adapted from Legislation of Interpol member states on sexual offences against children. Interpol Web site. Available at: https://www.interpol.int/Public/Children/SexualAbuse/NationalLaws/Default.asp. Accessed February 21, 2005.

the Internet follow a commonly accepted protocol that is specific to each service. New protocols are usually first described in Request for Comments (RFC) documents. These RFCs are formal papers that guide the evolution of the Internet upon their acceptance and adoption. The major services currently in public use on the Internet include the following:

— World Wide Web (WWW)

— Internet Relay Chat (IRC)

— Electronic mail (e-mail)

— Usenet newsgroups

— File Transfer Protocol (FTP)

— Web-based chat (WBC)

— Messengers

— Peer-to-peer (P2P) networks

Each of these areas facilitates different types of communication but all can foster child sexual exploitation. To investigators, the major difference between these areas is the information that must be obtained through interviews or physical evidence, which enables a suspect to be located. As the Internet evolves, these services will evolve, and others will be added. As a result, investigators must remain abreast of these changes to conduct investigations properly. To maintain compatibility among computer operating systems on the Internet, all existing and emerging services generally comply with the Transmission Control Protocol (TCP) and/or Internet Protocol (IP). Advanced Internet investigators should have a grasp of these TCP/IP concepts.

Regardless of the service used, an Internet user must connect to a point-of-presence (POP) and obtain an IP address, which is essentially a unique number that identifies a particular computer to others on the Internet. Users of the Internet primarily connect via one of the following 3 means (**Figure 26-2**):

1. A modem or cable modem and an ISP

2. An online service provider that allows an Internet connection

3. An Internet gateway provided by a corporate, government, library, education, or other computer network

All of these connection types have seen massive increases in bandwidth in recent years. Increased transmission speeds, resulting from broadband services, such as Digital Subscriber Lines (DSLs) and cable modems, have increased the potential damage that can be done to child victims. Greater numbers of child pornography images and even full-motion video images can be easily transmitted on the Internet, thereby creating permanent records of the child and causing repeated, perpetual victimization.

Fortunately, users of these connection methods, including broadband services, can usually be traced to their origin and identified to stop the abuse. When conducting such investigations, the primary concern is whether Internet records are available to follow the trail from the user's online identity to his or her true identity. Depending on which Internet service is being used, investigators need to obtain different information to begin this identification process (**Table 26-5**). Not all information is necessary to trace the offender successfully; however,

Figure 26-2. People connect to the Internet through a modem or cable modem and an ISP, an online service provider that allows an Internet connection, or an Internet gateway provided by a computer network.

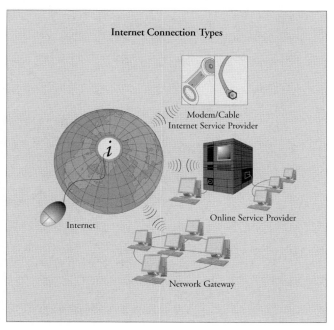

Internet Connection Types

Modem/Cable
Internet Service Provider

Online Service Provider

Internet

Network Gateway

Table 26-5. Information Necessary to Begin Tracing Offenders Identified Using Common Internet Protocols

WORLD WIDE WEB (WWW)

— Uniform Resource Locator (URL)
   (ie, Internet address)
— Domain name or Internet Protocol
   (IP) address
— Hosting
— Connection
— Domain name system (DNS) provider(s)

ELECTRONIC MAIL (E-MAIL)

— Complete Internet message headers
   (ie, full or advanced header, not just basic
   "To" and "From" lines)

FILE TRANSFER PROTOCOL (FTP)

— IP address
— Date
— Time
— Time zone
— Nickname
— Advertised location, if any

MESSENGERS

— Online identity (ie, screen name, identity
   name, or unique number)
— Chat room(s) used

INTERNET RELAY CHAT (IRC)

— IP address
— Date
— Time
— Time zone and/or nickname
— Server
— Channel(s) used

NETWORK NEWS TRANSFER PROTOCOL (NNTP)

— Complete Internet message headers (ie, similar
   to but different from e-mail headers)
— Posting nickname(s) and group(s)

PEER-TO-PEER (P2P) NETWORKS

— IP address
— Date
— Time
— Time zone
— Network, program, and online identity used

WEB-BASED CHAT (WBC)

— Online identity (ie, nickname) used by suspect
— Web site(s) and chat room(s) used

Table 26-6. "Traditional" Investigative Techniques

— Pretext calls	— Surveillance
— Phone records	— Trap and trace
— Interview/Interrogation	

the likelihood of success increases with more complete and accurate information.

Investigators must remember that the computer is an instrument used in this type of crime and not an end in itself. When the identification of a suspect through Internet means alone is unclear or needs further supporting evidence, investigators should rely upon more traditional investigative techniques to help identify the perpetrator behind the keyboard (**Table 26-6**).

WORLD WIDE WEB

The World Wide Web (WWW), or "Web" for short, is most users' introduction to the Internet. In fact, most people perceive that the Web is the entire Internet and remain oblivious to the other services available. The Web is easy to use, which has resulted in a high rate of use among all age groups; however, from an investigator's point of view, the Web can be difficult to master.

The Web is largely comprised of billions of pages of information that provide everything: basic text, images, movies, music, and even software. Usually, multiple pages are organized to form a Web site. Every page and element within the Web site has an Internet address, or Uniform Resource Locator (URL), that defines its location on the Web. By simply following a hyperlink on any page, users can be taken to other locations to view other Web content. This content can easily originate from a country other than that of the user even if the user is unaware. In fact, a single Web page is often comprised of content from multiple states or countries, thereby complicating Web site investigations.

HYPERTEXT TRANSFER PROTOCOL

A knowledgeable Internet user may recognize the commonly used term Hypertext Transfer Protocol (HTTP). Though often listed with a Web page address, HTTP means little to the average user even though HTTP is the essential means by which Web pages are transmitted for viewing. This is probably because the HTTP portion of a Web address does not usually need to be included in a Web browser to find the page and is often omitted. Likewise, the term WWW is often redundant, unnecessary, and unused. The information that flows over HTTP on the WWW includes the Hypertext Markup Language (HTML) programming code and the contents of other files related to the Web site being viewed (**Figure 26-3**). This code and all files related to the Web site can be useful to investigators as they search for the necessary information to trace the Web site and identify the responsible party.

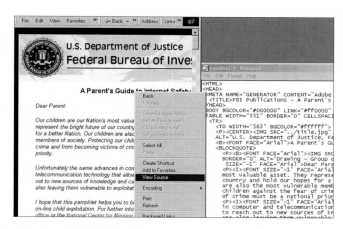

Figure 26-3. *Screen capture from the FBI Web site and the related HTML source code.*

PROBLEMS INVESTIGATORS CONFRONT

Previously, the Web was not widely used for child pornography because of the ease of determining the person(s) responsible for the content. Usually, this determination was not because of the HTML code but because of log files and billing records. Unfortunately, this has changed because of free Web hosting and the complexity of the Web pages themselves. Adding to the confusion is the process of Web page redirection. This redirection may cause an Internet user to be unaware that the Web page address selected for viewing is not the one being viewed. Another problem with Web site investigations is that multiple suspects can be responsible for a single page or site. This is especially true with a type of Internet service known as a virtual community, which is often referred to as a Web club, e-group, or Web community. In a virtual community, single Web sites can contain content posted by multiple members of the club who are usually offered free and unverified memberships. In other words, a single Web page may contain content originating from multiple domestic suspects or even suspects from other countries who have provided little or no true identity information.

INFORMATION HELPFUL TO INVESTIGATORS

The minimum information necessary to begin a Web site investigation includes the URL of the site, including the domain name and as much information about the content's actual location as possible. Investigators find a printout of the Web site contents helpful. Ideally, an investigator has a copy of the Web site contents saved to a diskette since the contents can provide useful information in the HTML code and related files. From this information, an Internet investigation specialist can locate the registrant of the domain name, the host of the content, the ISP providing the Internet connection to the content (often the same as the host), and the ISP providing the domain name system (DNS) entry for the Web site (**Figure 26-4**). Although these components are the keys to a successful Web site investigation, bogus registration information and frequently changing international hosts and connections have been a challenge in many attempts to dismantle child exploitation Web sites. Investigations of virtual communities have been more successful, mostly because the Web site host can provide other information that is useful in tracing the offenders.

Whether for basic Web site investigations or for an investigation of a Web site that hosts a virtual community, an accurate URL must be obtained in a timely fashion, or the investigation will be over before it has begun. The complexity of URLs can seem difficult to investigators, but this need not be the case. In the following examples, an

Figure 26-4. *Web site components help investigations by providing keys to identify the creator of a site.*

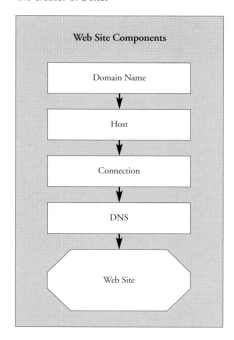

Table 26-7. Generic Top-Level Domains and Their Typical Uses	
.biz	Business
.com	Commercial
.edu	US educational institutions
.gov	US government
.info	Informational
.int	Established by treaty
.mil	US military
.net	Internet infrastructure
.org	Nonprofit organizations

Note: In the case of all but the ".edu," ".gov," ".mil," and ".int" domains, the use of the gTLD is generally at the discretion of the domain's registrant. This means that a Web site registered as ".org" may not be a nonprofit entity, one registered as ".net" may not be an Internet infrastructure component, and so on.

Table 26-8. Country Code Identifiers	
.au	Australia
.be	Belgium
.ca	Canada
.cc	Cocos (Keeling) Islands
.cr	Costa Rica
.de	Germany
.es	Spain
.fr	France
.ie	Ireland
.jp	Japan
.ky	Cayman Islands
.nl	The Netherlands
.nu	Niue Islands
.py	Paraguay
.ru	Russia
.se	Sweden
.tv	Tuvalu

investigator would be interested in the top-level domain (TLD), that is, "anyisp," as the proper ISP to begin the investigation:

— http://www.anyisp.com

— http://www.anyserver.anyisp.com

— http://clubs.anyisp.com/preteensex

— http://clubs.anyisp.com/html/93000673/73012486/club?target=preteensex

In each of these examples, "anyisp.com" is referred to in the domain name portion of the Internet address, which includes the ".com" portion [also known as the generic top-level domain (gTLD)]. For US domain names, the domain name is always the portion of the address directly before the gTLD and includes the gTLD itself. Current, common gTLDs and their typical uses are listed in **Table 26-7**.

Since the Internet is a global entity, a method is available to determine a Web site's possible country of origin. A domain can be registered with a country code top-level domain (ccTLD) in which the domain name is augmented with the 2-letter country identifier. For example, "http://www.anyisp.co.uk" would be the Internet address for "anyisp" in the United Kingdom; "anyisp. co.uk" is the ccTLD in this example. Country identifiers may or may not describe the country of origin, however. Since most Internet registrars do not verify registration information, a domain registrant can often choose to register in a country different than the ccTLD of the Web site's domain. As a result, ccTLDs may not be entirely useful in locating an offender, but a basic knowledge of ccTLDs is often helpful for investigators. **Table 26-8** lists examples of country code identifiers.

INTERNET RELAY CHAT

Internet Relay Chat (IRC) is accessible to all Internet users although many people may not be aware of this. By using appropriate software, users can connect to an IRC network server (**Figure 26-5**). Users then become connected to a particular network in which real-time "chats" with other users worldwide can be conducted in a "chat room." Thousands of Internet chat rooms exist. Each is referred to within IRC as a channel.

In addition to providing chat rooms, IRC allows for private conversations and the private exchange of files without the use of e-mail. Through a process known as a ***file server (f-serve)***, automated file exchanges can be accomplished.

As with all other Internet services, IRC can be used by legitimate users for legitimate means but can be abused by those seeking to exploit children. Major ISPs allocate server space to IRC and do not attempt to manage the content. As a result, no one owns IRC, and users are free to create whatever channels they wish to meet others, chat, and/or trade files. Unfortunately, IRC is perceived as a nearly risk-free environment for Internet users who believe they are free to do whatever they want, when they want.

For law enforcement officials to identify suspects on IRC, they must obtain a great deal of specific information. First of all, a user's IRC nickname, or the online identity of the user, should be obtained. This information alone is insufficient to determine a user's identity since IRC users can change their nicknames instantly. To be certain about a user's identity, an investigator must have the IP address of the user as well as the date, time, and time zone of the connection. Though such information is usually easily obtained via IRC software, complaining parties rarely have this information. As a result, investigators may need to obtain more general information (eg, IRC network and server to which the suspect was connected, the channel(s) used by the suspect) to locate the suspect. As with all Internet evidence, anything saved to disk will likely be more useful than printed items, so investigators should be sure to obtain disks from complainants and victims whenever possible. **Table 26-9** presents a sample of IRC channels and their descriptions, which are created by and available to IRC users.

ELECTRONIC MAIL

Electronic mail can be sent from and received within virtually any paid ISP account as well as via many free e-mail services (eg, Yahoo!, Hotmail), which are available to people who have an Internet connection. Although an increasing number of people are using free e-mail services and Web browsers to view their e-mail, this e-mail service is not really a Web function.

As with other Internet services, e-mail operates via its own set of protocols. The common protocols for e-mail are Simple Mail Transmission Protocol (SMTP) for sending e-mail and either Post Office Protocol (POP3) or Internet Message Access Protocol (IMAP) for receiving e-mail. Again, most users are unaware of the technical nature of e-mail; they view e-mail as only an exchange of text and files between the addressed Internet users.

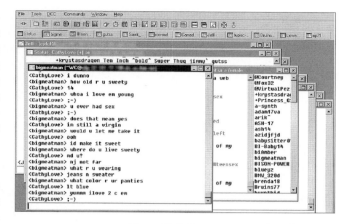

Figure 26-5. *Screen capture of a software program that is used to access IRC.*

Table 26-9. Sample Internet Relay Chat Channels and Their Descriptions

CHANNEL NAME	DESCRIPTION
#0!!!!!!!!!!!!!!12yroldsexx	[-Roleplay-Cybersex-&-Porno-]
#0!!!!!!!!!!!!!!preteen101	Welcome to 101—on-topic material
#0!!!!!!!!!!!!preteen00	We're open again, and doing great
#0!!!!!!!!!!!!littlekidsex	WelCome…16yo and younger cum play
#0!!!!!!!!!!!!mom'n'sonsex	#1 Place 4 Moms
#0!!!!!!!!!!!pedomoms	Men who love women and their kids
#0!!!!!!!!!!family_lovers	A Real family love channel
#0!!!!!!!!!dad&daughtersex	Come in and Chat…16+ Fantasy Only
#0!!!!!!!!!preteenrapesex	Roleplay-Cybersex-&-Porno
#0!!!!!!!!childslavesex	For those that love young slaves
#0!!!!!!!!forcedfamilysex	Fantasy Sex—Come in and play—16+
#0!!!!!!!!littleboysexchat	For boys and boy-lovers
#0!!!!!!!!ltlgirlsexchat	Where Young Girls get lots of loving
#0!!!!!!childsexchat	Where the kids are sexually active

Note: The exclamation points (or "bangs") in the channel names result in these channels being sorted to the top of a computer alphabetized list. Since this is an example, most IRC channels at the top of such a list are related to child sexual exploitation.

Investigators should note that e-mail information that is commonly seen by most users (eg, the "To" and "From" information) can be easily altered by using a spoof or remailer. Furthermore, most free e-mail accounts can be created using false user information or no information at all. Currently, e-mail "spam" exploits these vulnerabilities and has become a major scourge of the Internet; e-mail spam goes well beyond the simple annoyance of a clogged inbox. In fact, the use of spam e-mail as a delivery system for online security threats is considered a future threat to the Internet itself.

Tracking spam, which includes tracing messages that offer child pornography, has become incredibly difficult. In contrast, most personally addressed e-mail is easier to trace by using the more reliable information related to e-mail transmission, which is found in the message's header.

If a complainant or investigator has a copy of the message text but not the header information, then the entire message may be obtained if that message remains stored on the mail server of the user's ISP. When in doubt, investigators should contact a properly trained investigator to help save the e-mail message to a disk since a printout alone may be insufficient to trace the message.

Unfortunately, increased public knowledge regarding the ability of law enforcement officials to trace e-mail messages, in addition to the recent use of systems that can monitor e-mail in real time by law enforcement officials, has sparked a growing interest in "secure" e-mail services (eg, Hushmail, SafeMessage, ZipLip). The names of these services clearly indicate they are designed to ensure the privacy of e-mail, thereby complicating the investigator's role. These services are rarely used for child exploitation offenses, however, and most e-mail remains easily traceable if a true copy of the e-mail and the message's header information is obtained.

USENET NEWSGROUPS

Usenet newsgroups can be thought of as virtual bulletin boards on which messages containing text and computer files are posted for public exchange. Newsgroups are continuously updated by users worldwide and are usually not monitored by the ISPs that host them. More than 90 000 known newsgroups currently exist. These newsgroups serve legitimate and illegitimate topics. Because of the lack of monitoring and sheer volume of groups and postings, newsgroups are thought of as yet another "risk-free" Internet service for the posting and downloading of child exploitation materials.

Dedicated investigators can be on the winning side of this problem though. Newsgroup postings are maintained at ISPs for a matter of days or weeks and then may become available to download and trace to the user who posted the information, thereby providing valuable information to quick-acting investigators. Many ISPs will not carry some of the most heinous newsgroups; therefore, people interested in such groups must pay for a private newsgroup service. To conduct this type of investigation, investigators who want to fight members of such newsgroups must also pay for this private service.

As with other Internet services, posting and downloading content on newsgroups follows a protocol. In the case of newsgroups, the protocol is called Network News Transfer Protocol (NNTP).

As with e-mail, most newsgroup postings can be easily traced by careful analysis of message header information, which can be used to identify the authoring account (**Figure 26-6**). The analysis of newsgroup headers can be challenging, so investigators are urged to obtain a copy of the posting's complete message header for later analysis. Usually, if information such as the posting host and date, time, and time zone stamp are obtained from saved evidence, the user can be traced; however, various portions of a message header may be forged. For this reason, ISPs may use different portions of a message header to determine the authoring account. As a result, an investigator's best course of action is to provide the ISP with the entire message header if possible. Even if the suspect posting is no longer available to be downloaded and investigated, knowledge about the poster's online identity, the subject description of the postings, and the newsgroup to which the message is being posted can help locate the suspect. A small sample of child sexual exploitation-related newsgroups available on Usenet is presented in **Table 26-10**.

FILE TRANSFER PROTOCOL

Programs that use File Transfer Protocol (FTP) are still widely used by people who trade child pornography even though newer, more powerful programs exist. Users of any of the previously mentioned services (eg, World Wide Web, IRC, or newsgroups) may encounter Web pages, IRC messages, and newsgroup postings that offer FTP services (**Figure 26-7**). An FTP advertisement typically includes the IP address of the FTP server in addition to the username (ie, nickname) and password needed to connect to the server.

Like many Internet child exploiters, advertisers of FTP servers almost never charge for their services and are usually individual users operating an FTP program on their home, work, or school computer in an effort to propagate child pornography. Though this effort can require advertisement to others, hundreds and perhaps thousands of servers are probably operating secretly on the Internet at any given time.

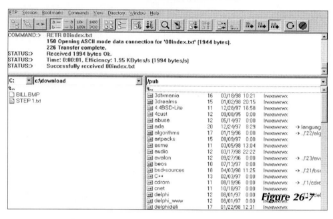

Figure 26-6.

Figure 26-6. Screen capture of a newsgroup posting with full headers displayed

Figure 26-7. Screen capture of a program that allows the use of FTP.

Table 26-10. Newsgroups Related to Child Sexual Exploitation

Newsgroup names are usually broken into segments that allow users to ascertain some information about the newsgroup's topic. The following provide examples:

— alt.binaries.pictures.erotica.age.13-17

— alt.binaries.pictures.erotica.child

— alt.binaries.pictures.erotica.child.female

— alt.binaries.pictures.erotica.child.male

— alt.binaries.pictures.erotica.lolita

— alt.fan.yardbird

— pedo.binaries.pictures.erotica.pre-teen

Newsgroups with clandestine names as well as privately circulated newsgroups also exist. For the descriptive newsgroups listed above, the following definitions are provided:

— alt	alternative
— binaries	binary data
— pictures	picture files
— erotica	erotic or sexual content
— pedo	pedophilic content

Once connected to an FTP server, users may upload and download files, including child pornography images. Similar in operation to an f-serve on IRC, FTP servers usually require users to upload images to receive credit to download others.

WEB-BASED CHAT

In recent years, many users have taken to Web-based chat (WBC), or chat, which functions within a Web browser. WBC is popular because it is easy to use when compared with paid services provided by online service providers (eg, America Online [AOL]) and free services like IRC chat. Chat within a Web browser is accomplished by using small programs (known as *applets* or *scripts*) downloaded by the user to the computer browser. As in IRC, Web-based chat online identities or nicknames are easily changed. Even more challenging for investigators, though, is that the evidence of chat rooms visited and messages sent and received are usually not logged because these chats occur within the Web browser. This means that though IRC and WBC have legitimate uses, some unscrupulous users have flocked to them in particular since a record of their communication is not maintained unless intentionally kept by the sender or receiver. In other words, the computers of many suspects and victims might not show obvious signs of them having used these services.

Web-based chat that incorporates Voice over IP (VoIP) further complicates this problem for investigators. As used in a Web browser, VoIP allows users to talk to one another rather than typing their chat. Whether via VoIP or regular chatting, tracing a user of WBC requires knowledge of the nickname or other online identity being used by the user as well as a specific location of the chat since one Web site can host thousands of different chat rooms. Investigators must work quickly on WBC cases because the logs to trace offenders may expire within hours or days if such logs are kept at all.

MESSENGERS

Another rapidly growing area of use on the Internet is that of **messengers**, which are free, standalone software programs offering users the ability to instant message one another, create private or multiuser chat rooms, and send messages to and from properly equipped cellular telephones. The most popular of these messengers are ICQ (also known as *I Seek You*), AOL Instant Messenger (AIM), Yahoo! Messenger, and Microsoft Network (MSN) Messenger (**Figure 26-8**). Millions of people use these products as online Internet "buddy" locators or as a way to find friends to chat with as well as powerful file transfer programs. Most people support some form of voice and video chat or VoIP. Many functions of the messenger programs are being built into Internet-based game software that include real-time chat between worldwide participants. Unfortunately, most parents will not realize the potential harm of such games since their sole understanding of the Internet is that of the Web browser. As a result, this concept will likely prove especially risky for unsupervised children.

Figure 26-8. The 4 primary messengers include AOL Instant Messenger, ICQ, Yahoo! Messenger, and MSN Messenger.

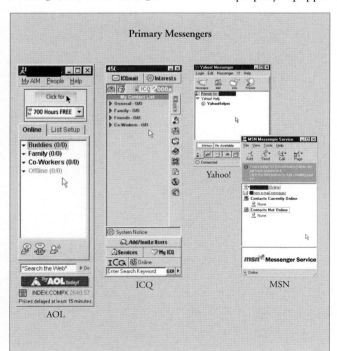

The information necessary to locate the user of a WBC or messenger program varies depending on the type of service used. Usually a nickname or other online identity (eg, a unique, identifying number) is sufficient; however, more specific information (eg, e-mail address, IP address) may be available. Investigators should be particularly specific and thorough when dealing with these services since one piece of information may be the difference between identifying or missing a targeted subject.

PEER-TO-PEER NETWORKS

Currently, a relatively new variant of Internet programs known as peer-to-peer (P2P) networks are some of the most hotly debated. The term **peer-to-peer network** refers to 2 or more computers directly connected to one another without the aid of a central server. However, P2P has become more widely associated with Internet P2P programs, which make file sharing easy for the masses.

Though most of the media rhetoric concerns on the protection of intellectual property rights and copyright enforcement are outside the scope of this chapter, investigators should be aware that, if left unchecked, no other area on the Internet seems to have as much future damage potential in terms of child pornography.

Programs such as Gnutella, WinMX, eDonkey, Morpheus, and KaZaA that run on the major P2P networks have the potential to propagate child pornography and frustrate even the most highly trained investigator. As parents strive to recognize the new "danger areas" for their children, these programs pose a great problem. This is because most of these programs show only an icon in the system tray on a Windows-based computer. This means that the program icon will show up only in the area near the computer's clock rather than on the taskbar at the bottom center of the screen where most users, including parents, expect to see icons.

When running a P2P program, users are not usually connected to other users via a central network; rather, they are directly connected to one another (hence the term *peer-to-peer*). All users can share files with one another, thereby allowing an unlimited ability to download and upload computer files, including software, music, images, and video. Since users have a direct connection to each other, criminal file transfers (eg, child pornography) are difficult to trace without a direct connection between an investigator downloading and the person uploading these file transfers. Furthermore, since file transfers can occur only when users are connected to the program (unlike a Web site or newsgroup posting that may remain up for days or weeks), the amount of time available to investigators to look into a P2P complaint may be small. Perhaps worst of all, the latest variants of these programs, known as **distributed P2P**, allow a user to simultaneously download a desired file from multiple users, thereby distributing the download among 2 or more computers. Distributed P2P greatly complicates investigations.

The description of this technology makes it seem impossible to investigate. However, successful investigative methods have been developed and are in use. Like most areas mentioned in this chapter, investigators are especially urged to leave active, online investigations of P2P to properly trained investigators. These trained investigators have the best chance of possessing the technical knowledge to solve such cases as well as a proper undercover computer and Internet connection with which to conduct such an investigation. Investigators seeking the ability to conduct P2P investigations should consult a properly trained online investigator who is currently working such cases for guidance in this important, emerging threat area.

The basic information needed to trace an offender includes the P2P network, program, and nickname used by the offender; however, this information can be used only to locate the offender when he or she is online. As a result, more useful information (eg, IP address information) can be obtained.

OTHER FUTURE THREATS

With such a large list of Internet concerns, it is difficult to imagine Internet investigations becoming more difficult, but that seems to be the case. The Internet is rapidly being integrated into all aspects of interpersonal communication. A convergence is occurring, and some services may be contracting or ceasing existence, but more continue to emerge (eg, P2P) and replace these services.

Another reemerging threat is use of VoIP for Web-to-telephone calls. With such calls, one user uses the computer to make a call to another user's telephone. Currently, many Web-based phone call service models are returning after losing their users in the shift from free-usage business models to fee-for-service models. Many users of such services chose not to pay for a service they perceived as free, but the technology has improved and become more reliable. This technology will likely be adopted in the future, thereby increasing the risk to children and hampering investigations.

Yet another concern is the rapid adoption of wireless technology. Improperly installed wireless home and business networks are ripe for unauthorized access and abuse by unintended users. Even a properly installed network is a threat because of the mobility this service provides an offender. The importation of the wireless feature into portable electronics (eg, mobile phones, personal digital assistants) exacerbates this problem.

Noteworthy is the integration of computers and other home media, such as television, music, and photography that combine Internet and other computer functions with a television. In the future, these devices will be potentially harmful since parents will be lulled into a false sense of safety and become more likely to allow children unsupervised Internet access.

ONLINE SERVICE PROVIDERS

Though most online service providers provide a connection to the Internet and the use of all other services mentioned in this chapter, an important and notable difference to investigators exists. Online service providers provide self-contained services exclusive to the subscribers. The 2 largest (AOL and MSN) provide services to more than 30 million users in the United States. Usually, online service providers offer the ability to create user "profiles" that may contain either true or false information about the user.

The real advantage to an investigator attempting to locate a suspect on an online service provider is that, unlike so many free services available on the Web (eg, free e-mail), these providers are usually paid services that provide some sort of verified information for investigators to use in locating a suspect. Investigators should be reminded, however, that maintaining the information is the services' prerogative and that few countries have laws requiring that these services maintain records useful to law enforcement officials. Some countries even have laws *preventing* the retention of such information or require the destruction of such information. This means that, as with ISPs, investigators should consider the long-term liaison relationship with online service providers and maintain decorum when dealing with them because a positive relationship may make the difference in developing an effective case.

INTERNET PROTOCOL ADDRESS "TRACING"

As previously described, the starting point for many Internet investigations is tracing an IP address or domain name to the responsible registrant. This information is usually available via public databases from organizations known as Regional Internet Registries (RIRs). The 3 major RIRs responsible for registration on the Internet include the following:

1. The American Registry for Internet Numbers (ARIN) is responsible for managing IP address numbers for the Americas and sub-Saharan Africa.

2. The Registrar for Internet Protocols in Europe (RIPE) is responsible for managing IP address numbers for Europe, the Middle East, the northern part of Africa, and parts of Asia.

3. The Asian-Pacific Network Information Center (APNIC) is responsible for managing IP address numbers for the Asian-Pacific region.

Each of these registries has its own Internet Web page for referencing the respective databases, so many investigators find it helpful to use the interface available at http://www.samspade.org, which was designed by security expert Steve Blighty. This site was originally set up to trace senders of spam and malicious computer hackers. In addition to a "whois" interface (ie, it identifies registration information provided by the owner of a second-level domain name who registered it with an RIR), this site also provides other tools to Internet investigators and hobbyists alike. A "whois" search performed on this site checks many international registries simultaneously for information about a given domain name or IP address.

Other ways exist to help track Internet information. For example, investigators can use third-party software to obtain IP address tracing and other Internet network information. For more technically minded investigators, some basic commands on a Windows-based computer can provide useful information.

Although locating IP and domain name information may appear easy when using Web sites, software, or even computer commands, investigators are warned that much of the information contained in the registry databases can be bogus and unreliable. Tracing Internet users is one of many technical challenges facing Internet investigators and is a primary reason for obtaining proper training before conducting such investigations.

THE IMPORTANCE OF TIME

Perhaps the most critical element and technical challenge of tracing offenders online is time. Just like any other crime, the chronology of events often links a particular suspect to a particular crime in Internet investigations. Investigators can rest assured that because of a system known as ***Network Time Protocol (NTP)***, a protocol used to synchronize computer clock times in a network of computers, most of the times provided from ISP logs are usually accurate. This may not be the case, however, when dealing with a victim's or suspect's computer, or even the investigator's own computer. Most times provided by the computer to files (eg, chat logs, image files) are based on the system clock of that computer.

The time of this clock may be set accidentally or intentionally by the user to display an incorrect time. This means that it is critical for investigators to note the time displayed on the computer clock as well as any difference from the accurate, current time as part of a complete investigation (eg, most self-timing cellular telephones display an accurate NTP time). This time correction as well as any correction based on time zone and possibly daylight savings time can be used to compare critical events.

OTHER TECHNICAL CHALLENGES

Starting or exiting Windows or any other operating system, or even viewing or printing a computer file, changes the integrity of the evidence. As a result, investigators are cautioned not to tamper with original evidence; rather, investigators are encouraged to use working copies for analysis.

Likewise, a competent team leader and properly trained assistants should lead the search of a premise for computer and other related evidence. If possible, a certified computer examiner should be a part of the search team. Even a "simple" computer search can become complicated by the discovery of a home or business network with more than one computer or a computer connected to other, unexpected or unrecognized devices.

Furthermore, with searches conducted at a place of business or anywhere else that may have other potential, innocent users using the same network should be conducted to obtain the necessary evidence from the suspect's computer while protecting the work and the privacy of the rest of the employees. In this regard, information technology professionals at the suspect's place of employment can often serve as valuable sources of information and assistance for the search team if those professionals are first ruled out as potential suspects or accomplices in the offense.

No matter what is searched and seized at the scene of a computer search, the evidence must be treated with caution and care. For proper analysis of computer evidence, seizure of the entire suspect computer system and related equipment is usually necessary to maintaining the chain of custody of all the seized items.

While investigators should strive to ensure that all technical matters are handled properly, they should not overlook other clues. Many successful cases have been made or assisted by the findings of such low-tech things as log books or notes containing online identities of the suspect or other victims, account numbers leading to additional evidence, or even printed images or chat logs kept by the suspect for reference or remembrance. Even if the offender does not make these mistakes and enlists the use of high-tech protections (eg, encryption or password protection), investigators should not rely on the hope that they may be able to "crack" or guess a password. Rather, these investigators should obtain the password from the suspect. No matter what the technical competence of the suspect, the most effective way to gain a confession and obtain other necessary information is with a thorough, well-conducted interview of the offender by an investigator familiar with all of the services and technology being used in the offense.

VICTIM IDENTIFICATION

During the past several years, an exciting development has been taking place with respect to identifying victims of Internet child pornography. In the past, if the previously described tracing techniques were used to identify a transmitter or possessor of child pornography but failed to identify the creator of the images, most investigators prosecuted the subject at hand and ignored the larger issue of identifying the producer. This worked fine to identify and prosecute many offenders but did little to help the victims being abused in the production of these images. Because of increased international cooperation and the proliferation of digitally produced child abuse images worldwide, many investigators find that it is rewarding to go beyond technical-tracing techniques and undertake the difficult work of using the clues provided in the images themselves.

Though this work can be technical and advanced at times, the work is based on the same 5 questions asked so often in any investigation (**Table 26-11**). Investigators can often find the answers to these questions in the child abuse images themselves.

The effectiveness of this investigative technique and the use of these clues depend upon several important assumptions. Most importantly, the assumption that national and international sharing of identified victim information will occur. If individual agencies and countries do not share this information, investigators will find themselves spending weeks analyzing the clues in a series of images to trace the offender and/or victim, only to find out that the victim is already safe. Though privacy issues need to be satisfied, all countries should find a law enforcement reason to share limited victim information such as the images themselves, the age of the child in the images, the name of the offender(s), and the circumstances of the abuse. Victim name information is not necessary and adds little or no value to subsequent investigative efforts, so the name should not be released or shared with others.

In the United States, the lead effort in victim identification is the multiagency National Child Victim Identification Program (NCVIP), which is a joint partnership among the Bureau of Immigration and Customs Enforcement (ICE), Federal Bureau of Investigation (FBI), US Postal Inspection Service (USPIS), US Secret Service, state and local police as represented by the Internet Crimes Against Children Task Forces, and the NCMEC, among other agencies. Members of the NCVIP partnership are coordinating their efforts with similar efforts being undertaken worldwide. These

Table 26-11. Primary Investigator Questions That Can Be Answered by Critically Observing an Image

QUESTION	POSSIBLE ANSWERS
Who	offender and victim face, gender, age, scars, marks, tattoos, jewelry
What	objects, logos, products, furniture, rooms
When	date and/or time on files or in images, seasonal clothing, calendars, decorations
Where	wiring, plumbing, language found on products, keyboards, clothing
How	one or more offenders, accomplice, use of self-timer

projects include work being done by the Trafficking in Human Beings Branch of the Interpol General Secretariat in Lyon, France, and a European Commission-sponsored project, which is bringing together representatives of Interpol, Europol, the European Commission, the Group of Eight Nations (G8), member nations, and several other countries known for expertise in victim identification (specifically, Sweden, Denmark, and the Netherlands). All of these efforts seek to build on the experiential knowledge of countries, such as Sweden, whose national police have led victim identification efforts worldwide and serve as the basis for the Interpol and G8 work in this area.

Regardless of the agency conducting the investigation, another important assumption in victim identification is that a sufficient number of images exist to be analyzed. Many of the stand-alone images contain few, if any, of the clues listed in **Table 26-11**; however, a series of images may develop many clues, especially when these images are reviewed as a related series.

To help relate one series to another, leading law enforcement agencies worldwide are working with state-of-the-art software to conduct automated, visual searches of these images. The combination of this software with the increased international sharing of information has led to a deluge of new cases fit for investigation. To select cases for investigation, many agencies prioritize by considering many factors, which include when the image was captured and whether the child victim(s) is in imminent danger.

The Danish National Police led one of the single most successful cases of victim identification, referred to as Operation Hamlet. Through a combination of technical Internet tracing techniques that used image clues to identify victims, this case identified more than 100 child victims worldwide.

Though the use of image clues and international sharing has increased the success of victim identification efforts, many heinous cases remain unsolved. To combat these cases, investigators in several countries have begun to use the mass media to help identify offenders and, in some countries, child victims. The German Federal Police, Bundeskriminalamt (BKA), is recognized worldwide as the pioneer of this technique. In at least 3 cases in which traditional and Internet tracing investigations failed to identify a child victim, the BKA successfully identified all of the victims by featuring them on a selected national crime television program. In the United States, the FBI has initiated similar efforts with the *America's Most Wanted* television program. With the help of this program, the FBI has had success in identifying the 3 offenders featured thus far. Further investigations revealed that each of these offenders had committed offenses against multiple child victims.

THE UNDERCOVER TECHNIQUE

Undercover (UC) operations have become a primary investigative strategy for dealing with Internet crime in countries in which the use of this technique is legally permissible; however, many countries do not allow the investigation of a suspect who lacks proper predisposition to commit a crime. Furthermore, an investigator who knowingly conducts unauthorized UC activity with subjects in countries in which such activity is illegal may be seen as infringing on national sovereignty. The bottom line is that investigators should carefully avoid issues of entrapment and remain cognizant of prevailing laws in the country or countries in which they conduct their investigative activities.

The good news is that if the UC technique can be used, UC officers and agents may pose as anyone on the Internet with relative ease and enjoy the same apparent anonymity craved by the offenders. In terms of child exploitation offenses, this may include posing as a child by standing in place of a would-be victim, proactively identifying suspects, assuming the role of a fellow trader interested in child pornography, or pretending to be a molester with access to children who are available for sex.

For UC investigations, investigators must only use computers set aside for these investigations that can not be traced to government agencies or compromise other computers or networks. All investigators, especially those conducting UC activity, should be keenly aware of the potential harm of a computer virus, Trojan, or worm. The occurrence of these threats, as well as their complexity and potential harm, continues to grow exponentially. At a minimum, online investigators should be proficient in using anti-virus software and a network with a proper firewall or, preferably, a stand-alone computer with a personal firewall. Investigators should be certain that such programs remain current.

One way to help prevent these harmful issues from arising is by understanding the use of a file name extension. Unfortunately, most Windows-based computers do not show file extensions for known file types. Therefore, investigators should learn ways to configure their computers to show all file extensions. Once this is done, investigators should remain aware of the many file name extensions that constitute a "danger list" (eg, .exe, .vbs, .js, .asp, .shs, .scr, .com, .bat, .sys, .ovl, .prg, .mnu).

The problem with identifying programs from this list is that each of these file types has a legitimate purpose but can be used to create harm. When considering whether a particular file may be harmful, investigators should consider the file's source, the context in which the file was found, and any messages or other files associated with the suspect file. In any case, all suspect files, especially those received via the Internet or from suspect evidence, should be scanned for viruses before opening. Whenever possible, a stand-alone computer that is *not* connected to the Internet or to another network should be used to open such files.

OTHER INTERNET CRIME CONCERNS

The world of Internet crime is not just that of child exploitation offenses. Terrorism, computer intrusion and hacking matters, Internet fraud and intellectual property violations, hate crimes and crimes of violence, and many other "traditional" crimes have found their way onto the Internet as well. This has led to great debate within larger agencies as to whether these investigations should be handled by cybercrime task forces, which work all types of computer crimes, or by more specialized teams, which treat the computer merely as a new instrument of the crime. Early experience has shown that both models can be used effectively.

TYPICAL INTERNET CHILD EXPLOITATION CASES

Case Study 26-1

In the United States, a 38-year-old civilian military contractor was running an automated file server from his home in an IRC channel named for a child pornography movie series. The subject appeared to be a serious distributor of child pornography because he allowed a massive amount of downloading per user. A UC FBI agent downloaded images of child pornography from the subject, who was found to have configured his computer to use an IP address other than the one assigned to him by his cable modem provider. By working with the network operations center of the cable modem provider, the UC agent was able to determine the true identity of the subject, and the subject's home was searched. The subject was charged with possession, advertising, and distribution of child pornography and was sentenced to 7 years in prison. As a result of his arrest, 2 of his cousins came forward to report that the subject had molested them when he was between 14 and 16 years old and they were between 6 and 8 years old.

Case Study 26-2

A successful 62-year-old Broadway music director who worked at a summer arts camp for kids was suspected of illicit contact with a minor. The local police department in New Hampshire contacted the FBI and supplied the subject's online identity. A UC FBI agent posed as a 13-year-old boy and sent a message to the subject to establish contact. The subject expressed a desire to meet the "boy," and he traveled to a mall in Maryland to meet the "boy" to have sex. A search executed at the subject's home revealed a victim logbook, which led to dozens of other possible victims. The subject was sentenced to a 41-month prison term.

Case Study 26-3

A 32-year-old man living in a suburb of Dublin, Ireland, was being monitored in the preteen channels on IRC. An Irish federal police official (or Garda) engaged him in conversation online in IRC after he requested a private chat. During the conversation, which continued over a number of nights, the suspect sent child pornography to the officer. A search of the subject's house revealed a huge collection of child pornography stored on disks kept under the floorboards in his bedroom.

Case Study 26-4

A 28-picture series showing the sexual abuse of an 8- to 10-year-old girl was detected during a routine Internet search by the computer crime squad of the German Federal Criminal Police Office at Interpol Wiesbaden. Identification of the person responsible for the postings was not possible because of the absence of log files. A shopping bag from a German supermarket was found in the background of some of the pictures, and other useful information was also found within the contents of the image files themselves. A difficult decision was made to publish and show on German television some selected, nonpornographic pictures that showed the abused girl. As a result, the girl and perpetrator were located a week later. The offender was a 26-year-old unmarried educator who specialized in caring for problem children and for individual cases, he did so in the child's home; he also volunteered as a Boy Scout leader. Investigators determined that he had abused 3 children, and he was sentenced to 4 years in prison. One accomplice was also identified.

Case Study 26-5

A 50-year-old man from Pamplona, Spain, who had police records for child abuse set up e-mail distribution lists for the purpose of distributing information and child pornography images. Even though the lists were in Spanish, English-speaking offenders joined the groups because of the amount of child pornography files available. The suspect was found to be the owner of a video club with child pornography videotapes available from Germany. At first, he used the distribution lists to offer and sell these tapes; however, portions of the movies were later digitized and posted within the groups. The Cuerpo Nacional de Policia first obtained access to the distribution list and then monitored 15 e-mail accounts. The investigation resulted in 8 arrests in Spain, and reports of other offenders were issued to law enforcement officials in the United States, Canada, Argentina, Mexico, Chile, Ecuador, Puerto Rico, Germany, Sweden, Serbia, the Netherlands, the United Kingdom, France, Denmark, Finland, Thailand, the Philippines, Korea, Malaysia, Australia, and New Zealand.

Case Study 26-6

In the Netherlands, a female Internet user reported to the local police that she had been chatting with a man on ICQ who sent her some child pornography images. He gave her his cell phone number and they arranged to meet each other on the Internet again the next day. The local police informed the Dutch national police which worked with the public prosecutor to trace the owner of the cell phone. The next day a police officer went to the woman's house and waited with the woman until the suspect was online again. At the same time, the public prosecutor and some police officers waited near the suspect's house. The moment the suspect sent another child pornography picture to the woman's computer, the officers arrested the man in his house since he was caught in the act. The man's computer was still online, and more child pornography pictures were found.

CONCLUSION

Regardless of the organizational model selected, communication among investigators and the sharing of knowledge and resources is the key to success. For this reason, investigators are cautioned *not* to investigate Internet crimes in isolation. Becoming involved in a task force (or at least seeking regular assistance), becoming trained, and sharing information are all necessary to conduct Internet investigations. Many domestic and international agencies, large and small, have such resources available and welcome contact from other investigators.

APPENDIX 26-1: GLOSSARY OF INTERNET-RELATED TERMS*

American Registry of Internet Numbers (ARIN)—The organization responsible for the management of Internet Protocol (IP) address numbers for the Americas and sub-Saharan Africa.

Anti-virus software—A program that can detect known or potential viruses found on hard drives, on floppy disks, or in Internet traffic.

Asian-Pacific Network Information Center (APNIC)—The organization responsible for the management of IP address numbers for the Asia-Pacific region. There are 62 economies within the Asia-Pacific region, from Afghanistan in the Middle East to Pitcairn in the Pacific Ocean.

Bandwidth—The potential speed of data transmission on a communication medium.

Broadband—A communication medium that provides a wide band of frequencies to transmit information.

Browser—A program that allows the user to look at and interact with all the information found on the World Wide Web (WWW).

Cable modem—A device that enables the connection of a computer to a cable television line to receive, and possibly transmit, data at higher speeds.

Channel—A specific chat group found on Internet Relay Chat (IRC) similar to a chat room on a Web site or an online service provider.

Chat room—A Web site or part of a Web site found on an IRC channel or as part of an online service provider. A chat room provides a venue for communities of users with a common interest to communicate in real time.

Country code top-level domain (ccTLD)—The top-level domain name of an Internet address that identifies that domain generically as associated with a country. For example, in the domain name, "police.se," Sweden (ie, ".se") is the chosen cc TLD. Some ccTLDs can be inaccurate and misleading.

Cyberspace—The global community created by the interconnectedness of people through computers and the Internet.

Domain name—The labeling system that locates an organization or other entity on the Internet by a name that corresponds to an IP address. For example, the domain name "www.klpd.nl" locates an Internet address for "klpd.nl," which is the Netherlands National Police Agency at IP address 193.178.243.72.

Domain name system (DNS)—The manner in which Internet domain names are located and translated into IP addresses.

---

* *Adapted from http://www.whatis.com.*

Download—The transmission of a file from one computer system to another, usually smaller computer system.

Digital Subscriber Line (DSL)—A broadband information system that brings high-bandwidth capacity to homes and businesses over ordinary telephone lines.

Electronic mail (e-mail)—The exchange of messages and sometimes file attachments via the Internet.

Encryption—The conversion of data into a form that can not be easily understood by unauthorized people.

File name extension—An optional addition to a computer file name that describes the file's format in a suffix that usually consists of 3 characters (eg, .pdf, .doc, .jpg, .mpg, .avi).

File Transfer Protocol (FTP)—The IP for downloading and uploading files.

Firewall—Hardware or software located at a network gateway server that protects the resources of a private network from users of other networks.

Gateway—A network point that acts as an entrance to another network.

Generic top-level domain (gTLD)—The top-level domain name of an Internet address that identifies that address generically as associated with some domain class (eg, .com, .net, .org, .gov, .edu, .int, .mil.). For example, in the domain name "www.fbi.gov," ".gov" is the chosen gTLD.

Header—In a newsgroup or e-mail message, the header is the portion of a transmission that is sent with the actual message and may identify the sender and other facts about the transmission.

Host—Any computer that has full, 2-way access (ie, transmit and receive) to other computers on the Internet.

Hosting—The business of housing, serving, and maintaining files for one or more Web sites. Also known as *Web site hosting* and *Web hosting*.

Hypertext Markup Language (HTML)—The set of symbols or codes inserted in a file that is intended for display on a Web browser.

Hypertext Transfer Protocol (HTTP)—The set of rules for exchanging files on the WWW.

ICQ—A program used to notify users when friends and contacts are online on the Internet and allows the sending of messages, files, audio, and video to other users. Also known as *I Seek You.*

Instant message—The exchange of real-time messages with chosen friends or co-workers on the Internet.

Internet—A worldwide system of computer networks. A network of networks in which users at any one computer can, if they have permission, obtain information or other services from any other computer. Also known as the *Net.*

Internet Assigned Numbers Authority (IANA)—The organization under the Internet Architecture Board of the Internet Society that, under a contract from the US government, oversaw the allocation of IP addresses to Internet Service Providers. Partly because the Internet has become a global network, the US government has withdrawn its oversight of the Internet, which was previously contracted to IANA, and has lent support to an organization with global, nongovernment representation. The Internet Corporation for Assigned Names and Numbers (ICANN) has assumed responsibility for the tasks formerly performed by IANA.

Internet Corporation for Assigned Names and Numbers (ICANN)—The private, nongovernment, nonprofit corporation with responsibility for the services previously performed by the IANA.

Internet Message Access Protocol (IMAP)—A standard protocol for receiving e-mail.

Internet Protocol (IP)—The protocol by which data are sent from one computer to another on the Internet.

Internet Protocol (IP) address—A 32-bit number, which is usually expressed as 4 decimal numbers. Each decimal number represents 8 bits, which are used to identify senders and receivers of information across the Internet.

Internet Relay Chat (IRC)—A system for chatting within stand-alone software or within a Web browser.

Internet Service Provider (ISP)—A company that provides individual and corporate access to the Internet and other related services (eg, Web site building, hosting).

Link—A selectable connection on a Web page from a word, picture, or other information to another Web page or Internet object.

Modem—A device that modulates outgoing digital signals from a computer or other digital device into analog signals for a conventional, copper-twisted pair telephone line and demodulates the incoming analog signal and converts that signal to a digital signal for the digital device.

Network—A number of host computers interconnected by communication paths.

Network News Transport Protocol (NNTP)—The protocol for managing the messages posted on Usenet newsgroups.

Network Time Protocol (NTP)—Protocol used to synchronize computer clock times in a network of computers.

Newsgroup—A discussion about a particular subject that consists of messages posted and propagated through Usenet.

Online service provider—A service (eg, America Online) that has its own online, independent content rather than connecting users directly with the Internet. Most online service providers provide an Internet connection, in which case these providers function as ISPs as well.

Password—A sequence of characters used to determine whether a computer user requesting access to a computer system is an authorized user.

Peer-to-peer (P2P)—A communications model in which each party has the same capabilities and either party can send or receive information.

Personal firewall—A software application used to protect a single computer from intruders outside the network. Also known as a *desktop firewall*.

Point-of-presence (POP)—An access point to the Internet.

Post Office Protocol (POP3)—The most recent version of a standard protocol for receiving e-mail.

Protocol—A special set of communication rules.

Redirection—A technique for moving visitors to a Web page that differs from the address entered or followed by the user.

Regional Internet Registries (RIRs)—Entities that provide IP registration services. The 3 current RIRs are the American Registry for Internet Numbers (ARIN), the Registrar for Internet Protocols in Europe (RIPE), and the Asian-Pacific Network Information Center (APNIC).

Registrar for Internet Protocols in Europe (RIPE)—The organization responsible for the management of IP address numbers membership in Europe, the Middle East, northern Africa, and parts of Asia.

Remailer—An Internet site to which e-mail can be sent for forwarding to an intended destination but conceals the sender's e-mail address.

Request for Comments (RFC)—A formal document from the Internet Engineering Task Force (IETF) that resulted from committee drafting and subsequent review by interested parties.

Server—A computer program that provides services to other computer programs in the same network or different computers. The computer that the server program runs on is also referred to as a server.

Simple Mail Transport Protocol (SMTP)—A protocol primarily used in sending e-mail.

Spam—Unsolicited e-mail or other unwanted communications received on the Internet.

Spoof—To deceive for the purpose of gaining access to someone else's resources. For example, if a user fakes an Internet address to appear to be a different kind of Internet user, the user is spoofing.

System tray—A section of the taskbar in the Microsoft Windows desktop user interface that is used to display the clock and icons of certain programs. Some running programs appear only in the system tray.

Top-level domain (TLD)—Identifies the general part of the domain name in an Internet address. A TLD is either a generic TLD (gTLD) (eg, .com for commercial, .edu for educational) or a country code TLD (ccTLD) (eg, .nl for the Netherlands, .ie for Ireland).

Transmission Control Protocol (TCP)—A protocol used along with the IP to send data in the form of message units between computers over the Internet.

Trojan—A program in which a malicious or harmful code is contained. A Trojan appears to be harmless programming or data so that it can gain control and do damage (eg, ruining a hard disk). A Trojan may be redistributed as part of a virus.

Uniform Resource Locator (URL)—The address of a file (ie, resource) that is accessible on the Internet. For example, "http://www.fbi.gov/hq/cid/cac/innocent. htm" describes the Federal Bureau of Investigation's Innocent Images Web page. This URL indicates the page to be accessed with an HTTP (ie, Web browser) application located on a server named "www.fbi.gov." The specific file is in the directories of "/hq/cid/cac" and named "innocent.htm."

Upload—Transmission from one, usually smaller, computer to another computer.

Usenet—A collection of user-submitted messages about various subjects that are posted to servers on a worldwide network in which each subject collection of posted notes is known as a *newsgroup*.

Virtual community—A community of people sharing common interests, ideas, and feelings via the Internet or other collaborative networks.

Virus—A program or piece of a program usually disguised as something else, which causes an unexpected and usually undesirable event, usually seeking to contaminate only the host machine.

Voice over IP (VoIP)—A protocol for managing the delivery of voice information using the IP.

Web site—A collection of Web files regarding a particular subject that includes a beginning file called a *home page*. For example, the Web site for Ireland's National Police Service, An Garda Síochána, has the home page address of "http://gov.ie/garda."

Whois—A program that identifies registration information provided by the owner of any second-level domain name who has registered it with a Regional Internet Registry. Whois information can be bogus or incomplete.

World Wide Web (WWW)—All the resources and users found on the Internet using the HTTP.

Worm—A self-replicating virus that resides in active memory and duplicates itself with the intent of sending itself to other users.

PROSECUTORIAL ISSUES IN THE CHILD PORNOGRAPHY ARENA

Susan S. Kreston, JD, LLM

Child pornography is the permanent recording of the sexual abuse and exploitation of a minor. The best approach to combating this crime is a multidisciplinary one, in which the investigator, prosecutor, and all other criminal justice professionals involved in the case work together to ensure that children abused in this way are assisted by the criminal justice system. Working together as a team also ensures the best chance for bringing justice to the perpetrators of this crime. Beginning with search and seizure issues and the case being assembled by the investigator coming to the prosecutor, this chapter will address charging and pretrial considerations, jury selection, and how untrue defenses can be met.

SEARCH AND SEIZURE ISSUES*

With the advent of computer technology, the production and storage of child pornography has changed radically. In the past, production and storage were expensive and technically difficult and often left a readily discernible trail for law enforcement to follow. With current computer technology, the creation of child pornography has been reduced to an easily accomplished exercise, needing only common video cameras, video capture boards, digital cameras, or scanners and software tools to record and edit the product inexpensively and easily. The computer's capacity to store images in digital form makes it an ideal repository for child pornography. A single floppy disk can store dozens of images and hundreds of pages of text. Hard drives can store hundreds of thousands of images at high resolution. Recordable compact discs, zip disks, and flash drives, which can be easily hidden due to their small size and shipped anywhere in the world, can also store thousands of images.

The communication between pedophiles engaging in the business of child pornography has been revolutionized by the nearly universal access to computers enjoyed in the United States. Communication links are established between computers in 1 of 3 ways: individual modems, which allow computers to connect to one another through telephone lines; large service providers (eg, America Online [AOL], Prodigy, Compu-Serve); or other Internet access providers (eg, universities, businesses, government agencies). In addition, many cable television companies offer Internet access. These communication links allow contact to be made around the world quickly, privately, and anonymously. These advantages to computer interaction are well known and serve as a foundation of trade among pedophiles.

---

* This section is adapted from Kreston S. Search and seizure in cases of computers and child pornography. National Center for the Prosecution of Child Abuse Update. 1999;12(9). Available at: http://ndaa-apri.org/ publications/newsletters/apri_update_vol_12_no_9_1999.html. Accessed September 1, 2004. For a fuller treatment of this topic, see Kreston S. Search and seizure issues in Internet crimes against children cases. Rutgers Comput Technol Law J. 2004;30:327.

The ability to produce child pornography easily, reproduce it inexpensively, and market it anonymously (through electronic communications) has drastically changed the distribution method. Child pornography can be electronically mailed to anyone with access to a computer and a modem. With the proliferation of commercial services that provide electronic mail, anonymous remailing, chat rooms, and off-site storage facilities, computers have become a favored medium among child pornographers. In view of the advancing technology available to those who traffic in child pornography, traditional tools used in criminal investigations, such as the search warrant, must be adapted to respond to the new and emerging facets of this crime. Prosecutors are specifically encouraged to review the recently enacted US Patriot Act of 2001.

SEARCH WARRANTS

A warrant must contain a detailed, specific description of the place to be searched and the person(s) or thing(s) to be seized and must be supported by probable cause. The items to be seized must be defined with sufficient detail so as to limit the executing officer's discretion in deciding what will be seized. These concepts will be discussed in detail in the following sections.

Background Information

A search warrant may begin with an introductory paragraph with a recitation of the affiant's (ie, a person who swears to an affidavit) training and experience in the area of investigating child sexual exploitation (CSE). An affiant's expertise may be established by listing the following: (1) present rank and assignment, (2) area(s) of responsibility, (3) length of experience as a law enforcement officer, (4) training and work experience received in the area of CSE, (5) training and work experience received in the area of computers, including conferring with other law enforcement officers trained in computer investigations, and (6) any other relevant information. The affiant may rely upon the expertise of others.

Information explaining the Internet, the World Wide Web, chat rooms, electronic bulletin boards, Internet Service Providers (ISPs), free e-mail programs (eg, Yahoo!), or other specialized online services relevant to the case should be included in the search warrant application. The affiant should not assume that the judge is up to date with the latest computer technologies or jargon. The terminology and descriptive explanations should be made easy to understand.

Probable Cause

Probable cause is established through an affidavit in support of the warrant, setting out the factual basis for the warrant application. In determining whether probable cause exists to issue a warrant, the issuing judge must decide whether, given the totality of the circumstances, there is a fair probability that contraband or evidence of a crime will be found in a particular place (*United States v Garcia*, 1993; *United States v Pitts*, 1993; *United States v Ricciardelli*, 1993; *United States v Simpson*, 1998). Affidavits supporting the warrant application should be specifically incorporated by reference into the warrant. Failing to do so may contribute to a warrant being held invalid (*Groh v Ramirez*, 2004).

In determining if a probable cause exists to seize and search a particular computer suspected of containing evidence of child sexual exploitation or having been used to facilitate the crime of child sexual exploitation, 2 facts must be established: (1) there is a computer physically located at a particular location and (2) the computer contains evidence of, or was used to commit, the crime. If this twofold test is not satisfied, the warrant will be invalidated (*Taylor v State*, 2001; *State v Nordlund*, 2002).

Recently, 2 federal circuits have reached differing opinions as to whether probable cause was present in child pornography cases involving fundamentally similar fact patterns. In *United States v Froman* (2004), the Fifth Circuit found probable cause present where an appellant had knowingly and voluntarily joined an online group that predominantly distributed child pornography, remained a member for approximately a month without canceling his subscription, and used screen names that reflected his interest in child pornography. This probable cause was bolstered by an expert's opinion that those who collect child pornography usually keep it. Using a "common sense" approach, the circuit found that probable cause existed for issuance of the search warrant.

In contrast, the Ninth Circuit in *United States v Gourde* (2004) failed to find probable cause where the appellant had (1) affirmatively subscribed to a pornography Web site that advertised over 1000 pictures of girls aged 12-17 and displayed several thumbnail images of girls who appeared to be at least prepubescent on the subscription page; (2) had unlimited access to hundreds of images, including past postings to the site, which could have been downloaded during his period of membership and would have included images of naked prepubescent females with captions describing them as girls aged 12-17; and (3) failed to unsubscribe to the site for at least 2 months. The affidavit provided expert opinion evidence of the proclivities of child pornography collectors and opined that Gourde's affirmative act of subscribing to http://www.Lolitagurls.com and failing to unsubscribe provided a sufficient basis to place Gourde in that category. The court found that an affidavit establishing that it is possible, with some straining, to infer that Gourde, "along with every other member of every site on the Internet containing what appears to be child pornography" (*United States v Gourde*, 2004) might possess child pornography is not enough to justify a warrant to search Gourde's home and seize his computer. This case, though some feel poorly reasoned, should be read to stand for 3 valid points. First, the government should employ the means to track the suspect's usage of the site to determine whether there are downloaded child pornography images. Second, the government should be careful not to rely solely on the Web site's personal and billing information to establish identity of the suspect. The government must take steps to ensure that the account(s) in question are not set up by someone impersonating the suspect. The e-mail account in *Gourde* was from a free Web-based provider, which could have been set up by anyone. Finally, the government must establish a nexus between the child pornography and the computer that is to be searched. The government should have case specific evidence linking the e-mail account to a person, and then from a person to a particular place and/or computer.

With this as a backdrop, the following discussion will address evidentiary issues that arise in particular investigations, issues that surround the acquisition and admissibility in court of different pieces of evidence.

Drafting the Warrant

In many cases, undercover communications with the suspect via the Internet furnish probable cause to believe that the suspect's computer contains child pornography and other evidence of distribution and receipt. An undercover agent, posing as a minor, may "meet" the suspect in a chat room or an Internet Relay Chat (IRC) channel that is dedicated to sexual activity with minors, such as "dad&daughtersex." Sometimes, the agent/minor receives child pornography image files from suspects after entering the "room" or IRC channel. In other cases, an actual minor may report receipt of child pornography image files to law enforcement agents, who then begin an investigation.

Many affidavits list the titles of each image and describe their contents so that the reviewing magistrate can make a determination as to the illegality of the images. When this practice is not followed, the warrant may be challenged, as in *United States v Brunette* (2001). In *Brunette*, the court held that "[w]here neither the magistrate judge nor the district court judge independently viewed the images, and because the affidavit did not adequately describe them, we conclude that the warrant was not supported by probable cause." The case was saved by applying a *Leon* good faith analysis (*United States v Leon*, 1984). Printed copies of the images can be placed in sealed envelopes, so they are available to the magistrate if he or she wants to review the images.

Accompanying e-mail messages, as well as the titles of the images, provide additional evidence as to the suspect's knowledge that they feature children engaged in sexually explicit conduct. In addition, IRC channels and newsgroups are typically named to correspond to the user's interest, as in "kinkypreteensex." This evidence is particularly important if the affidavit includes an expert opinion section discussing the behavioral characteristics associated with a child pornography collector. The affidavit should recite evidence demonstrating that the suspect is a candidate who is likely to fit the behavioral characteristics identified.

Child pornography warrants typically authorize the seizure of all images of child pornography. The affidavit and attachments should specifically define the meaning of the term "child pornography." If the warrant authorizes seizure of child pornography as referred to in Section 2252(a) of 18 United States Code (USC), there should be a reference to the definition found in Section 2256(8). This is especially true in light of the Supreme Court's ruling in *Ashcroft v Free Speech Coalition* (2002), which held that the definitions contained in Sections 2256(8)(b) and 2256(8)(d) of 18 USC are unconstitutional. In situations in which a suspect is downloading child pornography files from, or uploading such files to, a newsgroup, the affidavit should include descriptions and explanations for the reviewing magistrate.

Finally, the issue exists of whether the Fourth Amendment requires government investigators to follow a specific search methodology when searching a computer for evidence. Though there is some dissention, the overwhelmingly majority view is that the methodology of the search does not have to be spelled out in the warrant application (*United States v Hill*, 2004). The extreme minority view is that the Fourth Amendment may limit the particular way that government agents can examine a computer storage device for evidence pursuant to a warrant, and that a judge can impose these limits as a condition of issuing the warrant (*In the Matter of the Search of 3817 W WestEnd, First Floor, Chicago, Illinois*, 2004). Unless case law in a particular jurisdiction requires that a method of searching a computer be stated, the methodology (eg, locate the hard drive, make a duplicate of the original drive, search only the files marked "criminal evidence found here") does not have to be spelled out in the warrant application.

Expert Opinion

There is a division of opinion on the prudence of including an "expertise" component in a search warrant. *United States v Weber* (1991) stated that bare allegations from an expert in an affidavit are insufficient to support probable cause for a warrant, but *United States v Anderson* (1999a) and *United States v Lamb* (1996) held that a boilerplate expertise section is helpful and relevant when accompanied by case-specific information. Recent case law that has accepted expert testimony includes *United States v Long* (2003) and *United States v Romero* (1999), where testimony by a properly qualified expert as to methods and techniques of preferential child molesters was held admissible.

The key for investigators is to set forth in the affidavit the characteristics and mode of operation of pedophiles and specific facts as to how the defendant has demonstrated those characteristics and support for any conclusions that the suspect fits into that class of persons. When drafting an expertise component into a warrant, it should explain, in a *case-specific* manner, why or how the particular characteristics apply to the suspect (*United States v Lamb*, 1996). This component should be used to supplement the probable cause developed elsewhere in the affidavit or to address potential staleness issues (*United States v Anderson*, 1999b).

Additional Considerations in Description of Items to Be Seized

While the focus of this book is CSE, it must be stressed that these cases are a subset of all child abuse cases. As such, it is imperative that the "traditional" types of child molestation evidence not be forgotten when drafting a search warrant. If supported by the facts of the investigation, physical and forensic evidence should be sought from the victim, suspect, and crime scene. Examples of such evidence are listed in **Table 27-1**. It may be necessary to utilize special equipment, such as luminol lights, to search for some of these items properly and thoroughly. When executing the warrant, agents should be sure to look for any evidence, however small, that corroborates the child's account of the abuse.

Table 27-1. Physical and Forensic Evidence to Consider in Child Molestation Cases
PHYSICAL EVIDENCE
— Sexual devices
— Lubricants
— The child's clothing/underwear
— Bondage and discipline paraphernalia
— Adult pornography
— Any items that could be used to abuse or exploit the child sexually or physically
FORENSIC EVIDENCE
— Blood
— Blood spatter
— Semen
— Vaginal fluid
— Urine
— Hair
— Fiber evidence
— Chemical evidence

In addition, other items may be subject to seizure, depending upon the nature of the investigation. Examples of noncontraband evidence are listed in **Table 27-2** and should be considered as long as probable cause supports the seizure.

PARTICULARITY

Child pornography computer cases can present unique challenges when trying to describe the items to be seized with sufficient detail. For example, in *United States v Upham* (1999a), computer software and hardware, computer disks, and disk drives were ruled to be sufficiently specific. Additional examples are listed in **Table 27-3**. Affidavits in support of the warrant should be attached or incorporated by reference to cure any alleged lack of particularity in the warrant itself (*United States v Upham*, 1999a). Additionally, *United States v Simpson* (1998) held that even where an affidavit was neither attached nor incorporated into the warrant, the good faith exception established in *United States v Leon* (1984) may still allow for admissibility of the evidence.

Table 27-2. Examples of Noncontraband Evidence

— Child erotica

— Correspondence with other persons or groups interested in sexual behavior with children, eg, North American Man/Boy Love Association [NAMBLA]

— Diaries or other records of child sexual partners

— Phone or address books in which the suspect has recorded the name, address, and phone number of child sexual partners

— Camera equipment with which the suspect has taken photos of a child or children engaged in sexually suggestive poses or sexual activity

— Information concerning any safe deposit box or storage facilities used by the suspect to store records or personal belongings

— Computer hardware and software used by the suspect to store the personal records and information of his relationships with child victims

Table 27-3. Examples of Cases Illustrating Particularity

CASE	DESCRIPTION
United States v Kimbrough, 69 F3d 723,727 (5th Cir 1995)	Warrants authorizing search for materials related to child pornography sufficiently particular when language in warrants properly limited executing officers' discretion by informing them what items were to be seized
United States v Koelling, 992 F2d 817,821-822 (8th Cir 1993)	Sufficient particularity when warrant authorized seizure of materials depicting minors engaged in sexually explicit conduct as defined by statute
United States v Dornhofer, 859 F2d 1195,1198 (4th Cir 1988) *United States v Diamond*, 820 F2d 10,12 (1st Cir 1987)	Sufficient particularity when warrant authorized seizure of videotapes "depicting prepubescent children"

However, recently the limits of the particularity requirements were discussed in *Groh v Ramirez* (2004). In *Groh*, the agent drafting the warrant failed to identify any of the items intended for seizure. While the application did list the items to be seized, that application was not incorporated by reference. The Supreme Court held that under this fact pattern, the warrant was invalid and even the good faith exception could not apply here as the warrant was so obviously deficient that the executing officers could not reasonably believe it to be valid

An entire class of items may be seized if the warrant is sufficiently particular to establish probable cause to support the seizure of the entire class and a more precise description is not possible. Where detailed particularity is impossible, generic language, if it particularizes the types of items to be seized, would be permissible (*United States v Horn*, 1999; *United States v Layne*, 1995). Terminology used within the application should be defined. Any terms of "art" that are used in the application, such as explicit sexual conduct, may be defined by reference to the applicable statute's definitions of these terms (*United States v Kemmish*, 1997). Words must be defined with sufficient particularity to limit the executing officers' discretion in determining what to seize (*United States v Layne*, 1995). According to *United States v Koelling* (1993), typographical statutory citation errors may be rendered harmless if the full content of the statute is put in the warrant. Some courts have, however, held the warrant language to the higher "scrupulous exactitude" standard of particularity due to First Amendment/overbreadth concerns (*State v Perrone*, 1992). However, according to *United States v Rude* (1996), warrants must only be "reasonably specific, rather than elaborately detailed" and the specificity required "varies depending on the circumstances of the case and the type of items involved."

OVERBREADTH

Overbreadth issues arise when the warrant is too broad in the sense that it includes items that should not be seized. For example, *United States v Loy* (1999), stating that "children under the age of 18 engaging in sexually explicit conduct" was not considered to be overly broad. Additional examples are listed in **Table 27-4**. Deleted data that are recovered has been held to be within the scope of a warrant that authorized the search and seizure of "any and all visual depictions, in any format or media" (*United States v Upham*, 1999a).

Table 27-4. Examples of Cases Discussing Overbreadth	
CASE	DESCRIPTION
United States v Koelling, 992 F2d 817,821-822 (8th Cir 1993)	"[T]he fact that some adults look like children and some children look like adults does not mean that a warrant is overbroad. Most minors look like minors and most adults look like adults, and most of the time law enforcement officers can tell the difference."
United States v Upham, 168 F3d 532 (1st Cir 1999a)	"[A]ny and all visual depictions, in any format or media, of minors engaging in sexually explicit conduct [as defined by statute]" is not unconstitutionally broad.
United States v Lacy, 119 F3d 742,745,746 (9th Cir 1997) *United States v Layne*, 43 F3d 127 (5th Cir 1995)	Child pornography is not overly broad.

ANTICIPATORY WARRANTS

Anticipatory warrants (ie, warrants that become effective upon the happening of a future event) should be upheld where they are supported by probable cause and the conditions precedent are clearly set forth in the warrant and/or supporting affidavit. Anticipatory warrants differ from traditional warrants in that they are unsupported by probable cause to believe that the items to be seized are at the place to be searched at the time the warrant is issued (*United States v Loy*, 1999; *United States v Rowland*, 1998). They must, however, be supported by probable cause at the time of the issuance (*United States v Rowland*, 1998). Additionally, they must establish there is probable cause to believe that the contraband, which is not yet at the place to be searched, will be there when the warrant is executed. The "triggering event" is typically the future delivery, sale, or purchase of the contraband. If the triggering event does not take place, the warrant is void. A warrant that does not state, on its face or by reference and incorporation of the supporting affidavit, what the triggering event is, has been held fatally defective (*United States v Gendron*, 1994; *United States v Hotal*, 1998; *United States v Riciardelli*, 1993). If the place to be searched is not the place of the delivery (eg, residence versus a post office box), sale, or purchase of the contraband, additional facts must be offered to support probable cause to believe the contraband will be taken to the location to be searched. If no nexus (ie, link) between the place to be searched and the item to be seized is established, the anticipatory warrant is void.

GOOD FAITH

Even if no nexus is established, however, the good faith exception may allow for the admissibility of the seized item(s) (*United States v Loy*, 1999; *United States v Rowland*, 1998). The good faith exception requires that the officer acted in reasonable reliance upon a warrant issued by a detached and neutral magistrate and was unaware the warrant was unsupported by probable cause despite the magistrate's authorization. In both *United States v Loy* (1999) and *United States v Rowland* (1998), the courts held that where there was (1) more than a "bare bones" affidavit, (2) a specific condition placed on the execution of the warrant, and (3) reasonable reliance on the magistrate's authorization, the good faith exception applied and the seized items (child pornography delivered to a post office box but seized at a residence) were admissible. Similarly, *United States v Jasorka* (1998) held that the *Leon* good faith exception to the exclusionary rule applied to officers' reliance upon a search warrant for sexually explicit materials depicting minors that was issued in reliance on an affidavit describing an intercepted package of photographs. Though it was undecided whether sufficient basis existed for issuing a warrant without the magistrate judge viewing the photographs to determine whether they were "lascivious," the warrant was not so defective as to preclude reasonable reliance.

STALENESS

The expert should address whether the particular subject is likely to keep his or her contraband for long periods of time. For example, in *United States v Lacy* (1997), the court was "unwilling to assume that collectors of child pornography keep their materials indefinitely, but the nature of the crime, as set forth in this affidavit, provided 'good reason' to believe the computerized visual depictions downloaded by Lacy would be present in his apartment when the search was conducted ten months later."

The age of the information supporting a warrant application is a factor in determining probable cause. If the information is too old, it is stale and probable cause may no longer exist. Age alone, however, does not determine staleness. The nature of the crime and the type of evidence must be examined. For example, *United States v Lacy* (1997) held that 10-month-old information of receipt of child pornography was sufficient for probable cause, and *United States v Greany* (1991) held that 2-year-old evidence of marijuana growing activity at the defendant's residence was not too stale to support a search warrant. Rather, the question is whether "there is sufficient basis to believe, based on a continuing pattern or other good reasons, that the items to be seized are still on the premises" (*United States v Gann*, 1984). The lapse of time is least important when the suspected criminal activity is continuing in nature and when the property is not likely to be destroyed or dissipated (*United States v Horn*, 1999).

As noted, those who deal in pornography treat these materials as valuable commodities, sometimes regarding them as collections and retaining them in secure but available places for extended periods of time (Lanning, 2001). This is why an appropriate reference to expert opinion that child pornography collectors retain their collections for long periods of time can overcome staleness of the information. In *United States v Anderson* (1999c), the Ninth Circuit relied on expert testimony to that effect and held that an 11-month lapse between obtaining information on child pornography and the search did not render the information stale (See also *Lacy*, supra). The Eighth Circuit employed similar reasoning in *United States v Horn*

(1999) to allow for a 3-month lapse, and the Ninth Circuit followed its own precedent from *United States v Anderson* (1999c) in *United States v Hay* (2000) to allow a 6-month lapse before the search was executed.

EXCEPTIONS TO THE WARRANT REQUIREMENT*

Plain View Exception

The plain view exception applies to a seizure of electronic evidence if officers are in a lawful position to observe the evidence and its incriminating character is immediately apparent. For example, if officers were lawfully present in a target's house and observed child pornography on the computer screen, the officers could seize the computer under the plain view exception. The officers could not, however, search the computer based on their plain view seizure. The officers would be required to obtain a warrant, based on probable cause that the computer contained visual depictions of child pornography. They would then be allowed lawfully to search the entire hard drive and any relevant and material parts, peripherals, manuals, or other items identified in the warrant.

In *United States v Wong* (2003), the police executed a search with a warrant of the defendant's house looking for evidence that he had murdered his girlfriend. During the search of his computer, graphic files that contained child pornography were found. The police then obtained a supplemental warrant and found more child pornography. On appeal, the court held that the first image of child pornography was in plain view when the officer was legally searching for evidence in graphic files, and the supplemental warrant supported the introduction of all subsequent images found.

In *United States v Simmonds* (2001), a detective investigating a 14-year-old runaway entered the defendant's motel room and noticed a white piece of paper lying face-down on the edge of a nearby table. The detective could see through the sheet of paper an image of a child in a sexual pose. He turned over the paper and confirmed that it was indeed child pornography. The defendant subsequently pled guilty to receiving and distributing child pornography. In deciding the legality of the underlying search, the court held that "[a]lthough the paper was face-down against the table, Detective Washburn testified that he could see through the white sheet of paper an image of a child in a sexual position. In other words, the pornographic picture was in plain view, despite the paper being face-down. He, thus, had the requisite probable cause to turn over the sheet of paper and conduct a 'search' of it."

In *United States v Walser* (2001), police found a thumbnail sketch of child pornography while conducting a warrant search of the defendant's computer for drug information. The agent suspended the search and obtained a new warrant covering child pornography. The court upheld the search, emphasizing the appropriate restraint shown by the agent in obtaining the supplemental warrant. In *United States v Gray* (1999), federal agents seized Gray's computers to search for evidence of unauthorized computer intrusions at a library. During their routine search, agents came across pornographic pictures of minors. At that point, the agent ceased the search and obtained a second search warrant authorizing a search of the files for child pornography. The court ruled that the pornography was discovered under the plain view exception, reasoning that in searching for the items listed in the warrant, the agent was entitled to examine all of the defendant's files to decide whether they contained items that fell within the scope of the warrant. In doing so, the agent inadvertently discovered evidence of child pornography, which was incriminating on its face.

In contrast, in *United States v Carey* (1999), a police officer accidentally discovered child pornography on the defendant's computer while conducting a search for

---

* This section is adapted from Kreston S. Exceptions to the search warrant requirement in computer facilitated child sexual exploitation cases. National Center for the Prosecution of Child Abuse Update. 2000b;13(4). Available at: http://ndaa-apri.org/publications/newsletters/update_volume_13_number_4_2000.html. Accessed September 1, 2004.

evidence of drug transactions. Without obtaining another warrant, he downloaded and viewed more than 200 similarly labeled files in a search for additional images of child pornography. The court held that, though he discovered the first image of child pornography inadvertently, the officer exceeded the scope of the warrant because, after the accidental discovery of illegal pornography, "he expected to find child pornography and not material related to drugs" (*United States v Carey*, 1999). As a result, the panel concluded the officer had temporarily abandoned his search for drug trafficking evidence and intentionally commenced a search for more child pornography, which the existing warrant did not authorize.

Consent Exception

Consent from the party whose computer is being searched may eradicate the need for a search warrant, provided the consent is voluntary and not coerced. *United States v Salvo* (1998) held that voluntary consent was found when a suspect was told he was not under arrest and signed a consent form even when the agent stated a warrant would be obtained if consent was not given. The search must not exceed the scope of the consent given (*United States v Turner*, 1999). In this case, consent was granted to search for an intruder and evidence of an assault given, but computer files were searched as well. However, *United States v Lemmons* (2002) held that an initial consensual search can be expanded based on the defendant's actions.

A warrantless search must be executed with the permission of an authorized party. Consent searches can raise multiple issues depending on the parties involved. When a third party (eg, spouse, parent, employer, room/housemate) gives consent, the question becomes whether that party had common authority over the object of the search and, as a result, the authority to consent to the search. Generally, a spouse may consent to the seizure of a computer used by both spouses and a search for evidence. The exception to this rule is when one spouse has excluded the other from using the computer or from entering certain files within the computer by the use of encryption or passwords known only to one spouse. The critical case on this issue is *Trulock v Freeh* (2001), in which it was found that

the plaintiff and his co-habitant Linda Conrad both used a computer located in Conrad's bedroom and each had joint access to the hard drive. Conrad and Trulock, however, protected their personal files with passwords; Conrad did not have access to Trulock's passwords. The court held that although Conrad had authority to consent to a general search of the computer, her authority did not extend to Trulock's password-protected files.

Parents of minor children generally have the authority to consent to a search by law enforcement of a computer used by the minor. The exception to this rule would be if the minor maintained an expectation of privacy in the computer by virtue of being emancipated under state law for a particular purpose. Parents of adult children who still live with them generally do not have the authority to consent to a search of the adult child's computer by law enforcement absent the parent being a co-user of the computer. For example, *United States v Durham* (1998) ruled that a mother lacked the authority to consent to a search of her adult son's bedroom where he paid rent; she did not have a key to his locked room. Even if actual common authority does not exist, apparent authority of the consenting individual coupled with the police's reasonable belief in that apparent authority may suffice. *United States v Smith* (1998) held that the girlfriend/housemate of the defendant had the authority to consent to a search of the computer in her home, where all members of the household used the computer. Consent to search that is given after an illegal entry, however, is tainted and invalid under the Fourth Amendment (*United States v Hotal*, 1998).

Employees' expectation of privacy in their workplace computers depends on the notification given to the employees by management on this issue. If management has "spoken" to all employees through an employee handbook, general orders, a "splash" or banner page that specifically states the employee has no expectation of privacy, e-mail to the employees regarding the scope of their privacy rights, or other effective means of communication, then they should not expect privacy in the workplace computer (*United States v Slanina*, 2002; *United States v Bailey*, 2003; *United States v Angevine*, 2002). As a result, if at any time, and for any reason, management may enter an employee's computer, then the systems operator may allow law enforcement to search and seize evidence from any employee computer without a search warrant. Conversely, if management has failed to communicate what expectation of privacy their employees should have in workplace computers, employees may expect privacy, and the courts might require a search warrant to review employee computers (*United States v Simons*, 2000).

Exigent Circumstances Exception

Exigent circumstances are another exception to the search warrant requirement. Circumstances that comprise this exception would include urgency, amount of time needed to obtain a warrant under the particular facts of the investigation, likelihood that evidence would be destroyed, concealed, or altered, danger to officers or others, whether the target knows law enforcement is coming to the crime scene, the nature of the evidence and its susceptibility to destruction by remote "kill" switches or other means of destroying or concealing the evidence, or whether the target computer is a part of a network of computers that would facilitate the transfer of contraband to other computers outside the jurisdiction of the warrant (*United States v Reed*, 1991). This exception to the warrant requirement that allows police fearing the destruction of evidence to enter the home of an unknown suspect carries with it the following constraints: (1) requires clear evidence of probable cause, (2) is available only for serious crimes and in circumstances in which the destruction of evidence is likely, (3) is limited in scope to the minimum intrusion necessary to prevent the destruction of evidence, and (4) must be supported by clearly defined indications of an exigency not subject to police manipulation or abuse (*United States v Anderson*, 1998).

Even in exigent circumstances, a warrantless seizure may be permitted, and a subsequent warrant to search may still be necessary (*United States v David*, 1991; *United States v Grosenheider*, 2000). A "no-knock" warrant may also be sought if a factually particularized showing of imminent danger of destruction of the evidence can be made. ***No-knock warrants*** allow police to enter private premises without knocking and without identifying themselves. A showing is particularized when there is more than a suspicion or possibility that evidence will be destroyed; there must be particular, articulated facts to support that conclusion. However, finding computer equipment itself (instrumentality evidence) does not necessarily run the same risk of imminent destruction as other (documentary) evidence (*United States v Durham*, 1998).

Search and seizure questions commonly arise in Internet-based child exploitation investigations. Due to the constantly changing legal landscape in this area, search and seizure issues are of paramount importance, and prosecutors and investigators must stay abreast of recent case law in this area.

Private Searches

Private searches, most notably represented by the computer repair personnel cases, highlight the principle that the Fourth Amendment does not apply to nongovernmental actors, unless agency principles are present. Agency principles hold that law enforcement may not use civilians to act on behalf of law enforcement without making those persons subject to the same rules as law enforcement. If the agency is attached, so are the Fourth Amendment and issues of reasonable expectation of privacy (*United States v Barth*, 1998; *United States v Hall*, 1998). Law enforcement officials may obtain a warrant based on the private search, provided they do not expand the scope of the private search in the application for the warrant (*United States v Grimes*, 2001).

Probation and Parole Searches

Probationers enjoy conditional liberty, so the government may closely supervise probationers and impinge on their privacy to a greater extent than is allowed for the general public to ensure the probationer observes probation restrictions. The search of a probationer's home without a warrant and with less than probable cause does not violate the Fourth Amendment if the search is conducted under state probation regulations that satisfy the Fourth Amendment's reasonableness standard. A probationer can be subject to a warrantless search under a statutory scheme or pursuant to the findings of a sentencing court.

In *United States v Knights* (2001), a warrantless search of a probationer's house, supported by reasonable suspicion and authorized by a condition of his probation, was found reasonable within the meaning of the Fourth Amendment. Nothing in the defendant's conditions of probation limited searches to those with a probationary purpose. However, though probationers have a reduced expectation of privacy in their person and residency, a warrantless search of a probationer's residence may be problematic if conducted by the probation officer at the request of police or if directed by police. Factors to consider include if it was the probation officer's idea to conduct the search, if the search bears a direct relationship to the crime for which the defendant was convicted, and if the search is authorized by probation conditions (*United States v Oakes*, 2001).

An anonymous tip, suitably corroborated, may form the basis for a warrantless search of a parolee's residence by the parole officer. In *United States v Tucker* (2001), the search was held to be valid because the police were present, and the computer at the residence could be legally seized as evidence of a parole violation. Parolees' rights under the Fourth Amendment are satisfied if the parole officer who is investigating a parole violation has reasonable grounds to believe that a parole violation has occurred. Under these circumstances, the need for a search warrant is eliminated. *People v Slusher* (1992) held that where a convicted sex offender was on parole, corroborated allegations of sexual assault of a child and CSE supported a warrantless search of the parolee's house. Where the parolee consented to a search as a condition of parole, no warrant is required, so long as there is a reasonable suspicion, supported by specific and articulable facts, to believe that the parolee has committed a parole violation or crime (*People v Slusher*, 1992; *People v Tafoya*, 1999).

CHARGING AND PRETRIAL CONSIDERATIONS*

The case is now before the prosecutor. When determining what to charge, certain questions must be asked. Are the images child pornography? If so, in which jurisdiction should the defendant be charged? How many counts should be charged? Which specific images should be used? Are there additional charges that might be brought? If a victim is identifiable in the case, what special issues should the prosecutor be prepared to address? If there is not an identifiable victim, how will this have an impact on charging? What discovery motions should be filed, and what stand should the prosecution take on defense requests for discovery of the child pornography? These questions, and how charging decisions must incorporate and anticipate the defenses that will be raised, will be addressed in turn.

DEFINING CHILD PORNOGRAPHY

Federal law 18 USC § 2252 prohibits a minor from engaging in sexually explicit conduct. The term ***sexually explicit conduct*** is defined by 18 USC § 2256(2) as actual or simulated

---

* *This section is adapted from Astrowsky B, Peters JS. Charging decisions and trial preparation in child pornography cases. In: Peters JS, ed.* Prosecuting Internet Child Exploitation Crimes. *Washington, DC: US Dept of Justice; 2002b.*

— Sexual intercourse, including genital-genital, oral-genital, anal-genital, or oral-anal, whether between persons of the same or opposite sex

— Bestiality

— Masturbation

— Sadistic or masochistic abuse

— Lascivious exhibition of the genitals or pubic area of any person

The definition of a lascivious exhibition of the genitals is not always found in the visual depiction, but rather by putting the picture in context. The courts seem to agree that lasciviousness is not necessarily a characteristic of the child portrayed but is to be found in the intentions of the photographer (*United States v Wiegand*, 1987). Determining the intent of the photographer can be difficult if the photographer or the circumstances of production are unknown, as often happens in computer and Internet child pornography investigations. The *Dost* criteria attempt to discern the lascivious intent of the photographer by examining the visual depictions themselves. The court enumerated the following factors to assist in determining intent (*United States v Dost*, 1986):

— Whether the focal point of the visual depiction is on the child's genitalia or pubic area

— Whether the setting of the visual depiction is sexually suggestive, that is, in a place or pose generally associated with sexual activity

— Whether the child is depicted in an unnatural pose, or in inappropriate attire, considering the age of the child

— Whether the child is fully or partially clothed or nude

— Whether the visual depiction suggests sexual coyness or a willingness to engage in sexual activity

— Whether the visual depiction is intended or designed to elicit a sexual response in the viewer

The court acknowledged that this list of factors is not exhaustive and that a visual depiction need not involve all of the listed factors to constitute a lascivious exhibition of the genitals. The determination will have to be made based on the overall content of the visual depiction.

Even if a picture focuses on the clothed genitals of a minor, it may still be child pornography. This issue was considered in *United States v Knox* (1994). The *Knox* court refused to read a nude requirement into the statute, holding that though the genitals are covered, the display and focus on the genitals or pubic area still provides considerable interest and excitement for the pedophile. The court noted that the underlying rationale for the federal child pornography laws supports the position that a clothed exhibition of a child's genital area can be proscribed. The harm Congress attempted to eradicate by enacting the child pornography laws is present when a photographer unnaturally focuses on a minor child's clothed genital area with the obvious intent to produce an image sexually arousing to pedophiles. The child is treated as a sexual object, and the permanent record of this embarrassing and humiliating experience produces the same detrimental effects to the mental health of a child as would a nude portrayal.

State statutes vary in their definitions of child pornography. It will be necessary to review the state statute(s) to determine if the images conform to the state prohibitions. If the images fit under only one state or federal definition, charging is easily decided. If the images are contraband under the federal and state statutes, then statute of limitations and jurisdictional matters must be decided.

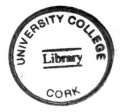

PROVING SCIENTER

The government must prove that the defendant knew that the person in a visual depiction was a minor. That issue was decided in *United States v X-Citement Video* (1994). The defendant challenged his conviction arguing that the federal child pornography statute, 18 USC § 2252, was facially unconstitutional because it lacked the necessary scienter requirement. The statute provides, in relevant part:

(a) Any person who:

(1) knowingly transports or ships in interstate or foreign commerce by any means including by computer or mails, any visual depiction, if:

(A) the producing of such visual depiction involves the use of a minor engaging in sexually explicit conduct; and

(B) such visual depiction is of such conduct.

The term "knowingly" appears in the statute only before the terms "transports" and "ships." Therefore, a literal reading of the statute would suggest that Congress intended to punish, for example, the mail carrier who knowingly transported in his mail truck a package that contained child pornography even though the mail carrier did not know the content of the package. The Supreme Court determined that Congress did not intend this result. Instead, it chose to interpret this criminal statute broadly to include applicable scienter requirements even where the statute by its terms does not contain them. The court considered the legislative intent and found that the age of the performers is the crucial element separating legal innocence from wrongful conduct. In addition, the court noted that "a statute completely bereft of a scienter requirement as to the age of the performers would raise serious constitutional doubts" (*United States v X-Citement Video*, 1994). Therefore, the court concluded that the term "knowingly" applied to the explicit nature of the material and to the age of the performers. Similarly, *United States v Esch* (1987) found that 18 USC § 2251(a) (1984 ed), which proscribed the employment or use of a minor for producing a visual depiction of that minor engaging in sexually explicit conduct, implicitly contains a scienter requirement.

More recently, *United States v Fabiano* (1999), involved a defendant who visited a private Internet chat room named "Preteen" using the Internet Service Provider AOL. Federal law enforcement agents monitored the chat room by participating in and logging the content of the conversations among the participants. It was soon clear to the agents that the participants used the chat room to trade child pornography. Over several months, the defendant was observed visiting the chat room often. This allowed the agents to obtain a search warrant for the defendant's home, where they found child pornography on the defendant's hard drive and on some computer diskettes. The defendant challenged the sufficiency of the evidence against him, arguing that the government did not prove that he knew that the files he received electronically contained child pornography. The court acknowledged that the government

must show that the Defendant had knowledge of the general nature of the contents of the material. The Defendant need not have specific knowledge as to the actual age of the underage performer. The Defendant must have knowledge or an awareness that the material contained a visual depiction of a minor engaging in sexually explicit conduct. Such knowledge may be shown by direct or circumstantial evidence, or both. Eyewitness testimony of the Defendant's perusal of the material is not necessary (*United States v Fabiano*, 1999).

This case is important if ever faced with the argument that a defendant can not be convicted because he or she did not know the exact age of the children depicted. It is important because it allows prosecutors to pursue cases against individuals though no one observed the person viewing the child pornography; circumstantial evidence suggesting that he or she had an awareness of the content of the material is enough.

Finally, it must be stressed that the government does not have to prove the particular identity of a child, only that the individual was a minor. Recent changes to the laws, specifically *Ashcroft v Free Speech Coalition* and the PROTECT Act, have not altered that basic premise. While proving identity of the child is one way to prove age, identification of any individual victim is not mandated by law, nor required for successful prosecution. Defeating the "virtual" defense in child pornography prosecutions post-*Ashcroft* will be discussed later in the chapter.

STATUTES OF LIMITATION ISSUES

One of the first matters to consider in making the charging decision for any case is if the case is stale, that is, whether the prosecutor will be violating any applicable statutes of limitation by filing the case. In child abuse and exploitation cases, a special statute of limitations may apply.

In April of 2003, the federal law was amended to eliminate the statute of limitations for child abuse. 18 United States Code Annotated (USCA) § 3283 now states "[n]o statute of limitations that would otherwise preclude prosecution for an offense involving the sexual or physical abuse, or kidnapping, of a child under the age of 18 years shall preclude such prosecution during the life of the child." Congress has defined child abuse as "the physical or mental injury, sexual abuse or exploitation, or negligent treatment of a child" (18 USC § 3509(a)(3)), thereby bringing exploitation cases within the coverage of this statute. Crimes against children committed after April 2003 have no statute of limitation, whereas those committed before the change are governed by the law in place at the time of commission of the act.

Prior to this change, the statute read "[n]o statute of limitations that would otherwise preclude prosecution for an offense involving the sexual or physical abuse of a child under the age of 18 years shall preclude such prosecution before the child reaches the age of 25 years." The general federal statute of limitations, referenced in the above statute, is found at 18 USC § 3282. It reads "[e]xcept as otherwise expressly provided by law, no person shall be prosecuted, tried, or punished for any offense, not capital, unless the indictment is found or the information is instituted within five years next after such offense shall have been committed." There is no death penalty for child exploitation cases; therefore, this 5-year time limit applied. The 5-year period begins to run the day after an offense is committed (*United States v Guerro*, 1983; *United States v Nappy*, 1995). However, there is an exception to the federal time limit for fugitives from justice. 18 USC § 3290 indicates there is no statute of limitations for any person who has fled from justice. Regarding the prior law, the federal statute of limitations ran though the identity of the offender was unknown (*Lee v State*, 1993).

Most states, like the federal government, have extended their statute of limitations for cases of child abuse. As such, the removal of this procedural barrier will now make it theoretically possible to prosecute even in cases where extremely delayed reporting of the abuse has occurred. A national survey of state statutes of limitations applicable to criminal child sexual abuse can be found in **Appendix 27-1**.

JURISDICTION

In the average child abuse case, there is one jurisdiction: the state in which the crime occurred. In a child pornography case, multiple jurisdictions are possible, particularly where the child pornography was distributed over the Internet. Factors to consider in deciding jurisdiction include the differences between federal and state child pornography laws, federal and state case law, and the varying penalties for the offenses. Experience of the prosecutor(s) and resources of their offices will play a part in jurisdictional decisions. The admissibility of prior uncharged acts should be considered.

Another factor to consider, particularly if the suspect is a repeat offender, is the existence of civil commitment statutes. Several states have passed civil commitment statutes, which provide for the commitment to a mental institution of certain sexual predators who have been convicted of a sex offense and have served their prison sentence but remain dangerous (Holmgren, 1998a,b).

Recently, in *United States v Cream* (2003), the court found that the Child Pornography Prevention Act (CPPA) applied to conduct that occurred on a US Naval station in Spain. The court stated that the nature of the offense and Congress' other legislative efforts in the area of child pornography suggested that the CPPA was intended to have broad application, implying extraterritorial application.

NUMBER OF COUNTS AND IMAGES TO CHARGE

Once state or federal jurisdiction has been established, the prosecutor must decide how many counts to charge and which images to select. As a rule, prosecutors should not charge more offenses than necessary to reflect the nature and extent of the criminal conduct and provide a basis for an appropriate sentence. Charges should not be filed to exert leverage in plea negotiations nor abandoned to reach a plea agreement. However, the state may charge offenses that will strengthen its case or provide a tactical advantage, if they meet all other charging criteria.

Congress has given prosecutors the authority to charge one count for each computer image file possessed by a defendant that contains a visual depiction of a minor engaged in sexually explicit conduct. Prosecutors, however, should be wary of overcharging these cases. In deciding how many counts to charge, it may be helpful to liken these cases to long-term intrafamilial abuse scenarios. Just as many cases of inhouse molestation involve many acts over many months, each of which could theoretically be charged separately, most cases of child pornography involve many images, each of which could be charged individually. However, there are a number of reasons to keep the number of counts under control. First, each count will have to be proven beyond a reasonable doubt. Prosecutorial economy may dictate that the number of images be kept to a reasonable number. It may be wise to group the images into classifications, such as by file name, or type of acts, or by status (eg, child with child, child with adult). Second, the jury may not be able to view hundreds, or even thousands, of images. Finally, charging a multiplicity of counts must eventually reach the zero sum gain point. Once the total sentencing potential reaches triple digits, it may be time to consider what is gained by additional counts. (Sample indictments are shown in **Appendix 27-2**.)

Concurrent with the number of counts is the decision as to which images to charge. Potential defenses, such as reasonable belief that the image was of an adult, must be considered at this juncture. Prosecutors should avoid, if possible, charging cases involving visual depictions of children with pubic hair development when there is a lack of extrinsic evidence that the child depicted is under age 18. Images of physically developed teenagers, whose identity is unknown, must be assessed before charging to make sure that a reasonable person would have no choice but to decide that the person depicted was under the age of 18 (*United States v Arvin*, 1990). Charging only images of prepubescent children will eradicate potential "mistake of fact" type defenses at trial, as well as reinforce to the jury that prosecutorial discretion is being properly exercised.

ADDITIONAL AND/OR ALTERNATIVE CHARGES

Though the focus of this chapter is child pornography, pornography is one type of child abuse. Traditional charges of molestation, rape, lewd and lascivious conduct, sexual battery, and any other factually appropriate sex crime charges should be considered. Other crimes might include kidnapping, custodial interference, and battery. Additionally, by focusing on the defendant, other charges may come to light. Is the defendant a nonregistered sex offender? Did he or she exhibit the child pornography to other victims? Did the defendant destroy or attempt to destroy evidence? Finally, in "sting" cases where the defendant believed he or she was dealing with another child pornography distributor or collector, consider charging attempt crimes, such as

Sample Protective Order

STIPULATION AND [PROPOSED] PROTECTIVE ORDER

In this case, the defendant is charged with [insert charges here] in violation of Penal Code § [___]. The People are prepared to disclose discovery documents (list type and nature of discovery), to counsel for the defendant in this case. Pursuant to *Westerfield v Superior Court Of San Diego County* (2002) __Cal App 4th __; 2002 WL 1384731, the parties jointly request that disclosure of these materials be subject to the following restrictions:

1. The above-described materials or their contents shall not be disclosed to anyone except the defendant, his counsel of record and any defense investigators working on the case, absent further order of the Court. These materials shall be used only in preparation of the defense in this proceeding. Any person to whom these materials or their contents are disclosed must be provided with a copy of this Stipulation and Order and must execute the Agreement in the form attached hereto as Exhibit A, which shall be served on the Court. While the defendant may review the materials, in the presence of counsel, for purposes of assisting counsel in preparing and presenting the defense in this proceeding, under no circumstances shall the defendant be given copies of any part of these materials to keep.

2. The above-described materials shall not be copied at all unless copying is necessary for preparation of the defense in this proceeding. Any copy of the materials that is made shall be accompanied at all times by a copy of this Stipulation and Order. The materials provided to defense counsel pursuant to this order, and any copies thereof, shall be returned to the court at the conclusion of this case.

3. The above-described materials shall not leave the confines of the county where this order was issued.

4. Failure to abide by this order will result in sanctions by this Court and may result in state or federal criminal charges for possession or dissemination of child pornography.

[attorney signatures here]

ORDER

In light of the stipulation and agreement of the parties to this action, and good cause appearing therefor, it is HEREBY ORDERED that disclosure of the above-described discovery materials shall be restricted as set forth in Paragraphs 1 through 4 above.

[judge's signature here]

EXHIBIT "A"

AGREEMENT TO BE BOUND BY PROTECTIVE ORDER

I, the undersigned, _____ (print or type name), hereby acknowledge that I have received a copy of the Protective Order (the "Protective Order") entered on _____, 2002, in that certain matter entitled People v Doe, Sacramento County Case No. 0000000, have read and understand the Order and agree to be bound by all the provisions thereof. My business/resident address is as follows:

_____
_____
_____

I consent to personal jurisdiction over me by the (Sacramento County Superior Court for purposes of enforcing the Order.

I declare under penalty of perjury under the State of California that the foregoing is true and correct, and that this Agreement was executed on the _____ day of _____, 2002, in _____.

Figure 27-1. *Protective orders like this are used so the materials are not altered, copied, or destroyed.*

Arizona courts embraced the same reasoning in *Cervantes v Cates* (2003). In *Cervantes*, the state was in possession of videotapes and photographs intended to be used as evidence that the defendant had possessed child pornography. The defendant requested copies of the items to be provided to his counsel. The state refused to copy, but offered the defendant and his counsel the opportunity to review the items. The trial court ruled the state could make the materials available for review provided defense counsel would be present and review could take place in one session. More than 12 hours were spent reviewing the materials, and a detective was posted outside of the reviewing room to avoid the destruction of the evidence and to protect the chain of custody. Defense was unable to complete the review within one session. Following this, the defendant filed a motion to compel the state to copy the videotapes and photographs. The trial court denied the motion to compel, and the matter was brought before the Court of Appeals. The Court of Appeals held that (1) under applicable rules of procedure, the defendant did not have the burden of showing why the state should be required to provide him with copies of requested materials; rather, burden was on the state to show good cause for a protective order excusing noncompliance with rules; (2) rules requiring disclosure of materials sought by the defendant did not exempt contraband; and (3) to the extent that the defense counsel used the materials in question solely for the purpose of providing a defense, the counsel would not be subject to criminal liability.

In *Taylor v State* (2002) in Texas, the defendant appealed convictions for 9 counts of possession of child pornography. The defendant argued that the trial court's refusal to order this to provide him with a complete copy of the hard drive as "material physical evidence" for inspection required reversal. The State argued that the images were contraband, and therefore, it could not provide the defendant with a complete copy of the hard drive.

The Texas Court of Appeals made an analogy to the right of a drug defendant to have an independent chemist review the make-up of the "contraband" with the right of the defendant to review the hard drive. The court found that

[i]t is no different in this instance to require the State to produce its evidence, ie, the hard drive, for independent review, subject to the State's right to have a representative present. Accordingly, at the very least, an exact copy of the duplicate of Taylor's hard drive should have been produced for review by an expert of Taylor's choosing, in the presence of a representative of the State. In so holding, we disagree with the State's position that such a review must be conducted at a State-controlled facility. We would not require a chemist to take a "porta-lab" with him or her into an evidence room to check alleged contraband drugs, and it is not appropriate to require a computer expert to carry his or her equipment into a State facility to review the documents. Under some circumstances, such as in this case where the accuracy of the copy itself is at issue, the duplicate and the original hard drive should both be produced for independent examination. The failure to produce the requested materials for independent review by defense counsel or his expert was error (*Taylor v State*, 2002).

JURY SELECTION

"The bottom line is that society condemns child molestation in the abstract, but how it responds to individual cases depends on who the offender is, who the victim is, and whether the case fits their stereotypical ideas" (Lanning, 2001).

Nowhere are the above words more true than in computer-facilitated child sexual exploitation cases. As "society" comprises the jury pool from which prosecutors must select the triers of fact in these cases, selecting the right jurors is of critical importance in the process of securing a conviction in these newest types of crimes against children. Effective ***voir dire*** (ie, the examination to determine if the juror is competent) is essential.

THE UNDERLYING CRIME

Though these cases involve computers, at their core they are child abuse cases and must address all the traditional components of such a case. In luring cases, the first questions should be about whether the potential juror has children or grandchildren, if those children use the Internet, and what type of supervision is provided during those sessions. Possible stereotypes surrounding offenders should be investigated, such as "Does anyone think they would recognize the type of person who engages in sexual conduct with children on sight?" and "Does everyone agree that this type of crime, like most crimes, can be committed by people from all walks of life?"

In most of the online luring cases, the victim will be a teenager and may have some emotional difficulties in testifying. The jury must be made aware of the child being an older child, and any problematic issues, such as recantation or behavioral troubles of the victim, must be dealt with as early as possible. If the victim was a boy, that should also be brought out immediately, as many jurors will automatically assume the victim was a girl. If the facts of the crime indicate that the child was a compliant victim (eg, did not fight back, did not immediately report the abuse, bonded with the perpetrator, initiated the contact), the jury must be questioned to discern how it feels about this and make certain that it understand this is not a defense. The law exists to protect children from adults and from themselves.

In child pornography cases, the jurors' attitudes toward child pornography *and* adult pornography should be explored. Prosecutors may inquire what, if any, media coverage of child pornography, or child sexual exploitation generally, potential jurors have been exposed to and how they feel about that issue. Most importantly, the jury must be informed that child pornography is not constitutionally protected.

COMPUTERS AND COMPUTER EVIDENCE

This area of questioning will deal with the potential juror's exposure to and comfort with computers. Questions in this area would cover the following: whether the person has ever used a computer, where, how often, and for what purposes. Prosecutors might ask if the potential juror accesses the Internet, how often, and for what purposes. Next, the juror's ability to listen to and understand computer evidence and forensic examiner's testimony must be assessed. While making certain that the jurors understand that they will be presented with forensic evidence, the technical nature of these cases should be underplayed to maximize jurors' comfort level at the start of the trial. It assists in making the point that this is a child abuse case, not a computer case.

GOVERNMENT REGULATION OF THE INTERNET

Most jurors will give broad theoretical support to the concepts behind the First Amendment. Prosecutors have to make certain jurors understand that these free speech interests must be counterbalanced against the government's compelling interest in protecting children and prohibiting crime. Not all Internet speech is protected, including libel, fraud, and child pornography. In fact, the government has regulated various media for decades, including television. Prosecutors must make certain jurors understand prohibiting child pornography (and other criminal activity) is not the same as regulating constitutionally protected free speech. Additionally, if potential jurors have children, inquiring as to what their practices are regarding allowing their children access to the Internet may speak volumes on their acceptance of regulation as a necessity in protecting children.

DIFFUSING POTENTIAL DEFENSES

There are a relatively small number of consistently raised potential defenses in these cases. These defenses are discussed in greater detail in the next section of the chapter. However, they are addressed here briefly, as it is important for the prosecutor conducting voir dire to assess potential jurors' knowledge in these areas.

The first type of defense is an attack on the police and their investigatory methods. Potential bias against undercover, proactive "sting" tactics should be examined. After asking about jurors' comfort level with these methods, it must be made clear to jurors these methods are legal, and they are used to put the officers in harm's way to block offenders successfully targeting real children. The fact that there is no "real" victim in a luring case should be addressed, stressing that because the police took on the persona of a child, does not mean that no crime occurred. In child pornography cases, that an image of a child being sexually violated was sent to a police officer rather than someone else, does not mean that the defendant is innocent.

The second type of defense is mistaken identity. This is simply a variation on the traditional defenses of "I've been framed" or "some other dude did it (SODDI)." As such, voir dire will cover what types of evidence or factors a potential juror would look to in determining identity in any case and then in a computer-facilitated case.

The third defense occurs when the defendant claims that the necessary element of intent is not present in his case. This may arise in any of the following forms: fantasy, good Samaritan accident, mistake of age, or deleted images. Questions along the following lines may help identify the jurors best suited to see through these types of untrue defense:

— "If 2 people agreed to the same set of facts or actions as being true (provide an example) but offered irreconcilably different explanations for these facts or actions, how would you go about deciding who was telling the truth?"

— "Intent is not a tangible thing, something you can hold in your hand or put up to the light to examine. How do you go about deciding what someone's intent is (provide an example)?"

— "Have you ever been on the Internet and had any sort of a pop-up appear? What sort of a pop-up was it? What did you do?"

— "If an individual claimed that something came into his or her possession accidentally (provide an example), how would you decide whether that was true or not?"

The fourth defense is loosely termed the "First Amendment" or privilege defense. This occurs where defendants admit to possession of child pornography, but claim they possess it in furtherance of activity protected by the Constitution or a legally viable reason. These include the reporter working on a story about child pornography, the medical practitioner who needs it for a book on child sexual abuse, or a "photographer" who claims the image is not child pornography but "nude art." In these cases, the prosecutor must stress, if applicable, the lack of any such exemption from the child pornography laws for people of the defendant's profession. If the defendant had a legitimate purpose for the contraband and the law allows for such possession, the state may still contend that the defendant was using it for purposes outside the prescribed exemption. The prosecutor must inquire how the juror would go about deciding if the defendant had a legitimate purpose.

Finally is the virtual child pornography defense. The recent decision in *Ashcroft v Free Speech Coalition* (2002) has resulted in the prosecution now having to prove that the image of child pornography is of a real child. The prosecution does not, however, have to prove the identity of the child. Questions regarding jurors' awareness of that case and their understanding of it should be scrutinized. Questions that might be asked might include

— "Are you familiar with any court decisions regarding pornography? Child pornography? What do you understand those decisions to say? What do you think of those decisions?"

— "Have any of you ever heard the term 'virtual child pornography'? What does that term mean to you?"

— "As part of its case, the state must prove that the images the defendant is charged with possessing/distributing/producing are images of real children. The state does not have to prove the identity of any particular child, only that the image is of a real child. Does everyone understand the state's burden on this point?"

If the defense is planning on calling an expert to testify that the images are completely computer generated and the state will call its own expert to testify to the contrary, additional questions should be asked. These might include

— "If you hear conflicting testimony from 2 experts, do you feel comfortable in the role of the decision maker who will resolve this? Do you understand that if there is a conflict among experts, this conflict is not the same thing as reasonable doubt? You, as the finder of fact, decide what weight to give each expert's testimony."

— "Do you understand that the testimony of an expert can be accepted or rejected, just like any other witness?"

In addition to the substantive issues and areas noted above, prosecutors should consider their own personality and courtroom persona style when conducting voir dire, as opposed to standing in front of a group of strangers and asking them questions. Not only is voir dire an opportunity to educate the jury, it is just as importantly an opportunity to gauge potential jurors' attitudes and beliefs about key aspects of these cases. One of the best techniques to get this information is to ask open-ended questions that ask for a juror to give more than a "yes" or "no" answer. The best voir dire incorporates personal style with the specific case, the potential jurors, the judge, local rules and practice, and other external factors, all coming together to yield a conducted and dynamic voir dire. Sample voir dire questions are provided in **Appendix 27-3**.

MEETING UNTRUE DEFENSES*

Many defenses are used in child pornography crimes. The facts and circumstances of each case, along with any statement(s) the defendant may have made, will limit plausible defenses. The defenses fall into 5 categories: mistaken identity, not a real child, lack of proof of age, lack of intent, and First Amendment.

MISTAKEN IDENTITY

One of the most difficult aspects of prosecuting computer-facilitated child pornography cases may be putting the perpetrator at the computer. The suspect may attempt to place blame on a roommate or a visitor, claim that the account was compromised and someone must have stolen the password(s) and screen name and accessed the Internet from another computer, or assert that he or she was the victim of a hacking or intrusion. These are all similar to the classic SODDI defense and may be met in various ways.

When an investigator is conducting an undercover sting operation or when there is a report of sexually exploitive conduct involving computers, connecting the screen or user name of the perpetrator to a real person is crucial for the investigator. This may be done by identifying the suspect's ISP, using header information on the suspect's e-mail or other electronic communications, and then obtaining subscriber information from the ISP. (For more information, see Kreston, 2000a.) Using a search warrant, subpoena, or court order, prosecutors may obtain subscriber information such as the name, address, and billing information associated with the person who pays for the account associated with that screen name or user name. Prosecutors should note that the person who pays for the account may not be the same person who engaged in the criminal activity and that the address where the bill is sent may not be the same as the location of the computer used in that activity. The account could belong to a parent, relative, or friend of the suspect or could have been created using the stolen credit card information or identity of another.

Investigative Techniques to Prove Identity

Prosecutors should always keep in mind conventional investigative techniques when attempting to prove the identity of the perpetrator in a computer crime case. They should not overlook investigative techniques common to all cases, including surveillance of the suspect's home, observing who enters and departs from the home, talking to the neighbors, and interviewing the suspect. If the investigation determines that the suspect lives alone and has no regular guests, it will be difficult to argue that someone else was using the suspect's home computer.

If others live with the suspect, he or she may argue that he or she allows the others in the home to use his or her account to access the Internet, and that he has no knowledge of the unlawful activity. When multiple people live at the location and have

---

* This section is adapted from Astrowsky B, Peters J. Anticipating and meeting defenses. In: Peters JS, ed. *Prosecuting Internet Child Exploitation Crimes. Washington, DC: US Dept of Justice (2002a)*.

access to the computer, investigate the schedules of all the occupants of the house and compare those schedules against the time and date printouts from the ISP for when the relevant transmissions were made or when the online sessions took place.

When the subject is believed to be using a home computer, a recorded pretext telephone call (where authorized by law) may yield information about who is at the terminal at a particular time and whether anyone else has access to the computer. Posing as a start-up ISP doing a market survey, for example, investigators could offer a free trial account. Then, they could ask the suspect how many computers he or she has, whether he or she has a desktop computer at home, and whether he has a laptop computer. They could ask about Internet access, the name of his or her ISP, how many people access the Internet using the account, and how often the suspect goes online. If the person says that he or she is the only one who uses his ISP account, it will go a long way toward combating the defense argument that someone else was using his or her account.

When billing information from the ISP shows that the criminal activity originated at a public access terminal such as a library or school, investigators may review sign-on logs or engage in covert surveillance and video monitoring to help in identifying the subject. Once the suspect is identified, good interview techniques (preferably recorded or reduced to writing and signed) can produce corroboration of essential elements, including identity. The subscriber information from the ISP, together with facts gathered using conventional investigative techniques, may be enough to obtain a search warrant of the subscriber's home and computer or other locations where there is probable cause to believe evidence will be found.

Another conventional technique to verify the identity of an anonymous online "chatter" is a face-to-face meeting in a public location. The Internet allows individuals to communicate with other people from all over the world, and some suspects in undercover operations may reside in another jurisdiction or country. However, eager perpetrators will sometimes travel great distances in hopes of obtaining child pornography. In these cases, the investigator can suggest that he or she has nondigital pictures, videos, or magazines that he is willing to trade for the suspect's digital images. If the suspect appears in person to conduct the transaction, it will be difficult for him or her to contend that he or she was not the person who engaged in the online conversations.

Finally, no-knock warrants should be considered. In *People v Foley* (2000), the police executed a no-knock search warrant at the defendant's house and found him engaging in the crime as he was typing at his computer. The no-knock warrant, like no other investigative technique, permits agents to catch the perpetrator in the act and verify his identity.

Forensic Examination

In addition to these traditional techniques, other ways of proving identity may be present. The suspect may claim that he or she gave someone else his or her user/screen name and password to go online, and that person must have used his account from another computer. While such a defense may be true, forensic evaluation of the suspect's computer may be able to verify or refute this claim. Even if the examiner does not find child pornography on the suspect's computer, incriminating evidence may be found such as saved online chats with minors, or incriminating evidence in the cache, history files, temporary Internet files, bookmarks, or file slack that the prosecutor can use to show that the suspect's story was a fabrication.

Defeating Hacker/Intrusion Defenses

Another variation of the identity defense is the claim that child pornography or other evidence "mysteriously appeared" on the suspect's computer, the work of an anonymous hacker who took control of the computer over the Internet (*United States v*

Hay, 2000). Prosecutors should recognize that it is at least theoretically possible for this to occur, using one of several so-called Trojan horse type programs, such as Back Orifice (BO), Netbus, Brown Orifice, and others. Basic knowledge of computer operating systems and other computer basics can help overcome such a defense. One important point is that BO works only on computers running the Windows 95, Windows 98, or Windows 2000 Operating System (OS). Thus, Macintosh or Linux users, or users with other versions of the Windows operating system are not susceptible to BO, so the first thing to do is check which OS the defendant was using. Once BO or other Trojan horses are installed in the target's computer, a hacker can run the BO client program and control the user's computer remotely. The operations that the client application can perform on the target machine (eg, the machine running the server application) include executing commands, listing files, logging keystrokes, restarting the target machine, viewing the contents of files, and uploading and downloading files to and from the target machine. It is the last function that leads to the potential for a hacker intrusion defense. Forensic examiners can detect the presence or absence of BO, manually or with software. Even if a Trojan horse is detected, however, that is not the end of the inquiry. The question is then whether the target is a dupe who accidentally installed the Trojan horse and opened himself up to a hacker or whether he or she installed it himself, in a preemptive attempt to lay the groundwork for raising the hacking/intrusion defense at a later time if and when he or she was caught.

PROVING THE IMAGE DEPICTS A "REAL" CHILD AFTER *ASHCROFT V FREE SPEECH**

In the recent Supreme Court decision of *Ashcroft v Free Speech Coalition* (2002), the Supreme Court held that the Child Pornography Protection Act was unconstitutional to the extent that it prohibited computer-generated, or "virtual," child pornography, that is, images created solely by technology. The court held that where no real children were used to create the child pornography, no harm to real children was present. This factually distinguished it from the concerns voiced in *New York v Ferber* (1982), which struck down any First Amendment protection for child pornography based on the state's compelling interest in protecting children from the immediate physical and psychological harm visited on the child by the production. In so doing, the court ignored the role that child pornography, real or virtual, plays in the grooming process of the next generation of real child victims. The court ignored congressional findings of a link between child pornography and child abuse and that virtual child pornography feeds into the marketplace for child pornography. In summary, the court looked only to the circumstances surrounding the *creation*, but not the *consequences*, of child pornography. In the aftermath of *Ashcroft*, it now falls to the state to prove that the image is that of a real child who is underage. The state need only prove that the image is of a real child and not that it is of any particular, identifiable child. The following are ways in which to prove the child is real, a minor, or both.

Testimony of the Child or Someone Who Knows the Child
The best method to prove age and status (a real child) is to present testimony from the child depicted or someone competent to testify as to the age of the actual child depicted. This may be possible in cases in which a child has been identified and prosecutions have taken place. One such recent example is the "Helen & Gavin" case, in which the 2 children exploited in a child pornography series of photos were identified by Scotland Yard. The detectives who handled the case and testified in the prosecutions are providing affidavits to prosecutors throughout the world as to the identities and ages of the children and that they are real children. The detectives further assert that they are prepared to come to court to testify under oath to the

---

* For a fuller treatment of this topic, see Kreston S. Defeating the virtual defense in child pornography prosecutions. *High Technol Law J. 2004;3:49.*

Figure 27-2. *Having a detective or other competent person provide an affidavit is one way to prove a child is real.*

same. **Figure 27-2** shows a copy of one such affidavit. Recognizing, however, that such testimony will only rarely be available, other methods will have to be utilized in the majority of cases to prove that the child was real and a minor.

Affidavit Proving Age

Form MG 11

Witness Statement
(CJ Act 1967, s.9;MC Act 1980, ss.5A(3)(a) and 5B;MC Rules 1981, r.70)

Statement of	Sharon G.

Age if under 18
(if over 18 insert 'over 18') Over 18 Occupation Police Officer

This statement (consisting of: 2 pages each signed by me) is true to the best of my knowledge and belief and I make it knowing that, if it is tendered in evidence, I shall be liable to prosecution if I have wilfully stated anything which I know to be false or do not believe to be true.

Dated: 11th July 2002

Signature: Sharon G.

I am a Police Officer serving with the National Crime Squad of England and Wales based in the United Kingdom.

Since May 1998 I have been a case officer responsible for conducting investigations into a worldwide paedophile organisation. Part of these investigations is to identify and locate the children subject to abuse on the images and video clips seized throughout the world.

On the 29th March 2000 I removed from our exhibits store two compact disks named Hercules1. These disks were recovered from the computer of a male named Gary SALT and formed part of a bestcrypt container. Bestcrypt is a program that creates a container or a strongbox to hold images and other sensitive material. Access can be gained only if the correct password or passphrase is known. The passphrase was supplied to Law Enforcement by Gary SALT.

I examined the disk marked 1 of 2 and made a copy of it which, I produce as my exhibit SAG/128. Upon the examination of the CD I found a file path directory which I copied and produce as my exhibit SAG/129.

I viewed that file path and found Six Hundred and Six paedophilic images all of which are exhibited and produced by me as exhibits SAG/130 to SAG/735.

All of the children from these images have been identified.

Lisa Parsons, a Deputy County Attorney of the Technology and Electronic Crimes Bureau in the Maricopa County Attorneys Office in the United States of America, has sent me sixteen images in an effort to identify the children in those images. Having viewed them I am able to identify as follows:

Hel&g012 is identical to image hel&gav012.jpg which is produced by me as exhibit SAG/412.
Hel&g014 is identical to image hel&gav014.jpg which is produced by me as exhibit SAG/414.
Hel&g015 is identical to image hel&gav015.jpg which is produced by me as exhibit SAG/415.
Hel&g016 is identical to image hel&gav016.jpg which is produced by me as exhibit SAG/416.
Hel&g020 is identical to image hel&gav020.jpg which is produced by me as exhibit SAG/420.
Hel&g026 is identical to image hel&gav001.jpg which is produced by me as exhibit SAG/401.
Hel&g029 is identical to image hel&gav029.jpg which is produced by me as exhibit SAG/429.
Hel&g049 is identical to image hel&gav049.jpg which is produced by me as exhibit SAG/449.
Hel&g13 is identical to image hel&gav009.jpg which is produced by me as exhibit SAG/409.
Hel&ga11 is identical to image hel&gav011.jpg which is produced by me as exhibit SAG/411.
Hel&gav0 is identical to image hel&gav040.jpg which is produced by me as exhibit SAG/440.
Hel_gav0 is identical to image hel&gav015.jpg which is produced by me as exhibit SAG/415.

The male child in these pictures are:
Gavin **M**. born 22nd April 1988. I produce his birth certificate as exhibit SAG/96.

Hel_rob2 is identical to image hel_rob02.jpg which is produced by me as exhibit SAG/499.
Hel_rob03 is identical to image hel_rob03.jpg which is produced by me as exhibit SAG/500.

The male child in these pictures are:
Robert **M**. born 22nd October 1986. I produce his birth certificate as exhibit SAG/95.

Hel-cum0 is identical to image hel-cum02.jpg which is produced by me as exhibit SAG/518.
Hel-lo04 is identical to image hel-lo04.jpg which is produced by me as exhibit SAG/534.

The female child in all of these sixteen pictures is:-
Helene **M**. born 9th May 1989. I produce her birth certificate as exhibit SAG/97.

I have seen and met Robert, Gavin and Helene on numerous occasions and can confirm that without doubt they are the three children subjected to sexual abuse in the images produced.
The adult male responsible for the abuse of the named children is Gary SALT. SALT has been convicted in England with the assault of these children and I produce the certificate of his conviction as exhibit SAG/126.

On Tuesday 4th April 2000 I took these sixteen images to Wandsworth Prison, London, and showed them to Gary SALT. He identified them as being a true and accurate copy of the photographs taken by him of Robert **M**., Gavin **M**. and Helene **M**. Both Gary SALT and myself signed them to that effect.

All of the original exhibits have been retained by me and will be made available at any court appearance.

I am prepared to attend court and give any evidence if necessary.

Child Pornography Historian

One method of proving the child is real involves the use of an expert in the history of child pornography. Prosecutors and investigators involved in many child pornography cases see the same images repeatedly. Often, offenders have scanned these images into the computer from a child pornography magazine or other printed publication. Investigators and prosecutors who are familiar with these printed publications may recognize the original source of a computer image of child pornography. In fact, these child pornography history experts can probably obtain, via a library of materials that they have kept themselves or via the FBI Innocent Images Task Force or the United States Customs Service (which has a large library of child pornography magazines), the original magazine that contained the same picture that has been distributed in electronic form over the Internet. The magazines and publications chronicled by these historians may have been published many years before the commercial availability of the personal computer. They may also have been printed many years before the commercial availability of computer graphics software that allows for the altering of computer images. Therefore, if a prosecutor can present a witness who can testify that the computer image that a defendant distributed came from a magazine printed in the early 1970s, years before any individual could create or alter such an image on a personal computer, that prosecutor will have proven that the picture is of an actual child and not a virtual one.

One recent case to employ such an expert was *United States v Guagliardo* (2002), where a government witness testified that he had worked as a mail inspector for the Customs Service during the mid-1980s and that he had personally encountered magazines that contained copies of Guagliardo's images. The United States Customs Service Cyber Smuggling Center maintains the world's largest reference collection of child pornography materials. To find an expert in any given United States jurisdiction, contact the local FBI field office, the local customs agent, the FBI's Innocent Images Task Force, the United States Postal Inspection Service, Criminal Investigations/Child Exploitation program, or the Child Exploitation of Obscenity Section of the Department of Justice.

Computer Graphics Expert

Another method to establish that the child is not a "virtual" child is to use a computer graphics expert. By looking at the pixels, or by looking for shading differences in an image, an expert can determine whether the image has been altered in any way. The prosecutor should find an expert who is familiar with commercially available computer graphics software and how it works. That person would then educate the jury concerning how images are created and/or altered using these programs. This person can testify as to when morphing software became available, how images are altered or created, and how difficult such alteration or creation is, particularly when a series of photos is involved. The expert can then render an opinion as to whether the images had been morphed, altered, or created.

PROVING AGE

In child pornography prosecutions involving images of physically developed but unidentified teenagers, the defense may argue that the government has failed to prove beyond a reasonable doubt that the persons depicted are under the age of 18. Title 18 USC § 2256(1) defines minor as "any person under the age of eighteen years." The federal statute requires the visual depiction to be actionable and be of a minor under the age of 18. It does not require that the government prove the exact age of the child. Therefore, all that the government must do is prove that the person depicted is not an adult (*United States v Freeman*, 1987). In state statutes, the age requirement may vary, but the same principles apply.

The court in *United States v Villard* (1988) suggested 4 methods of proving the age of depicted individuals:

1. The minor, or someone who knows him or her, testifies as to his or her age at the time the photos were taken.

2. An expert (eg, a pediatrician) offers an opinion as to the age of the depicted individual.

3. A lay witness gives an opinion as to the age of the depicted individual.

4. The members of the jury decide.

These and other methods of establishing age will now be addressed.

Proving Minority Through Computer Forensics

Since most Internet child pornography cases include images of children who are minors, the defense of mistake of age will rarely apply. If, however, a defendant offers the defense that he or she thought the image portrayed an adult, beyond examination of the images, examination of the defendant's computer may reveal electronic footprints, including the cache, cookies, history file, bookmarks, and temporary Internet files, which may lead to circumstantial evidence rebutting the defense. If these areas of the computer reveal files and other indications of an interest or obsession with underage children, this can be used to help prove that the defendant knew what he or she was looking at. Indeed, the computer history shows that he or she specifically sought images of children.

Proving Age Through Expert Testimony

Another method of proving age involves the use of expert testimony. A pediatrician may testify that, based upon training and experience, the person depicted is under the age of 18. The prosecutor should select a pediatrician with substantial experience in child physical development and lay the foundation for the expert's training and experience. In *United States v Bender* (2002) and *United States v Pollard* (2001), medical experts testified that the characteristics of a subject image were consistent with an actual child, noting such factors as proportions, distribution of body fat, and "typical pre-pubertal spontaneous movements and behaviors" of the subjects.

In cases in which the depicted children have reached puberty, the government can call expert witnesses to testify as to the physical development of the depicted person and present testimony regarding the way the creator, distributor, or possessor labeled the disks, directories, or videos (*United States v Anderton*, 1998; *United States v Robinson*, 1998).

In United States v Long (1997), a Cincinnati pediatrician offered an opinion as to one child seen in a pornographic video being under age 18. A forensic psychiatrist offered a second opinion using the Tanner scale. The court held that expert testimony on the ages of the video participants does not invade the province of the jury, and the forensic psychiatrist (who taught human sexuality at the University of Kentucky Medical School) had sufficient qualifications to testify regarding methodology used to give his opinion. The court further found that "the jury itself, of course, might make its own determination of age based on the evidence and on the juror's own experience in a case of this type" (*United States v Long*, 1997).

Expert Testimony Regarding the Tanner Scale

Dr. James Tanner of the University of London developed "Tanner staging" to be used by doctors to help them determine the stages of a child's sexual maturation. Tanner stages range from 1 (preadolescent) to 5 (adult) and are based on pubic hair development (both sexes), penis and scrotum size (males), and breast development (females) (Seidel et al, 2003). Many prosecutors have used medical experts familiar with Tanner staging to testify in their child pornography cases. If the expert determined that the person depicted was in Tanner stage 1, 2, or 3, that meant the child had not begun puberty and was under the age of 13. However, Tanner stages 4 and 5 refer to children who had begun puberty, developed pubic hair, and were aged 13 or older.

In *United States v Katz* (1999), Arnold Katz sent a videotape to an undercover agent that the government concluded contained child pornography. Before trial, Katz filed a *Daubert* motion to exclude all expert witness testimony purporting to set the age of the persons depicted in the videotape via application of the Tanner scale (*Daubert v Merrell Dow Pharmaceuticals, Inc*, 1993). The trial court held a *Daubert* hearing "wherein it was developed that the Tanner Scale of Human Development for females is the recognized scientific test used for determining the age of postpubescent Caucasian females and consists of separately rating, on scales 1 to 5, breast development and pubic hair development, with Stage 1 being preadolescent and Stage 5 being adult" (*United States v Katz*, 1999). Further testimony revealed that the Tanner scale "is valid as to Caucasians, but it is not valid as to all ethnic groups" (*United States v Katz*, 1999). Ultimately, the trial court allowed the government's expert to testify regarding his conclusions concerning the age of the children depicted in the videotape based upon the Tanner scale.

Unfortunately, Tanner has called for experts to cease using the Tanner scale to decide the approximate age of children depicted in pornography. In a letter to the editor of *Pediatrics*, Tanner, along with Dr. Arlan L. Rosenbloom of the University of Florida, wrote that estimating probable chronologic age in a child pornography case is a "wholly illegitimate use of Tanner staging" (Rosenbloom & Tanner, 1998). For this reason, pediatricians should refrain from using Tanner staging, and prosecutors should avoid basing a prosecution solely on the expert opinion of someone using the Tanner scale (Rosenbloom & Tanner, 1998). Controversy over use of the Tanner scale continued in 3 letters to the editor in the October 1, 1999, issue of *Pediatrics*, and in the surrebuttal from Rosenbloom, all seeking to clarify the issue. The 3 letters presented cogent arguments that Tanner staging remains useful in child pornography cases, along with the clinical experience of physicians, in giving the courts valuable and accurate information whether an individual has the appearance of a child (Kutz, 1999). Dr. Rosenbloom clarified that the letter he and Tanner wrote was in response to several cases in which Tanner staging had been misused to determine chronological age. He explained that there was nothing in their original letter that would preclude testimony based on sound clinical judgment by expert pediatricians relying on their experience in examining children.

Proving Age Through Lay Opinion

An additional useful tool for prosecutors was suggested in *United States v Stanley* (1990). The government offered a postal inspector's testimony as to the ages of the children in the images as lay opinion under Federal Rule of Evidence 701, which allows for lay opinion testimony if such testimony is limited to those opinions or inferences which are (a) rationally based on the perception of the witness and (b) helpful to clear an understanding of the witness testimony or the determination of a fact in issue.

In *Stanley*, the first requirement of Rule 701 was met since the postal inspector had personally viewed the child pornography. However, the defendant argued that the jury was able to judge the age of the persons depicted on its own, and the inspector's opinion concerning the age of the persons was not helpful to an understanding of his testimony nor to the determination of any fact at issue. The court disagreed, showing that the inspector's opinion was important to explain his reason for seizing the photographs. In addition, the court determined that the age of the persons depicted in the photographs was a fact at issue in the trial. Therefore, the inspector's testimony concerning his opinion as to the age of the children depicted was properly admitted. A more recent, post-*Ashcroft* example of this can be found in *United States v Richardson* (2002). In this case, a Special Agent of the Innocent Images Task Force testified that, based on his training and extensive experience as a member of the task force, the images depicted actual children, not what simply appeared to be children.

Proving Age Through the Defendant

Proving age can be as simple as having an investigator question the defendant about his or her belief concerning the age of the persons in the photos. Other times, language used by the defendant in correspondence can be used to prove this element. For example, in *United States v Broyles* (1994), the persons shown were described as "teenies," "between the ages of eleven and fifteen," "just developing," and "range could be as low as six to eight but no higher than fifteen." In cases in which the depicted children have reached puberty, the government can call expert witnesses to testify as to the physical development of the depicted person and present testimony regarding the way the creator, distributor, or possessor labeled the disks, directories, or videos (*United States v Anderton*, 1998; *United States v Robinson*, 1998).

In *United States v Broyles* (1994), the defendant challenged the sufficiency of the evidence supporting a finding that the individuals depicted were younger than 18. The standard of review is whether any rational trier of fact (eg, the judge in a bench trial or jury in a jury trial) that carries the responsibility of determining the issues of fact in a case could have found the essential elements of the crime beyond a reasonable doubt. Factors the *Broyles* court used to support its finding that the government met its burden included the following:

— Defendant used specific language in describing his interest while ordering the material, such as the word "teenies," and ordered a video described as 11- and 12-year-olds having sex

— Defendant pointed out the location of the "child porn" during the search

— Defendant stated that he knew the tape contained girls aged 13 and 15

— Postal inspector gave lay opinion as to age of individuals depicted

— Pediatric endocrinologist gave expert opinion as to the individuals' ages

— Jury, which saw parts of the tape, was in a position to draw its independent conclusions as to the age of the performers.

Age as a Question for the Trier of Fact to Decide

The triers of fact may be presented with an image and have it left up to them to draw their own conclusion as to the age of the children depicted. There is no requirement that the government present expert testimony on this issue. In *United States v Gallo* (1988), the court held that "[e]xpert testimony as to age, while perhaps helpful in some cases, is certainly not required as a matter of course." Similarly, *United States v Lamb* (1996) declined to require the government to prove the age of the persons depicted by expert testimony, and *United States v Villard* (1988) noted that "the jury can examine the photographs in question and determine for itself whether the individual is under eighteen years of age." The pictures need only be shown to the jury, and if the child is under the age of 18, the jury should be able to make that factual finding on its own. When the facts permit, prosecutors using this technique should be careful to select for charging only those images that are minors, such as images of prepubescent children. Examples of post-*Ashcroft* cases supporting this rationale include *United States v Deaton* (2003), *United States v Hall* (2002), and *United States v Lee* (2002).

The Mistake-of-Age Defense for Producers of Child Pornography

A photographer named Gilmour photographed a 17-year-old girl he thought to be 22 years old engaging in various sexual acts with her boyfriend (*Gilmour v Rogerson*, 1997). When the girl requested the photos and negatives, Gilmour agreed to release them provided she engage in a scenario involving the seduction of a pizza deliveryman. The young woman complied, but Gilmour did not honor his part of the agreement and sought to modify it by requiring the girl to have sex with him to obtain the photos and negatives. The girl complained, and Gilmour was convicted under an Iowa state statute prohibiting sexual exploitation of minors. He asserted as a defense that he had asked for her age and was told 22 and that he verified the information by inspecting her driver's license. He reasoned that his mistaken belief as to the girl's age should operate as a defense to the charge. The trial court refused to admit any evidence dealing with Gilmour's mistake-of-age defense. Gilmour was convicted and appealed to the Iowa Supreme Court, which affirmed.

The Eighth Circuit began its opinion by explaining *mens rea*, a culpable mental state, and its relation to nefarious crimes. The court noted that an exception to the required proof of *mens rea* arises in protecting minors from sexual exploitation. Specifically, proof of *mens rea* is not required in connection with a minor's age. The court held the mistake-of-age defense to be the antithesis of the state's interest in protecting minors from sexual exploitation (*Gilmour v Rogerson*, 1997). It drew a distinction between producers and distributors of child pornography, holding that a *producer* such as Gilmour may easily obtain and corroborate the age of the model since he is dealing personally with the minor model. A *distributor*, on the other hand, deals with the minor in image form only, thus greatly increasing the opportunity of mistake as to the subject's age. The court held that deprivation of the mistake-of-age defense did not constitutionally infringe upon Gilmour's First Amendment rights because he was a producer.

Lack of Intent

Entrapment

An entrapment defense is often raised when law enforcement agents engage in undercover sting operations. All jurisdictions in the United States allow the defense of entrapment, but the definition and application of the defense vary considerably. Some states view the entrapment defense as a curb on overly aggressive law enforcement and use an "objective" standard to evaluate the police action. The objective standard focuses on how the tactics of the agency would affect the hypothetical "reasonable law-abiding citizen." Other jurisdictions are more concerned with the mental state of the charged individual and focus on the defendant's intent, or predisposition, to commit the crime charged. This is the so-called subjective standard. This defense has been a basis for reversal in several federal child pornography cases.

For the entrapment defense to be successful, the objective and subjective formulations require that the crime be induced, or encouraged, by government agents. The objective test asks, "Did the government's encouragement of the crime exceed acceptable limits?" The subjective test asks, "Was the defendant predisposed to commit the crime when he was approached by the government agent?" The subjective test has prevailed in federal criminal law (Allen et al, 1999). The key concepts within entrapment are inducement and predisposition.

The Requirement of Inducement

To establish the first element of entrapment, the defendant must show the government agents induced him or her to commit the crime. In *United States v Stanton* (1992), the court approved of an undercover child pornography operation conducted by the United States Postal Inspection Service in which the defendant ordered child pornography after receiving a questionnaire and catalog containing descriptions of available photographs and videos. The court noted that the 2 mailings exerted no pressure upon the defendant and merely allowed him to commit the crime. **Inducement** is government conduct that "creates a substantial risk that an undisposed person or otherwise law-abiding citizen would commit the offense" (*United States v Mendoza-Salgado*, 1992). Inducement can include pressure, assurance the person is doing nothing wrong, persuasion, fraudulent representations, threats, coercive tactics, harassment, promises of reward, or pleas based upon need, sympathy, or friendship. The focus of the inquiry is whether the defendant stood eager or reluctant to participate in the alleged criminal conduct (*United States v Mendoza-Salgado*, 1992).

That the government offered a defendant an opportunity to commit a crime, coupled with mild inducement, does not support a claim of entrapment (*United States v Thoma*, 1984). The concept of inducement was the crux of the case of *United States v Poehlman* (2000). In *Poehlman*, charges were brought against a self-described cross-dresser and foot-fetishist who sought the company of like-minded adults on the Internet and found himself the target of a government sting. Poehlman's wife had divorced him and taken custody of his 2 children, and he had been discharged from the Air Force after he admitted that he could not control his compulsion to cross-dress. Lonely and depressed, he began to search through Internet discussion groups seeking a suitable companion. Most often, women rejected him after they learned of his sexual interests. Eventually, in the summer of 1995, Poehlman saw a message posted by a woman named Sharon suggesting that she was looking for someone who understood her family's "unique needs." Poehlman answered the ad and said that he was looking for "a long-term relationship leading to marriage," "didn't mind children," and "had unique needs too." In a series of e-mail messages, Sharon explained that she had 3 children and that she wanted "someone to help with their special education." At one point, she said that she was looking for "a special man teacher" for her children. Poehlman told Sharon that he did not understand what this meant, but said that he would teach the children "proper morals," and he repeated his interest in Sharon.

"Sharon," who was the alter ego of an undercover investigator, rebuffed Poehlman's interest in her and indicated more directly that she was really interested in a special teacher for her kids. Poehlman "finally got the hint," and expressed his willingness to play sex instructor to Sharon's children. In later e-mail messages, Poehlman graphically described to Sharon his ideas, which included "various acts too tasteless to mention." Poehlman and Sharon eventually planned for him to travel to California. After arriving at a hotel room where he met a woman who said she was Sharon, he entered an adjoining room where he was to meet her children. Instead, he was arrested. Poehlman was convicted by a federal jury of crossing state lines to engage in sex acts with a minor. He was sentenced to 10 years in prison.

In making its determination regarding the propriety of the agent's inducement, the court wrote

where government agents merely make themselves available to participate in a criminal transaction, such as standing ready to buy or sell illegal drugs, they do not induce commission of the crime. An improper "inducement" goes beyond providing an ordinary "opportunity to commit a crime." An "inducement" consists of an "opportunity" plus something else, typically, excessive pressure by the government upon the defendant or the government's taking advantage of an alternative, non-criminal type of motive (*United States v Poehlman*, 2000).

The court found that the undercover agents did a great deal more than provide Poehlman with an opportunity to commit a crime. By playing on his obvious need for an adult relationship, for acceptance of his sexual proclivities, and for a family, the agents acting as Sharon exerted excessive pressure on Poehlman, drew him deeper into a fantasy world, and induced him to commit a crime. "Sharon did not merely invite Poehlman to have a sexual relationship with her minor daughters, she made it a condition of her own continued interest in him" (*United States v Poehlman*, 2000). However, if a court finds that the state did not induce the defendant, then the court need not consider whether the defendant lacked the predisposition to commit the crime (*United States v Stanton*, 1992).

Proving Predisposition
Whether a defendant is predisposed to commit a crime requires an analysis of the following 5 factors:

1. The character or reputation of the defendant

2. If the suggestion of criminal activity was originally made by the government

3. If the defendant was engaged in criminal activity for a profit

4. If the defendant evidenced reluctance to commit the offense, overcome by government persuasion

5. The nature of the inducement or persuasion offered by the government

The most important element is whether the defendant was reluctant to commit the offense. Reluctance does not necessarily negate a finding of predisposition. A certain amount of reluctance can be attributed to "the natural savvy of one versed in the ways of the pornography trade" (*United States v Thoma*, 1984).

In *United States v Gendron* (1994), the court noted that the defendant met with enthusiasm an initial opportunity to buy child pornography, responded to each further government initiative with a purchase order, and showed no particular interest in an anticensorship campaign. As a result, the court concluded that "Gendron would have responded affirmatively to the most ordinary of opportunities" (*United States v Gendron*, 1994) to commit the crime and was not entrapped. In *United States v Gamache* (1998), the First Circuit elaborated upon its opinion in *Gendron* and stated that though ready commission of the criminal act can show an individual's predisposition, eagerness alone, when coupled with "extra elements," may require that a defendant's predisposition be gauged by the jury. The court suggested that "psychologically graduated" responses, appeals to alternative motives (ie, anti-censorship), and lengthy investigations may constitute improper inducement.

Some courts have found that a suspect's collection of child erotica can be valuable in proving a predisposition (*United States v Byrd*, 1994). Child erotica is "any material relating to children that serves a sexual purpose for a given individual" (Lanning, 2001) and includes items such as toys, games, children's clothing, sexual aids, manuals, drawings, catalogs, and nonpornographic photographs of children (Brown, 2001; Lanning, 2001).

Responding to an Entrapment Defense
The first question a prosecutor should ask when confronted with an entrapment defense is whether the defense is entitled to an instruction on entrapment. For tactical reasons in certain situations, the government may want to propose an instruction to reduce the likelihood of jury nullification when the jury acquits the defendant in disregard of the judge's instructions and contrary to the jury's findings of fact because they have sympathy for the defendant or regard the law under which the defendant is charged with disfavor. There is a difference between legally defined entrapment and what may be referred to as "street-level" entrapment. Most nonlawyers have a liberal definition of entrapment; for example, if the police are involved in the discussions about committing the crime, lay jurors may perceive it as entrapment. As a result, prosecutors must be careful when handling this issue at trial. One way to handle this potential problem is not to object to a defendant's request for an entrapment instruction or even to ask for one. If the judge has given a proper jury instruction, the prosecutor can educate the jurors as to the legal definition of entrapment and steer them away from using notions of entrapment from what they have learned "on the street."

A claim of entrapment by an accused person may allow for the introduction of character evidence by the prosecution that may otherwise be inadmissible. Proof of prior crimes, prior bad acts, bad reputation, or other evidence of bad character, particularly as to child molestation, exploitation, or any related matter, may be admissible to prove predisposition. Evidence of hearsay, suspicion, and rumor—all of which would be inadmissible in most other contexts—may be admissible to prove the defendant's predisposition.

Internet Addiction

The following signs have been posited as symptoms of the "disorder" of Internet addiction:

— Using the computer for pleasure, gratification, or relief from stress

— Feeling irritable and out of control or depressed when not using it

— Spending increasing amounts of time and money on hardware, software, magazines, and computer-related activities

— Neglecting work, school, or family obligations

— Lying about the amount of time spent on computer activities

— Risking loss of career goals, educational objectives, and personal relationships

— Failing at repeated efforts to control computer use

There are no published cases in which Internet addiction has been presented successfully as a substantive defense in a criminal case. However, the issue has been presented at sentencing. In *United States v McBroom* (1997), the defendant's therapist testified that the defendant exhibited obsessive and compulsive behaviors, of which viewing pornography was a manifestation, and that his childhood sexual abuse led to his mental condition. The fact that McBroom was found to be suffering from a mental disorder that prevented him from controlling his behavior should have been considered when he was sentenced. He was granted a one-point downward departure—giving the defendant less of a sentence than is normally called for under the sentencing guidelines—for diminished capacity. In *United States v Motto* (1999), the defendant unsuccessfully sought a downward departure for allegedly suffering from a "compulsive personality disorder [that] prevented him from exercising volitional controls over a behavior he knew was wrong." Similarly, *State v Osborn* (1998) held that a child pornography defendant suffering from "avoidant personality disorder" and "dysthymic disorder" should receive downward departure from the recommended guidelines sentence.

Upon first notice that the defense will be seeking to present expert testimony about Internet addiction, a prosecutor should file a motion *in limine* to preclude it and request a *Daubert* hearing. Research on Internet addiction to date has been composed exclusively of exploratory surveys by clinicians, not researchers. These surveys can not establish causal relationships between specific addictive behaviors and their cause. Though surveys can help establish descriptions of how people feel about themselves and their behaviors, they can not draw conclusions about whether a specific technology, such as the Internet, has caused those behaviors. The clinicians have drawn purely speculative and subjective conclusions from their observations which existing data can not support and thus probably can not survive a vigorous challenge during a *Daubert* hearing. (See http://psychcentral.com?netaddiction, which contains further links on this issue.) For example, a civil case held that testimony from a licensed professional counselor regarding Internet addiction and Internet pornography was inadmissible where the counselor was not qualified as an expert in either Internet pornography nor Internet addiction, but only as a lay witness (*Bower v Bower*, 2000).

Next, prosecutors should argue that the defendant being addicted to the Internet is irrelevant to any issue before the trier of fact. If the addiction is to the Internet, that does not explain why the defendant would obtain, maintain, and meticulously organize child pornography.

Accident

Spam is unsolicited e-mail that usually involves an advertisement or solicitation. Defendants may claim that the child pornography the defendant is alleged to have possessed was received in unsolicited e-mail or was accidentally downloaded from unsolicited e-mail. This may be refuted in a number of ways. A complete forensic examination of the suspect's computer could reveal what Web sites the suspect had been visiting. If the suspect had visited a child pornography Web site, it will be difficult for him or her to use the defense of accident, as his or her visits to those sites demonstrate an interest in child pornography or sex with children. In addition, the examiner can probe for evidence of the Usenet newsgroups to which the suspect has subscribed. If the suspect had subscribed to the newsgroup "alt.binaries.pictures. teens," it would be difficult for him or her to argue that he or she accidentally came into possession of child pornography. A computer-savvy investigator could prepare a "Screen Cam" to illustrate to the jury the steps one must go through to subscribe to a newsgroup and to download graphic images from them to rebut the claim that the defendant came across the material accidentally.

A variation on the accident theme is "it just appeared, as if out of nowhere." This can be overcome by asking the jurors to consider how many times they have ever experienced computers generating new data, as opposed to losing or destroying the data. In sum, accidents destroy evidence; they do not create it. Asking jurors to reflect on how many times they have ever experienced a computer crashing, and then, when rebooted, having thousands of child pornography images appear, will under-score the ridiculous and counterintuitive nature of this defense.

"Deleted" Computer Images

Defendants may assert that they did not "know" they possessed child pornography because they thought they had deleted the images from their computer's hard drive. Most recently, *United States v Tucker* (2001) held that under the theory of constructive knowledge, a defendant may still knowingly possess an image after deletion. The court held that the ability to destroy evidence is definitive evidence of control. It further held that destruction of contraband does not logically lead to the conclusion that one never possessed it; rather, it leads to the opposite.

Earlier, in *United States v Simpson* (1998), the court found that though the specific files that were downloaded over the Internet had apparently been deleted, the government sustained its burden of proof by introducing unrebutted expert testimony that deletion of files obtained via the Internet is common if the computer user finds that he or she already has a copy of the file. The court held that a defendant deleting (or destroying) evidence does not eliminate his or her culpability for engaging in the conduct related to that evidence.

In *United States v Hathcock* (1999), the defendant had "downloaded hundreds of images from the Internet, kept some and deleted others, then used the floppies to transfer the files to a new computer in hidden file subdirectories." He "argu[ed] that his possession of the material on floppy disks was only 'fleeting' as the floppies were merely used to transfer files from one computer to another and were then erased" (*United States v Hathcock*, 1999). This argument was rejected based on extrinsic proof that Hathcock had "at least three floppies, unerased, in his possession during [at least part of the] period covered by the indictment" (*United States v Hathcock*, 1999). Though he deleted the pornography from the disks later, that did not negate that he possessed these matters or that he did so with knowledge of their contents.

"Mere Viewing"

Having determined that deletion of images does not necessarily void possession, the next question must be asked: Can "mere viewing" constitute possession? The court in *United States v Tucker* (2002) answered that question in the affirmative as well. The court held that even as a defendant views the images on the computer monitor, the defendant has the power to print, enlarge and zoom in, and copy the image(s) to another directory. Even where the defendant did not personally download the images, he or she still had control over them and that is the core of possession. Though this sort of case may not be prosecuted as often as other types where the defendant exerts more traditional control over the image, proceeding with such a case is possible should the underlying facts mandate.

FIRST AMENDMENT

One of the more challenging defenses for prosecutors to evaluate is the so-called First Amendment defense. This may be raised by persons being investigated for possessing child pornography who claim a legitimate professional use for possessing such materials. This could include reporters, researchers, social workers, scientists/doctors, individuals conducting training for law enforcement, artists, and therapists who use child pornography with phallometry testing. Some jurisdictions specifically allow for certain categories of individuals to possess child pornography pursuant to statute. Aside from these specific grantings of immunity, there is no recognized exception to the rule of not being legally allowed to possess child pornography.

Lanning (2001) suggests that the test for those claiming a professional use defense for the possession and use of otherwise prohibited child pornography should be twofold: Do they have a professional use for the material, and were they using it professionally. The first prong of this test can be determined on a factual basis; that is, is the person a journalist, researcher, or author. This determination would then be coupled with such facts as disclosure, or failure to disclose, to others what activities the individual was engaged in. The second prong can be decided on a number of issues. Most pragmatically, a good forensic crime scene workup of the area in which the child pornography was found will often divulge the presence of copious quantities of seminal bodily fluids, thereby rebutting any legitimate claim to professional usage. The following cases highlight the types of individuals who have attempted to invoke this defense and why they have been unsuccessful.

Social Worker Claimed He Was Researching the Internet for Therapeutic Material

The First Amendment defense was raised in *People v Fraser* (2000). There, a licensed social worker downloaded child pornography from the Internet in connection with research he claimed he was conducting to develop therapeutic treatment methods for Internet child pornographers and was convicted of a criminal offense. According to the published opinion, the social worker

testified that he was a member of a task force made up of mental health professionals and formed by the Oneida County Department of Mental Health, with encouragement from the Oneida County District Attorney's Office, to develop such treatment programs. He further testified that he had informed other members of the task force, including the Deputy Commissioner of the Oneida County Department of Mental Health, that he was engaged in research concerning persons who deal in child pornography on the Internet. According to the testimony of other members of the task force, including the Deputy Commissioner, the social worker indicated to them that he was conducting research concerning child pornography on the Internet and sending questionnaires to persons he identified as disseminators of child pornography on the Internet. He never informed them, however, that he was downloading child pornography from the Internet nor had anyone in the task force given the defendant permission to do so (*People v Fraser*, 2000).

The court held that "it is no less traumatic for an innocent child to be sexually abused in front of a camera when the images produced are allegedly used for a 'scientific' purpose than when the images are used to satisfy the prurient desires of the possessor" (*People v Fraser*, 2000). Given the nature and extent of the harm to children who are involved in the production of pornography, the compelling interest of the state in eradicating the market for that despicable material and less than minimal value of child pornography for scientific or educational purposes, the court decided that it is a reasonable determination by the legislature not to allow a person charged with possession of child pornography to assert the "scientific" defense.

Journalist Claimed He Was Researching an Article on Child Pornography

Another case is *United States v Matthews* (2000), in which a journalist was convicted for receiving and transporting child pornography via a computer. In pretrial motions, Matthews moved to dismiss the indictment, and the government filed a motion *in limine* to prevent him from raising his First Amendment defense. The district court held, as a matter of first impression, that the defendant's activities did not enjoy First Amendment protection afforded news-gathering activities of the press and that his activities did not enjoy the First Amendment free speech protection. The district court granted the government's motion *in limine* that forbade the defendant from arguing to the jury that it may find him not guilty if it were to find that his acts were committed as part of news-gathering activity. The trial judge addressed the First Amendment issue this way:

The examples given in Ferber, medical textbooks, and the National Geographic contain depictions whose production and dissemination does not involve the sexual exploitation of children. In contrast, the Court does not believe that the First Amendment protects pictures that are undisputably hardcore child pornography, even if the pictures are used in an arguably productive manner. Because the production and dissemination of the pictures involves the sexual exploitation of children, even well-intended uses of the images are unprotected (United States v Matthews, 1998).

In weighing the significance of this decision, the defendant in Matthews downloaded images and uploaded images of child pornography, thus raising concerns about the legitimacy of his journalistic purpose claim.

"Author" Claimed He Was Researching a Book on Child Abuse

Troy Upham was found guilty of 4 counts of transmitting child pornography over the Internet and 1 count of possession of child pornography after he transmitted pictures via AOL to a United States Customs undercover operation (*United States v Upham*, 1999b). Forensic work on diskettes and the hard drive of the computer Upham used recovered more than 1400 images of children engaged in sexually explicit conduct, including several images that Upham had sent to the undercover agents. Upham offered what he characterized as a First Amendment defense by testifying that he had been a victim of childhood sexual abuse and was collecting child pornography as research for a serious book on child abuse that he was writing. Upham testified that he had written a few pages over many years as part of this project. The jury was given the following special interrogatory: "Was the defendant's sole purpose in committing the offense or offenses to produce a serious literary work?" "The jury answered the question in the negative" (*United States v Upham*, 1999b). Though his defense was unsuccessful, on appeal, Upham objected to the district judge's refusal to afford him a downward departure adjustment for acceptance of responsibility. Upham argued that he had gone to trial only so he could assert the First Amendment defense. Affirming the district court's refusal to grant the reduction, the First Circuit found that the jury's answer to the special interrogatory supported the trial judge's ruling that the factual premise of the First Amendment defense was untrue, and that sexual gratification, rather than literary ambition, was the central aim of his actions.

Conclusion

This chapter has dealt with some of the primary issues of concern to prosecutors of child pornography. One final note should be made regarding an evidentiary question: What should be done with a computer that contains child pornography when the case is either no-billed, where the prosecutor decides not to bring a bill of indictment, or results in an acquittal? Should such a situation arise, some jurisdictions have adopted a protocol that though they will return the computer, they will not return the hard drive within it or they will delete the images of child pornography and then return the hard drive. Whatever a particular jurisdiction decides to do, it is necessary to have a policy and practice in place to address this situation and be ready to implement it uniformly when confronted with such a fact scenario.

REFERENCES

Allen RJ, Luttrell M, Kreeger A. Clarifying entrapment. *J Crim L Criminology.* 1999;89(2):407-431.

Ashcroft v Free Speech Coalition, 535 US 234 (9th 2002).

Astrowsky B, Peters J. Anticipating and meeting defenses. In: Peters JS, ed. *Prosecuting Internet Child Exploitation Crimes.* Washington, DC: US Dept of Justice; 2002a.

Astrowsky B, Peters J. Charging decisions and trial preparation in child pornography cases. In: Peters JS, ed. *Prosecuting Internet Child Exploitation Crimes.* Washington, DC: US Dept of Justice; 2002b.

Bower v Bower, 758 So2d 405, 413 (Miss 2000).

Brown D. Developing strategies for collecting and presenting grooming evidence in a high tech world. *Update.* 2001;14(11). Available at: http://www.ndaa-apri.org/publications/newsletters/update_volume_14_number_11_2001.html. Accessed September 2, 2003.

Brown D. Pornography after the fall of the CPPA: strategies for prosecutors. *Update.* 2002;15(4). Available at: http://www.ndaa-apri.org/publications/newsletters/update_volume_15_number_4_2002.html. Accessed September 2, 2003.

Cervantes v Cates, 76 P3d 449 (Az App Div 1, 2003)

Daubert v Merrell Dow Pharmaceuticals, Inc, 509 US 579 (1993).

18 USC § 1460 et seq.

18 USC § 2251.

18 USC § 2252.

18 USC § 2256.

18 USC § 3282.

18 USC § 3283.

18 USC § 3290.

18 USC § 3509(a)(3).

Fed R Crim P 16(d)(1).

Fed R Evid 403.

Federal R Evid 701.

Gilmour v Rogerson, 117 F3d 368, 369 (8th Cir 1997), *cert denied,* 522 US 1122 (1998).

Groh v Ramirez, 124 S Ct 1284 (2004).

Holmgren B. Sexually violent predator statutes: implications for prosecutors and their communities. *The Prosecutor.* 1998a;32(3):20-41.

Holmgren B. Structuring charging decisions, plea negotiation and sentencing recommendations for sex offenders in the wake of sexual predator statutes. *Update.* 1998b;11(5). Available at: http://www.ndaa.org/publications/newsletters/apri_update_vol_11_no_5_1998.htm. Accessed September 2, 2003.

In the Matter of the Search of 3817 W West End, First Floor, Chicago, Illinois, 321 F Supp 2d 953 (ND Ill 2004).

Kreston S. Alphabet soup: ECPA, PPA and privacy protection issues in computer facilitated child sexual exploitation cases. *Update*. 2000a;13(11). Available at: http://www.ndaa-apri.org/publications/newsletters/update_volume_13_number_11_2000.html. Accessed September 1, 2004.

Kreston S. Defeating the virtual defense in child pornography prosecutions. *High Technol Law J*. 2004;4:49.

Kreston S. Exceptions to the search warrant requirement in computer facilitated child sexual exploitation cases. *Update*. 2000b;13(4). Available at: http://www.ndaa-apri.org/publications/newsletters/update_volume_13_number_4_2000.html. Accessed September 1, 2004.

Kreston S. Search and seizure in cases of computers and child pornography. *Update*. 1999;12(9). Available at: http://ndaa-apri.org/publications/newsletters/apri_update_vol_12_no_9_1999.html. Accessed September 1, 2004.

Kreston S. Search and seizure issues in internet crimes against children cases. *Rutgers Comput Technol Law J*. 2004;30:327.

Kutz TJ. Tanner staging and pornography (reply). *Pediatrics*. 1999;104(4 pt 1):995-997.

Lanning K. Law enforcement perspective on the compliant child victim. *The APSAC Advisor*. Spring 2002;14(2):4-9.

Lanning K. *Child Molesters: A Behavioral Analysis for Law Enforcement Officers Investigating the Sexual Exploitation of Children by Acquaintance Molesters*. 4th ed. Arlington, Va: National Center for Missing & Exploited Children; September 2001.

Lee v State, 438 SE2d 108,112 (Ga Ct App 1993).

New York v Ferber, 458 US 747 (1982).

People v Arapahoe County Court, 74 P3d 429 (Colo App 2003).

People v Foley, 731 NE2d 123 (NY 2000).

People v Fraser, 704 NYS2d 426 (NY App Div 2000).

People v Slusher, 844 P2d 1222 (Colo App 1992).

People v Tafoya, 985 P2d 26 (Colo App 1999).

Rosenbloom AL, Tanner JM. Misuse of Tanner puberty stages to estimate chronologic age. *Pediatrics*. 1998;102(6):1494.

Seidel HM, Ball JW, Dains JE, Benedict GW. *Mosby's Guide to Physical Examination*. 5th ed. St. Louis, Mo: Mosby; 2003.

State v Nordlund, 53 P3d 520,525 (Wash Ct App 2002).

State v Osborn, 707 So2d 1110-1111 (Fla Dist Ct App 1998).

State v Perrone, 834 P2d 611 (Wash 1992).

Taylor v State, 93 SW3d 487 (Tex App Texarkana 2002).

Taylor v State, 54 SW3d 21,24 (Tex Ct App 2001).

Trulock v Freeh, 275 F. 3d 391 (4th Cir 2001).

United States v Anderson, 97-10498, 97-10499, 1999 WL 459586 (9th Cir 1999a).

United States v Anderson, 154 F3d 1225 (10th Cir 1998).

United States v Anderson, 187 F3d 649 (unpublished) (1999b).

United States v Anderson, 187 F3d 649 (9th Cir 1999c).

United States v Anderton, 136 F3d 747 (11th Cir 1998).

United States v Angevine, 281 F3d 1130 (10th Cir 2002).

United States v Arvin, 900 F2d 1385,1390, n4 (9th Cir 1990).

United States v Bailey, 2003 US Dist LEXIS 12691 (Neb).

United States v Barth, 26 F Supp 2d 929 (WD Tex 1998).

United States v Bender, 290 F3d 1279 (11th Cir 2002).

United States v Broyles, 37 F3d 1314 (8th Cir 1994).

United States v Brunette, 256 F3d 14 (1st Cir 2001).

United States v Byrd, 31 F3d 1329, 1337 (5th Cir 1994).

United States v Carey, 172 F3d 1268 (10th Cir 1999).

United States v Cream, 58 MJ 750 (NM Ct Crim App 2003).

United States v David, 756 F Supp 1385 (D Nev 1991).

United States v Deaton, 308F, 3d 454 (8th Cir 2003).

United States v Diamond, 820 F2d 10, 12 (1st Cir 1987).

United States v Dornhofer, 859 F2d 1195, 1198 (4th Cir 1988).

United States v Dost, 636 F Supp 828 (SDCA 1986).

United States v Durham, 1998 US Dist LEXIS 15482.

United States v Esch, 832 F2d 531,536 (10th Cir 1987).

United States v Fabiano, 169 F3d 1299 (10th Cir 1999).

United States v Freeman, 808 F2d 1290,1292-1293 (8th Cir 1987).

United States v Froman, 355 F3d 882 (5th Cir 2004).

United States v Gallo, 846 F2d 74 (unpublished) (4th Cir 1988).

United States v Gamache, 156 F3d 1,12 (1st Cir 1998).

United States v Gann, 732 F2d 714,722 (9th Cir 1984).

United States v Garcia, 983 F2d 1160 (1st Cir 1993).

United States v Gendron, 18 F3d 955, 963 (1st Cir 1994).

United States v Gourde, 382 F3d 1003, WL 1945321 (9th Cir 2004).

United States v Gray, 78 F Supp 2d 524 (ED Va 1999).

United States v Greany, 929 F2d 523, 525 (9th Cir 1991).

United States v Grimes, 244 F3d 375 (5th Cir 2001).

United States v Grosenheider, 200 F3d 321 (5th Cir 2000).

United States v Guagliardo, 278 F3d 868 (9th Cir 2002).

United States v Guerro, 694 F2d 898 (NY 1983).

United States v Hall, 142 F3d 988 (7th Cir 1998).

United States v Hall, 312 F3d 1259 (11th Cir 2002) *cert denied.*

United States v Hathcock, 172 F3d 877 (unpublished) (9th Cir 1999).

United States v Hay, 231 F3d 630, 2000 WL 1593400 (9th Cir 2000).

United States v Hill, 322 F Supp 2d 1081 (CD Cal 2004).

United States v Horn, 187 F3d 781 (8th Cir 1999).

United States v Hotal, 143 F3d 1223 (9th Cir 1998).

United States v Husband, 246 F Supp 2d 467, ED VA 2003

United States v Jasorka, 153 F3d 58 (2d Cir 1998).

United States v Katz, 178 F3d 368 (5th Cir 1999).

United States v Kemmish, 120 F3d 937 (9th Cir 1997).

United States v Kimbrough, 69 F3d 723, 27 (5th Cir 1995).

United States v Knights, 534 US 112 (2001).

United States v Knox, 32 F3d 733 (3rd Cir 1994).

United States v Koelling, 992 F2d 817,821-822 (8th Cir 1993).

United States v Lacy, 119 F3d 742,745,746 (9th Cir 1997).

United States v Lamb, 945 F Supp 441 (NDNY 1996).

United States v Layne, 43 F3d 127 (5th Cir 1995).

United States v Lee, 57 MJ 659 (AF Ct Crim App 2002).

United States v Lemmons, 282 F3d 920 (7th Cir 2002).

United States v Leon, 468 US 897,922 (1984).

United States v Long, 108 F3d 1377 (unpublished) (6th Cir 1997).

United States v Long, 328 F3d 655 (DC Cir 2003).

United States v Loy, 191 F3d 360 (3rd Cir 1999).

United States v Matthews, 11 F Supp 2d 656 (D Md 1998).

United States v Matthews, 209 F3d 338 (4th Cir 2000).

United States v McBroom, 124 F3d 533 (3d Cir 1997).

United States v Mendoza-Salgado, 964 F2d 993,1004 (10th Cir 1992).

United States v Motto, 70 F Supp 2d 570 (ED Pa 1999).

United States v Nappy, 1995 US Dist LEXIS 17677 (NY 1995).

United States v Oakes, 2001 WL 30530 (D Me 2001).

United States v Pitts, 6 F3d 1366 (9th Cir 1993).

United States v Poehlman, 217 F3d 692 (9th Cir 2000).

United States v Pollard, 128 F Supp 2d 1104 (ED Tenn, 2001).

United States v Reed, 935 F2d 641 (4th Cir), *cert denied*, 112 S Ct 423 (1991).

United States v Ricciardelli, 998 F2d 8 (1st Cir 1993).

United States v Richardson, 304 F3d 1061 (11th Cir 2002), *cert denied*.

United States v Robinson, 137 F3d 652,653 (1st Cir 1998).

United States v Romero, 189 F3d 576 (7th Cir 1999), *cert denied*.

United States v Rowland, 145 F3d 1194 (10th Cir 1998).

United States v Rude, 88 F3d 1538 (9th Cir 1996).

United States v Salvo, 133 F3d 943 (6th Cir1998).

United States v Simmonds, 262 F3d 468 (5th Cir 2001).

United States v Simons, 206 F3d 392 (4th Cir 2000).

United States v Simpson, 152 F3d 1241 (10th Cir 1998).

United States v Slanina, 283 F3d 670 (5th Cir 2002).

United States v Smith, 27 F Supp 2d 1111 (CD IL 1998).

United States v Stanley, 896 F2d 450 (10th Cir 1990).

United States v Stanton, 973 F2d 608, 610 (8th Cir 1992).

United States v Thoma, 726 F2d 1191,1198 (7th Cir 1984).

United States v Tucker, 150 F Supp 2d 1263 (D Utah 2001); affd 305 F3d 1193 (10th Cir 2002).

United States v Turner, 169 F3d 84 (1st Cir 1999).

United States v Upham, 168 F3d 532 (1st Cir 1999a).

United States v Upham, 168 F3d 532 (1st Cir 1999), *cert denied*, 527 US 1011 (1999b).

United States v Villard, 700 F Supp 803,814 (DNJ 1988).

United States v Walser, 275 F3d 981 (10th Cir 2001).

United States v Weber, 923 F2d 1338 (9th Cir 1991).

United States v Wiegand, 812 F2d 1239,1244 (9th Cir 1987).

United States v Wong, 334 F3d 831 (9th Cir 2003).

United States v X-Citement Video, 513 US (1994).

Westerfield v Superior Court, 99 Cal App 4th 994 (2002).

APPENDIX 27-1: LEGISLATION EXTENDING OR REMOVING THE STATUTES OF LIMITATION FOR OFFENSES AGAINST CHILDREN*

STATE LEGISLATION

Alabama

Ala Code § 15-3-5 (a)(4)

There is no limitation of time within which a prosecution must be commenced for any sex offense involving a victim under 16 years of age, regardless of whether it involves force or serious physical injury or death.

Alaska

Alaska Stat § 12.10.010 (a)(2) & (4)

Prosecution for felony sexual abuse of a minor or for an unclassified felony sexual assault, when committed against a person who, at the time of the offense, was under 18 years of age, may be commenced at any time.

---

* *Kentucky, Maryland, North Carolina, South Carolina, Virginia, West Virginia, and Wyoming have no statute of limitations for criminal felony prosecutions. Arizona and Ohio have general time limitation statutes. California's statute, Cal Penal Code § 803, has been held unconstitutional by Stogner v California, 123 SCt 2446 (2003). (Legislation to amend the statute is currently pending.)*

Arkansas
Ark Code Ann § 5-1-109 (h)
(h) If the general time limitation period has expired, a prosecution may nevertheless be commenced for violations of the following offenses if, when the alleged violation occurred, the offense was committed against a minor, the violation has not previously been reported to a law enforcement agency or prosecuting attorney, and the general time limitation period has not expired since the victim has reached the age of eighteen (18):

(1) Battery in the first and second degrees as prohibited in §§ 5-13-201 and 5-13-202;

(2) Aggravated assault as prohibited in § 5-13-204;

(3) Terroristic threatening in the first degree as prohibited in § 5-13-301;

(4) Kidnapping as prohibited in § 5-11-102;

(5) False imprisonment in the first degree as prohibited in § 5-11-103;

(6) Permanent detention or restraint as prohibited in § 5-11-106;

(7) Rape as prohibited in §§ 5-14-103;

(8) Sexual assault in the first degree as prohibited in § 5-14-124;

(9) Sexual assault in the second degree as prohibited in § 5-14-125;

(10) Sexual assault in the third degree as prohibited in § 5-14-126;

(11) Sexual assault in the fourth degree as prohibited in § 5-14-127;

(12) Incest as prohibited in § 5-26-202;

(13) Endangering the welfare of a minor in the first degree as prohibited in § 5-27-203;

(14) Permitting child abuse as prohibited in § 5-27-221(a)(1) and (3);

(15) Engaging children in sexually explicit conduct for use in visual or print medium, transportation of minors for prohibited sexual conduct, use of a child or consent to use of a child in sexual performance, and producing, directing, or promoting sexual performance by a child, as prohibited in §§ 5- 27-303, 5-27-305, 5-27-402, and 5-27-403.

Colorado
Colo Rev Stat § 16-5-401(6) & (7)
(6) The period of time during which an adult person or juvenile may be prosecuted shall be extended for an additional seven years as to any offense or delinquent act charged involving wrongs to children, unlawful sexual behavior, or enumerated child prostitution, as they existed prior to July 1, 2000, when the victim at the time of the commission of the act is a child under fifteen years of age, or charged as criminal attempt, conspiracy, or solicitation to commit any of the acts specified in any of said sections.

(7) When the victim at the time of the commission of the offense or delinquent act is a child under fifteen years of age, the period of time during which an adult person or juvenile may be prosecuted shall be extended for an additional seven years as to a felony charged for keeping a place of child prostitution, under section 18-3-404, CRS, or criminal attempt, conspiracy, or solicitation to commit such a felony, and such period shall be extended for an additional three years and six months as to a misdemeanor charged under section 18-3-404, CRS, or criminal attempt, conspiracy, or solicitation to commit such a misdemeanor.

Connecticut

Conn Gen Stat Ann § 54-193a

Notwithstanding the provisions of section 54-193, no person may be prosecuted for any offense, except a class A felony, involving sexual abuse, sexual exploitation or sexual assault of a minor except within thirty years from the date the victim attains the age of majority or within five years from the date the victim notifies any police officer or state's attorney acting in such police officer's or state's attorney's official capacity of the commission of the offense, whichever is earlier, provided if the prosecution is for a violation of subdivision (1) of subsection (a) of section 53a-71, the victim notified such police officer or state's attorney not later than five years after the commission of the offense.

Delaware

Del Code Ann tit 11, § 205(e)

(e) Notwithstanding the period prescribed by subsection (b) of this section, a prosecution for any crime that is delineated in Subpart D of Subchapter II of Chapter 5 of this title, or is otherwise defined as a 'sexual offense' by § 761 of this title except § 763, § 764 or § 765 of this title, or any attempt to commit said crimes, may be commenced at any time. No prosecution under this subsection shall be based upon the memory of the victim that has been recovered through psychotherapy unless there is some evidence of the corpus delicti independent of such repressed memory. This subsection applies to all causes of action arising before, on or after July 15, 1992, and to the extent consistent with this subsection, it shall revive causes of action that would otherwise be barred by this section.

If any provision of this Act or the application of any such provision to any person or circumstance should be held invalid by a Court of competent jurisdiction, the remainder of this Act, or the application of its provisions to persons or circumstances other than those to which it is held invalid shall not be affected thereby.

Approved June 24, 2003.

Florida

Fla Stat Ann ch 775.15(7)

(a) If the victim of sexual assault, indecent exposure, or incest is under the age of 18, the applicable period of limitation, if any, does not begin to run until the victim has reached the age of 18 or the violation is reported to a law enforcement agency or other governmental agency, whichever occurs earlier. Such law enforcement agency or other governmental agency shall promptly report such allegation to the state attorney for the judicial circuit in which the alleged violation occurred. If the offense is a first or second degree felony of sexual assault, and the crime is reported within 72 hours after its commission, paragraph (1)(b) applies. This paragraph applies to any such offense except an offense the prosecution of which would have been barred by subsection (2) on or before December 31, 1984.

(b) Notwithstanding the provisions of paragraph (1)(b) and paragraph (a) of this subsection, if the offense is a first degree felony violation of sexual assault and the victim was under 18 years of age at the time the offense was committed, a prosecution of the offense may be commenced at any time. This paragraph applies to any such offense except an offense the prosecution of which would have been barred by subsection (2) on or before October 1, 2003.

This act shall take effect October 1, 2003.

Georgia

Ga Code Ann § 17-3-1(c)

(c) Prosecution for felonies other than those specified in subsections (a), (b), and (c.1) of this Code section must be commenced within four years after the commission of the crime, provided that prosecution for felonies committed against victims who are at the time of the commission of the offense under the age of 18 years must be commenced within seven years after the commission of the crime.

(c.1) A prosecution for enumerated violent and sexual offenses may be commenced at any time when deoxyribonucleic acid (DNA) evidence is used to establish the identity of the accused provided, however, that a sufficient portion of the physical evidence tested for DNA is preserved and available for testing by the accused and provided, further, that, if the DNA evidence does not establish the identity of the accused, the limitation on prosecution shall be as provided in subsections (b) and (c) of this Code section.

Hawaii

Haw Rev Stat Ann § 701-108(6)(c)

The period of limitation does not run for any felony offense under chapter 707, regarding sexual offenses and child abuse, during any time when the victim is alive and under eighteen years of age.

Idaho

Idaho Code § 19-402

1) A prosecution for any felony other than murder, voluntary manslaughter, rape, or any felony committed upon or against a minor child, or an act of terrorism, must be commenced by the filing of the complaint or the finding of an indictment within five (5) years after its commission. Except as provided in subsection (2) of this section, a prosecution for any felony committed upon or against a minor child must be commenced within five (5) years after the commission of the offense by the filing of the complaint or a finding of an indictment.

(2) A prosecution for the offense of sexual abuse of a child or lewd conduct with a minor child must be commenced within five (5) years after the date the child reaches eighteen (18) years of age.

(3) A prosecution for the offense of ritualized abuse of a child must be commenced within three (3) years after the date of initial disclosure by the victim.

Illinois

720 Ill Comp Stat Ann § 5/3-6

(c) Except as otherwise provided in subdivision (i) or (j) of this Section, a prosecution for any offense involving sexual conduct or sexual penetration, as defined in Section 12-12 of this Code, where the victim and defendant are family members, as defined in Section 12-12 of this Code, may be commenced within one year of the victim attaining the age of 18 years.

(d) A prosecution for child pornography, indecent solicitation of a child, soliciting for a juvenile prostitute, juvenile pimping or exploitation of a child may be commenced within one year of the victim attaining the age of 18 years. However, in no such case shall the time period for prosecution expire sooner than 3 years after the commission of the offense. When the victim is under 18 years of age, a prosecution for criminal sexual abuse may be commenced within one year of the victim attaining the age of 18 years. However, in no such case shall the time period for prosecution expire sooner than 3 years after the commission of the offense.

(j) When the victim is under 18 years of age at the time of the offense, a prosecution for criminal sexual assault, aggravated criminal sexual assault, predatory criminal sexual assault of a child, or aggravated criminal sexual abuse or a prosecution for failure of a person who is required to report an alleged or suspected commission of any of these offenses under the Abused and Neglected Child Reporting Act may be commenced within 10 years after the child victim attains 18 years of age.

Indiana

Ind Code § 35-41-4-2

(e) A prosecution for the following offenses is barred unless commenced before the date that the alleged victim of the offense reaches thirty-one (31) years of age:

(1) IC 35-42-4-3(a) (Child molesting).

(2) IC 35-42-4-5 (Vicarious sexual gratification).

(3) IC 35-42-4-6 (Child solicitation).

(4) IC 35-42-4-7 (Child seduction).

(5) IC 35-46-1-3 (Incest).

(f) Notwithstanding subsection (e)(1), a prosecution for child molesting under IC 35-42-4-3(c) or IC 35-42-4-3(d) where a person who is at least sixteen (16) years of age allegedly commits the offense against a child who is not more than two (2) years younger than the older person, is barred unless commenced within five (5) years after the commission of the offense.

Iowa

Iowa Code § 802.2

1. An information or indictment for sexual abuse in the first, second, or third degree committed on or with a person who is under the age of eighteen years shall be found within ten years after the person upon whom the offense is committed attains eighteen years of age.

2. An information or indictment for any other sexual abuse in the first, second, or third degree shall be found within ten years after its commission.

Kansas

Kan Stat Ann § 21-3106

(2) Except as provided by subsections (7) and (9), a prosecution for any of the following crimes must be commenced within five years after its commission if the victim is less than 16 years of age: (a) Indecent liberties with a child as defined in KSA 21-3503 and amendments thereto; (b) aggravated indecent liberties with a child as defined in KSA 21-3504 and amendments thereto; (c) enticement of a child as defined in KSA 21-3509 and amendments thereto; (d) indecent solicitation of a child as defined in KSA 21-3510 and amendments thereto; (e) aggravated indecent solicitation of a child as defined in KSA 21-3511 and amendments thereto; (f) sexual exploitation of a child as defined in KSA 21-3516 and amendments thereto; or (g) aggravated incest as defined in KSA 21-3603 and amendments thereto.

(7) (a) Except as provided in subsection (9), a prosecution for any offense provided in subsection (2) or a sexually violent offense as defined in KSA 22-3717, and amendments thereto, must be commenced within the limitation of time provided by the law pertaining to such offense or one year from the date on which the identity of the suspect is conclusively established by DNA testing, whichever is later.

(9) The period within which a prosecution must be commenced shall not include any period in which:

(a) The accused is absent from the state;

(b) the accused is concealed within the state so that process can not be served upon the accused;

(c) the fact of the crime is concealed;

(d) a prosecution is pending against the defendant for the same conduct, even if the indictment or information which commences the prosecution is quashed or the proceedings thereon are set aside, or are reversed on appeal;

(e) an administrative agency is restrained by court order from investigating or otherwise proceeding on a matter before it as to any criminal conduct defined as a violation of any of the provisions of article 41 of chapter 25 and article 2 of chapter 46 of the Kansas Statutes Annotated which may be discovered as a result thereof regardless of who obtains the order of restraint; or

(f) whether or not the fact of the crime is concealed by the active act or conduct of the accused, there is substantially competent evidence to believe two or more of the following factors are present: (i) The victim was a child under 15 years of age at the time of the crime; (ii) the victim was of such age or intelligence that the victim was unable to determine that the acts constituted a crime; (iii) the victim was prevented by a parent or other legal authority from making known to law enforcement authorities the fact of the crime whether or not the parent or other legal authority is the accused; and (iv) there is substantially competent expert testimony indicating the victim psychologically repressed such witness' memory of the fact of the crime, and in the expert's professional opinion the recall of such memory is accurate and free of undue manipulation, and substantial corroborating evidence can be produced in support of the allegations contained in the complaint or information but in no event may a prosecution be commenced as provided in this section later than the date the victim turns 28 years of age. Corroborating evidence may include, but is not limited to, evidence the defendant committed similar acts against other persons or evidence of contemporaneous physical manifestations of the crime. "Parent or other legal authority" shall include but not be limited to natural and stepparents, grandparents, aunts, uncles or siblings.

Louisiana

La Code Crim Proc Ann art 571.1
The time within which to institute prosecution of the following sex offenses: sexual battery (RS 14:43.1), aggravated sexual battery (RS 14:43.2), oral sexual battery (RS 14:43.3), aggravated oral sexual battery (RS 14:43.4), carnal knowledge of a juvenile (RS 14:80), indecent behavior with juveniles (RS 14:81), molestation of a juvenile (RS 14:81.2), crime against nature (RS 14:89), aggravated crime against nature (RS 14:89.1), incest (RS 14:78), or aggravated incest (RS 14:78.1) which involves a victim under seventeen years of age, regardless of whether the crime involves force, serious physical injury, death, or is punishable by imprisonment at hard labor shall be ten years. This ten- year period begins to run when the victim attains the age of eighteen.

La Code Crim Proc Ann art 573
The time limitations established by Article 572 shall not commence to run as to the following offenses until the relationship or status involved has ceased to exist when the offense charged is with aggravated battery (RS 14:34) and the victim is under seventeen years of age.

Maine

Me Rev Stat Ann Tit 14, § 752-C
Actions based upon sexual acts toward minors may be commenced at any time.

As used in this section, "sexual acts toward minors" means the following acts that are committed against or engaged in with a person under the age of majority: Sexual act, as defined in Title 17-A, section 251, subsection 1, paragraph C; or Sexual contact, as defined in Title 17-A, section 251, subsection 1, paragraph D.

Massachusetts

Mass Gen Laws Ann ch 277, § 63
If a victim of a crime set forth in enumerated sections regarding sexual offenses perpetrated on children, assault, or kidnapping of a child, prostitution of a child, obscene materials, unnatural or lascivious acts, or incest, is under the age of sixteen at

the time such crime is committed, the period of limitation for prosecution shall not commence until the victim has reached the age of sixteen or the violation is reported to a law enforcement agency, whichever occurs earlier.

Michigan
Mich Stat Ann § 767.24
An indictment for a violation or attempted violation of rape or child sexually abusive activity may be found and filed as follows: (a) Except as otherwise provided in subdivision (b), an indictment may be found and filed within 10 years after the offense is committed or by the alleged victim's twenty-first birthday, whichever is later.

An indictment for kidnapping, extortion, assault with intent to commit murder, attempted murder, manslaughter, conspiracy to commit murder, or first-degree home invasion shall be found and filed within 10 years after the offense is committed.

Minnesota
Minn Stat Ann § 628.26(d) & (e)
(d) Indictments or complaints for criminal sexual conduct if the victim was under the age of 18 years at the time the offense was committed, shall be found or made and filed in the proper court within nine years after the commission of the offense or, if the victim failed to report the offense within this limitation period, within three years after the offense was reported to law enforcement authorities.

(e) Notwithstanding the limitations in paragraph (d), indictments or complaints for criminal sexual conduct may be found or made and filed in the proper court at any time after commission of the offense, if physical evidence is collected and preserved that is capable of being tested for its DNA characteristics. If this evidence is not collected and preserved and the victim was 18 years old or older at the time of the offense, the prosecution must be commenced within nine years after the commission of the offense.

Mississippi
Miss Code Ann § 99-1-5
A person shall not be prosecuted for any offense, with the exception of murder, manslaughter, aggravated assault, kidnapping, arson, burglary, forgery, counterfeiting, robbery, larceny, rape, embezzlement, obtaining money or property under false pretenses or by fraud, felonious abuse or battery of a child as described in Section 97-5-39, touching or handling a child for lustful purposes as described in Section 97-5-23, sexual battery of a child as described in Section 97-3-95(1)(c) or (d) or exploitation of children as described in Section 97-5-33, unless the prosecution for such offense be commenced within two (2) years next after the commission thereof, but nothing contained in this section shall bar any prosecution against any person who shall abscond or flee from justice, or shall absent himself from this state or out of the jurisdiction of the court, or so conduct himself that he can not be found by the officers of the law, or that process can not be served upon him.

This act shall take effect and be in force from and after July 1, 2003.

Missouri
Mo Rev Stat § 556.037
The provisions of section 556.036, to the contrary notwithstanding, prosecutions for unlawful sexual offenses involving a person eighteen years of age or under must be commenced within ten years after the victim reaches the age of eighteen.

Montana
Mont Code Ann § 45-1-205
A prosecution a felony offense of sexual assault, sexual intercourse without consent,

or incest may be commenced within 10 years after it is committed, except that it may be commenced within 10 years after the victim reaches 18 years of age if the victim was less than 18 years of age at the time that the offense occurred. A prosecution for a misdemeanor offense under those provisions may be commenced within 1 year after the offense is committed, except that it may be commenced within 5 years after the victim reaches 18 years of age if the victim was less than 18 years of age at the time that the offense occurred.

Nebraska
Neb Rev Stat § 29-110(2)
No person or persons shall be prosecuted for sexual assault in the first degree, second degree, or third degree pursuant to section 28-319 or 28-320, sexual assault of a child pursuant to section 28-320.01, kidnapping pursuant to section 28-313, false imprisonment pursuant to section 28-314 or 28-315, child abuse pursuant to section 28-707, pandering pursuant to section 28-802, debauching a minor pursuant to section 28-805, or an offense pursuant to section 28-813, 28-813.01, or 28-1463.03 when the victim is under sixteen years of age at the time of the offense (a) unless the indictment for the same shall be found by a grand jury within seven years next after the offense has been committed or within seven years next after the victim's sixteenth birthday, whichever is later, or (b) unless a complaint for the same shall be filed before the magistrate within seven years next after the offense has been committed or within seven years next after the victim's sixteenth birthday, whichever is later, and a warrant for the arrest of the defendant shall have been issued. The limitations prescribed in this subsection shall include all inchoate offenses pursuant to the Nebraska Criminal Code and compounding a felony pursuant to section 28-301.

Nevada
Nev Rev Stat § 171.095
An indictment must be found, or an information or complaint filed, for any offense constituting sexual abuse of a child before the victim of the sexual abuse is:

(1) Twenty-one years old if he discovers or reasonably should have discovered that he was a victim of the sexual abuse by the date on which he reaches that age; or

(2) Twenty-eight years old if he does not discover and reasonably should not have discovered that he was a victim of the sexual abuse by the date on which he reaches 21 years of age.

New Hampshire
NH Rev Stat Ann § 625:8
If the general time limitation has expired, a prosecution may nevertheless be commenced if the offense is sexual assault, where the victim was under 18 years of age when the alleged offense occurred, within 22 years of the victim's eighteenth birthday.

NH Rev Stat Ann § 639:2
In cases of alleged incest where the victim is under the age of 18 when the alleged offense occurred, the statute of limitations shall run pursuant to RSA 625:8, III(d).

New Jersey
NJ Stat Ann § 2C:1-6(b)(4)
A prosecution for an offense of criminal sexual conduct or endangering the welfare of a child, when the victim at the time of the offense is below the age of 18 years, must be commenced within five years of the victim's attaining the age of 18 or within two years of the discovery of the offense by the victim, whichever is later.

New Mexico

NM Stat Ann § 30-1-9.1

The applicable time period for commencing prosecution shall not commence to run for an alleged violation of abandonment or abuse of a child, criminal sexual penetration, or criminal sexual contact of a minor until the victim attains the age of eighteen or the violation is reported to a law enforcement agency, whichever occurs first.

New York

NY Crim Proc Law § 30.10(3)(f)

Notwithstanding the provisions of subdivision two, the periods of limitation for the commencement of criminal actions are extended as follows in the indicated circumstances:

For purposes of a prosecution involving a sexual offense as defined in article one hundred thirty of the penal law committed against a child less than eighteen years of age, incest as defined in section 255.25 of the penal law committed against a child less than eighteen years of age, or use of a child in a sexual performance as defined in section 263.05 of the penal law, the period of limitation shall not begin to run until the child has reached the age of eighteen or the offense is reported to a law enforcement agency or statewide central register of child abuse and maltreatment, whichever occurs earlier.

North Dakota

ND Cent Code § 29-04-03.1

A prosecution for the offense of gross sexual imposition, sexual imposition, corruption or solicitation of a minor, sexual abuse of wards, sexual assault, fornication, or incest, where the victim was under eighteen years of age at the time the offense was committed must be commenced in the proper court within seven years after the commission of the offense or, if the victim failed to report the offense within this limitation period, within three years after the offense was reported to law enforcement authorities.

ND Cent Code § 29-04-03.2

If the victim the enumerated offenses is under the age of fifteen, the applicable period of limitation, if any, does not begin to run until the victim has reached the age of fifteen.

Oklahoma

Okla Stat Ann tit 22, § 152

Prosecutions for the crime of rape or forcible sodomy, sodomy, lewd or indecent proposals or acts against children, involving minors in pornography, shall be commenced within seven (7) years after the discovery of the crime.

However, prosecutions for the crimes listed in paragraph 1 of this subsection may be commenced at any time after the commission of the offense if:

a. the victim notified law enforcement within seven (7) years after the discovery of the crime,

b. physical evidence is collected and preserved that is capable of being tested to obtain a profile from deoxyribonucleic acid (DNA), and

c. the identity of the offender is subsequently established through the use of a DNA profile using evidence listed in subparagraph b of this paragraph.

As used in paragraph 1 of subsection C of this section, "discovery" means the date that a physical or sexually related crime involving a victim under the age of eighteen (18) years of age is reported to a law enforcement agency, up to and including one (1) year from the eighteenth birthday of the child.

Oregon
Or Rev Stat § 131.125

A prosecution for any of the following felonies may be commenced within six years after the commission of the crime or, if the victim at the time of the crime was under 18 years of age, anytime before the victim attains 24 years of age or within six years after the offense is reported to a law enforcement agency or other governmental agency, whichever occurs first:

Criminal mistreatment in the first degree, rape in any degree, sodomy in any degree, unlawful sexual penetration in the first or second degree, sexual abuse in the first or second degree, using a child in a display of sexual conduct, encouraging child sexual abuse in the first degree, incest, compelling prostitution, or promoting prostitution.

A prosecution for any of the following misdemeanors may be commenced within four years after the commission of the crime or, if the victim at the time of the crime was under 18 years of age, anytime before the victim attains 22 years of age or within four years after the offense is reported to a law enforcement agency or other governmental agency, whichever occurs first:

Sexual abuse in the third degree, furnishing obscene materials to minors, exhibiting an obscene performance to a minor, or displaying obscene materials to minors.

Notwithstanding subsection (2) of this section, a prosecution for rape in the first or second degree or sodomy in the first or second degree may be commenced within 12 years after the commission of the crime if the defendant is identified after the period described in subsection (2) of this section on the basis of DNA (deoxyribonucleic acid) sample comparisons.

Pennsylvania
42 Pa Cons Stat § 552(c)(3)

If the general time limitation has expired, a prosecution may nevertheless be commenced for any sexual offense committed against a minor who is less than 18 years of age any time up to the period of limitation provided by law after the minor has reached 18 years of age. As used in this paragraph, the term "sexual offense" means a crime under the following provisions of Title 18 (relating to crimes and offenses):

Section 3121 (relating to rape).

Section 3122.1 (relating to statutory sexual assault).

Section 3123 (relating to involuntary deviate sexual intercourse).

Section 3124.1 (relating to sexual assault).

Section 3125 (relating to aggravated indecent assault).

Section 3126 (relating to indecent assault).

Section 3127 (relating to indecent exposure).

Section 4302 (relating to incest).

Section 4304 (relating to endangering welfare of children).

Section 6301 (relating to corruption of minors).

Section 6312(b) (relating to sexual abuse of children).

42 Pa Cons Stat § 5554

Except as provided by section 5553(e) (relating to disposition of proceedings within two years), the period of limitation does not run during any time when a child is under 18 years of age, where the crime involves injuries to the person of the child caused by the wrongful act, or neglect, or unlawful violence, or negligence of the child's parents or by a person responsible for the child's welfare, or any individual residing in the same home as the child, or a paramour of the child's parent.

Rhode Island

RI Gen Laws § 12-12-17
There shall be no statute of limitations for rape, first degree sexual assault, first degree child molestation sexual assault, or second degree child molestation sexual assault.

South Dakota

SD Codified Laws § 22-22-1
A charge of rape may be commenced at any time prior to the time the victim becomes age twenty-five or within seven years of the commission of the crime, whichever is longer.

SD Codified Laws § 22-22-7
A charge of sexual contact with a child under the age of 16 may be commenced at any time before the victim becomes age twenty-five or within seven years of the commission of the crime, whichever is longer.

SD Codified Laws § 22-22-19.1
A charge of incest may be commenced at any time prior to the time the victim becomes age twenty-five or within seven years of the commission of the crime, whichever is longer.

Tennessee

Tenn Code Ann § 40-2-101(f)
Prosecutions for any offense committed against a child on or after July 1, 1997, that constitutes a criminal offense for aggravated rape, sexual battery, rape of a child, incest, and the production and distribution of obscenity, commence no later than the date the child reaches twenty-one (21) years of age; provided, that if the general time limitations provide a longer period of time within which prosecution may be brought than this subsection, the general time limitation periods shall prevail.

Texas

Tex Code Crim P Ann § 12.01
Felony indictments for sexual assault, if during the investigation of the offense biological matter is collected and subjected to forensic DNA testing and the testing results show that the matter does not match the victim or any other person whose identity is readily ascertained may be presented without limitation.

Felony indictments for indecency with a child, sexual assault, or aggravated sexual assault may be presented within 10 years from the 18th birthday of the victim of the offense and not afterward.

Utah

Utah Code Ann § 76-1-303.5
If the general time limitation period has expired, a prosecution may nevertheless be commenced for rape of a child, object rape of a child, sodomy upon a child, sexual abuse of a child, or aggravated sexual abuse of a child within four years after the report of the offense to a law enforcement agency.

Vermont

Vt Stat Ann tit 13, § 4501
Prosecutions for aggravated sexual assault, murder, arson causing death, and kidnapping may be commenced at any time after the commission of the offense.

Prosecutions for sexual assault, lewd and lascivious conduct and lewd or lascivious conduct with a child, alleged to have been committed against a child 16 years of age or under, shall be commenced within the earlier of the date the victim attains the age of 24 or six years from the date the offense is reported, and not after. For purposes of this subsection, an offense is reported when a report of the conduct constituting the offense is made to a law enforcement officer by the victim.

Washington
Wash Rev Code Ann § 9A.04.080(c)
Prosecutions for rape, when the victim is under 14 years of age when the rape is committed and the rape is reported to a law enforcement agency within one year of its commission, may by presented up to three years after the victim's 18th birthday or ten years after the rape's commission, whichever is later. If it is not reported within one year, the rape may not be prosecuted: (A) More than three years after its commission if the violation was committed against a victim fourteen years of age or older; or (B) more than three years after the victim's eighteenth birthday or more than seven years after the rape's commission, whichever is later, if the violation was committed against a victim under fourteen years of age.

Prosecution for the rape of a child, child molestation, indecent liberties with a child, or incest shall not be presented more than three years after the victim's eighteenth birthday or more than seven years after their commission, whichever is later.

Wisconsin
Wis Stat Ann § 939.74(c)
A prosecution for enumerated offenses against children shall be commenced before the victim reaches the age of 31 years, or be barred. However, a prosecution for the physical abuse of a child or child enticement shall be commenced before the victim reaches the age of 26 years or be barred.

FEDERAL LEGISLATION
18 USCA § 3509(k)
If, at any time that a cause of action for recovery of compensation for damage or injury to the person of a child exists, a criminal action is pending which arises out of the same occurrence and in which the child is the victim, the civil action shall be stayed until the end of all phases of the criminal action and any mention of the civil action during the criminal proceeding is prohibited. As used in this subsection, a criminal action is pending until its final adjudication in the trial court.

18 USCA § 3283
No statute of limitations that would otherwise preclude prosecution for an offense involving the sexual or physical abuse, or kidnapping, of a child under the age of 18 years shall preclude such prosecution during the life of the child.

APPENDIX 27-2: SAMPLE INDICTMENTS

INDICTMENT 1

RICHARD M. ROMLEY
MARICOPA COUNTY ATTORNEY

Joe Smith
Deputy County Attorney
Bar ID No.: 2525
301 West Jefferson, 6th Floor
Phoenix, AZ 85003
Telephone: (602) 506-1000
MCAO Firm No.: 00032000
Attorney for Plaintiff

QUADRANT UA – **COMPLEX CASE**

DR 20012680316 - Police Dept.

IN THE SUPERIOR COURT OF THE STATE OF ARIZONA

IN AND FOR THE COUNTY OF _____

THE STATE OF ARIZONA,	)
Plaintiff,	)
vs.	)
L D F (001),	)
Defendant.	) 305 GJ 74
	)
	) INDICTMENT
	)
	) COUNTS 1 – 7: SEXUAL EXPLOITATION OF A
	) MINOR, CLASS 2 FELONIES AND DANGEROUS
	) CRIMES AGAINST CHILDREN

The Grand Jurors of Maricopa County, Arizona, accuse LDF, on this 16th day of January, 2003, charging that in Maricopa County, Arizona:

COUNT 1:
    LDF, on or about the 25th day of September, 2001, knowingly distributed, transported, exhibited, received, sold, purchased, electronically transmitted, possessed, or exchanged any visual depiction in which a minor under fifteen years of age is engaged in exploitive exhibition or other sexual conduct (to-wit: This refers to "M1HHM02K.jpg"), in violation of ARS §§ 13-3553, 13-3551, 13-3821, 13-604.01, 13-702, 13-702.01, and 13-801.

COUNT 2:
    LDF, on or about the 25th day of September, 2001, knowingly distributed, transported, exhibited, received, sold, purchased, electronically transmitted, possessed, or exchanged any visual depiction in which a minor under fifteen years of age is engaged in exploitive exhibition or other sexual conduct (to-wit: This refers to "ps1587713so0.jpg"), in violation of ARS §§ 13-3553, 13-3551, 13-3821, 13-604.01, 13-702, 13-702.01, and 13-801.

COUNT 3:
    LDF, on or about the 25th day of September, 2001, knowingly distributed, transported, exhibited, received, sold, purchased, electronically transmitted, possessed, or exchanged any visual depiction in which a minor under fifteen years of age is engaged in exploitive exhibition or other sexual conduct (to-wit: This refers to "11.jpe"), in violation of ARS §§ 13-3553, 13-3551, 13-3821, 13-604.01, 13-702, 13-702.01, and 13-801.

COUNT 4:
    LDF, on or about the 25th day of September, 2001, knowingly distributed, transported, exhibited, received, sold, purchased, electronically transmitted, possessed, or exchanged any visual depiction in which a minor under fifteen years of age is engaged in exploitive exhibition or other sexual conduct (to-wit- This refers to "M13BEF2I.jpg"), in violation of ARS §§ 13-3553, 13-3551, 13-3821, 13-604.01, 13-702, 13-702.01, and 13-801.

COUNT 5:

LDF, on or about the 25th day of September, 2001, knowingly distributed, transported, exhibited, received, sold, purchased, electronically transmitted, possessed, or exchanged any visual depiction in which a minor under fifteen years of age is engaged in exploitive exhibition or other sexual conduct (to-wit: This refers to "ps1586569so0.jpg"), in violation of ARS §§ 13-3553, 13-3551, 13-3821, 13-604.01, 13-702, 13-702.01, and 13-801.

COUNT 6:

LDF, on or about the 25th day of September, 2001, knowingly distributed, transported, exhibited, received, sold, purchased, electronically transmitted, possessed, or exchanged any visual depiction in which a minor under fifteen years of age is engaged in exploitive exhibition or other sexual conduct (to-wit: This refers to "ps1591313so0.jpg"), in violation of ARS §§ 13-3553, 13-3551, 13-3821, 13-604.01, 13-702, 13-702.01, and 13-801.

COUNT 7:

LDF, on or about the 25th day of September, 2001, knowingly distributed, transported, exhibited, received, sold, purchased, electronically transmitted, possessed, or exchanged any visual depiction in which a minor under fifteen years of age is engaged in exploitive exhibition or other sexual conduct (to-wit: This refers to "ps1625601so0.jpg"), in violation of ARS §§ 13-3553, 13-3551, 13-3821, 13-604.01, 13-702, 13-702.01, and 13-801.

_____
("A True Bill")

RICHARD M. ROMLEY   Date: January 16, 2003
MARICOPA COUNTY ATTORNEY

_____   _____
JOE SMITH   CARRIE JONES
DEPUTY COUNTY ATTORNEY   FOREPERSON OF THE GRAND JURY

BHA/kj/OK

INDICTMENT 2

UNITED STATES DISTRICT COURT

FOR THE CENTRAL DISTRICT OF CALIFORNIA

February 2001 Grand Jury

UNITED STATES OF AMERICA,   )   CR No. 01-_____
)
)   I N D I C T M E N T
                  Plaintiff,   )
)   [18 USC § 2251(c)(1)(A): Publishing an Advertisement to
                  v.   )   Receive, Exchange, and Distribute Child Pornography; 18
)   USC § 2252A(a)(1): Transportation and Shipping of Child
E.G.,   )   Pornography; 18 USC § 2(b): Causing an Act; 18 USC §
)   2252A(a)(5)(B): Possession of Child Pornography; 18 USC §
)   2253: Forfeiture]
                  Defendant.   )
_____   )

The Grand Jury charges:

COUNT ONE
[18 USC § 2251(c)(1)(A)]

On or about October 31, 1999, in Ventura County, within the Central District of California, and elsewhere, defendant E.G. knowingly made and published, and caused to be made and published a notice and advertisement seeking and offering to receive, exchange, and distribute visual depictions the production of which involved minors engaged in sexually explicit conduct, knowing and having reason to know that such notice and advertisement would be transported in interstate and foreign commerce by any means including by computer and such notice and advertisement was transported in interstate and foreign commerce by any means including by computer.

COUNT TWO
[18 USC § 2252A(a)(1) and 18 USC § 2(b)]

On or about October 31, 1999, in Ventura County, within the Central District of California, and elsewhere, defendant E.G. knowingly transported and shipped and caused to be transported and shipped in interstate and foreign commerce by any means, including by computer, an image of child pornography, as defined in Title 18, United States Code, Sections 2256(8)(A) and (8)(C), entitled "hea_004.jpg", knowing that the image was child pornography.

COUNT THREE
[18 USC § 2252A(a)(1) and 18 USC § 2(b)]

On or about October 31, 1999, in Ventura County, within the Central District of California, and elsewhere, defendant E.G. knowingly transported and shipped and caused to be transported and shipped in interstate and foreign commerce by any means, including by computer, an image of child pornography, as defined in Title 18, United States Code, Sections 2256(8)(A) and (8)(C), entitled "hea_026.jpg", knowing that the image was child pornography.

COUNT FOUR
[18 USC § 2252A(a)(1) and 18 USC § 2(b)]

On or about October 31, 1999, in Ventura County, within the Central District of California, and elsewhere, defendant E.G. knowingly transported and shipped and caused to be transported and shipped in interstate and foreign commerce by any means, including by computer, an image of child pornography, as defined in Title 18, United States Code, Sections 2256(8)(A) and (8)(C), entitled "hea_029.jpg", knowing that the image was child pornography.

COUNT FIVE
[18 USC § 2252A(a)(1) and 18 USC § 2(b)]

On or about October 31, 1999, in Ventura County, within the Central District of California, and elsewhere, defendant E.G. knowingly transported and shipped and caused to be transported and shipped in interstate and foreign commerce by any means, including by computer, an image of child pornography, as defined in Title 18, United States Code, Sections 2256(8)(A) and (8)(C), entitled "hea_028.jpg", knowing that the image was child pornography.

COUNT SIX
[18 USC § 2252A(a)(5)(B)]

Between on or about October 31, 1999, and on or about February 15, 2000, in Ventura County, within the Central District of California, defendant E.G. knowingly possessed three computer hard drives that contained more than three images of child pornography, as defined in Title 18, United States Code, Sections 2256(8)(A) and 2256(8)(C), that had been mailed, shipped and transported in interstate and foreign commerce by any means, including by computer, and that had been produced using materials that had been mailed, shipped and transported in interstate and foreign commerce by any means, including by computer, namely, approximately 525 images of child pornography, knowing that the images were of child pornography.

COUNT SEVEN
[18 USC § 2253]

As a result of the foregoing offenses in Counts One through Six of this indictment, namely: Title 18, United States Code, Sections 2251(c)(1)(A); 2252A(a)(1); and, 2252(A)(a)(5)(B), E.G. shall forfeit to the United States all property, real or personal, used or intended to be used to commit or promote the commission of such offenses, which property is more specifically identified as follows:

1. one computer CPU, no brand, no serial number, containing three hard drives bearing the brands and serial numbers: Fujitsu, serial # 01012728; Conner, serial # CFS425AERBD6QA; Samsung, serial # 0100J1FK210754;

2. one Nimble brand keyboard, no serial number;

3. one computer monitor, CTX brand, 14", serial # ACE15104371;

4. one Logitech brand computer mouse, serial # LZA82003179;

5. 147 3 1/2" floppy diskettes;

6. eighteen Zip disks; and,

7. all visual depictions contained in the above media the production of which involved minors engaged in sexually explicit conduct as provided in Title 18, United States Code, Section 2253.

A TRUE BILL

_____

Foreperson

ALEJANDRO MILLER
United States Attorney

JOHN S. GENIN
Assistant United States Attorney
Chief, Criminal Division

SALLY L. CONTI
Assistant United States Attorney
Chief, Major Crimes Section

APPENDIX 27-3: VOIR DIRE IN COMPUTER-FACILITATED CRIMES AGAINST CHILDREN

SAMPLE QUESTIONS

Comfort Level with Computers

1. I would like to start by asking some questions about your familiarity with computers. On a scale of 1 to 5, with 1 being no usage or familiarity and 5 being an expert, where would you rank your knowledge of computers? How many of you consider yourself to be completely computer illiterate with absolutely no computer experience at all?

2. How many of you consider yourself to be a computer expert based on your work experience, education, or self taught by the time you spend using the computer?

3. How many of you feel comfortable enough with your computer knowledge that you can help other people if they have trouble?

4. Are you more likely to be asked to help with a computer question or to ask for help with a computer question?

5. Do you use a computer at either your home or work?

6. At home, what do you use your computer for?

7. At home, what sorts of accessories do you have on your computer (eg, scanner, zip drive, camera, color printer, laser printer)?

8. At work, what is the nature of your computer use: E-mail? Spreadsheets? Internet? Word processing?

9. Have you ever "password protected" any of your files?

10. Have you ever used or tried to use encryption?

11. Do you rely on computers or computer-based information to get your job done?

12. How reliable do you find computers to be?

13. Do you consider information that comes from a computer more reliable or less reliable than information you get from other sources? Why?

14. Does anyone not own a home computer?

15. Does anyone not know how to use e-mail?

16. Is there anyone who does not know how to send or open an attachment to e-mail?

17. Does anyone not know how to access and use the Internet?

18. Which operating system(s) do you use or are you familiar with (eg, Linux, Mac, Windows, UNIX)?

19. Do you use a commercial online service, such as America Online, Yahoo!, or CompuServe?

20. Do you use the Internet? For approximately how much time on a weekly basis? Doing what (eg, browsing, e-mail)?

21. What software programs do you use for: e-mail, WWW, newsgroups, discussion groups?

22. Do you visit chat rooms on either the Internet or an online service?

     a.   If so, which chat rooms do you frequent?

     b.   How often do you visit chat rooms?

     c.   When in chat rooms, do you participate in the discussions?

     d.   Do you ever visit "unmonitored" chat rooms?

23.   Have you ever been contacted online by someone you didn't know? How did you respond?

24.   Are you familiar with IRC (Internet Relay Chat)?

25.   If so, have you ever used a fileserver (or f-serve)?

26.   Are you familiar with UseNet?

27.   Do you ever read the news online?

28.   Do you own a digital camera?

29.   If so, do you store your digital photographs on your computer?

30.   Did your camera come with image-correction software? Have you ever used it?

31.   Have you ever used any type of image-correction software?

32.   Do you have any experience with digital video?

33.   If so, have you ever created a digital video clip?

34.   How many of you know how to download something off the Internet?

35.   How many of you know how to find it and open it once you download it?

36.   How many of you would know how to retrieve it and rename or refile it in another file or directory or on a floppy disk, CD-ROM, or zip drive?

37.   How many of you think that if you delete a file from your computer by hitting the "delete" button, it is gone? What about after you empty the trash or recycle bin? How many of you think a trained computer examiner could not find the deleted file?

38.   Depending on the facts of the case and the defense(s) raised, the following may be asked:

     a.   Have you ever heard of the term "Trojan Horse?" What is your understanding of that term?

     b.   Have you ever heard of the term "e-mail spoofing?" What is your understanding of that term?

     c.   Have you ever heard of the phrase "wiping" a hard drive? What is your understanding of that term?

Computer Forensic Examiner/Expert Testimony/Computer Evidence

39.   Have you ever heard of Computer Forensic Examiners? If so, what does that term mean to you?

40.   Do any of you have any education or background experience in computer forensics? Do any of you know anyone with such a background?

41.   If you hear conflicting testimony from 2 experts, do you feel comfortable in the role of the decision maker who will resolve this? Do you understand that if there is a conflict among experts, this conflict is not the same thing as reasonable doubt? You, as the finder of fact, decide what weight to give each expert's testimony.

42. Do you understand that the testimony of an expert can be accepted or rejected, just like any other witness?

43. On a scale of 1 to 5, how would you rate your ability to follow computer-based evidence and testimony?

44. On a scale from 1 to 5, how would you rate your comfort level in discussing computer-based evidence or testimony?

45. Are you able to rely on computer evidence to find someone guilty?

46. What sort of factors would you look to in determining whether to believe one expert rather than another?

    a. Profession and position

    b. Education (formal [degrees] and informal [seminars and trainings])

    c. Work experience

    d. Teaching experience

    e. Publications

    f. Honors and awards

    g. Memberships and associations

    h. Prior testimony and qualification recognition

    i. Potential bias, motive for testifying or personal agenda

    j. Whether what the expert is saying makes sense

Government Regulation of the Internet

47. Do you have any opinions or feelings about government regulation of the Internet or commercial online services?

48. There are people who believe that the government has no business regulating what people do or say online. How do you feel about that?

49. Are your feelings about free speech the same when what's being sent over the Internet is a picture of a child being sexually violated?

50. Would you agree that it's acceptable for the government to block some types of communications, but not others?

51. Do you have any opinions or feelings about whether law enforcement officers should police the Internet or commercial online services?

Bias Regarding "Sting" Tactics

52. Sometimes police officers conduct undercover investigations, sometimes called "stings," in which an officer makes people believe he or she is not a police officer. Do you have any opinions or feelings about undercover investigations, where an officer assumes or creates another identity?

53. Some people believe it is wrong for a police officer to impersonate someone else. How do you feel about that?

54. In this state, it is not against the law for police officers to conceal their identity during the course of an investigation. How do you feel about that?

Attempt and Factual Impossibility

55. In this case, the defendant is charged with attempt (fill in the charge). It is only an attempt because the minor in this case was a police officer. The law says a person can be convicted of an attempt when the victim is not actually a minor, assuming all the other elements are proven. How do you feel about that law?

56. Would the fact that it was a police officer, rather than a real child, who was sent the pictures in this case prevent you from finding the defendant guilty, provided that the evidence was sufficient to convict under the instruction that will be given to you by the judge?

Children on the Internet

57. Do you have children?

58. Do you have any opinions or feelings about whether children should be allowed to use the Internet or commercial online services?

59. Do you have children who use the Internet or online services?

60. Do you have any rules in your household that your children must follow when using the Internet or online services?

61. Do you have any friends or relatives whose children use the Internet or online services?

62. Have your children or any children you know ever gotten into "trouble" online?

63. Have they ever had contact online with anyone you were not comfortable with?

Problematic Victims

64. The law of this state prohibits adults having sex with children? Does anyone disagree with this law?

65. The evidence in this case will reveal that the victim is a troubled child/teenager. You may or may not like this victim, his or her conduct, attitudes or behavior. In light of this, would you find it more difficult to judge the evidence fairly to determine if the defendant is responsible for his or her criminal conduct with this victim?

66. Would you excuse the defendant's criminal conduct simply because of the victim he chose?

67. Does anyone feel that the State does not have an interest in protecting troubled children?

68. You may approve or disapprove of the victim's background, lifestyle, conduct, or character. Regardless of your feeling do you accept the fact that your judgment or opinion of the victim can not affect your decision regarding whether the defendant committed the offense(s) for which he or she is on trial?

69. Would you disbelieve the testimony of a witness solely because you did not like the witness' appearance, attitude, background, or lifestyle?

70. The laws against child exploitation exist to protect children not only from adults, but also from themselves. The evidence in this case will reveal that

   a. It was the child who initiated contact with the defendant.

   b. The child did not fight back.

   c. The child did not say no.

   d. The child actively cooperated with the defendant.

   e. The child did not tell.

   f. The child accepted gifts/money.

   g. The child enjoyed the sexual activity and attention.

   The judge will instruct you that none of these acts or omissions by the child constitutes a defense because children can not give consent to the types of acts that the defendant is charged with committing. Can you evaluate and decide this case on the defendant's conduct, and the defendant's conduct alone?

71. Does anyone here think that a child should be held to the same conduct and judgment standards as an adult, or that we should judge a child's conduct or behavior in the same way we judge an adult's?

72. Do all of you understand that this trial is about the defendant's criminal acts and culpability, not the child's, and that the child's conduct is not on trial alongside that of the defendant?

73. Does anyone think they would recognize the type of person who engages in sexual conduct with children if they saw him or her?

74. Does everyone agree that this type of crime, like most crimes, can be committed by people from all walks of life?

75. Do you think that sexual exploiters target popular, happy, self-confident, loved, and supported children?

76. Can you think of any reasons that an exploiter would target children with family problems, emotional difficulties, or low self-esteem?

77. Do you have any preconceived ideas about how a child might react to being abused or exploited?

78. Would you feel that the defendant should not be held accountable for his or her criminal conduct simply because the victim did not want him or her prosecuted, or did not want to come to court?

79. Do you believe that victims of abuse promptly report their abuse?

80. Can you think of any reasons why a child might not promptly report?

81. Can you think of any reasons why victims would deny that they had been abused or exploited, even if it were true?

82. Can you think of any reasons why children would recant, or "take it back," that they had been abused or exploited, even if it were true?

83. Can anyone think of reasons that a child victim might want to protect the exploiter or abuser?

84. Do you have any ideas, expectations, or beliefs as to how victims of sexual exploitation will act or react when they testify in court?

85. Would you expect them to exhibit any particular emotion? For example, act fearful, tearful, angry, or withdrawn.

86. Could you understand how 3 different victims could react completely differently to the same set of circumstances? For example, one victim of armed robbery could be terrified, another furious, and a third stunned at being the victim of a crime. Can you accept that there is no one, correct way for a person to react to being victimized?

87. Do you understand that although the court will instruct you that demeanor of a witness during testimony should be considered in evaluating his or her testimony, your expectations, beliefs or ideas about how he or she should act on the witness stand may not be realistic or appropriate for this particular victim?

88. Do you understand that because a victim is gullible or "should have known better," that does not mean the perpetrator did commit a crime. The law protects the savvy as well as the naïve. For example, if someone sends a cashier's check for $45 000.00 to an online seller for a car, but no car is delivered, that does not mean that the "seller" has not committed fraud.

Attitudes Toward Adult Pornography

89. Do you have any opinions or feelings about a person's right to possess or distribute pornography?

90. Do you have any opinions or feelings about whether pornography should be available on the Internet or commercial online services?

91. Some types of pornography are legal, some are illegal. Do you believe all pornography should be illegal?

92. Do you believe children should be protected from pornography?

Attitudes Toward Child Pornography

93. Have you watched, read or heard any media reports on the sexual exploitation of children? What were you told? What did you think of that?

94. The Defendant has been charged with and plead not guilty to sending pictures of children who are being sexually exploited. Is there anything about these charges that will affect your ability to sit as a juror on this case?

95. Will you have any difficulty viewing pictures of sex acts?

96. Will you have any difficulty viewing pictures of children being sexually exploited?

97. Have you ever been exposed to child pornography?

98. Some people have the mistaken belief that possessing, transmitting, or trading child pornography, including possession in your own home or trading by computer, is an activity that is protected by the First Amendment to our Constitution, or may otherwise be Constitutionally protected activity. The court will instruct you that—as a matter of law—this is not the case, that Congress and our own State Legislature has passed laws which make it a criminal offense to receive, transmit, and possess child pornography, and such activity is not protected by the First Amendment, nor by any other Constitutional right.

99. Before I informed you just now that the receipt, possession, or transmission of child pornography was not Constitutionally protected conduct, did any of you believe that it was?

100 Do you believe that child pornography *should* be protected by the First Amendment or by any other provision of the Constitution?

101. Would you have any difficulty accepting and following my instruction to you that such activity is not—as a matter of law—Constitutionally protected?

102. Have any of you [or your relatives or close friends] ever been involved in any incident in which there was sexual contact, sexual abuse, sexual molestation, or sexual assault between an adult and a child?

    a. Nature and circumstances of the situation (including ages of persons involved)

    b. When and where

    c. Outcome (Police involved? Went to court?)

    d. Your feelings about it (Satisfied with the outcome? Why or why not?)

    e. Whether it affects in any way your ability to be fair to both sides

103. Have any of you (or your relatives or close friends) ever been involved in any way in any incident similar to the one charged in this case? Details regarding:

  a. Nature and circumstances of the situation

  b. When and where

  c. Outcome (Police involved? Went to court?)

  d. Your feelings about it (Satisfied with the outcome? Why or why not?)

  e. Whether it affects in any way your ability to be fair to both sides

Virtual Child Pornography

104. Are you familiar with any court decisions regarding pornography? Child pornography? What do you understand those decisions to say? What do you think of those decisions?

105. Have any of you ever heard the term "virtual child pornography"? What does that term mean to you?

106. As part of its case, the State must prove that the images the defendant is charged with possessing/distributing/producing are images, in whole or in part, of real children. The State does not have to prove the identity of any particular child, only that the image, or any part thereof, is of a real child. Does everyone understand the State's burden on this point?

Fantasy/Good Samaritan/Cyber Vigilante/First Amendment Defenses

107. If two people agreed to the same set of facts or actions as being true (provide an example), but offered irreconcilably different explanations for these facts or actions, how would you go about deciding who was telling the truth?

108. Intent is not a tangible thing, something you can hold in your hand or put up to the light to examine. How do you go about deciding what someone's intent is (provide an example)?

Accident

109. Have you ever been on the Internet and had any sort of a pop-up appear? What sort of a pop-up was it? What did you do?

110. If an individual claimed that something came into his or her possession accidentally (provide an example), how would you decide whether that was true or not?

111. If someone claimed to have accidentally accessed an adult pornography Web site, how would you expect to react?

112. If someone claimed to have accidentally accessed a child pornography Web site, how would you expect him or her to react?

SAMPLE FORMAT OF STATE'S REQUESTED VOIR DIRE QUESTIONS

RICHARD M. ROMLEY
MARICOPA COUNTY ATTORNEY

LISA PENTEL
Deputy County Attorney
Technology & Electronic Crimes Bureau
Bar No. 3939
MCAO Firm No. 00032000
301 W. Jefferson St., 5th Floor
Phoenix, AZ 85003-2143
Telephone: (602) 506-1000
FAX: (602) 506-8173
Attorney for Plaintiff

IN THE SUPERIOR COURT OF THE STATE OF ARIZONA
IN AND FOR THE COUNTY OF MARICOPA

THE STATE OF ARIZONA, Plaintiff, vs. STEVEN SCOTT, Defendant.	CR2001-018097 STATE'S REQUESTED VOIR DIRE QUESTIONS Honorable Crane McClennen

The State of Arizona, by undersigned counsel, hereby submits the attached requested voir dire questions and also requests appropriate follow up questions, pursuant to Rule 18.5(c) and (d), Arizona Rules of Criminal Procedure. These questions are in addition to the usual standard questions asked by the Court.

The undersigned respectfully requests that she be allowed to ask the attached computer related questions, rather than the Court, as this will facilitate more meaningful and quicker follow up questions as the need for follow up arises, rather than waiting and coming back to the subject later.
Respectfully submitted January 22, 2002.

RICHARD M. ROMLEY
MARICOPA COUNTY ATTY

BY_____
   LISA PENTEL
   Deputy County Attorney

Copy delivered/mailed _____ to:

Donna Ellis
Deputy Public Defender

Honorable Crane McClennen
Judge of the Superior Court
Central Court Bldg.

By: _____

STATE'S REQUESTED VOIR DIRE QUESTIONS

1. Some people have the mistaken belief that possessing, transmitting or trading child pornography, including possession in your own home or trading by computer, is an activity that is protected by the Free Speech Clause of the First Amendment to our Constitution, or may otherwise be a Constitutionally protected activity. I tell you that—as a matter of law—this is not the case. Congress and our own State Legislature have passed laws which make it a criminal offense to receive, transmit and possess child pornography, and such activity is not protected by the First Amendment or by any other Constitutional right. Before I informed you just now that the receipt, possession or transmission of child pornography was not Constitutionally protected conduct, did any of you believe that it was? Do you believe that such activity should be protected by the First Amendment or by any other provision of the Constitution? Would you have any difficulty accepting and following my instruction to you that such activity is not—as a matter of law—Constitutionally protected?

2. As I am certain you have guessed, part of the evidence in this case will be the images themselves, which the State alleges: (a) constitute child pornography, and (b) that the defendant had something to do with, either by receiving, possessing, transmitting or some other involvement in violation of the law. These images may be distasteful, offensive and unpleasant to view. However, the prospect of having to see distasteful, offensive or unpleasant evidence is not a basis to avoid the responsibility of jury service. Many cases, both criminal and civil, involve unpleasant things. If we excused prospective jurors on the ground that jury duty makes demands—including some unpleasant demands—then we could not function. Moreover, the parties have the right to expect that prospective jurors will not seek to avoid jury service simply because they would rather not serve or because they would like to avoid some unpleasantness. We are certainly not asking that you be "in favor" of child pornography or that you must guarantee us that you will have absolutely no reaction to it, but you must look at it if offered in evidence during the trial. Having said that, is there anyone who honestly believes there is some compelling reason why he or she could not be an impartial juror—that is to consider all of the evidence and follow the law—simply because images depicting child pornography will be presented as evidence in the trial?

3. Have any of you [or your relatives or close friends] ever been involved in any way in any incident similar to the one in this case? Details regarding:

    — Nature and circumstances of the situation
    — When and where
    — Outcome (police involved? go to court?)
    — Your feelings about it (satisfied with the outcome? why or why not?)
    — Whether it affects in any way your ability to be fair to both sides

4. Have any of you [or your relatives or close friends] ever been accused of, arrested for, or convicted of any crime? Details regarding:

    — Nature and circumstances
    — When and where
    — Outcome (police involved? go to court?)
    — Your feelings about it (satisfied with the outcome? why or why not?)
    — Whether it affects in any way your ability to be fair to both sides

5. Is there anyone on the panel who has had an unpleasant experience with a *[police officer, prosecuting attorney, defense lawyer]*? If so, please describe the nature of the experience. Does your experience affect your ability to be fair and impartial to both sides in this case?

6. Is there anyone on the panel who feels that he or she could not, or might not, be able to vote a person guilty of a crime *even if the State has proven its case against him*? (Any personal, political, religious, philosophical or other beliefs or problems with judging a person?)

7. At the time of his arrest, the defendant was a Glendale police detective. Is there anyone on the panel who can not be fair and impartial because of this fact alone? Is there anyone who feels that you will either hold it against him or be sympathetic to him because of the fact that he was a police detective?

Computer-Related Questions

8. How many of you consider yourself to be completely computer illiterate—absolutely no computer experience at all?

9. How many of you consider yourself to be a computer expert—based on your work experience, education, or self-teaching?

10. So everyone else is somewhere between being computer illiterate and an expert?

11. How many of you feel comfortable enough with your computer knowledge that you can help other people if they have trouble?

12. How many of you work with a computer at your work? Describe the nature of your work with computers (ie, what do you use it for and how often—word processing, e-mail, Internet, etc?)

13. Does anyone not own a home computer?

14. Does anyone not know how to use e-mail?

15. Is there anyone who does not know how to send or open an attachment to e-mail?

16. Does anyone not know how to access and use the Internet?

17. How many of you know how to download something off the Internet?

18. How many of you know how to find it once you downloaded it?

19. How many of you would know how to retrieve it and re-name or re-file it in another file or directory?

20. How many of you think that if you delete a file from your computer by hitting the "delete" button, it is gone? What about after you empty the trash or recycle bin? How many of you think I couldn't find the deleted file?

21. How many of you have accessed or used "chat rooms" on the Internet? How often, to what extent, and which chat rooms?

Childhood Victimization and the Derailment of Girls and Women to the Criminal Justice System

Cathy Spatz Widom, PhD

Female crime is generally perceived as not representing a serious threat to the social functioning of society and as being primarily sexual in nature. In addition, people believe the female offender to be an exception—someone who manifests extreme forms of psychological deviance. Furthermore, these beliefs lead to a perception that society does not need to understand or intervene to prevent female crimes. Historical perspectives regarding female crime first illustrated these notions. For example, Glueck & Glueck (1934) referred to female offenders as "themselves on the whole a sorry lot" (ie, not a serious threat), Smith (1962) focused on the "precocious sexual development" of the female offenders as the root cause of their delinquency, and Lombroso & Ferrero (1895) described the criminal woman as "a monster ... whose wickedness must have been enormous before it could triumph over so many obstacles ... put in the path of normal women."

Female offending continues to be perceived as relatively nonthreatening. For example, Steffensmeier & Broidy (2001) concluded that "[t]he girls and women who make up the bulk of the criminal justice workload involving the female offender (and are the grist of the female offender programs) commit ordinary crimes—mostly minor thefts and frauds, low-level drug dealing, prostitution, and simple assaults involving their mates or children ... They are *not* career criminals" [emphasis added].

This chapter focuses on the role of childhood victimization in the development of criminal behavior for girls and women. In addition, this chapter argues that childhood victimization experiences derail the normal developmental processes experienced by girls and young women and that this derailment has consequences for their ability to cope with the demands of life and adulthood. The chapter is divided into 3 major sections. First, it focuses on 4 key questions about abused and neglected girls and women. Second, it examines some of the possible mechanisms whereby young girls may become derailed. Third, it concludes that the picture of female criminality is substantially more complex than depicted in most of the literature and that delinquent and criminal girls and women may best be viewed as *both* victims and offenders.

Numerous reports describe the extent of childhood sexual and physical abuse in the backgrounds of incarcerated women (Browne et al, 1999; Harlow, 1999). It is tempting to conclude from these reports that the childhood abuse experiences somehow played a role in causing these women to become offenders; however, the best way to answer questions about the role of child abuse and neglect in the development of criminal behavior is through prospective, longitudinal studies that follow abused and neglected girls into adolescence and adulthood. In this way, one could determine the percentage of girls who go on to become offenders as adolescents and adults as well as learn about their criminal careers. In addition, this research strategy would also permit knowledge of what happens to the abused and neglected girls whose careers might not have taken this trajectory. Unfortunately, most of the existing large, longitudinal studies, which have provided much of the information for the field of criminology, have involved males who are most often of Caucasian decent. Fortunately, studies are currently underway that may redress some of these limitations in the future when the subjects of these studies, who are currently young girls, grow into adulthood.

The material presented in this chapter draws on the findings of research involving a study of a large number of abused and neglected children and a matched comparison group who were followed into young adulthood (Maxfield & Widom, 1996; Widom, 1989). In this study, criminal histories of women were gathered at 2 times—once when they were about 26 years old and again when they averaged age 33. Thus, these women had sufficient opportunity to offend and be arrested for their criminal behavior over the years.

Although numerous advantages and strengths are associated with this study's design, it has important limitations to bear in mind. First, these samples represent documented court cases of abuse and neglect, and they are skewed toward the lower end of the socioeconomic spectrum. Second, generalizations can not be made about middle-class and upper-class cases of abuse and neglect or about cases of abuse and neglect that do not come to the attention of the authorities. Finally, the consequences of childhood victimization may differ for abused and/or neglected girls from middle-class or upper-class backgrounds as well as for those whose cases did not come to the attention of the authorities and the courts.

QUESTIONS ABOUT CRIMINAL BEHAVIOR AMONG ABUSED AND NEGLECTED GIRLS AND WOMEN

Considering whether childhood victimization derails the normal development processes of girls and young women and whether this derailment affects their ability to cope with the demands of life and adulthood, the following 4 key questions about criminal behavior among abused and neglected girls and women were identified:

1. Is criminal behavior among abused and neglected girls and women rare?

2. Is criminal behavior among abused and neglected girls and women predominantly sexual?

3. Do abused-status and neglected-status offenders escalate to criminal offending?

4. Do abused and neglected girls develop antisocial and/or delinquent lifestyles that persist into adulthood, and do they become chronic, persistent offenders with serious criminal careers?

IS CRIMINAL BEHAVIOR AMONG ABUSED AND NEGLECTED GIRLS AND WOMEN RARE?

In childhood and adolescence, abused and neglected girls are nearly twice as likely to be arrested as juveniles (20% vs. 11.4%), twice as likely to be arrested as adults (28.5% vs. 15.9%), and 2.4 times more likely to be arrested for a violent crime (8.2% vs. 3.6%). All 3 types of childhood victimization (physical abuse, sexual abuse, and neglect) lead to an increased risk of arrest for violence among these women. Despite this increased risk, childhood victimization does not inevitably lead to later arrests. The majority (about 70%) of abused and neglected females do not become offenders.

IS CRIMINAL BEHAVIOR AMONG ABUSED AND NEGLECTED GIRLS AND WOMEN PREDOMINANTLY SEXUAL?

Although abused and neglected females are at an increased risk for prostitution (as defined by arrests and/or self-reports), they also engage in various other criminal behaviors. Of the females in the study's sample, 248 had an arrest as a juvenile or as an adult. Of those who had been arrested, only 40 females (16.1% of those with an arrest) were arrested for a sex-related crime. The remaining females were arrested for various other crimes. Interestingly, the majority (80%) of the 40 females arrested for sex crimes were disproportionately the abused and/or neglected females rather than the nonabused and non-neglected females in the study's sample.

Do Abused-Status and Neglected-Status Offenders Escalate to Criminal Offenses?

Despite the belief that status offenders do not escalate in their offending (Chesney-Lind, 1989), the results from the present research indicate that an escalation of status offenders to other offenses does occur. Nearly half (49%) of the abused and neglected girls who had a status offense (ie, an arrest as a juvenile for an offense that would not be considered criminal if committed by an adult) went on to have arrests as adults. In comparison, 36% of the control females escalated from status offenses as juveniles to adult criminal behavior. Therefore, a substantial portion of the girls with status offenses engaged in crime and were arrested as adults. These results suggest that girls who are status offenders tend to escalate their criminal behavior. In addition, these results lead to additional questions, such as the following:

— What is it about status offenses that enable these offenses to serve as precursors for adult criminal activity among these girls?

— What are the best ways (ie, most helpful and least harmful ways) to respond to these offenses so that the girls do not persist in these behaviors?

Do Abused and Neglected Girls Develop Antisocial and/or Delinquent Lifestyles That Persist Into Adulthood, and Do They Become Chronic, Persistent Offenders With Serious Criminal Careers?

A series of further analyses of these data have recently led to the examination of developmental trajectories of criminal offending (Widom et al, 1998c). Counter to the notion that female offenders are not serious, chronic, or career criminals, these new analyses have identified a group of abused and neglected female offenders who can be characterized as "high-rate, chronic" or "persistent" offenders. This group represents about 8% of the abused and neglected females in the study's sample; a similar group does not exist among the control females. These "high-rate, chronic" abused and neglected young women showed peaks of offending around the ages of 26 and 27. These women averaged slightly more than 1 arrest every 2 years (0.6 arrests per year) until the age of 35. About 38% of the women in this group had been arrested as girls for status offenses, but 54% also had arrests for property crimes, 76% had arrests for order offenses, 46% had arrests for violent crimes, and 32% had arrests for drug offenses. In addition, the women in this "high-risk, chronic" offender group have criminal histories that are similar in the types of crimes committed as those committed by "mid-rate, chronic" offenders among males. These results suggest that there is a subset of abused and neglected females who develop antisocial and delinquent lifestyles that persist into adulthood and who become chronic, persistent offenders with serious criminal careers.

POTENTIAL MECHANISMS IN THE DERAILMENT OF ABUSED AND NEGLECTED GIRLS AND WOMEN

RUNNING AWAY

Girls who have been abused and neglected may become derailed through the experience of running away from home. Chesney-Lind & Shelden (1992) assert that victimization triggers the entry of girls "into delinquency as they try to escape abusive environments." Further,

[s]ince adolescent females are unable to end this abuse through legal channels, they run away and end up on the streets with few legitimate survival options—unable to enroll in school or take a job to support themselves because they fear detection. Here they engage in panhandling, petty theft, and occasional prostitution in order to survive. Young women in conflict with parents (often for very legitimate reasons) may actually be forced by present laws into petty criminal activity, prostitution, and drug use (Chesney-Lind & Shelden, 1992).

Kaufman & Widom (1999) found that abused and neglected children are at an increased risk for running away from home and that running away is associated with an increased risk for being arrested as juveniles and as adults; however, nonabused and non-neglected children who ran away from home were also at an increased risk of being arrested.

Bracey (1983) described juvenile prostitutes as neglected at home. She quoted 1 young woman who reported "[my] parents didn't tell me to get out, but they didn't come looking for me when I did." Neglected young children who are on the streets alone are at risk of being victimized or enticed into prostitution. Runaways may come under the control of pornographers and pimps as well as become susceptible to subsequent physical and sexual victimization experiences by pimps and customers. Given the lack of adequate medical care experienced by runaway youth and the high occurrence of risky lifestyles (eg, prostitution, alcohol, drugs, smoking), these children may be at risk for multiple problems, which include those of public health concern (eg, sexually transmitted diseases [STDs]).

DEFICITS IN IQ OR COGNITIVE ABILITY

Perez & Widom (1994) found that abused and neglected women tend to have lower average scores on IQ tests and tests of their reading ability than nonabused and non-neglected women. Abused and neglected women also reported having done more poorly in school (ie, received poor grades, misbehaved, were expelled) and, on average, completed 1 year less of school than their counterparts.

The origin of these academic-performance and intellectual-performance deficits among abused and neglected females remains unknown; however, 2 possibilities may exist. One possibility is associated with physical abuse, while the other is concerned with neglect. For example, physical abuse (eg, battering) or severe neglect (eg, dehydration, diarrhea, failure to thrive) may lead to developmental retardation, which, in turn, may affect school performance and behavior.

Deficits in IQ or cognitive ability during early childhood may lead to impaired performance in elementary and/or secondary school, which, in turn, may lead to impaired functioning as a young girl. As a result of decreased cognitive functioning, a lowered self-esteem may result. A lower self-esteem, or the lack of a sense of mastery and control over one's life, may directly result from childhood victimization (ie, since the child feels somehow responsible for the abuse or neglect and/or was unable to prevent or stop the abuse) or be a by-product of lowered cognitive functioning and poor social and interpersonal skills.

Furthermore, since expectations for early academic skills are often higher for girls than for boys (Keenan & Shaw, 1997), these types of deficits in girls may elicit more negative responses from teachers and caregivers. These negative responses may, in turn, place girls at risk for developing behavior problems and antisocial behavior (Keenan et al, 1999).

LACK OF TRADITIONAL SOCIAL CONTROLS

Traditionally, females are closely supervised and antisocial behavior is discouraged through negative sanctions especially during the formative years. As Steffensmeier & Broidy (2001) point out, risk-taking behavior among girls is discouraged, whereas such behavior is encouraged and often rewarded among boys. In addition, the friends of girls tend to be more carefully monitored, thereby decreasing the likelihood of influence by delinquent peers (Giordano et al, 1986).

Life for abused and neglected young girls does not necessarily reflect this traditional socialization, however. While these mechanisms for social control may encourage girls and women to behave properly in general, the situation in which abused and neglected girls find themselves is often quite different. Most neglected children and often abused children are not reared in households characterized by traditional social controls. The barriers that Lombroso & Ferrero (1895) referred to as holding the "normal woman in the path of virtue" are not in place for many abused and neglected females who grow up in multiproblem homes with parents who often suffer from alcohol or other drug problems and/or other social maladies. Perhaps the "lucky" abused and neglected females are those who are placed in foster care and develop relationships with their foster parents at an early age or those who have grandparents or other relatives who rear them successfully.

RELATIONSHIPS WITH DEVIANT AND/OR DELINQUENT FRIENDS AND/OR RELATIVES

Another possibility is that abused and neglected girls are derailed into delinquency and crime through relationships with deviant and/or delinquent friends and/or relatives. Abused and neglected individuals are more likely to report that someone in their family was arrested (ie, a parent or sibling) than nonabused and non-neglected individuals. Cloninger & Guze (1973) reported high rates of psychopathology among the families of female delinquents and felons. Robins' (1966) work indicates that antisocial women and men often engage in assortative mating (ie, nonrandom mating resulting from the selection of similar partners).

If behavioral preferences are indeed a function of the networks in which a person is embedded (Smith-Lovin & McPherson, 1993), then it would not be surprising that abused and neglected girls and women tend to engage in deviant or criminal behaviors since their networks oftentimes offer models or support for such behavior. Since many abused and neglected girls are more likely to grow up in "criminogenic" homes (ie, likely to lead to criminal behavior) and in neighborhoods characterized by high rates of crime and violence, they may have more opportunities to learn and model aggressive and antisocial behavior. This picture contrasts sharply with the explanations typically offered for the generally low rates of female crime.

FAILURE TO LEARN THE SOCIAL AND PSYCHOLOGICAL SKILLS NECESSARY FOR SUCCESSFUL ADULT DEVELOPMENT

Derailment may also occur because child abuse and neglect prevents girls from learning the social and psychological skills needed for successful adult development. Abused and neglected girls and women have multiple problems: lower academic and intellectual performance; more stressful life events; more suicide attempts (Widom, 1998a); an increased likelihood of abusing alcohol (Widom et al, 1995); higher levels of hostility and sensation-seeking; and lower levels of self-esteem, mastery, and sense of control (Widom, 1998b) than nonabused and non-neglected girls and women.

In unpublished research, Chavez & Widom found that abused and neglected females are more likely to report using alcohol and other drugs, and turn to criminal and violent criminal behaviors, when coping with stressful life events. Some writers suggest that the patterns of problems experienced by women lead to noncriminal forms of coping with strain rather than actions likely to lead to aggressive or violent behavior, but the findings of Chavez & Widom suggest otherwise.

CONCLUSION

Three general conclusions can be drawn regarding the relationship between childhood victimization and the derailment of girls and women to the criminal justice system. First, commonly used assumptions and explanations used to describe female crime and the often nonthreatening nature of these crimes remain inadequate when explaining the development and derailment of abused and neglected girls to the criminal justice system. From a public health perspective, the consequences of childhood abuse and neglect are particularly important in terms of potential STDs and the potential to facilitate a young girl's transition into prostitution.

Second, a small subset (approximately 8%, which is about the same percentage of nonabused and non-neglected males identified in other studies) exists among abused and neglected girls who become chronic, persistent offenders who engage in violence and other forms of troublesome behavior that persists into adulthood. Rather than denying that some women are serious offenders, there is a need to understand what it is about the experiences of these women, about their families, and about their characteristics that leads them down these nontraditional, criminal paths.

Third, women play a unique role in our society in that they bear children. Between 80% and 85% of the females in this sample have children. The at-risk behavior of and health risks taken by these young adult women directly impact the health and development of their children, which is especially disconcerting given the increased risk for serious alcohol problems among the abused and neglected females. The environments will affect the physical and psychosocial development of their children.

In the past, criminologists concentrated their efforts and resources on male offenders to the general neglect of the female. Two reasons have typically been offered for the neglect of research on female crime: the nature of female offenses and the number of female offenders involved. Not only is there evidence of considerable delinquency and adult criminal behavior among female offenders, but little knowledge exists regarding how best to intervene and treat abused and neglected females. There is a need for more research about women and girl offenders in general and about abused and neglected girls and women in particular. Interventions are needed when these children first come into contact with the system as runaways and status offenders. These should be the first steps undertaken to prevent the derailment of young abused and neglected girls and to enhance the likelihood of their leading more healthy and successful lives.

REFERENCES

Bracey D. The juvenile prostitute: victim and offender. *Victimology.* 1983;8:151.

Browne A, Miller B, Maguin ET. Prevalence and severity of lifetime physical and sexual victimization among incarcerated women. *Int J Law Psychiatry.* 1999;22(3-4): 301-322.

Chesney-Lind M. Girls' crime and woman's place: toward a feminist model of female delinquency. *Crime Delinq.* 1989;35:5-29.

Chesney-Lind M, Shelden RG. *Girls, Delinquency, and Juvenile Justice.* Pacific Grove, Calif: Brooks/Cole; 1992.

Cloninger CR, Guze SB. Psychiatric illness in the families of female criminals: a study of 288 first-degree relatives. *Br J Psychiatry.* 1973;122:697-703.

Giordano PC, Cernkovich SA, Pugh MD. Friendships and delinquency. *Am J Sociol.* 1986;91:1170-1202.

Glueck E, Glueck S. *Five Hundred Delinquent Women.* New York, NY: AA Knopf; 1934.

Harlow CW. *Prior Abuse Reported by Inmates and Probationers.* Washington, DC: US Dept of Justice, Bureau of Justice Statistics; 1999. NCJ 172879.

Kaufman JG, Widom CS. Childhood victimization, running away, and delinquency. *J Res Crime Delinq.* 1999;36:347-370.

Keenan K, Loeber R, Green S. Conduct disorder in girls: a review of the literature. *Clin Child Fam Psychol Rev.* 1999;2:3-19.

Keenan K, Shaw DS. Developmental and social influences on young girls' early problem behavior. *Psychol Bull.* 1997;121:95-113.

Lombroso C, Ferrero W. *The Female Offender.* London, England: Fisher Unwin; 1895.

Maxfield MG, Widom CS. The cycle of violence: revisited six years later. *Arch Pediatr Adolesc Med.* 1996;150:300-395.

Perez CM, Widom CS. Childhood victimization and long-term intellectual and academic outcomes. *Child Abuse Negl.* 1994;18:617-633.

Robins LN. *Deviant Children Grown Up.* Baltimore, Md: Williams & Wilkins; 1966.

Smith AD. *Women in Prison.* London, England: Stevens and Sons; 1962.

Smith-Lovin L, McPherson JM. You are who you know: a network approach to gender. In: England P, ed. *Theory on Gender/Feminism on Theory.* New York, NY: Aldine de Gruyter; 1993:223-254.

Steffensmeier D, Broidy L. Explaining female offending. In: Goodstein L, ed. *Women, Crime and Criminal Justice: Contemporary Issues.* Los Angles, Calif: Roxbury Press; 2001.

Widom CS. Childhood victimization: early adversity and subsequent psychopathology. In: Dohrenwend BP, ed. *Adversity, Stress, and Psychopathology.* New York, NY: Oxford University Press; #1998a:81-95.

Widom CS. The cycle of violence. *Science.* 1989;244:160-166.

Widom CS. Motivation and mechanisms in the cycle of violence. In: Hansen DW, ed. *Nebraska Symposium on Motivation.* Vol 46. Lincoln, NE: University of Nebraska Press; 1998b.

Widom CS, Ireland T, Glynn PJ. Alcohol abuse in abused and neglected children followed-up: are they at increased risk? *J Stud Alcohol.* 1995;56:207-217.

Widom CS, Nagin D, Lambert L. Does childhood victimization alter developmental trajectories of criminal careers? Paper presented at: American Society of Criminology, annual meeting; November 11-14, 1998c; Washington, DC.

Chapter 29

Juvenile Courts and Sexual Exploitation: A Judge's Observations

The Honorable Ernestine S. Gray

When I was first asked to write a submission for this book, I was excited about the prospect. The longer I contemplated the end product, however, I became increasingly worried. Partly because I was concerned about the possibility of writing a piece that was critical of the courts' handling of these cases, and partly because I am not sure that I have any concrete ideas or "best practices" to offer as a solution. I eventually realized that most of my concern arose out of my recognition of the difficulty of the problem itself, that of sexual exploitation of minors in the specific form of juvenile prostitution. This problem is difficult to deal with psychologically, socially, and judicially. Consequently, I decided to provide some background regarding the juvenile courts, both historically and as presently constituted. I follow this background with discussion of juvenile prostitution in which I attempt to give some idea of the extent and pervasiveness of the problem of juvenile prostitution. I end with discussion of the judicial response to the issue of juvenile prostitution and some suggestions for improvement.

The History of Juvenile Courts

In preparation for writing this chapter, I reread some of the history of the juvenile justice system, including the philosophy that supported the founding of the juvenile court. Though there has been much debate in recent years about whether or not there is a continued need for a juvenile court, largely because of the concern about violent juvenile crime, my rereading of the history and thinking about juvenile prostitution again led me to the conclusion that the juvenile court as an institution continues to be relevant in our work with young people in our communities. The adult criminal system is not equipped to deal with the special, new, or youthful offenders, nor has it done a good job with the adults who have gone through that system.

The first juvenile court in the United States was established in 1899 in Illinois. The juvenile court was founded on philosophies quite different from the adult criminal court. The first of these courts were established to protect children and provide them with the treatment they needed so that they could return to society as productive adults. The philosophy of the early court was based on the belief that, because children are not fully developed physically or mentally, they are not accountable for their behavior in the same way as adults. In fact, adolescent psychology has come to the same conclusions. This philosophy was based partially on prior common-law presumptions of the incapacity of young children. Generally speaking, under the common law, children under the age of 7 were deemed incapable of violating the criminal law because of their inability to form the requisite criminal intent, and children up to the age of 14 were presumed incapable in the same way, though this presumption could be rebutted. In any case, all but 2 states had established juvenile courts by 1925.

It was originally thought that the criminal behavior by children resulted from external influences such as parental neglect and impoverished living conditions. If criminality was believed to be a youthful illness, that illness might be cured by moving the child to a better family life in a rural setting.

The first juvenile court judge, a Cook County, Illinois judge, set the court's primary responsibilities as the welfare of the child and the welfare of the community. Therefore, the early courts focused on the individual offender and not on the offense. In addition, these courts ascribed the doctrine of state as parent (ie, *parens patriae*). Under this doctrine, the state is placed in the position of a surrogate parent to the delinquent or abused child, and the child becomes a ward of this state and/or "parent." Such doctrine is still codified in many modern juvenile statutes, such as the following language from Article 801 Louisiana Children's Code, which states the purpose of the delinquency provisions of this code: "… in those instances when [the juvenile] is removed from the control of his parents, the court shall secure for him care as nearly as possible equivalent to that which the parents should have given him." The main goal was not to determine guilt or innocence, but rather what the child is, how has the child become what he or she is, and what is in the best interest of both the child and the state to keep the child from entering a downward spiral.

THE MODERN JUVENILE COURT

The main participants and their roles in the modern juvenile court process are detailed in **Table 29-1**. The modern juvenile court process in which these participants work is supposed to protect the interests of the child and society just as the statutes creating the first juvenile courts envisioned. The same philosophy of *parens patriae* as well as the incapacity of children and the inability of children to protect themselves underlies the modern juvenile court. Such an approach still has direct relevance for the problem of teenage prostitution.

JUVENILE PROSTITUTION

Prostitution is the practice of engaging in sexual relations, especially for money. It has often been dubbed the "oldest profession in the world." Recent trends indicate that there is a noticeable increase in teenage prostitution and that the majority of street prostitutes are children. Children involved in prostitution are getting younger;

Table 29-1. Participants and Their Roles in the Modern Juvenile Court

— *The judge.* Generally has more power, by tradition and law, than judges in other arenas, granting the judge freedom to craft decisions that are creative and appropriate

— *The child's attorney.* Charged with advancing the best legal interest of the child, whether the case involves a delinquency (ie, criminal) charge or an abuse and/or neglect situation

— *A guardian ad litem, a court-appointed special advocate (CASA), or another person charged with a similar role.* Looks after the child's general interest (ie, social, psychological, and so on) more broadly than the child's attorney

— *The parents' attorney.* Looks after the parents' interest in an abuse and/or neglect case

— *The prosecutor.* Performs the role of prosecuting the accused juvenile (ie, in a delinquency case) or of petitioning for the child's removal from the home or for the termination of the parents' parental rights (ie, in an abuse and/or neglect case)

the average age of juvenile prostitutes is 13, but some are as young as 9 years old. A growing number of these children come from middle-class homes. In fact, juvenile prostitutes come from every economic, social, and ethnic background. Also, recent trends indicate that juvenile prostitutes may not just be running away from physical or sexual abuse at home. Teenage prostitutes are recruited in shopping malls, movie theaters, community centers, schools, fast-food establishments, clubs, sporting events, concerts, arcades, amusement parks, transportation centers, and the Internet. Girls are now the fastest-growing segment of the juvenile justice system, a trend that perhaps is not unrelated to the growth of teenage prostitution. Teenage girls are arrested more often than teenage boys (with a ratio of almost 3:2). Consistent with the adult world, the prostitute gets arrested, and the john does not.

JUVENILE PROSTITUTION CASES

The juvenile court system, as presently constituted, is ill-equipped to deal with the problem of child prostitution. Many of these deficiencies are the result of the adult system's failure to use the legal tools that already exist, such as the enforcement of laws in situations that involve child prostitution since these laws were designed to protect minors from sexual mistreatment. For instance, laws criminalize sexual conduct with children based on the ages of the offender and victim. In Louisiana, for example, laws that could be used to charge an adult who engages in sexual conduct with a child prostitute, depending on the specific fact pattern, include Louisiana Revised Statutes 14:80 and 14:80.1, felony and misdemeanor carnal knowledge of a juvenile; 14:81, indecent behavior with juveniles; 14:81.2, molestation of a juvenile; 14:92, contributing to the delinquency of a juvenile; 14:43.1, sexual battery; and 14:43.3, oral sexual battery. Louisiana Revised Statute 14:42.1, aggravated rape, is committed when anyone has sex with a child under the age of 12, whether that child is a prostitute or not. Crimes specifically relating to the criminal liability of adults involved in child prostitution include: Louisiana Revised Statute 14:82.1, prostitution of a person younger than age 17, which criminalizes the act of a person who is older than age 17 having sex with a prostitute who is younger than age 17, or the act of a parent "consenting to…the entrance" (into prostitution of a person younger than age 17); and 14:86, enticing persons into prostitution, which is committed by a person older than age 17 who "entices, places, persuades, encourages, or causes" a person under the age of 21 to engage in prostitution. Again, aggressive enforcement of such laws in the child prostitution arena may discourage adults from exploiting children in this way.

Such children may come before a juvenile court judge themselves because they are runaways or in the context of a child abuse case. Unfortunately, oftentimes the judicial response to children who have engaged in prostitution is insufficient or inappropriate. Judges and others often throw up their hands and ask, "Why don't you just get out of it?" Service providers commonly feel that these girls are difficult to work with. Judges often believe that they have no choice but to incarcerate runaway children who are involved in child prostitution: "I had to lock her up for her own safety; she kept running away." The perception also exists that a child involved in the "adult" behavior of prostitution is no longer a child worthy of the same level of protection accorded other children. Generally, the laws designed to protect children from sexual abuse, such as those previously noted, are not applied to child prostitution cases. Although they are victims under the law, prostitutes are seen as bad people, outcasts, and people who make poor choices, rather than as victims. Teen-agers who are involved in prostitution are seen as bad or different. While the sexually abused child in another context is seen as a victim, the juvenile prostitute is not seen by society as a worthy victim. We must realize that these victims are one and the same.

This acknowledgment and realization that child prostitutes are indeed victims would then require a different approach by everyone with respect to the growing problem of juvenile prostitution in order to remain consistent with the early and continued philosophy of the juvenile courts protecting children. The following is needed:

— Enforcement of existing criminal law against the customers of and other adults that benefit from child prostitutes, and the creation of model statutes to address the insufficiencies in the law related to the definitions of crime and their punishment so that johns and pimps face significantly more severe consequences for the devastation they perpetuate

— Expanded treatment services that are culturally competent and developmentally appropriate

— An increase in the number of shelters for runaway and homeless youth as well as greater options for placement

— Community awareness and intolerance for the sexual abuse of children in situations involving prostitution that equals society's outrage directed at child sexual abuse in other situations

— Mentors to provide healthy role models to enable these children to perceive alternatives for their lives

— Opportunities for these children to participate in athletic events

— Work opportunities for these children

CONCLUSION

The social and judicial response to the issue of teenage prostitution has to embody the idea that these children are exploited victims, not criminals, who need and deserve effective interventions, supports, and services. Unfortunately, significant changes in juvenile courts are necessary for this acknowledgement to occur.

REFERENCES

La Children's Code § 801.

La Rev Stat Ann § 14:42.1, 14:82.1, 14:86.

years. Her mother acted caring and concerned, always giving the impression of being a doting caretaker. Lauren graduated from using marijuana to using intravenous drugs and began having unprotected sexual encounters with multiple partners. By age 13, Lauren had more sexual experience than most grown women. The path of exploitation created a path of self-destruction.

Shortly before her 18th birthday, Lauren was found unconscious and taken to a local hospital. She had experienced multiple strokes caused by endocarditis, a serious infection of the heart valve. Lauren would later explain that she was at the end of a methamphetamine binge in a stage called tweaking. **Tweaking** is considered by medical and law enforcement personnel to be the most dangerous stage of methamphetamine abuse. It is characterized by feelings of emptiness, anxiety, and uneasiness, leading to use of another depressant, often alcohol. The user becomes sleep deprived, possibly causing paranoia—which is exactly what happened to Lauren. The paranoia caused her to search for any form of the drug, which she found in a used needle on the floor. The contaminated needle introduced a bacteria into her system that consequently caused endocarditis and the strokes. Lauren spent 20 days in the hospital undergoing valve replacement surgery to save her life. Chemically paralyzed to help her heal, Lauren could not move or function independently. Her estranged mother came to see her in the intensive care unit, where she saw her daughter obscured by multiple tubes, cords, and medical devices. Though unconscious and unable to move, the monitors showed an intense increase in Lauren's blood pressure, and she vomited. When her mother left, Lauren's blood pressure returned to normal.

Today, Lauren bears the physical and emotional scars of her sexual and physical abuse. As is common among exploited and abused children, Lauren had an affinity for the source of her abuse. This explains why, at age 17, after having been deemed an "adult" by juvenile authorities, Lauren did not leave her mother to pursue a better life. Instead, she and her mother became inseparable. This fact led to the abuse continuing undetected for several years and is an example of the reason exploitation is so difficult to eradicate. It is a secret crime, one that occurs worldwide and takes many different forms.

BACKGROUND INFORMATION

Child prostitution is big business. The organization End Child Prostitution, Child Pornography and Trafficking of Children for Sexual Exploitation (ECPAT) estimated that in 1996, between 100 000 and 300 000 children were sexually exploited through prostitution and pornography in the United States (1996). The reason is simple: The market for child prostitution exists. People are willing to pay to have sex with children. Reportedly, more than a half million children in the world have become prostitutes as a means to survive. Child exploitation occurs in all types of societies, from the richest cities to the poorest corners of the earth.

The statistics regarding the exploitation of children in the sex trade are staggering. Updates are posted on the Internet daily, and the numbers continue to increase at alarming rates. The predators and pimps have become more sophisticated in their recruitment methods. They use power and control to force children into prostitution. In the United States, victims are often moved from state to state and are forced to work as prostitutes on the outskirts of larger metropolitan areas or in small towns where police and social workers have little or no experience with child prostitution.

Prostitution is a seasonal problem. It is most prevalent during the warmer months and in cities with warmer climates. During the peak seasons for prostitution, as many as 500 prostitutes may be found on the streets of the larger cities in the United States. At least 25% to 30% of the prostitutes are children younger than 18 (Haggarty, 1997).

Recruiting children for the sex trade has become easier. As parents become less involved with their children and sexuality becomes a more socially acceptable topic, the numbers of susceptible children increase; they can be recruited almost anywhere. Any place where children frequent and adult supervision is inadequate can become a recruiting area. Malls, entertainment arcades, carnivals, tourist attractions, concerts, and clubs are prime examples of environments in which children are recruited into the sex trade. The pimp grooms and then seduces a child or an adolescent with promises of wealth, luxury, designer clothing, expensive vehicles, and an exciting life. Victimology makes some children and adolescents prime targets. Children who are alone, troubled, desperate, and unsupervised are often targets. The pimps manipulate their victims in an atmosphere of alienation and isolation. A child is taken from familiar surroundings to areas that are new, increasing dependence on the pimp. At this point, the previously made promises become meaningless words. The child is in a strange city, far away from the protection of family and friends, and dependent on a controlling person. The child loses all self-worth and self-esteem and is forced into prostitution or pornography as a means of survival. The captor becomes the savior and the person who provides food and shelter. Child prostitutes are lost children, and tens of thousands of children worldwide are brainwashed into prostitution every year.

Several target groups have been identified by the US Department of Labor *Report on Child Prostitution as a Form of Forced Labor*. Examples of children who are at high risk for becoming involved in child prostitution include the following (Saikaew, 2001):

— A child who has been expelled from school or is no longer interested in pursuing an education but still wants the money and material items popular in a peer group

— A child who has an older sister or another relative involved in prostitution

— A child whose parents are separated or divorced or whose parents are deceased and who is living with a relative or friend

— A child whose parents are drug addicts, alcoholics, or compulsive gamblers

— A child whose family is living in extreme poverty and needs the child to make money in any way possible

Though several organizations worldwide have been established to combat the problem of child sex rings, the prostitution of children remains a devastating problem the majority of society fails to acknowledge. No one in the mainstream press seems to report stories about the topic, so it remains blanketed in a veil of secrecy. In addition, many consider child prostitutes to be criminals rather than victims of exploitation. Many child prostitutes are the focus of pornographic images that appear in child pornography magazines and are often downloaded and traded on the Internet. Exploitation is a cycle.

Many child prostitutes were and are victims of sexual, physical, or emotional abuse, some of which occurred when they were young. Without intervention, these children often escape to the streets during their adolescence to get away from their abusers. Some children are on the streets long enough before being recruited into prostitution that they become somewhat street toughened or at least perceive themselves to be street tough. In reality, they are children, and beneath the street hardened surface they are troubled children reaching out for help. Other children seem defenseless and lack the internal fortitude and aggression required for survival on the streets. They are more vulnerable to being manipulated by pimps and other people. Unfortunately, both types of children find "help" in the wrong people.

CONSEQUENCES

The most tangible consequence of involvement in juvenile prostitution is the extremely high probability of being assaulted. The majority of female prostitutes are beaten by their pimps and abused repeatedly by their customers. Rape is common among girls involved in prostitution; up to 70% of juvenile female prostitutes say that they have been raped by customers an average of 31 times (Saikaew, 2001).

Many prostitutes, especially those between the ages of 14 and 17, can make $500 to $600 dollars a night (Saikaew, 2001). This money is often used to bail their pimps out of jail. Child prostitutes rarely get more than a $25 allowance from their earnings (Saikaew, 2001).

Countless stories such as Christine's and Lauren's are played out every year. Every day, children in all walks of life become victims of exploitation. Many investigators fail to note that delinquency, drug use, promiscuity, alcoholism, truancy, and running away from home are often linked to previous or current abuse or exploitation.

INCARCERATED PEDOPHILES*

In 2003, interviews were conducted and information was collected on 48 incarcerated male pedophiles to gain insight and understanding about their thought processes and methods of operation. Information was obtained on a wide range of topics: offender childhood and background; sexual history; victim preference; selection, grooming, and seduction of victims; personal habits; and offender experiences with the police and criminal justice system. The hope is that data collected in this study can be used to educate people and prevent child sexual abuse. Perhaps it will benefit the law enforcement community and other professionals who are involved in the investigation and prosecution of child sexual abuse cases.

MEN WHO MOLEST BOYS

In February 2003, Alan[†] was interviewed in a Missouri prison. A 62-year-old man serving 7 years in prison for molesting a 9-year-old boy, he was serving his third prison sentence for child molestation, 2 of which he served in another state. This 3-hour interview was conducted to understand how and why he had committed the crimes, how and why he had selected and groomed these particular children, and how long his activities had gone undetected.

During the course of the interview, Alan said that in his lifetime he had molested 35 to 40 children, all between the ages of 8 and 12. He even admitted that he had once married a woman so that he could have a relationship with her 8-year-old son. He molested the boy before and during the 18-month marriage. The marriage ended when he was arrested and convicted of molesting another boy who lived in their neighborhood. Though Alan has been convicted of molesting 3 children, he will never be prosecuted for molesting any of the 35 or so other children. Too much time has elapsed, and the statute of limitations has expired. At the time of the interview, Alan was nearing the end of his 7-year prison sentence, and he had recently been terminated from (ie, failed to complete) a sex offender treatment program that was offered in the prison.

The state of Missouri has a sexual predator law that allows for the civil commitment (ie, mental health commitment rather than criminal incarceration) of certain sex offenders who are considered to be a threat to the community after release from prison. Alan is an ideal candidate, but nothing ensures his commitment. He could be released back into the community in the near future.

Unfortunately, society is filled with men like Alan. Some are in prison, but most are not. They are in communities throughout the world, actively molesting children. Some of the men will be arrested one day, but most will never be caught. Regardless, a tremendous amount of information can be learned from child molesters that *have* been caught.

The following section is a summary of the findings from a research study on a specific type of child molester: pedophiles who target young boys. As mentioned, Alan was one of 48 convicted child molesters who were studied for this project.

DEFINITIONS

The words *pedophile* and *pedophilia* are frequently used in the United States and throughout the world. Though most people have seen or heard these words, many

---

* *Study conducted by the author, Lt William D. Carson.*
† *Name has been changed.*

can not define them. Even professionals can not agree on one definition of pedophilia. The terms have slightly different meanings depending on the context in which they are used. Technically, pedophilia is a psychiatric diagnosis and not a legal term. A well-accepted definition of pedophilia and pedophile is found in the fourth edition (text revision) of the *Diagnostic and Statistical Manual of Mental Disorders*, or the DSM-IV-TR (American Psychiatric Association, 2000):

A. Over a period of at least 6 months, recurrent, intense sexually arousing fantasies, sexual urges, or behaviors involving sexual activity with a prepubescent child or children (generally age 13 years or younger).

B. The person has acted on these urges, or the sexual urges or fantasies caused marked distress or interpersonal difficulty.

C. The person is at least age 16 years and at least 5 years older than the child or children in Criterion A.

Three other issues are addressed in this definition: (1) determining whether the person is sexually attracted to boys, girls, or both; (2) determining whether the behavior is limited to incest; and (3) determining whether the person is an ***exclusive type*** (ie, attracted only to children) or a ***nonexclusive type*** (ie, occasionally attracted to adults).

In other words, pedophilia is a state of mind, a sexual orientation. An individual who obsesses and fantasizes about having sex with prepubescent children is a ***pedophile***, regardless of whether the person ever acts on the thoughts and fantasies. A person can be a pedophile and never molest a child, just as any person can choose to be celibate (sexually abstinent). It does not change the person's basic sexual orientation.

In comparison, the term ***child molester*** is a broad term. It describes any person who has ever molested a child, regardless of whether the person is attracted to children. A person can be a child molester and not be a pedophile. Some child molesters are ***situational offenders***; they do not prefer children but may still molest a child given the right set of circumstances.

This was not a research study of all types of child molesters. It was a study of a specific category of child molester: a person who has molested a child *and* has a sexual preference for prepubescent children. Some refer to this type of person as a *preferential child molester*, but here the term *pedophile* is used. The DSM-IV-TR definition of pedophilia fits the type of offenders who were sought out for this research project. Pedophilia is the only term that addresses the preference of the person and includes individuals who have never molested a child. Therefore, when someone is referred to as being a *pedophile* in this chapter, it is not a psychiatric diagnosis. This is only a category based on experience with sex offenders and an understanding of the definition and terminology.

Male-Target and Female-Target Pedophiles

This study focused only on pedophiles who were attracted to prepubescent boys, the exclusive and nonexclusive types. This study concentrated on this group for several reasons. Pedophiles who are attracted exclusively to boys (***male-target pedophiles***) have been shown to be different from pedophiles who are attracted only to girls (***female-target pedophiles***). Previous studies have shown they are dissimilar in many ways.

In 1983, Gene Abel and his colleagues studied 561 sex offenders, 232 of which were child molesters. They found that fewer men were male-target offenders though those who were had a significantly higher number of victims than men who were female-target offenders. The female-target offenders averaged 20 victims each, whereas the male-target offenders averaged 150 victims each (Abel et al, 1987).

A later study by Abel involved 3952 child molesters and yielded lower average numbers but similar basic findings. More men molest girls than boys, but those who molest boys have many more victims (Abel & Harlow, 2001). It follows that another significant difference between male-target and female-target pedophiles is the recidivism rate. According to the DSM-IV-TR, "the recidivism rate for individuals with Pedophilia involving a preference for males is roughly twice that for those who prefer females." Kenneth Lanning wrote that "men that are sexually attracted to young adolescent boys are the most persistent and prolific child molesters known to the criminal justice system," adding that they usually begin molesting as teenagers and continue throughout their lives as long as they are physically able (2001).

Boys may be more reluctant to report being sexually abused because of embarrassment and the stigma associated with "homosexual" activities. They may feel guilty and ashamed because they were aroused by the contact or think of themselves as having been willing participants. The pedophiles may give them normally off-limit items such as cigarettes, alcohol, drugs, or pornography, telling the boys that they could get into trouble if they report the molestation because people will find the items. In some instances, the grooming and seduction of victims is so complete that it wears down their inhibitions and creates a strong bond and loyalty between the victim and the offender. Some molested children may not consider themselves victims. For these and other reasons, the sexual molestation of boys tends to be underreported, which allows the offenders to continue molesting other children without being discovered.

A prime example involves an Australian man named Clarence Osborne. He recorded in great detail sexual contacts with more than 2500 boys. Osborne lived in a middle-class suburb of Brisbane, Australia, and was a court recorder who worked with juvenile offenders. His life started to unravel when the state police began investigating a child pornography complaint. In 1979, at the age of 61, Osborne committed suicide.

Only after his death did police realize the magnitude of Osborne's criminal activity. In his house, they found names, photographs, tape recordings, and written documentation by Osborne describing more than 20 years of sexual encounters with teenage boys. Osborne was obsessive about his records, and everything was recorded in great detail. He had hidden recorders in his house and car so that he could record conversations and sexual activities. Some of his victims were later interviewed and confirmed the incidents that Osborne had documented. Osborne met his victims in many different environments. Some of the boys were neighbors, some were picked up while hitchhiking, and others were picked up at local parks and shopping centers. His victims came from all parts of the community, and many of his victims were from wealthy, prominent families (Wilson, 1981).

Osborne is usually referred to as a pedophile though he was probably more of an *ephebophile* (ie, a person who is attracted to adolescent children). Regardless, he molested more than 2500 boys, and not a single child ever reported him to the police. It is difficult to understand how anyone could molest so many children and go undetected for so long, but Osborne is not the only example. Many other men have molested numerous children and have never been discovered.

THE PEDOPHILE POPULATION
To study pedophiles, pedophiles who are willing to be studied must be located. This is difficult because pedophiles tend to live a secretive lifestyle.

Some pedophiles have never molested a child. Some may be married, have a family, and have a successful business or career and simply fear the consequences of acting out their secret desires. The fear of getting caught and losing everything is strong enough to keep some from acting out sexually. Some pedophiles may struggle throughout their lives to suppress their sexual urges. They may have strong religious convictions that directly conflict with their sexual desires, or they may have moral convictions that are stronger than their sexual inclinations. As explained later in the chapter, some men with deep moral or religious convictions are not able to suppress their desires, but it is likely that others have done so.

Some pedophiles may seek out sexual partners who look young but are of legal age. They may prefer younger children but settle for substitutes. Other pedophiles live a life of fantasy and masturbation. They may collect child erotica or pornography and work with or associate with children in a nonsexual way but have never had sexual contact with the children.

Other pedophiles act out sexually with children but never get caught or exposed. They may molest a few children or hundreds, but their crimes are never disclosed, so they are never held accountable for their actions. Most sex crimes go undetected. According to Abel, sex offenders only have a 3% chance of being caught (Abel et al, 1987).

Some pedophiles are discovered but not reported to law enforcement officials for various reasons. Many child molestation issues are handled informally within families, neighborhoods, and organizations. The police are never notified, and the incidents are never officially documented. Pedophiles have been allowed to resign from positions and permitted or forced to move from one community to another in return for not being reported to the authorities. Some of the current scandal in the US Roman Catholic Church involves allegations that pedophile priests were transferred from parish to parish and never reported to law enforcement officials. This problem is not unique to the Catholic church. Many other religious denominations, schools, and organizations have been accused of covering up pedophiliac behavior and essentially moving the problem elsewhere.

Other pedophiles are reported to the police but are not prosecuted. Many legitimate reasons can make it impossible to prosecute a case, including lack of corroborating physical evidence, uncooperative victims or witnesses, and a statute of limitation expiration. Previously available evidence may have become unobtainable, or the offender, victims, or witnesses may have moved from the area, all of which could hamper efforts to prosecute the offender. Pedophiles may be arrested but never convicted of any crime.

Another group of pedophiles are exposed, arrested, and prosecuted. Regardless, even after being prosecuted, a convicted pedophile may not serve time in prison. Some pedophiles receive probation, and others may receive some form of "shock time" (ie, a short sentence, usually 90-120 days, to let the offender experience incarceration).

RESEARCH METHODS

This study focuses on incarcerated pedophiles. Incarcerated pedophiles do not necessarily represent all pedophiles. They were caught and imprisoned, so they are different from pedophiles who have never molested and may be different from those who have never been caught. Still, much information can be learned from them.

All of the men studied in this research project were in prison because they had been convicted of molestation crimes involving children. Though they were studied in Missouri prisons, these offenders are certainly not unique to a particular state. The men who were interviewed for this study had molested children throughout the United States. Some of the men had served prison sentences in other states, including California, Florida, Texas, Illinois, Maryland, South Carolina, Kansas, Indiana, and Oklahoma.

Data developed in this research study have been derived from 2 distinct groups: The interview group consisted of 23 offenders and the archival file review group consisted of 25 offenders.

The offenders were identified as *potential* candidates for this study if they met the following selection criteria:

1. The offender is an adult male, having been convicted and imprisoned in the state of Missouri for a child molestation offense.

2. The conviction involved an underage male victim, who was likely prepubescent.

3. Some other factor indicates the offender is a preferential child molester rather than a situational child molester (eg, the offender had multiple or previous victims).

Prepubescence is not based solely on age. Children develop and reach puberty at different ages. One boy may be prepubescent at age 14, whereas another boy may have already reached puberty by age 11. Therefore, general assumptions have been made about whether victims were prepubescent. This study involved offenders whose victims were age 14 and younger.

Offenders who met the criteria were contacted and asked if they would be willing to participate in this research study. The offenders were told that the interviews would be for research and training purposes. They were promised confidentiality in return for their cooperation; specifically, they were told that they would not be identified by their name in any written or oral form. Numerous offenders refused to participate but ultimately, 23 men agreed to be interviewed; they became the interview group. Each man signed a waiver form indicating that he understood the guidelines and was willing to participate in the study.

The interviews took place over 6 months at 5 different Missouri prisons. An interview questionnaire was developed specifically for this project, so each offender was asked the same set of 66 basic questions. The questions covered a wide range of topics. Initial questions asked about the offender's childhood, family and caretakers, siblings, birth order, history of childhood abuse, history of domestic violence, history of family drug and alcohol abuse, and education. Questions addressed the offender's education, work history, organized youth affiliations, adult relationships, marriage, children, personal habits, and arrest history. Of course, much of the questionnaire was devoted to the offenders' sexual history, including their views concerning their own sexuality; their first awareness of their pedophilia; their first experience as a perpetrator; victim preferences; victim selection, grooming, and seduction; sexual acts preferred; the use of aids such as pornography, alcohol, and drugs; the use of computers; and an estimated number of victims. The final section addressed their discovery, arrests, and prosecutions; experiences with law enforcement, interviews, and admissions of guilt (or, in many cases, denials of guilt); criminal convictions; and finally, opinions regarding their own treatment and rehabilitation. Though the interviews began with the same 66 initial questions, they were not limited or restricted to those questions. Answers to certain questions often segued into additional questions not on the questionnaire.

The second group studied was the archival file review group, which consisted of 25 offenders. They were selected based on the same criteria as the interview group but were not interviewed. Instead, the prison files of each of the offenders were reviewed. The prison files usually consisted of police reports, criminal record checks, court records, presentence investigation reports, and the Hare Psychopathy Checklist (PCL) questionnaire (Hart et al, 1995). The PCL questionnaire screens offenders before they are placed in sex offender treatment programs. The PCL interviews are conducted by social workers who are staff members at the Missouri Sex Offender Treatment Program. Though not identical, many of the questions asked on the PCL questionnaire are the same basic questions asked on the interview group questionnaire.

A second questionnaire was developed for the archival file review group. This questionnaire was a shorter version of the interview group questionnaire and eliminated questions that could not be answered through a file study. The object of the file study was to review the entire file and answer as many of the questions that could be addressed based on the information documented in the prison files.

Most of the offenders in the interview group and all of the offenders in the archival group had been screened for placement in a sex offender treatment program. Those who had been screened usually had a written diagnostic impression in their prison files that had been submitted by a licensed therapist. A diagnostic impression might read as follows: "Axis I 302.2 Pedophilia, sexually attracted to males, exclusive type" (the number is one found in the DSM-IV-TR). This documentation served as additional confirmation that the offenders being studied were pedophiles.

FINDINGS

Both groups of pedophiles were diverse in terms of age, education, occupation, appearance, and life experiences. Though similarities were found among many of these offenders, no one profile or description characterized all of them. The following sections contain some of the observations and findings from this study.

Age and Race

The 23 men in the interview group ranged in age from 20 to 69 at the time of their interviews, with the average age being 44. The archival group had a similar range: ages 23 to 67 at the time their files were studied.

Twenty of the men (87%) in the interview group were white and 3 (13%) were African-American. Twenty-four men (96%) in the archival group were white and 1 (4%) was African-American.

Criminal Convictions and History

The men in the interview group had been in prison an average of 7 years at the time of their interviews. The 23 offenders were serving prison sentences for the molestation of a total of 40 victims, with sentences ranging from 5 years to life in prison. Thirteen (57%) of the men had been convicted of molesting a single victim, whereas 10 (43%) had been convicted of molesting 2 or more victims.

Men in the archival group were serving prison sentences for the molestation of 36 total victims, with sentences ranging from 3 to 28 years. Eighteen (72%) of the men had been convicted of molesting a single child, whereas 7 (28%) had been convicted of molesting 2 or more victims.

Twelve (52%) of the men in the interview group had been previously convicted of sex crimes involving children. Of the 11 men that had not been convicted of sex crimes, 5 (22%) had no arrest record before their first offense, and 6 (26%) had arrest records for crimes other than sex offenses.

At least 12 (48%) of the 25 men in the archival group had been previously convicted of sex crimes involving children. Five men (20%) had no arrest record, 4 (16%) had arrest records for crimes other than sex offenses, and 4 men had unknown arrest records.

Offender Childhood and Background

Of the 23 men in the interview group, 13 (57%) were the products of broken homes (ie, both biological parents were not present), whereas 10 (43%) grew up in families with both biological parents. The offenders had various numbers of siblings ranging from none to 11. Four men were the oldest children in their families, 9 were middle children, 6 were the youngest children, and 1 was an only child. Sibling and birth order information was not recorded on the remaining 3 men.

Thirteen (57%) of the men in the interview group reported that they had experienced physical abuse or emotional neglect in their families while growing up, and 9 (39%) reported having had an alcoholic parent. Seven (30%) reported that they had a personal history of drug abuse, alcohol abuse, or both.

Eight men (32%) in the archival group reported experiencing physical abuse or neglect in their families while growing up, 7 (28%) reported having had an alcoholic parent, and 8 (32%) reported having a personal history of drug abuse, alcohol abuse, or both. Several men in the archival group did not make any disclosures on these issues.

Childhood Sexual Abuse

Many child molesters were molested as children. However, a wide disparity in the actual proportions exists among studies. Studies show that the percentages of child molesters who were molested as children range from 22% to 82% (Knopp, 1984). A later study of child molesters shows that 47% had been sexually abused as children (Abel & Harlow, 2001).

In the interview group, 18 (78%) of the 23 men reported that they had been sexually molested as children. Three (13%) others reported that they had not been molested though they had been involved in sex play with male peers before reaching puberty. Only 2 (9%) of the men reported no history of sexual abuse or sex play with peers in their childhood. One of these 2 men said that his childhood was completely non-sexual, adding that he did not even discover masturbation until he was in college.

Results regarding childhood sexual abuse were similar in the archival group. Information in the files revealed that 20 (75%) of the 25 men had reported being molested as children. Two (8%) said that they had never been molested, and the remaining 3 did not know (**Figure 30-1**).

Of the 18 men in the interview group who had been molested, many reported quite extensive sexual abuse. Some of the men had been violently sodomized, molested over long periods of time, or molested by multiple perpetrators. It was determined that 7 (30%) had been molested by older children (who were unrelated), 4 (17%) by older siblings, 4 (17%) by older cousins, 2 (9%) by a stepfather, 6 (26%) by other adult acquaintances, and 4 (17%) by complete strangers. One man said that he had been molested at age 10 but refused to disclose who had molested him. Some of the men reported being molested by several different people. For example, one man reported that over the course of several years, he had been molested by 4 people: his stepfather, an older brother, an older cousin, and the boyfriend of an aunt.

Of the 20 men in the archival group who reported being molested, 7 (28%) had been molested by older children (who were unrelated), 3 (12%) by older siblings, 8 (32%) by other relatives (cousins and uncles), 1 (4%) by a stepfather, 2 (8%) by biological fathers, 7 (28%) by other adult acquaintances, and 1 (4%) by a complete stranger.

Though the sampling is too small to be statistically significant, it was interesting to find a correlation between the age at which the perpetrators were molested and the age of their victims. Five pedophiles in the archival group molested young boys ages 2 to 5; all 5 of the pedophiles were molested at a young age (4 to 5 years old).

Being sexually molested as a child does not cause pedophilia. Most sexually abused children do not grow up to become pedophiles, and many pedophiles were never sexually abused as children. Most of the previous theories regarding the cause of pedophilia have attributed it to single factors, and they have proven to be inadequate. Research suggests that the cause of pedophilia is complicated and involves an integration of multiple factors (Finkelhor & Araji, 1986). For example, a person who was molested as a child may have the potential to become a pedophile depending on the presence or absence of other moderating factors. Common characteristics among pedophiles include social competence deficits such as inadequate social and interpersonal skills, lack of assertiveness, and low self-esteem (Prentky et al, 1997). Other common traits include lack of impulse control, obsessive-compulsive tendencies, lack of empathy toward children, depression, and poor family relationships (Lowenstein, 2001).

Figure 30-1. Comparison of offenders in interview and archival groups as related to their own molestation as a child.

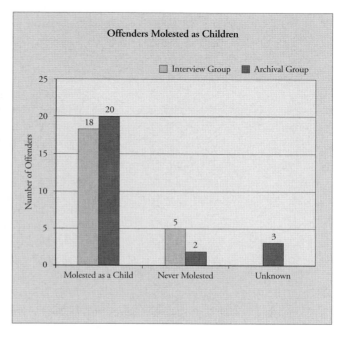

Though this particular study did not involve specific questions used to identify each of the mentioned traits, some of the offenders did mention that they had difficulty relating to adults. One man stated that he was "intimidated by adults" and was much more comfortable in the presence of children. This theme seemed fairly common though some did not have any difficulties with adults. Five men disclosed a history of severe depression, and others spoke of loneliness and frustration.

Marriage and Adult Relationships

Fourteen (61%) men in the interview group had been married at least once in their lifetime. Three of the men had been married twice, and 1 had been married 3 times. Only 1 offender was still married though 5 of the men had been in marriages that lasted 10 years or longer. Nine offenders (39%) had never married. The marriage numbers were similar in the archival group. Twelve (48%) of the men had been married (and at least 3 had been married twice), 8 (32%) had not been married, and the marital history of 5 offenders was unknown. At least 14 (29%) of the 48 men in both of the groups combined reported having fathered children of their own.

Many pedophiles are referred to as either homosexual or heterosexual pedophiles based on their preferred targets. Regardless, more than half of 48 pedophiles preferred boys but had been married to women and most of the men did not consider themselves to be homosexual. When offenders in the interview group were asked about their own sexual orientation, 9 (39%) were heterosexual, 6 (26%) were homosexual, 5 (22%) were bisexual, and 3 (13%) did not respond. Seven men reported having pedophile tendencies. It appears that some of the men were sexually attracted to prepubescent boys but simultaneously were attracted to and maintained sexual relationships with adult women.

In the study by Abel & Harlow (2001) of 1038 men who had molested boys, 70% described themselves as exclusively or predominantly heterosexual in their adult sexual preferences. Only 8% of the men reported that they were exclusively homosexual.

Offenders in the interview group were asked if they had ever had sexual relationships with other adults, whether male or female. Twenty (87%) of the 23 indicated that they had, 2 (9%) stated that they had not, and 1 (4%) stated that he had not had an adult sexual relationship before going to prison.

Education, Employment, and Volunteer Affiliations

No significant findings regarding education were found. Ten (43%) of the 23 men in the interview group had only a high school diploma or an equivalent, whereas 13 (57%) had at least a partial college education. Six men (26%) had a college degree, and 3 (13%) had a master's degree.

The interview group had a wide range of occupations. Six (26%) of the 23 men had previously been employed in occupations that gave them access to children: 2 as high school teachers, 1 as a sixth-grade school teacher and youth pastor, 1 as a school bus driver, 1 as a childcare worker at a children's home, and 1 as a manager of a youth sports club. The remaining 17 (74%) were not employed in occupations that involved children.

In the archival group, fewer men (3 of 25, or 12%) had been employed in settings that gave them access to children: 1 as a sixth-grade school teacher, 1 as an elementary school librarian, and 1 as a youth pastor. Employment information was unknown for 2 men in the group. The remaining 20 men (75%) reported having had a wide range of occupations that did not involve children.

Nine (39%) of the men in the interview group reported having volunteer affiliations with youth groups or organizations such as the Boy Scouts, Big Brothers Big Sisters, the YMCA, church youth groups, or youth sports clubs. Five of the 9 men did not have occupations that involved children, but 11 (48%) had access to children through their occupations, volunteer work, or both.

First Experiences as a Perpetrator

Each man in the interview group was asked about his age during his first experience as a perpetrator, which was defined as a sexual experience in which he was "significantly older" than the victim. Thirteen (57%) of the 23 reported that they were in their teens, 4 (17%) were in their 20s, 2 (9%) were in their 30s, 2 (9%) were in their 40s, and 1 man (4%) was in his 50s.

In the archival group, 9 men (36%) were unsure of when their first experience occurred. Thirteen (52%) indicated that their first experience as a perpetrator occurred during their teen years. One man (4%) reported that it was during his 20s, 1 (4%) during his 30s, and 1 (4%) during his 40s. These results are summarized in **Figure 30-2**.

Victim Preferences

Men in the interview group were asked questions about their victim preferences. Most of the men had a clear preference for certain age groups. The preferences varied but included children ages 7 to 9, ages 8 to 12, ages 9 to 12, ages 11 to 13, and ages 11 to 14. The man who preferred boys ages 7 to 9 explained that "after 9, they start losing their cuteness."

All of the white men in the interview group stated that they had a preference for white boys, and one of the African-American men preferred white boys. All 3 African-Americans in the interview group had molested white victims at some point. Only 1 white man reported having any nonwhite victims. He said that most of his victims were white though he had molested "a couple of blacks and one mulatto."

At least 6 men in the interview group specifically used the word "attractive" when describing appearances they preferred. Preferred physical features included being tall and thin, having a smooth face, being clean cut and neat, having no body hair, having a high voice, and having fair skin. Pedophiles are attracted to children who have not reached puberty, which explains why they prefer boys without pubic hair and who have high voices.

Men in the interview group were asked about characteristics or personality traits that they were attracted to or looked for in a boy. The most common response was that they sought out boys who were lonely, needy, vulnerable, seeking attention, or looking for a friend. Other specific adjectives used by the offenders to describe potential victims included passive, quiet, naïve, loving, weak, innocent, poor, neglected and with low self-esteem. Only 2 men stated that they were attracted to boys who were popular and confident and had high self-esteem.

The men in the interview group were asked about traits or characteristics that might cause them to avoid molesting a particular child. Some men mentioned physical char-

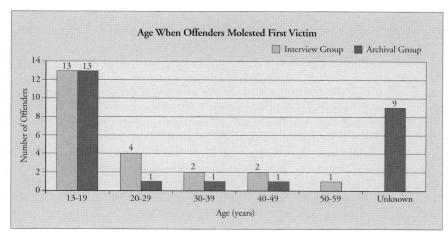

Figure 30-2. *Comparison of offenders in interview and archival groups as related to when they molested their first victim.*

acteristics such as obesity, but the most common response was that they would not choose children who had actively involved parents. The offenders did not want to approach children who communicated well with their parents, and most tended to avoid selecting children with confidence, good self-esteem, an outgoing personality, and a lack of interest in sex talk. In one area of victim selection, a definite difference in preference was found. Some men avoided children who had a "bad" attitude, were rebellious, or were sarcastic, whereas other men considered these types of children to be easy targets.

All 23 of the men in the interview group stated that they had molested boys they knew and with whom they had some type of relationship. Only 2 (9%) of the men reported that they had had sexual encounters with boys who were complete strangers.

Men in the interview group were asked how they first met their victims. Eight men (35%) reported meeting victims through friends, 8 (35%) met victims through organizations such as church and school, 8 (35%) met victims in their neighborhood, 7 (30%) had victims who were relatives, 5 (22%) had victims who were the children of girlfriends, and 3 (13%) molested children they were babysitting. The 2 men who reported molesting complete strangers stated that they had met the victims in malls, in parks, or on city streets.

Similarly, Abel & Harlow (2001) found that 68% of molesters sexually abuse children in their own families, including their own children, grandchildren, nieces, and nephews. He found that 40% molest children in their social circle, and only 10% molest children they do not know.

Victim Grooming and Seduction

Most pedophiles engage in a seduction, or grooming process, that can last for months or years before any sexual abuse occurs. The offender cultivates a relationship with the child and gains trust. The grooming may include special attention, affection, favors, money, and gifts. The offender and child may share intimate or personal secrets or have sexual conversations that the offender disguises as educational. A pedophile can assess a child's vulnerabilities and weaknesses. He knows how to take advantage of a child's natural curiosity about sex and then lower inhibitions.

Often the grooming process involves borderline, or "accidental," touching to assess the child's reaction. The process of moving from normal physical touching to overt sexual acts can be gradual. It can be so subtle that the child may not even realize what is happening. The grooming process may include rationalizations and assurances that the sexual activities are natural and acceptable. Pedophiles who molest boys minimize the homosexual aspect of their activities, making them seem like experimentation and play. They may reassure the boys that performing the sexual acts does not mean they (the boys or the offenders) are homosexuals.

Only 2 men (9%) in the interview group and 2 men (8%) in the archival group reported using force to molest a child. Most pedophile offenders clearly prefer using the grooming and seduction process. Fifteen (65%) of the men in the interview group said that they groomed their victims before molesting them. Eight men (35%) did not consider their behavior to be grooming. Regardless, review of the responses seems to indicate that all the offenders were somehow involved in grooming behaviors. The 15 men who acknowledged grooming their victims described the process, which included spending time with the child, becoming the child's friend, gaining the child's trust, isolating the child, going places with the child, buying the child gifts, providing false praise to the child, and making the child feel special and unique. Some of the men stated that their grooming behavior included talks about sexuality and feelings. Several stated that they talked about sex and masturbation but disguised it as sex education. Some of the men in the interview group said that as part of the grooming process, they allowed children to engage in "forbidden" activities, such as smoking, drinking, or viewing pornography.

The length of the grooming process ranged from a few minutes to a few years, but most of the men reported grooming children for weeks or months before molesting them. Two of the men reported that they had each groomed a boy for 3 or more years before molesting the child.

Men in the interview group were asked how they determined whether a child might be receptive to sexual advances. Eight (35%) of the men said that they first used non-sexual touches such as hugs, back rubs, or tickling to determine how the boys reacted to being touched. Four men (17%) said that they playfully wrestled with the boys and at some point touched the children's groin while wrestling. If a particular boy had a negative reaction, it was easy for the man to claim it was accidental. Three men (13%) said that they determined whether a child might be receptive through sexual conversations. Most of the men observed their victims carefully by paying attention to body language and gauging their reactions to touch and conversation, they determined if it was safe to proceed or if they should retreat.

Seven (30%) of the men in the interview group mentioned that they had misjudged boys, assuming that the children were receptive to their sexual advances when they were not. All 7 men said that when they realized their mistake, they quickly stopped. Some made excuses or claimed it was an accident and others apologized, but they all changed what they were doing once they determined that a boy was not interested.

Men in the interview group were asked if they had used any aids to lower the inhibitions of potential victims. Fourteen (61%) said that they had, 8 (35%) said that they had not, and 1 man did not respond to the question. Eight men (35%) said that they had used pornographic photographs or magazines, 7 (30%) used pornographic movies, 6 (26%) provided victims with alcohol, 1 (4%) gave his victims cigarettes, and 2 men (9%) mentioned using sex education material that was not pornographic.

Miscellaneous Findings

Although it was mentioned previously that 12 (52%) of the 23 men in the interview group had been previously convicted of sex crimes involving children, others had been discovered but not prosecuted. Eight men (35%) in the interview group reported that their sexual abuse of a child had been discovered in the past, but the crimes were not reported to the authorities or the men were not prosecuted for various reasons. Five of the men said they were told they would not be prosecuted or reported if they began therapy (or, in one man's case, remain in therapy). One man said that he was forced to resign from his job as a youth pastor and move out of the state in exchange for not being reported to the authorities. One man said that his wife discovered him sexually abusing a child, but she did not report him because she depended on his income.

Men in the interview group were asked if they had ever associated with other pedophiles or pedophile organizations or ever used the Internet to meet victims, meet other pedophiles, or collect child pornography. The overwhelming majority—21 (91%)—said that they had not. Only 1 man (4%) reported that he had used the Internet, stating that he had communicated with other pedophiles while searching for child pornography sites. He had downloaded thousands of pornographic images of children. One man did not answer the question.

Only 1 man in the interview group reported using the computer for pedophila purposes. Eight men (32%) said that they had owned a computer but did not have Internet access, and 13 (52%) of the men said that they had never owned a computer. Initially, these numbers seem surprising, but it could be related to many of the men having been in prison since the early to mid 1990s, which is before Internet use became widely popular. It is likely that sex offenders entering prison today are much more knowledgeable about computers and the Internet than those in this study.

Men in the interview group were asked if they had ever taken nude or sexually explicit photographs or video of their victims. Nineteen (83%) said that they had not, and only 3 men (13%) stated that they had. The numerous unknowns in the archival group made it impossible to draw any conclusions, though 4 (16%) of the men were known to have taken sexual photographs, videos, or both of children.

Including prior convictions, the 23 men in the interview group had been convicted of molesting a total of 51 children. When asked to estimate the total number of children they had molested in their lifetime, the men had molested between 282 and 319 children among them. In other words, they averaged about 13 victims each and were only convicted of molesting approximately 1 of every 6 victims.

In the archival group, the 25 men had been convicted of molesting a total of 49 children. Because the archival group was a file study, it was harder to determine the number of children molested in their lifetime. However, 7 men in the group admitted they had molested a total of 77 children but had only been convicted of molesting 15.

Men in the interview group were asked questions about their experiences with the police and the entire criminal justice system. Sixteen men (70%) reported that when they were arrested and interviewed by the police, they confessed. Seven men (30%) said that they did not confess. Additional questioning revealed that 8 (50%) of the 16 men who claimed to have confessed withheld significant information when questioned by the police. Six of these men said that they did not disclose additional victims and details, 1 did not disclose a collection of child pornography that was never found by the police, and 1 did not disclose accurate details concerning the molestation.

The 16 men who said they had confessed were asked what had led them to confess. Two men were relieved they had been apprehended, 2 men knew it was over and gave up, 2 men did not want their victims to have to testify, 2 men were afraid, 2 men had been given false promises by the police, 1 man felt guilty, and 1 man wanted to get help.

Those who did not confess were asked the reason. Two of them said that they did not cooperate because the police had treated them poorly, 2 others felt that they had not been asked the right questions, and 2 men refused to confess because of embarrassment and humiliation.

Though many of the offenders seemed to be predatory and have little concern for their victims, some of the men explained that they loved and cared deeply for their victims. Two men considered their relationships to be long-term love affairs and their victims to be lovers. They justified their victim's ages (10 and 11), suggesting that the boys were different than others of the same age and were mature enough to make the right choices. Both men said that the boys were willing participants, and they often initiated the sexual activity. The offenders seemed to believe what they were saying. Both of the men confessed to the police and later pled guilty so that their victims would not have to testify.

Several of the men minimized their behavior and blamed others for their actions. One man, who had been convicted of molesting 4 children, claimed that his victims had initiated the sexual activity. He suggested that the boys had become sexually active with one another and had initiated him into their group. His victims were 6 to 10 years old when the abuse started. Another man complained about the length of his prison sentence and blamed it on "election-year politics." He also stated, "All I did was have consensual oral sex with two boys." His victims were 8 and 9 years old. Several other men blamed drugs and alcohol for their behavior, suggesting that the molestations happened because they were under the influence of a particular substance.

Most of the men in the interview group considered themselves to be pedophiles and were realistic about their need for therapy though 5 men claimed they were not pedophiles. One of these men claimed that he was not even a sex offender and did not need therapy despite being convicted twice of molesting children.

The men who recognized a need for therapy believed that they could learn to manage their impulses and behavior through treatment. No one felt that they could be "cured," but most believed that they could be treated or rehabilitated. One man said that it would be difficult for him to change because his behaviors had been "ingrained since early childhood." Another man stated, "30 years of having sex with boys—you're not going to cure that in a couple of months."

CONCLUSION

The 48 offenders who were studied for this project do not necessarily represent all pedophiles in society. These pedophiles were arrested and sent to prison, which puts them in a small subgroup of all pedophiles. Several other studies of pedophiles have been done that were not carried out in correctional or clinical settings. An article, published in 1999, documented a study of 41 admitted pedophiles who had been identified in a "boy-love" computer forum discussion group (Durkin & Bryant). However, most of the existing knowledge of pedophilia comes from individuals who have been caught and successfully prosecuted.

The 23 men in the interview group cooperated without any compensation or reward. Many of these men disclosed information that they had never told anyone. As stated previously, a few men denied that they were pedophiles, withheld details, minimized their conduct, and blamed others for their problems, but overall, the men were very cooperative volunteers.

The hope is that information obtained in this study can benefit professionals who perform child sexual abuse investigations. It will help them recognize and identify specific traits sought out by pedophiles. They will better understand the grooming and seduction process, recognizing the significance of "accidental" touches often used by perpetrators. They will understand how perpetrators can lower the inhibitions of children to encourage them to participate in the abuse. They will understand how a long grooming process can result in a victim-offender bond, making a victim reluctant to disclose anything that would harm the offender.

Information obtained in this study can assist law enforcement officials who interview perpetrators. A key to interviewing sex offenders is having a basic understanding of their thought processes. An investigator needs to be able to empathize with the person being interviewed and recognize the importance of certain disclosures. For example, a suspect may disclose a personal history of childhood sexual abuse. This type of revelation should prompt the interviewer to address related issues, such as how that sexual abuse affected the suspect's own sexual development and orientation. Many offenders admit that their own victimization resulted in confusion and sexual experimentation during their teenage years. This line of questioning may help an offender feel more comfortable admitting to any crimes that he has committed.

The section of the study regarding police contacts, interviews, and confessions should be of particular interest to investigators. The pedophiles' reasons for confessing, or in some cases, not confessing, can be useful when developing interview strategies. Investigators can learn from the previous mistakes of other investigators and should use interview techniques that have worked in the past. A nonintimidating, counselor-style interview can be very effective with pedophiles.

Police officers often assume molestation cases involve just one victim. This study has shown that few offenders have only molested once. Most pedophiles have a long molestation history that dates back to their own childhood. A good investigator can reveal many other crimes by being thorough during the interview process and not quickly accepting a suspect's assertions that only one victim was involved.

Offenders in this study revealed a great deal that can be used for education and prevention purposes. Many people believe that child molesters are strangers—men in raincoats, prowling the playgrounds and offering candy to unsuspecting children. The reality is that most child molesters are friends, relatives, neighbors, and acquaintances. They are the people who parents trust with their children: teachers, coaches, youth ministers, and family members.

Material from this study can be used to educate parents about characteristics targeted by pedophiles, the reasons they focus on certain children, and how they groom and eventually seduce their victims. A parent who understands the grooming process may recognize possible danger signs, such as when an adult begins showing an excessive interest in one of their children by spending inordinate amounts of time with the child, buying gifts for the child, or frequently offering to babysit or go on camping or overnight trips with the child.

One of the most interesting and helpful things parents can learn from this study is the power of the word "no." Few of the men interviewed in this study ever used force to molest their victims. They seduced their victims and, from their own perspective, committed only those acts that the victims allowed them to commit. Generally, the men said that they stopped pursuing a child if they thought that the child would resist them in any way. Many pedophiles stated that "no" was enough to cause them to stop what they were doing, apologize, make excuses, or claim that what happened was an accident. Several offenders said that there had been times when they had misjudged a potential victim, and upon being told "no," the offenders stopped and did not make any additional attempts to molest the child.

Another piece of information learned in this study is worth repeating: Pedophiles tend to avoid children with actively involved parents. Children who communicate well with their parents are not attractive targets for pedophiles. Parents need to have frank discussions with their children about sexual abuse and inappropriate touching. Children need to be told that when any person does anything inappropriate, they are to tell them "no, stop, leave me alone" and immediately tell a parent or other adult. Being incapable of telling an adult "no" does not necessarily make a child a willing or receptive victim.

Additional studies can continue to provide valuable insights into the minds of pedophile offenders. For example, studies of female-target and mixed-target pedophiles would be helpful. In addition, it would be helpful to study the way computer use among pedophiles has changed in the last decade. Additional studies about the minds of pedophiles will better help law enforcement officials, investigators, and parents understand and therefore prevent this form of sexual abuse.

REFERENCES

Abel GG, Becker JV, Mittelman MS, Cunningham-Rathner J, Rouleau JL, Murphy WD. Self-reported sex crimes of nonincarcerated paraphiliacs. *J Interpers Violence.* 1987;2(1):3-25.

Abel GG, Harlow N. *The Stop Child Molestation Book.* Philadelphia, Pa: Xlibris Corp; 2001.

American Psychiatric Association. *Diagnostic and Statistical Manual of Mental Disorders.* 4th ed. Text revision. Washington, DC: American Psychiatric Association; 2000.

Durkin KF, Bryant CD. Propagandizing pederasty: a thematic analysis of the on-line exculpatory accounts of unrepentant pedophiles. *Deviant Behav.* 1999;20(2):103-127.

End Child Prostitution, Child Pornography, and Trafficking of Children for Sexual Purposes (ECPAT) International. Europe and North America regional profile.

Regional report prepared for: the World Congress Against Commercial Sexual Exploitation of Children; August 1996, Stockholm, Sweden.

Finkelhor D, Araji S. Explanation of pedophilia: a four factor model. *J Sex Res.* 1986; 22(2):145-161.

Haggarty J. Material presented at: Prostitution and Related Offenses Workshop; October 15, 1997; Washington, DC.

Hart SD, Cox DN, Hare RD. *The Hare PCL: Screening Version Interview and Information Schedule.* North Tonawanda, NY: Multi-Health Systems Inc; 1995.

Knopp FH. *Retraining Adult Sex Offenders: Methods and Models.* Orwell, Vt: Safer Society Press; 1984.

Lanning KV. *Child Molesters: A Behavioral Analysis.* 4th ed. Alexandria, Va: National Center for Missing & Exploited Children; 2001.

Lowenstein LF. The identification and diagnosis of alleged victims and alleged pedophiles (what to do and what to avoid doing.) *Police J.* 2001;74(3):237-250.

Prentky RA, Knight RA, Lee AF. *Child Sexual Molestation: Research Issues.* Washington, DC: National Institute of Justice; 1997.

Saikaew L. *The Report on Child Prostitution as a Form of Forced Labor: A Non-Governmental Organization Perspective.* Washington, DC: Bureau of International Labor Affairs; 2001.

Wilson P. *The Man They Called A Monster.* New South Wales, Australia: Cassell Australia Limited; 1981.

Chapter 31

HUMAN TRAFFICKING FOR SEXUAL EXPLOITATION: THE ROLE OF INTERPOL

Sharon W. Cooper, MD, FAAP*

The first International Criminal Police Congress was held in Monaco in 1914. Legal experts and police officers from 14 countries gathered together to study the possibility of establishing an international criminal record office and coordinating extradition procedures. The outbreak of World War I halted progress until 1923, when the second International Criminal Police Congress met in Vienna, Austria, and set up the International Criminal Police Commission (ICPC), establishing its headquarters in Vienna. The ICPC, which was essentially a European organization, operated successfully until World War II.

In 1946, a conference was held in Brussels, Belgium, to revive the ICPC. New statutes were adopted, the commission's headquarters was moved to France, and "INTERPOL" was chosen as the telegraphic address of the headquarters. Interpol, a contraction of "international police," is the current name of what was formerly called the ICPC. In the year 2004, it had 182 member states.

The principles and procedures governing police cooperation in Interpol have been established over the years. According to Article 2 of the organization's constitution, Interpol's aims are as follows:

(1) To ensure and promote the widest possible mutual assistance between all criminal police authorities within the limits of the laws existing in the different countries and in the spirit of the 'Universal Declaration of Human Rights';

(2) To establish and develop all institutions likely to contribute effectively to the prevention and suppression of ordinary law crimes (ICPO-Interpol Constitution and General Regulations, 2004).

According to Article 3 of its constitution, Interpol is forbidden to be involved in "any intervention or activities of a political, militaristic, religious or racial character" (ICPO-Interpol Constitution and General Regulations, 2004).

HUMAN TRAFFICKING

The role of Interpol in the international community is of an educator and facilitator of crime investigations. Interpol is an international source of perhaps the most comprehensive array of information about child sexual exploitation, especially of crimes against children, trafficking of women, and human smuggling. As a gatekeeper of controlled information for the law enforcement agencies of its 182 member countries, Interpol plays a crucial role in the struggle against exploitation.

For example, Interpol provides a complete list of international legislation regarding missing children, important information in human trafficking situations. If a child

---

* A significant portion of this text was contributed by Hamish McCulloch, Assistant Director, Trafficking in Human Beings Sub-Directorate of the International Criminal Police Organization (ICPO)-Interpol

were taken from one country to another to be sexually exploited, the child's home country would need assistance with performing an investigation in another country and managing the complex legal maneuvers needed to extradite the offenders and rescue the child. Interpol provides missing children posters to help investigators identify victims. In addition, Interpol maintains a Web site of legislation information (http://www.interpol.int/Public/Children/missing/NationalLaws/mcFirst Page.asp). Information regarding commonly used trafficking routes for the smuggling of people, drugs, and other contraband is available through the Web site.

Interpol makes a clear distinction between the smuggling of migrants and trafficking of people. According to Interpol, the smuggling of migrants "shall mean the procurement, in order to obtain, directly or indirectly, a financial or other material benefit, of the illegal entry of a person into a State Party of which the person is not a national or a permanent resident" (Children and human trafficking, 2004). In contrast, trafficking of persons

shall mean the recruitment, transportation, transfer, harboring or receipt of persons, by means of the threat or use of force or other forms of coercion, of abduction, of fraud, of deception, of the abuse of power or of a position of vulnerability or of the giving or receiving of payments or benefits to achieve the consent of a person having control over another person, for the purpose of exploitation. Exploitation shall include, at a minimum, the exploitation of the prostitution of others or other forms of sexual exploitation, forced labour of services, slavery, or practices similar to slavery, servitude or the removal of organs (Children and human trafficking, 2004).

INTERPOL STRUCTURE AND ADMINISTRATION

Interpol has 2 governing bodies that meet periodically: the General Assembly and the Executive Committee. The General Assembly is composed of delegates from member countries and has the most authority as a governing body. The Executive Committee is a much smaller group that verifies the execution of the various decisions of the General Assembly. The organization's General Secretariat, which comprises the secretary general and technical and administrative staff members, is headquartered in Lyon, France. The General Secretariat is responsible for implementing the decisions and recommendations adopted by the governing bodies, maintaining close contacts with the Interpol national central bureaus (NCBs) in the various member countries and for providing the framework for daily international police cooperation. Numerous Interpol subregional bureaus coordinate regional activity and are located in Harare, Zimbabwe; Abidjan, Ivory Coast; Nairobi, Kenya; and Buenos Aires, Argentina. In addition, a European liaison bureau is based within the General Secretariat. Interpol has created a number of expert working groups who specialize in various fields to establish best practices in criminology. These specialist groups provide training as well. The specialist group (the Interpol Specialist Group on Crimes Against Children) is coordinated by the Trafficking in Human Beings branch within the Criminal Intelligence Directorate of the General Secretariat.

NATIONAL CENTRAL BUREAUS

Experience has shown that the following 3 factors tend to hamper international cooperation among police agencies:

1. The varying structures of the different national law enforcement agencies often make it difficult for others outside their country to know which department has the power to handle a case or supply information.

2. Different languages in the various countries can be a barrier to communication.

3. Legal systems vary throughout the world, as do ages of consent.

To solve these problems, it was decided that the government of every Interpol member state should appoint 1 permanent police department to serve as its country's Interpol NCB and act as a contact point for international cooperation. Each country's

NCB is staffed solely by the country's own police officers or government officials, and they always operate within the limits set by that country's laws.

NCBs carry out numerous tasks, including the following:

— NCBs collect documents and criminal intelligence that have a direct bearing on international police cooperation from sources in their countries and pass this material to the other NCBs and the General Secretariat.

— NCBs transmit requests for international cooperation made by their country's courts or police departments to the NCBs of other countries.

— NCBs ensure that police action or operations requested by another country's NCB are carried out.

— NCBs receive requests for information, background checks, and other tasks from other NCBs and reply to such requests.

— The heads of NCBs attend the Interpol General Assembly sessions as members of their countries' delegation and subsequently ensure that the assembly's resolutions are implemented.

The NCBs communicate directly among themselves, however, they keep the General Secretariat informed of investigations so that the Secretariat can perform its task of centralizing information and coordinating cooperation.

INTERPOL TOOLS FOR THE PROTECTION OF CHILDREN

Numerous documents are published by Interpol to circulate information through the NCBs to the police forces of the member states. The documents are prepared by the notices group and often contain information collected from several countries. The various documents and information relevant to the Interpol Specialist Group on Crimes against Children include the following:

— Individual notices

— International yellow notices and the Interpol poster on missing children

— International green notices

— Computer systems

— Data entry, electronic archiving, and automatic consultation

INDIVIDUAL NOTICES

Individual notices provide specific information about a person who has committed a crime, who is missing, or whose body can not be identified. The notices include details about a person's identity and include a physical description and the individual's photographs and fingerprints if they are available. Five types of individual notices are issued:

— *Wanted*, or *red*. These are notices issued about people whose arrest is requested so they can be extradited. They contain full details of the arrest warrant and offenses committed.

— *Enquiry*, or *blue*. These notices are published to collect additional information about a particular person. For example, blue notices can help locate an offender who may not have a prior criminal record or who has not yet had an official arrest warrant issued.

— *Warning*, or *green*. These notices give information about professional offenders who operate in several countries. In the United States, this offender would be one who is possibly connected with organized crime or who is well known for criminal activity over a prolonged period of time in numerous international jurisdictions.

— *Missing persons*, or *yellow*. These notices are issued when a person, especially a child, is reported missing from his or her usual place of residence, and the person needs to be found.

— *Unidentified body*, or *black*. These notices contain a description of a body that has been discovered and includes the fingerprints if available.

In addition, the Children and Human Trafficking branch produces a periodic newsletter specifically intended for law enforcement officials. This newsletter includes information about current crime trends, international yellow notices, and the Interpol poster about missing children.

INTERNATIONAL YELLOW NOTICES AND THE INTERPOL POSTER ON MISSING CHILDREN

Locating missing children is a particularly important task of the General Secretariat. The yellow notices received by the NCBs are usually circulated to the police departments that handle disappearances and to departments in border regions.

Since 1994, Interpol has circulated the Interpol poster on missing children. These special posters have 12 photographs of children who have been missing for as long as five years or longer. Some children's photographs are age progressed to represent their likely current appearance. This type of poster is intended to be circulated and is not restricted to police departments. The posters are intended for the general public and can be displayed in railway stations or airports, published in the press, or even distributed to nongovernmental organizations (NGOs), which are known to help search for missing persons. The posters for missing children are published periodically. Their success in helping people find the children depends on 2 factors: (1) that the NCBs of Interpol member countries ensure they report all missing minors and (2) that the NCBs distribute the posters in their countries. The establishment of these posters in 1994 was an important step for the General Secretariat because until that time, the public had only been notified about the most wanted criminals and stolen works of art, not of child victims.

INTERNATIONAL GREEN NOTICES

The purpose of the green notice is to provide information about offenders who are likely to commit additional crimes in various countries. The publishing of such notices is normally subject to the following criteria:

— The person concerned has convictions for offenses committed in at least 3 different countries, including the country of the person's habitual residence, or the person's criminal activities or connections have been revealed in an inquiry during an investigation or court case regarding someone else.

— The person has proven links with organized crime.

Green notices apply to perpetrators of crimes against children, including traveling pedophiles and international traffickers of child pornography, and are an important working tool for combating the sexual abuse of children by individuals who operate in more than one country. NCBs must report such offenders and request the General Secretariat to issue green notices. The use of the information provided by the green notice varies according to the existing national legislation, regulations, or both. For example, some countries will do the following:

— Prevent the offender from entering its territory

— Begin discreet surveillance of the offender

— Take note of the information and use it in their documentation and databases

COMPUTER SYSTEMS

The computer systems used at the General Secretariat have made it possible to provide the technical and professional assistance required by member nations. This assistance was needed to implement the automated search facility (ASF), which has played an essential role in the fight against international crime since its introduction in the early 1990s.

State-of-the-art technology is used in 2 main sectors of the Interpol headquarters: the electronic criminal information system (CIS) and office automation, electronic mail, and archiving systems. The CIS has been expanded to improve methods of storing and retrieving data regarding crimes and criminals, thereby substantially reducing the time it takes to answer enquiries from NCBs and giving the police division rapid access to data sent in by member states. Office automation, electronic mail, and archiving systems have been installed, making it possible to work in all 4 of the organization's languages (ie, Arabic, English, French, and Spanish) and greatly facilitating communication within Interpol headquarters.

DATA ENTRY, ELECTRONIC ARCHIVING, AND AUTOMATIC CONSULTATION

The different departments responsible for processing criminal intelligence maintain the following data entry, electronic archiving, and automatic consultation records:

— A computer record of the names and aliases of people implicated in international crime cases

— A computer record of offenses, which are classified by type of offense, place of commission, and modus operandi

— A computer record of identification numbers noted during the course of police investigations

— A *10-print file*, which contains the prints of all 10 fingers of various international offenders

— A photograph file for specialized and habitual offenders as well as missing persons

— A system of electronic archiving with computerized indexing

— An electronic text and image server allowing NCBs to instantly and remotely consult a database of selected information

INTERPOL ACHIEVEMENTS AND COOPERATION AMONG AGENCIES

Since 1991, cooperation among law enforcement agencies has increased regarding international aspects of crimes committed against children. Advances include the establishment of national police liaison officers and increased cooperation with NGOs.

In 1989, Interpol inaugurated a new General Secretariat headquarters in Lyon, France, at the 58th General Assembly session. In his inaugural speech, the president of the French Republic denounced all forms of exploitation of children and called for the elimination of this "unspeakable suffering" by all possible means. A resolution was adopted, and for the first time, Interpol became actively involved in exploitation cases.

In 1990, little information regarding child exploitation crimes was being exchanged among countries, so Interpol prepared and circulated a questionnaire to all its members. Though many crimes against children, such as physical, sexual, and emotional abuse and neglect, are not necessarily international crimes, such offenses occur in all countries, so members would benefit from exchanging information regarding good working practices and training. For other offenses such as child pornography and sex tourism, the benefits from greater international police cooperation and exchange of information were obvious.

In May 1991, a specially selected group of experts with various backgrounds was invited by Interpol to study with officers from the Interpol General Crime Group the replies to the questionnaires, which were received from more than 50 member countries. The group met at the General Secretariat headquarters in Lyon and was subdivided into 2 sections—one concentrating on international policing aspects and another on training and cooperation with the United Nations (UN) and NGOs.

The group produced a set of recommendations based on the answers to the questionnaires and their own specialist knowledge and experience. The study group believed that their proposals could serve as a guide and would support the efforts of member countries attempting to combat crimes against children more effectively, whether by reviewing existing methods or introducing new measures. In April 1992, the First Interpol Symposium on Offences Against Children and Young Persons was held in Lyon. The symposium members gave general approval to the recommendations proposed by the expert group.

In November 1992, the members of the 61st General Assembly of Interpol meeting in Dakar, Senegal, approved the resolution based on the conclusion of the April symposium. The members recommended that participating countries review their legislation and practices relating to offenses against children and, if necessary, introduce the recommendations of the April symposium. This meeting decided that an Interpol specialist group comprising police officers and experts working in relevant fields should be created to follow up on the conclusions and coordinate subsequent actions by member countries.

The Interpol Specialist Group on Crimes Against Children meets twice a year in Lyon and in many other host countries. As the specialist group's reputation has grown, so have the numbers of regular participants. At the first meeting of the new millennium, held in May 2000, 40 countries were represented by almost 100 high-ranking police and customs officials who specialize in combating crimes against children. As the group has developed, the structure has also changed. Initially, the specialist group was subdivided into 2 basic groups, but it is now divided into 4 groups: (1) child prostitution and sex tourism, (2) child pornography, (3) missing and trafficking in children, and (4) management of sex offenders. Each subgroup has a chairperson, and the meetings are structured so experts and practitioners from many parts of the world can share their knowledge and experiences with all members of the specialist group.

Since the Interpol specialist group's inception, the General Secretariat members have coordinated meetings and followed up the specialist group's initiatives, resulting in intense and active collaboration between Interpol and UN ad hoc committees and divisions, particularly with the UN Crime Prevention and Criminal Justice Division in Vienna and the UN Committee on the Rights of the Child. In recent years, the General Secretariat has been involved in UN work by drafting the rules of evidence and procedure for the international criminal court, where the UN specifically advocates the victim rights of children who have been involved in war crimes (eg, children as soldiers, sexual crimes against children in a time of war, child massacres in war zones).

In 1994, the Interpol Working Party reaffirmed its desire to combat crimes against children by asking the 176 member countries to appoint a specialized liaison officer dedicated to this issue, in the hopes that it would facilitate the international exchange of information. Many countries responded and expressed their concern and desire to cooperate. Because most of the appointed officers were not specialists, the Working Party decided, in accordance with their credo concerning training, to collaborate with the General Secretariat to organize the training needed.

In April 1995, the General Secretariat hosted the first training seminar for specialized liaison officers dealing with offenses against children. The seminar was favorably received by the 38 member countries represented and was a great success. Lack of training is a key problem for police departments in different countries, regardless of how modern or developed their departments may be. At this time, few police officers are capable of approaching, handling, and solving cases involving child victims. To address these crimes, understanding the psychology of children is essential, which changes according to age and intellectual maturity.

Other than medical information about children's physical condition, in most cases of sexual abuse the only evidence is provided by the children themselves. It is easy to manipulate this sort of evidence by asking child victims, who are understandably psychologically fragile and severely traumatized, questions in a way that elicits answers that are not admissible as evidence.

In 1996, Interpol was involved as a specialist in the first World Congress Against the Commercial Sexual Exploitation of Children, which was organized by the United Nations Children's Fund (UNICEF); End Child Prostitution, Child Pornography and Trafficking of Children for Sexual Purposes (ECPAT); and the NGO group working with the UN Committee for the Rights of the Child under the auspices of the Swedish government. Interpol members were in charge of the legal and law enforcement aspects of the commercial sexual exploitation of children and used their expertise to help draft a background document and the declaration and plan of action that was adopted by the 120 represented countries. Members of the Interpol Specialist Group on Crimes Against Children served as chairpersons and conducted different workshops regarding law enforcement issues. Moreover, the 8th meeting of the specialist group was held in Stockholm, Sweden, at the same time as the World Congress and was hosted by the National Swedish Police Board, which highlights Interpol's support for the World Congress. Interpol is now welcomed at many important international conferences and has become a natural partner for training programs and advisement on matters of legislation and law.

After the World Congress, the 65th Interpol General Assembly met in Antalya, Turkey, and adopted 3 resolutions involving trafficking of women and children for sexual exploitation, child pornography, and the improvement of international police cooperation regarding offenses committed against children. The detailed recommendations updated by the specialist group were appended to the last resolution and received enthusiastic support from all the participants at the General Assembly. In keeping with the second resolution, in 2004, Interpol assumed the responsibility of maintaining the child sexual abuse image database of Combating Paedophile Networks in Europe (COPINE). Until COPINE began work on this database in 2001, law enforcement officials worldwide were overwhelmed with images of abused children and had no source to identify the children or determine whether an image was new or had been circulated previously.

While developing its own much smaller database that was combined with the COPINE database, Interpol worked with member states, the G8 law enforcement project sun group (ie, a cyber crime and cyber law group), the European Commission, NGOs, and academic institutions, including the University College Cork, Ireland, which had undertaken extensive research on images within their COPINE project under the direction of Max Taylor and Ethel Quayle of the Department of Applied Psychology. The database involved several software programs, including image comparison software capable of matching crime scenes.

During the 7 years that the COPINE Project existed, in cooperation with police agencies around the world, it clarified the degree to which children were being victimized and was instrumental in identifying numerous abuse victims. When the project ceased due to funding issues, the images and information collected were passed through the Irish Garda to Interpol.

Great progress has been made since the 1989 adoption of Interpol's first resolution to eradicate all forms of exploitation of children. Interpol now plays an international role in protecting children from all forms of abuse. Topics such as child sex tourism and child pornography are still unmentionable issues in many countries and receive less media attention than other crimes. In addition, some police officers still do not recognize the significance of such crimes. The achievements of the Interpol specialist group improve the future of the world's children and, therefore, the future of society.

INFLUENCE OF INTERPOL IN THE INTERNATIONAL COMMUNITY

REPUBLIC OF MACEDONIA

Interpol maintains a world focus, which is essential when addressing child abductions and trafficking among countries. It has had a positive impact on numerous countries throughout the world, such as the Republic of Macedonia. During a report on prostitution in Macedonia to the Interpol Specialist Group on Crimes Against Children, the Macedonian investigator described the 3 types of prostitution that had been identified by law enforcement officials: (1) street prostitution, (2) high-style prostitution involving escort women, and (3) import prostitution. The presenter explained that individuals involved in street prostitution were citizens of the Republic of Macedonia, and no cases involving foreign citizens had been registered. Street prostitution involved pimps who in some instances lived with their prostitutes to avoid criminal prosecution. This type of prostitution was associated with a high risk for sexually transmitted diseases.

The presence of foreign soldiers, missionaries, and other organizations had brought foreign prostitutes to the republic who worked with the domestic prostitutes in rented apartments shared among 3 or 4 women. This form of prostitution occurred in what was referred to as a *massage saloon* and was a relatively new phenomenon in the Republic of Macedonia. In comparison to street prostitution, this more established high-style prostitution was less obvious to the general public. The investigator reported that no problems seemed to stem from this form of prostitution because the women and girls were educated, often had their own business, and did not seem to be forced to provide the sexual services.

However, import prostitution had become the most severe prostitution problem in the Republic of Macedonia because of its clear link with illegal trafficking of human beings. The existing Macedonian law, the Law on Public Order and Peace in the Criminal Code, cited prostitution as a misdemeanor. As a result of the education by and assistance of Interpol and other members of the international community, the Republic of Macedonia began establishing a new criminal code that would bring harsher penalties to any person who recruited, instigated, or enticed another into prostitution, thereby resulting in a potential penalty of 6 months to 5 years in prison. If a person were found to have sexually exploited women and children within the context of organized crime, the punishment would be imprisonment for 1 to 10 years.

INTERNATIONAL HUMAN TRAFFICKING AND SMUGGLING

Interpol is a consistent source of information about human trafficking and smuggling. Interpol has chosen to use the definitions for human trafficking as is included in the United Nations Convention Against Transnational Organized Crime. This treaty uses the terms smuggling of migrants and trafficking in persons. The former term involves illegal entry into a state of which a person is not a citizen or resident and results in financial or material gain for the smuggler. The international criminal smuggling networks are increasing in sophistication, moving more people daily, and receiving higher profits. Such smuggling entails aspects of international human migration because of the recent unprecedented migration from the least developed countries of Asia, Africa, South America, and Eastern Europe to Western Europe, Australia, and North America. Smuggling of migrants often involves inhumane conditions, with migrants being placed in overcrowded trucks or boats and often dying as a result. Migrants who survive the journey and arrive at their destination country are illegal immigrants and are completely dependent on the smugglers. The migrants often become indentured servants for years, being told that they are paying off the debts related to their transportation. If the migrants are unable to pay their debts, their family members in their home countries are threatened and often forced to pay to save their smuggled relative's life

Trafficking in persons is specific to the recruitment, transportation, transfer, or receipt of persons for the purpose of exploitation. Exploitation includes prostitution or other forms of sexual exploitation, forced labor, slavery, and servitude.

Though the trafficking routes have been carefully defined, when people are preparing to reach western countries, land travel is forfeited for the more expensive but successful air travel. Interpol has noted that trafficking networks are tending to focus more on Central and South America, where they can maintain the necessary links to Mexico and an ability to move women and children into North America.

The Eastern European trafficking route, which ultimately leads to Mexico and into the United States, was the subject of a compelling and controversial article by Peter Landesman in the *The New York Times Magazine* (2004). The author spent several months performing a covert journalistic investigation and discovered that thousands of women and children were sold into sexual slavery in the United States from countries such as Moldova, Russia, and Ukraine, often through Mexico. He discovered that several sex trafficking ring organizers were advertising in local newspapers for American nanny positions or model and actress jobs and were then bringing the women and children into the United States to be sexual slaves. Landesman helped to explain the important distinction between sexual slavery and prostitution. Prostitution, though usually associated with coercion and intimidation, left the victims with some sort of living arrangement and some small amount of actual income; however, the women, teenagers, and toddlers who became sexual slaves were in chains, figuratively and literally. They were forced to cooperate or be killed, as were their families in the villages from which they came. The victims earned no money whatsoever. Landesman discussed the Mexican traffickers of Los Lenones, a well-organized group of pimps operating as wholesalers, "collecting human merchandise and taking orders from safe houses and brothels in the major sex-trafficking hubs in New York, Los Angeles, Atlanta, and Chicago" (2004). The first transporter who is often in the country of origin of the trafficked person might purchase a girl for as little as $60. However, every subsequent transfer into another country would be associated with a price increase, with the final cost for an Eastern European girl topping out at almost $2500, paid by the organization that would ultimately control her. Landesman found that the process of "breaking in" new victims is particularly inhumane and involved forcing them to perform sexual acts as often as 20 to 30 times per day for weeks or months—as long as it took for the victims to become completely compliant. The women and girls were eventually smuggled across the Mexican-American border through vehicles and on foot with final transport to various large American cities.

Landesman's article also cited Gary Haugren of the International Justice Mission, an NGO that fights sexual exploitation in South and Southeast Asia. Haugren discussed the corruption rampant in the international sex industry: "Sex trafficking isn't a poverty issue but a law enforcement issue. You can only carry out this trade at significant levels with the cooperation of local law enforcement. In the developing world, the police are not seen as a solution for anything. You don't run to the police; you run from the police" (Landesman, 2004). According to estimates by the Central Intelligence Agency (CIA), between 18 000 and 20 000 people are trafficked annually into the United States. John Miller of the US State Department's Office to Monitor and Combat Trafficking in Persons stated, "[t]hat figure could be low. What we know is that the number is huge" (Landesman, 2004). Laura Lederer, a senior advisor on trafficking for the US State Department, stated, "[w]e're not finding victims in the United States because we're not looking for them" (Landesman, 2004).

Interpol continues to lobby politically for stronger international legislation on human trafficking. Consistent arrests and prosecutions are a goal of the international community through the structure provided on a global basis by Interpol and other policing and advocacy agencies such as ECPAT.

One of the missions of an American grassroots NGO, The Polaris Project, is to assist with legislation development and public education in the area of human trafficking and sexual slavery. The Polaris Project notes that not only do international law enforcement agencies need education and sensitivity training regarding the plight of victims, but the military helps propagate this form of sexual exploitation. They stress that though foreign national trafficking is an immense problem, national domestic trafficking among states is an even greater concern in the United States. The Polaris Project provides model legislation for states that desire to strengthen their laws and the penalties for individuals involved in human trafficking for sexual exploitation.

CONCLUSION

The 182 countries that are members of Interpol have the opportunity to benefit immensely from the expertise of excellent investigators who are adroit in addressing crimes against children, which include child pornography, prostituted children and youth, human trafficking for sexual exploitation and slavery, and Internet recruitment of children for sexual exploitation. This landmark agency provides the greatest ability to link many countries together in its battle against the exploitation of children.

REFERENCES

Children and human trafficking. Interpol Web site. Available at: http://www.Interpol.int/Public/THB/default.asp. Accessed December 31, 2004.

ICPO-Interpol Constitution and General Regulations. Interpol Web site. Available at: http://www.interpol.com/public/ICPO/LegalMaterials/constitution/constitution GenReg/constitution.asp. Accessed November 22, 2004.

Landesman P. The girls next door. *New York Times Magazine*. January 25, 2004.

INVESTIGATION AND PROSECUTION OF THE PROSTITUTION OF CHILDREN

Susan S. Kreston, JD, LLM

"Sympathy for victims is inversely proportional to their age and sexual development."
Kenneth Lanning (2001)

INTRODUCTION

The statistics regarding prostituted children abound. Although an estimated 325 000 children are considered "at risk" in the United States (Estes & Weiner, 2001), the estimates regarding the number of prostituted children vary drastically and range from 1700 (Hammer et al, 2002) to 400 000 (Spangenberg, 2001) children.

Prostituting children may take many forms: domestic prostituting of children, domestic and international trafficking of children for the purpose of prostitution, or child sex tourism. Since each type of exploitation has a unique dynamic, initially each will be presented separately and followed by an assessment of the best practices of the criminal justice system in responding to the specific challenges incurred in investigating and prosecuting the domestic prostitution of children. Issues surrounding trafficked and tourism-targeted children are discussed in other chapters of this book.

All prostituted children are already marginalized, if not alienated, from society. They begin with 3 strikes against them: they are children, they are designated as prostitutes, and they often engage in criminal activities (eg, drug usage, theft, immigration violations, and other crimes). Many people condemn or dismiss these children; few ask what could have happened to these children to force them into this life.

THE CRIMES

PROSTITUTION OF CHILDREN

Child prostitution is defined as the act of engaging or offering the services of a child to perform sexual acts for money or other consideration (**Table 32-1**). The prostitution of children usually involves an extrafamilial "pimp," which is an acronym for "*p*rofiting from the *i*ncome of *m*anaging *p*rostitutes," and in this chapter includes female exploiters called ***madams***; however, the prostitution of children also includes factual situations in which parents offer their children to third parties for money or anything of value. Such cases are referred to as ***charm school cases***.

Laws and Penalties

The federal government and most states have laws against prostituting children (**Appendix 32-1**). In most cases, these laws target the conduct of the economic exploiter and/or pimp but ignore the culpability of the sexual molester and/or john.

In identical, factual scenarios involving an adult who has sexual intercourse with an underage child, the penalty difference between the crime labeled "prostitution" and the crime labeled "child sexual abuse" is significant. *Patrons*, as they are euphemistically called, are often specifically excluded from the coverage of child prostitution

Table 32-1. Factors Contributing to the Prostitution of Children

— The laws primarily target the exploiter and/or pimp but ignore the culpability of the sexual molester and/or john.

— There are predictable situations that make children more at risk to becoming victims of prostitution. Most are runaway, "thrownaway," or deserted children who have experienced sexual abuse, physical abuse, emotional abuse, and/or domestic violence before leaving home. Many become sexually exploited as a result of family dysfunction, familial drug abuse, and recurrent school and other social failures.

— The "infantilization" of prostitution because of the increased demand for "virgins" by molesters and/or johns.

— The laws pertaining to the prostitution of children are not enforced as often or as stringently as they could be.

legislation. For example, Minn Stat Ann § 609.322 (West Supp, 2000) specifically exempts criminal liability for patrons who exploit children between the ages of 16 and 18 years old. Even when included, the penalty generally pales compared to that of the molester prosecuted under traditional child sexual abuse laws. For example, La Rev Stat Ann § 14:42(D)(2)(a) makes the act of having sex with a child younger than 12 years old a death penalty eligible offense, but La Rev Stat Ann 14:82.1 (West, 1986; Supp, 1999) sets the penalty between 2 and 10 years of imprisonment for an individual who has sex with a prostituted child of any age, including children younger than 12 years old.

Since the prostitution of children does not conform to traditional sexual abuse dynamics (Willis & Levy, 2002), the exploitation of prostituted children by a patron is generally not prosecuted under child abuse laws. These cases may be shuffled among the juvenile, vice, family, and criminal divisions of a police department because the sexual molester is usually extrafamilial and the victims tend to be teenagers against whom the defense of consent may be raised (Walsh & Fassett, 1994). Unfortunately, many cases and children are lost in this shuffle.

State laws pertaining to prostituted children can be broken down into laws that deal with the criminal liability for individuals who patronize prostituted children and individuals who operate or manage the prostitution of children. Though most state laws do not specifically focus on patrons, the criminal liability of patrons may be addressed in general prostitution statutes, in which such a crime tends to be handled as a summary or misdemeanor offense (Klain, 1999). States with laws that deal with individuals who manage the prostitution of children address the crime in terms of pimping, pandering, procuring, profiting, or promoting prostitution. These laws also reflect a varying degree of protection for children based on the child's age, in that younger children receive the greatest protection as reflected by stiffer penalties for their exploitation (Klain, 1999). Additional state laws may impose penalties on individuals who aid or abet the prostitution of children, that is, people who attempt to prostitute children and parents who allow their children to engage in prostitution (Klain, 1999).

Federal laws that specifically apply to the prostitution of children are found in the Mann Act, found at 18 USC section 2421, et seq. Section 2423 (**Appendix 32-1**). These laws specifically address the prostitution of children as well as transportation and travel with the intent to engage in criminal sexual activity. Section 2423(a) targets the criminal culpability of the pimp and allows for the prosecution of offenders who knowingly transport a minor across state lines with the intent to prostitute the child;

section 2423(b) allows for prosecution of patrons when they cross state lines with the intent of prostituting a child, regardless of whether the actual exploitation takes place:

(a) Transportation with intent to engage in criminal sexual activity. A person who knowingly transports an individual who has not attained the age of 18 years in interstate or foreign commerce, or in any commonwealth, territory, or possession of the United States, with intent that the individual engage in prostitution, or in any sexual activity for which any person can be charged with a criminal offense, shall be fined under this title and imprisoned for not less than 5 years and not more than 30 years.

(b) Travel with intent to engage in illicit sexual conduct. A person who travels in interstate commerce or travels into the United States, or a United States citizen or an alien admitted for permanent residence in the United States who travels in foreign commerce, for the purpose of engaging in any illicit sexual conduct with another person shall be fined under this title or imprisoned not more than 30 years, or both.

Reasons Children Become Victims of Prostitution

While many victims of prostitution are teenagers, children of all ages are victimized. Children become victims of prostitution in depressingly predictable ways. The majority are runaway, "thrownaway," or deserted children. Usually sexual abuse, physical abuse, emotional abuse, and/or domestic violence existed in the homes of these children before they left.

Once the dynamics are known and acknowledged regarding the ways children come to be prostituted, better investigation and prosecution of the prostitution of children will be possible.

Though poverty is often posited as a major force behind the prostitution of children, poverty is *not* a primary factor; rather, family dysfunction (eg, violence, mental illness, sexual victimization), familial drug abuse, and recurrent school and social failures are more often identified as the factor(s) that contribute to the sexual exploitation of children (Estes & Weiner, 2001). Another factor is the presence of a pre-existing, adult prostitution market. A recent study that cites links found in Chicago, Honolulu, Las Vegas, New Orleans, New York, and San Francisco between adult prostitution and the prostitution of children, succinctly summarized the relationship between the 2 types of prostitution:

Without equivocation … the presence of pre-existing adult prostitution markets contributes measurably to the creation of secondary sexual markets in which children are sexually exploited. [W]e find no support for the legalization of prostitution in the U.S., especially given the relationship that we can confirm to exist between adult and juvenile sexual exploitation(Estes & Weiner, 2001).

Infantilization of Prostitution

Though prostitution of children has been documented as young as 9 years old (Brinkley, 2000; Klain, 1999), the average age when children enter into prostitution is 14 years old (Klain, 1999; Whitcomb & Eastin, 1998). In addition, the **infantilization** of prostitution is a trend that continues to grow. This means that the demand for "virgins" continues to increase as a result of the risk of contracting acquired immunodeficiency syndrome (AIDS), a potentially lethal sexually transmitted disease (STD). This demand exists because of the molester's and/or john's belief that virgins (ie, prepubescent children) will not have STDs since they have not been exposed through prior sexual intercourse. Some abusers even believe that sex with a virgin will cure STDs. In reality, prostituted children have usually been sexually abused and exploited by their parent(s), their pimp, or others long before they were lured or forced into prostitution. Ironically, prepubescent children are some of the most at-risk people for AIDS and STDs because the likelihood of anal or vaginal tearing resulting during intercourse is greatest with small children. By choosing the youngest of victims, criminals may unwittingly be signing their own death warrants.

Enforcement of the Laws

Another contributing factor to an environment in which the prostitution of children is allowed to exist intentionally unnoticed and willfully unchecked is the laxity of the enforcement of laws pertaining to the prostitution of children among law enforcement agencies, social service agencies, and health care professionals (Estes & Weiner, 2001). This is especially true with respect to older victims.

Prostituted children present special challenges to the criminal justice system. These children are often hostile toward law enforcement and social service personnel, and they do not believe that either group is genuinely interested in helping them. The mistaken societal attitude that prostituted children, particularly teenagers, are somehow responsible for their exploitation and, therefore, are unworthy of the protection the law affords to other victims of child sexual abuse does nothing to alter this view. In fact, the US Department of Justice's Office of Juvenile Justice and Delinquency Prevention (OJJDP) notes that even when adjusting for all other variables, crimes against teenagers receive lighter sentences than crimes committed against other victims (Finkelhor & Ormrod, 2001). In addition, an attachment to their pimps and the resulting noncooperation from victimized children create untold difficulties at the investigative stage. These problems become magnified at the prosecution stage, should the case get that far.

TRAFFICKING IN CHILDREN

Sex trafficking is defined as the recruitment, harboring, transportation, provision, or obtaining of a person for the purpose of a commercial sex act (22 USCS § 7102(9)). An estimated 20 000 people are trafficked into the United States annually (US Dept of State, 2003). ***Coercion***, which is defined by threats of serious harm to or physical restraint against any person, is often used in these crimes (22 USCS § 7102(2)(A)). In a small number of cases, parents are tricked into believing that their child(ren) will be placed in a good job (eg, becoming a nanny) or will receive a good education, only to have their child(ren) forced into prostitution upon entering the United States. In a far greater number, children are sold by parents or other family members.

The causes of this crime are greed, moral turpitude, political instability, social and/or cultural practices that systematically devalue women and girls, and the concealment of incest (ECPAT International, 2004; US Dept of State, 2003). Many traffickers are involved in other transnational crimes (ECPAT International, 2004; US Dept of State, 2003), and the profits from trafficking in human beings makes this the fastest growing source of profits for organized criminal enterprises worldwide (22 USCS § 7101, et seq.). Traffickers engage in this crime because it yields a high profit, requires relatively low risk, does not require a large capital investment, and because people can be used repeatedly unlike other commodities such as guns and drugs (US Dept of State, 2003). The risk of detection is relatively low because many of the victims come from countries where the authorities are a source of fear rather than assistance (US Dept of State, 2003). In addition, as with all types of child abuse, the children may not wish to disclose what happened to them, which may result from their understandable reluctance to relive the abuse or from cultural taboos that were broken by the abuse.

In 2000, federal law established the crime of sex trafficking of children whether by force, fraud, or coercion (18 USCS § 1591). This law increased the penalty to include life in prison for the worst traffickers and allotted money for antitrafficking enforcement and victim assistance programs. The Victims of Trafficking and Violence Protection Act of 2000 (22 USCS § 7101, et seq.) established new protection and assistance for these targeted individuals. The act grants eligibility to these victims to receive benefits, services, programs, and activities to the same extent as legally admitted refugee aliens (22 USCS § 7105(b)(1)(A)). In addition, the act establishes T-visa (8 USCS § 1101(a)(15)(T)(i)) status for victims to allow them to stay legally in the United States in order to effectuate the prosecution of the criminal case (22 USCS §

7105 (b)(1)(E)(i)(I)). Within any fiscal year, 5000 T-visas are available (8 USCS § 1184 (n)(2)).

CHILD SEX TOURISM

Child sex tourism occurs when an individual from one country enters another, usually less developed country with the intent to sexually abuse or exploit children in that foreign land. The intent to exploit can be the primary motive for travel or in conjunction with a legitimate reason to travel, which is best illustrated by the business traveler and/or sex tourist scenario. These abusers justify their exploitation as "culturally acceptable" in the foreign land or as helping to provide the children and their families with money (ECPAT International, 2004). In reality, these abusers are simply morally and sexually indiscriminate child abusers (Collins, 2001).

According to ECPAT-USA (2004), 25% of child sex tourists are American, thereby making the United States the number 1 exporter of sex tourists worldwide. As a response to this, the United States has chosen to exercise extraterritorial jurisdiction over its nationals when they commit crimes against children abroad. (The United States is 1 of 32 countries to exercise this option.) In the United States, these cases are prosecutable under the relatively new federal child sex tourism statute enacted in 1994 (18 USC § 2423(b)). This statute allows for extraterritorial jurisdiction to be exercised by the United States where the intent to commit the crime was formed in this country. (See also *Child Sex Tourism Action Survey* [ECPAT International, 2001], which cites Australia, Canada, Ireland, and the United Kingdom as countries that have enacted special laws forbidding travel with the intent of abusing children and allowing for punishment of the offender at home.) The crime is defined by US law rather than the law of the foreign country. There is currently discussion of removing the intent formation requirement and simply prosecuting these crimes in the United States regardless of where the intent was formed. Thus far, there have been only a small number of prosecutions under this statute, but these prosecutions have been successful, and they disclose another dimension to this type of exploitation: These perpetrators are serial abusers and usually have a number of victims. For example, Nobel Prize winner Daniel Carleton Gajdusek, a pediatrician and researcher, was jailed in 1997 for molesting a 16-year-old boy, 1 of 56 Micronesian children he molested (Under plea deal, *Washington Post,* 1997).

THE INVESTIGATION

There must be an orchestrated and coordinated response from law enforcement officers, prosecutors, and other criminal justice professionals involved in the investigation of this problem. All criminal justice professionals need to recognize that prostituting children is, quite simply, child sexual abuse.

Law enforcement personnel need to become educated about prostituted children. Ideally, law enforcement offices should have specialized staff members (ie, a multidisciplinary staff comprised of investigators, prosecutors, victim advocates, social workers, and other allied professionals) who are specifically trained for and who dedicate time to child exploitation cases. In smaller jurisdictions, one officer who has expertise and a commitment to working in this field could be designated. (Vieth [1998] discusses ways to use available resources to develop expertise in a smaller jurisdiction.) All the investigative techniques used in other felony investigations are applicable to these cases, but these cases place a premium on suspect interrogation.

This phase of the investigation is important because the information gathered at this stage may prove critical at the charging phase and during the trial itself. Investigators must obtain training in best practices for interviewing intrafamilial and extrafamilial child abusers and exploiters. Witness interviews and informants' statements are also important. Surveillance of the scene(s) where the prostitution takes place (eg, on the street, at escort services, in massage parlors, through computer "dating" services) should be explored. Videotaping of these scenes may help bring the jury into the world of the exploited child during the trial. Subpoenas and search warrants should be used to gain information and evidence pertinent to the cases. Pretext calls, in states where this is allowed by law, may be a strategy worth considering; however, careful consideration must be given to the victim's psychological ability to perform this task, as well as to the possibility that the victim may use this opportunity to alert the target. Reverse sting e-mails, in which the investigator takes over an existing e-mail correspondence with the defendant, may be used. Sting operations and undercover investigations are also successful, proactive approaches to this crime (*United States v Spruill*, 2002). **Table 32-2** lists specific questions and issues that should be addressed during the investigation phase.

When talking to the victim, do not use the word "pimp" unless the victim does; use whatever name or description the victim uses, such as "friend" or "boyfriend." Similarly, if the child refers to himself or herself as a "hustler" or "escort," reflect that language back to the child. Above all, do not convey a judgmental attitude.

These children may be noncooperative, sullen, recalcitrant, and emotional. Many of the children who are being prostituted are difficult for law enforcement officers to detect because they may appear older than their age and may view police officers as the enemy. In light of these dynamics, these children should be immediately interviewed, and the interview should be recorded. If possible, videotape the interview. The use of

---

Table 32-2. Issues to Be Addressed During the Investigation

1. How was the victim recruited? At what age was the victim recruited?

2. What is the name of the pimp and his or her street name(s) or alias(es)?

3. Did the pimp provide instructions to the victim about the way the process worked?

4. Did the pimp receive the money directly, indirectly, or in another manner?

5. Did the pimp use or threaten violence?

6. Did the victim ever receive medical treatment?

7. Can the victim identify any other victims and adult prostitutes with whom the victim had contact? If so, what were their street names, aliases, or stage names? Were any of these other victims and/or adults ever arrested? Did any of them show the victim the way the process worked?

8. What mode of prostitution was used (eg, track, services, front companies)?

9. If travel was involved, what mode of transportation was used? Who paid for the transportation? Was it by bus or air carrier? If so, what were the dates?

10. If hotels were used, what were their names and descriptions? Who paid for these hotels?

11. Identify the victim's terms (eg, define "sex") during the forensic interview.

12. Did the victim have sex with the pimp?

13. Did the victim ever become pregnant? If so, what happened to that pregnancy? If the pregnancy was terminated, when, where, and by whom did this occur?

a forensic interview specialist is encouraged because these specialists have training and expertise regarding how best to interview the victims in these cases, particularly teenage victims. Since these victims may be "cooperating" or "compliant" victims (Lanning, 2002) and may not be in active disclosure regarding their abuse, the use of a child interview specialist is highly advised. For example, the Federal Bureau of Investigation's (FBI) Innocent Images National Initiative (IINI) program uses these child interview specialists.

If the case falls across police departmental divides (eg, vice, juvenile, child abuse), the units must coordinate their efforts to best investigate the case and assist the child. The decisions regarding who will lead the investigation should be based on the probable charges and available penalties within each area, the personnel and economic resources available in each department, and the amount of experience each department has with these cases. The priority and importance allotted to these cases should be no different from other sex crimes committed against children.

One of the newer avenues in investigatory practices is the search and seizure of computer evidence in these cases. After drafting a search warrant, seizing computers used by the molester and/or john, the exploiter and/or pimp, and the victim(s) may yield the following types of evidence: address books; biographies; calendars; customer database and/or records; e-mail, notes, and/or letters; false identification; financial asset records; Internet activity logs; medical records; and World Wide Web page advertising. (For a more complete discussion of drafting search warrants for computers and computer evidence, see Kreston, 1999.)

Individuals who engage in this criminal conduct should be arrested for prostituting a child, molestation, rape, or other factually appropriate child sexual abuse violations. The crime(s) for which the defendant is arrested will directly affect the amount at which bail is set before formal charging by the prosecutor's office. The children who have been violated should be taken into mandatory protective custody and then released into the custody of protective services. Prostituted children should be treated as victims, *not* as criminals.

THE TRIAL

CHARGING AND PRETRIAL DECISIONS

Once the investigation is completed, the following 3 crucial decisions must be made:

1. Does sufficient, admissible evidence exist to prove the defendant's guilt beyond a reasonable doubt?

2. Who will be charged for this crime? What safeguards must be put in place to ensure that the defendant(s) do(es) not leave the jurisdiction?

3. If prosecution is possible, should prosecution take place in the federal system, state system, or both?

The prosecutor must first determine if prosecution is possible based on an analysis of whether sufficient, admissible evidence exists to prove the defendant's guilt beyond a reasonable doubt. Any foreseeable or anticipated problem with the victim's testimony should be thoroughly addressed at this time. Victims in these cases are generally reluctant to testify, and this situation may be exacerbated if the victim still retains any feelings of loyalty or fear of the pimp. These victims may also not wish to go to court if they think that their sexual history will be opened up in the court of law. As a result, a rape shield hearing should be requested first in order to obtain a ruling from the court to restrict the evidence to include only the victim's sexual history that is relevant to the case (Federal Rule of Evidence 412; Myers, 1997, suppl 2002). In addition, a victim witness advocate may be useful to serve as a bridge and buffer between the victim and the prosecutor since the victim may have hostile feelings toward law enforcement officers and prosecutors.

Next, the prosecutor must determine who will be charged. Choices must be made regarding whether it is necessary to consider granting the molester and/or john or exploiter and/or pimp immunity or another type of compensation in exchange for his/her/their testimony against the other. As previously discussed, one of the most egregious problems with state laws is that, as a rule, patrons (or johns) are seldom specifically encompassed by the existing laws and are sometimes specifically exempted from state law coverage (Klain, 1999). As a result, prosecutors may not be able to prosecute the john for his and/or her actions under the state's prostitution statute. Under these circumstances, charging the molester with the sex crime applicable to the fact-specific case must be considered. Alternatively, the possibility of federal involvement should be assessed. Another difficulty with the law is that coverage varies from state to state based on the victim's age (eg, NY Penal Code § 230.04-06) (Klain, 1999) and, in some cases, on the age of the molester and/or pimp (La Re Stat Ann § 14.86). This preferential coverage is, in turn, reflected in the penalties, which vary according to the age of the child (La Re Stat Ann § 14.86).

In addition to determining who will be charged with the crime, a decision should be made regarding what safeguards the prosecutor should put in place to counter attempts by the defendant(s) to flee the jurisdiction. The likelihood of the victim and potential witnesses leaving should also be assessed at this time.

Finally, if prosecution is feasible, the prosecutor should determine whether the trial should take place in the federal system, the state system, or both. For federal jurisdiction to attach, there must be an activity that involves interstate or foreign commerce. If there is no "interstate nexus," then the case must be prosecuted at the state or local level. If the case could be prosecuted in the state or federal system, a decision regarding where best to bring charges must be made. Note that while prosecution is theoretically possible in federal and state court, if the state case is tried first, the federal prosecutor may need to obtain special permission to pursue the federal case thereafter.

The decision-making process begins by assessing the possible charges and penalties available under either system, as well as any other relevant factors that affect prosecution. For example, the federal laws, sometimes referred to collectively as the Mann Act (18 USCA § 2422(b)), assess a penalty of up to 15 years upon conviction and have provisions that target the pimp (18 USCA § 2423(a)) and the patron (18 USCA § 2423(b)). It is important to consider other attendant crimes as well as the obvious state or federal prostitution-based charges (18 USCA § 2422(b);18 USCA § 2423(a), 2423(b)). (See **Appendix 32-1** for a listing of state charges.) Other crimes might include prosecution under traditional state law child abuse or sex crimes statutes, including statutory rape laws (NCPCA, 2004). If violence was present, charges reflecting that may arise. If the production or distribution of pornography occurred, this could be charged federally or at the state level (NCPCA, 2004). Possible federal charges include aggravated sexual abuse (18 USC § 2241(c)), sexual abuse of a minor or ward (18 USC § 2243), Racketeering Influenced and Corrupt Organization (RICO) (18 USC § 1952; Tyrangiel & Bonesteel, 2001; Opening (US) Session Statement for the Second World Congress Against Commercial Sexual Exploitation of Children, 2001), money laundering (18 USC § 1956 (a)(1)), and tax fraud. Accessory and/or accomplice liability should be considered if factually appropriate. Other relevant factors might include convenience of the victim and witnesses, docket load and speed of trial, and which jurisdiction has the best resources, including specialized personnel and economic considerations, to most effectively handle the prosecution.

JURY SELECTION
Jury selection is important. This is one of only 3 opportunities the prosecutor has to speak directly to the jury, the others being the opening and closing statements. This is

the only time there are any dialogue and exchange of ideas between the counselors and the jurors. During this crucial stage of the trial, gaining a rapport with the jurors and getting a feel for the people in whose hands the decision of guilt or innocence will be placed is paramount. While each jurisdiction has specific local or court rules regarding the type of allowable *voir dire*, this article addresses the widest possible scope of *voir dire*.

In selecting a jury for these cases, certain concepts apply across the board. First, prosecutors should envision an ideal individual whom they would like to see as a juror. This individual should empathize with children, feel comfortable with hearing and believing the testimony of a child, hold adults accountable for their actions, have some awareness of this type of child abuse, and be committed to the rule of law. Second, prosecutors should develop a theme that will be carried throughout the trial. Third, prosecutors need to decide on which points they want to educate the jury during *voir dire*. Issues of witness credibility; questions related to the appearance, conduct, and/or character of a state's witness; questions related to expert testimony; and potential juror biases or prejudices should all be explored. Fourth, case-specific facts (eg, the victim being male, the victim having drug or behavior problems, the victim having engaged in criminal behavior) should be introduced by the prosecutor at this stage. Another problem area would be victim recantation (Marx, 1999). Each juror's attitude toward adult prostitution should be explored. The prosecutor can be in the best position to determine who the best jurors for the state would be to hear this case only if the potential juror has as full a picture of the case as the particular jurisdiction allows.

In order to prosecute these cases, prosecutors must disabuse jurors of the widespread myths about children forced or drawn into prostitution (**Table 32-3**). These myths allow and encourage the exploitation of children. Society must become aware of the true profile of the prostituted child and understand the reasons children are brought into prostitution.

Individuals who prostitute children generally use these commonly accepted myths about prostitution to justify their abuse. The abusers distort reality to claim that the child consented, and therefore, no harm has been done. Unfortunately, abusers are not alone in holding these views. Public acceptance of prostitution as a "legitimate" business or an unavoidable evil is widespread. The erroneous tendency to regard sexually exploitative johns as human beings with human needs rather than as child abusers further undermines the ability of the criminal justice system to safeguard against the prostitution of children. Until prosecutors are able to refute the myths that surround prostitution, children will continue to be victimized by its practice.

The following refutes the common myths about the prostitution of children that are listed in **Table 32-3**.

Prostitution is a Victimless Crime

When an adult uses a prostituted child for sexual gratification, it is called ***child sexual abuse***. The fact that the abuser gives the child money does not alter the fact that child abuse occurred. If the child is younger than the legally recognized age of consent, the fact that the child "consented" is equally irrelevant. The consent of the abused child is never a legally recognized defense in child sexual abuse cases because the child can not give meaningful consent (Phipps, 1997). The presence of money merely allows perpetrators to engage in rationalizations that eradicate personal responsibility for their own actions.

Immediate harm to the prostituted child is blatantly apparent and comes in many forms. Degrading and humiliating sexual encounters, muggings, severe beatings, rape, and even death are the reality of prostituted children. Unwanted pregnancy, human immunodeficiency virus (HIV) and/or AIDS as well as other STDs are also constant

---

> **Table 32-3. Myths about the Prostitution of Children**
>
> — Prostitution is a victimless crime.
>
> — Children freely choose prostitution.
>
> — Prostitution can be an exciting and glamorous life and can offer wealth and independence to the children.
>
> — Prostitution is a deterrent to sex crimes.

facts of life for these children. Long-term physical and psychological health problems can also be expected (WHO, 1996).

Children Freely Choose Prostitution

Minors are most frequently driven to prostitution to escape abusive and/or neglectful homes. These children are not running *to* prostitution; they are running *from* dysfunctional authority figures who emotionally, physically, and/or sexually abused them. For many of these children, the only way to escape the abuse is to run away from it. Unfortunately, they jump out of the frying pan and into the fire. Young and frightened children who possess limited or no skills and who are unable to find shelter become easy prey for pimps or johns. Once involved in prostitution, both pimps and johns replicate the abuse the children endured in their home life. Eighty percent of all adult prostitutes began as prostituted children (Davidson, 1996).

Prostitution Can Be an Exciting and Glamorous Life

Cultural mythology regarding prostitution is built on intentionally distorted misinformation. The typical depiction of the prostitution lifestyle in movies, on television, on video, and in printed material is far from the truth. The movie *Pretty Woman* is an example of one of the worst offenders, while *Leaving Las Vegas* is one of the few high-profile films that offers a far more accurate portrayal of the bleak realities of the lifestyle. The truth is that prostituted children suffer immediate harm in the form of physical, sexual, and/or emotional degradation and humiliation, as well as longterm physical and psychological effects (Estes, 2001; Davidson, 1996). There is nothing glamorous about the reality of prostitution.

The economics of prostitution are complex. If a child is controlled by a pimp, most or all of the money earned by the child will go to the pimp. If the child works independently for a house of prostitution, a large percentage of that child's earnings are given to the house. The child's ability to set up independent funds is carefully guarded because economic dependence is part of the pimp's strategy. Any profit made by the child is often spent as rapidly as it is obtained, thereby perpetuating the need for continued participation in the system.

The reality is that prostituted children are controlled by their johns and/or their pimps. Once involved with a pimp, the child loses autonomy. The more involved a child becomes, the more difficult it is to get out of prostitution. Pimps demand money from the children; shortfalls often result in punishment. If a child balks at performing the acts demanded by the abuser, this can result in violence. The exploiter and the abuser choose children because children are easier to physically assault and intimidate into doing as they are told. These assaults are rarely reported to the police, which further reinforces the child's feelings of isolation and powerlessness.

Prostitution Is a Deterrent to Sex Crimes

There is no methodologically sound evidence whatsoever that prostitution deters sex crimes. Rapists and child molesters commit their crimes out of a desire to control and exert power over their victims or to humiliate and degrade their victims. While sex offenders use prostituted children as additional victims, this only strengthens their belief that sexual violence and exploitation are acceptable. The fact that these crimes often go unreported allows the perpetrator to gain confidence and strike again. Prostitution does *not* deter sex crimes; rather, it promotes them (Kreston, 2000).

OPENING STATEMENT

This is the prosecutor's second opportunity to speak to the jury directly and the first opportunity the prosecution has to present its theory of the case as well as provide the jury with a theme that the prosecution can return to throughout the trial and again during the closing argument. Such themes for these cases might include the following: "catastrophically misplaced love" (ie, if the victim is "in love" with the pimp); "out of the frying pan and into the fire" (ie, if the child ran away from home to escape sexual violence and/or physical abuse); or "sex with a child is sex with a child" (ie, if the defense runs along the lines of "no harm, no foul" or otherwise tries to attack the victim). At this point in the trial, the prosecutor must begin the personalization of the victim. The prosecutor should refer to the victim by name and take every opportunity to show the child as a unique human being who has been violated by the defendant.

Brevity is the soul of wit and the essence of a good opening. The rules of primacy and latency hold that people tend to remember what they hear first and last. Prosecutors should keep their opening statements brief and merely provide a blueprint of the evidence the State will present. If there are problems with the case, such as recantation or drug usage by the victim, discuss them now; do not allow the defense to broach these subjects first. Do not oversell the case or promise more than can be delivered. Finally, ask for the jury to return the only just and true verdict possible after the presentation of all the evidence, which is guilty as charged.

CASE IN CHIEF

Prosecutors need to recognize prostitution of children for what it is: child abuse. The fact that the defendant does not present himself or herself as the stereotypical child molester does not justify a failure to prosecute other types of child sexual abuse, so it should not be used as a justification in cases in which children have been prostituted either. Case acceptance rate should reflect this even with the difficulties surrounding a case with a less than sympathetic victim. Strategies must be created to deal with the child's lack of credibility in front of the jury. The dislike jurors initially feel for the child may be successfully shifted to the defendant through the use of expert witnesses to show that the pimp and/or molester made the child who he or she is today. Expert witnesses may be used to bolster the child's credibility by confirming the existence and reality of prostituted children's experiences.

Victim Testimony

A number of issues must be addressed regarding the victim's testimony. First, determine whether the victim is cooperative. If the victim will not cooperate, the reasons why must be understood so these reasons can be explained to the jury. Determine whether the victim fears the defendant or sees the defendant as a boyfriend or girlfriend. Either way, the motivation for the victim to deny events that occurred, refuse to testify, or claim memory loss must be dealt with for the trier of fact.

If the victim denies previously acknowledged events, prosecutors may attempt to impeach the victim's denials with prior inconsistent statements. If the child is simply refusing to testify, hearsay exceptions may allow for the admission of prior statements, such as excited utterance (Federal Rule of Evidence 803 and its state equivalents), prior identification (Federal Rule of Evidence 803 and its state equivalents), present sense impression, or medical diagnosis and treatment. If the victim has a genuine loss of memory, standard hearsay exceptions may allow for the admissibility of previous statements. If the victim is feigning memory loss, impeachment with prior inconsistent statements is allowed. The need to consider supplementing the child's testimony with that of an expert to explain to the jury the reasons the child is not cooperating will be addressed later.

If the victim is going to testify, the child's statement concerning the way he or she became involved in prostitution *must* be explored. If the child was a runaway, why did he or she run? How did the child meet the pimp? Did the pimp approach the child directly or did the first contact occur through a "runner" or agent of the pimp? How did the prostitution begin? Why did the child not leave the pimp? Did the child fear the pimp? Did the child feel loyal to or have feelings for the pimp? Was the child ever subjected to violence? All these issues need to be dealt with, because the jury requires a full picture of what happened to the victim in order to understand many of the dynamics at work in these cases.

Law Enforcement Testimony

The testimony of law enforcement officers should fulfill 3 tasks in the prosecution of these cases: to provide background information regarding the prostitution of children, to explain the details of this particular case and, to assure the jurors that the law enforcement officers involved took this case seriously while investigating. Upon taking the stand, the prosecutor should first ask the investigator to discuss his or her qualifications and background and should then seek to qualify the law enforcement officer or detective as an expert in the field of prostituted children and the investigation of such cases (eg, as is done to qualify a drug officer in that specialty). After providing background regarding the dynamics of the prostitution of children, the prosecutor should then lay out the specific details of the case. The prosecutor should especially provide jurors with a complete picture of the child's life, the facts of the case, and the evidence amassed against the defendant. The final task required of the investigator is referred to as ***impression management***. This means that the investigator must inform the jurors about the time and effort put forth by law enforcement officers while investigating this case. The investigator conveys that commitment through the testimony's style and substance so that the jury is left without doubt that this case is taken seriously by the police and is viewed in the same light as other types of crimes against children and violent crime.

Additional Expert Testimony

In jurisdictions that allow syndrome or typology evidence, 2 additional types of expert witnesses should be considered: a child sexual abuse accommodation syndrome (CSAAS) expert (Summit, 1983) and an offender typologist. Both expert witnesses should be presented as "pure" experts; that is, they have no knowledge of the facts regarding this particular case and do not have a stake in the trial's outcome (eg, *State v DeCosta*, 772 A 2d 340, 343 [NH 2001]). Rather, their testimony is about the various behaviors exhibited by the victims or the offenders.

The CSAAS expert would be called to educate the jury about the counterintuitive aspects of the sexually exploited child's behavior. Most children become victims of prostitution through deceit and manipulation. As with the preferential child molester, the pimp seduces these children (Lanning, 2001; Walsh & Fassett, 2001). The pimp gains the child's trust and then exploits that trust. The child perceives that the pimp provides comfort, affection, understanding, and protection. In addition, the pimp makes the child feel loved and, initially, asks nothing in return, much as the traditional parent would do within a family.

The CSAAS expert could explain to the jury such issues as entrapment and accommodation, recantation, and the child's feelings of helplessness to help jurors understand the psychology of the child victim and the reason the child could not simply leave the situation. Especially since the issue of recantation is so prevalent in these cases, the expert's testimony can assist the trier of fact in understanding an area of special knowledge well outside that of the average juror (Myers, 1997, suppl 2002).

The State may also wish to call an offender typologist, who will testify to the way that the exploiter selects a victim and looks for a child who will not tell or who is unlikely to be believed even if he of she does disclose what is happening. The expert can also testify to the way the exploiter initially engages a child and then grooms that child for abuse by lowering the child's inhibitions toward sexual matters and breaking down emotional barriers. Exploiters do this either by seducing and grooming the child for prostitution or by exerting violence or blackmail over the child to ensure compliance. Finally, the expert can discuss the ways the exploiter gets the child to conceal their "secret" or goes about discrediting the child so that if the secret is disclosed, the likelihood of the child being believed is noticeably lowered (*United States v Long*, 2003; *United States v Romero*, 1999).

Usually, these experts should be placed on the stand before the child testifies. The prosecutor must show the way that the child's behaviors are consistent with the testimony of the CSAAS and the way the general grooming cycle was reflected in the actions of this particular offender when exploiting this particular victim.

Meeting Untrue Defenses
Mistake of Age
Untrue defenses may be divided into 2 major camps: those attacking criminal intent and those attacking the relevant law or law enforcement practices. The first kind of untrue defense is typified by the "mistake of age" defense. State laws are divided on this issue; some allow the defendant to raise such a defense and others specifically preclude it within their statutes (Klain, 1999). Mistake of age should only be raised if the term "knowingly" is present in the state statute. If the law does not specifically address this issue, case law should be examined for precedent excluding this defense. If this defense is raised, it should be combated with a series of questions designed to show how impossible such a defense is in this case. The prosecutor needs to present information to prove that there is no way this defendant could have genuinely believed this child was an adult (eg, the length of time the defendant and victim have known each other, the circumstances under which they met, the child's appearance if factually appropriate, the child's maturity level, the child's intellectual development, the child's voice and conversational ability). In the federal system, while 18 USC § 2242(b) does require the State to show proof of knowledge of the minor's age (ie, "[*k*]*nowingly* persuade, induce, entice or coerce a minor to travel in interstate commerce to engage in prostitution or any criminal sexual act"), 18 USC § 2423(a) and (b) do not have any such requirement. In *United States v Taylor* (2001), "[i]gnorance of age provides no safe harbor from the penalties in § 2423(a)," and in *United States v Griffith* (2002), the government is not required to prove that the defendant knew the child's age.

Factual or Legal Impossibility
The second type of untrue defense is one used when law enforcement officers employed undercover techniques and the defendant thought he or she was going to have sex with a child but, in fact, no child was involved. This has been rejected at the federal level with one circuit ruling that the defendant unquestionably intended to engage in illegal conduct but failed only because of circumstances unknown to him, that is, a 14-year-old girl turned out to be an FBI agent (*United States v Farner*, 2001). Another circuit followed that same rationale and held that the existence of a minor is not required in order to convict (*United States v Root*, 2002). When state courts have addressed the issue, some have specifically precluded it by statute while others allow it. Even in those jurisdictions that do allow this defense, it should stand if the charge of attempt and analogies to drug cases in which undercover agents sell fake drugs may be used. In both cases, undercover law enforcement officers put themselves in harm's way in order to protect real victims from the defendant.

Other Untrue Defenses
These defenses tend to fall under the rubric of consent (or "it was her idea"), the

Good Samaritan, and "the victim is lying." These should be dealt with along the lines of traditional child abuse cases. Any allegation of consent should be excluded through pretrial motions because no such defense to charges of sex crimes against children exists. Children can not consent to an illegal act. If, somehow, this defense does manage to be raised during the case, the defense may be refuted by arguing that the law exists as much to protect children from themselves as from adults.

If the molester defendant attempts to transfer responsibility to the child for what occurred and claims that the child was the aggressor, then, because the child is a child, even if the child was the aggressor, that fact is irrelevant and does not erase the adult defendant's culpability for his or her acts.

If the pimp defendant argues that he or she was unaware of the victim's activities and was merely acting as a Good Samaritan by providing food, clothing, and shelter, common sense impossibilities can be used to dispute this allegation. The prosecutor can ask the following questions:

— Where did the pimp think the child went when he or she left?

— Did the pimp ever leave with the child?

— At what times did the child leave?

— Did the child ever have any extra spending money, new clothes, and so on?

— How did the pimp think the child obtained this extra money, new clothes, and so on?

This overlaps with the defense that the child is lying. This defense can be raised by either the molester and/or john or the exploiter and/or pimp. Basically this defense can be reduced to the victim's credibility and the police investigation vs. the self-serving story put forward by the defendant(s). Since prostituted children generally do not enter the courtroom cloaked in an aura of trustworthiness, all aspects of the investigation must be documented and, if at all possible, corroborated. Emphasize the child has no motive to lie, and explain any negative consequences that have followed the victim's disclosure of what happened. Any information obtained during the suspect interrogation should be used to expose the defendant as the one with the real motive to lie.

CLOSING

The closing arguments may be broken down into 2 parts—opening close and rebuttal argument. Some states (eg, Minnesota) do not allow rebuttal close, but most state and federal courts do. The first line of opening close should reference the theme and theory of the case, which the prosecutor began developing during jury selection. After reiterating the theme, the prosecutor summarizes the evidence and the way that evidence proves each element of the case beyond a reasonable doubt. The State's strongest points should be presented first, but the prosecutor should address any weaknesses (eg, a difficult or uncooperative victim). Next, the prosecutor needs to dispose of the defenses by assessing claims of innocence in light of the evidence and common sense.

While the defense gives its closing argument, the prosecutor should note the arguments being made and be ready to respond to them point by point. The prosecutor should address these points in order of their importance, that is, dispose of the strongest point first and work down to the trivial or ridiculous.

A number of things must be covered during closing. The prosecutor must correct misstatements of fact. In addition, any question the defense has raised regarding the way certain things were or were not done during the investigation must be addressed. At this time, the prosecutor should expose the defense strategy. This is the time for righteous indignation. For example, if the defense tries to attack the victim's character, the prosecutor can turn this around by discussing the way the defendant is using the "Dixie" defense; that is, "look away" from the charged offense and try the child instead. The prosecutor should reinforce and recapitulate the State's strong points (eg, the vulnerability of an unstable child, the cynical, calculating nature of the defendant) and conclude the closing statement with a definitive concluding sentence. This concluding sentence should be delivered with confidence (eg, "Sex with a child is sex with a child" or "No child is disposable").

Finally, the prosecutor should refer to the jury instructions that the judge is about to read. These instructions will usually reinforce a lack of legal defenses as well as the status of the child victim (*United States v Lawrence*, 1999 US App LEXIS 16967 in § 2423 (a) and (b)).

SENTENCING

At the time of the offender's sentencing, the judge's pronouncement should reflect the community's feelings of revulsion toward child abuse as well as the seriousness and harm of the defendant's conduct. From a sentencing perspective, the defendant who sexually exploited a prostituted child must be punished as severely as all other child molesters. If the defendant has been charged and convicted of child abuse, the punishment should be consistent with the punishments for other types of child sexual abuse. If the defendant has been found guilty or pled guilty to a prostitution-related charge, the sentence should still reflect the seriousness of the underlying reality that child abuse has occurred. The prosecutor should be prepared to refute dubious claims in mitigation. For example, the defendant may claim to have suffered enough through the public humiliation of a trial. This point can be refuted by arguing the trial was necessary because of the defendant's refusal to accept responsibility for his or her actions and the child is actually the person who endured the ordeal of testifying, thereby acting as aggravating factors. The prosecutor must create and protect a record that will support sentencing.

Another possible avenue to explore during sentencing is the designation of the defendant and/or molester as a sexual offender for purposes of community registration and notification under the local equivalent of Megan's law. This would entail designating a conviction for prostituting a child as a predicate offense to trigger registration under sex offender statutes and/or community notification.

Other sentencing options include restitution to the victim to help defray the costs of counseling and other attendant rehabilitation expenses. In addition, the defendant could be made to forfeit any property that was used in this criminal activity (eg, cars, houses).

VICTIM ASSISTANCE

Prosecutors and other members of the multidisciplinary team should explore the availability of specialized treatment and/or reintegration programs provided by social services or not-for-profit organizations that can assist the child victims. (Two programs that may be contacted for assistance in instituting such treatment are Children of the Night and the Paul & Lisa Program). Many children who are targeted for this type of exploitation may be able to obtain Victims of Crime Assistance, which is usually a monetary award that can be used toward counseling and long-term rehabilitation needs. This is easiest to effectuate in cases in which the child is designated a victim. In other cases, it may be necessary to style the child's criminal justice role as that of a material witness to activate eligibility for such funding. The source of such funding may come from the federal Office of Victims of Crimes monies, if the crime is pursued in federal court, or from state and local victim restitution funding, which may be administered through the local prosecuting attorney's office. These funds are most often used for counseling and other restitutional expenses incurred by the victim and perhaps even the victim's family.

Other victim needs must be met. A transitional living program must be created for the child. The exact goals of such a program will vary with the child's age. For the youngest victims, the child's return to the home or to members of the extended family may be one goal. If the child should not or can not be returned, then placement through local social services would be another option. This option, however, may be problematic since the child may suffer severe behavioral difficulties as a result of the exploitation.

For older children, group homes, family host homes, foster care, or institutional placement may be the most appropriate. Some unique issues must be addressed when assisting older children. If the child has left the street involuntarily (eg, through police and social service intervention), that child may need to be segregated from other children to avoid putting those children at risk of being recruited. Long-term, residential treatment centers may be the most appropriate transitional environment for some children, but the number of such facilities is low and the expense is high. Regardless of whether the child is in transition voluntarily or not, the child should be relocated from the geographical area in which the victimization occurred to deter the pimp attempting to reassert control. Intensive counseling to address the child's anxieties to help the child and learn new behaviors must be provided.

A successful transition to a safe and supportive environment can not be accomplished overnight; merely taking the child off the streets is not enough. Best practices indicate that, at a minimum, 18 months of transition are necessary to accomplish any significant change in the child's life. These children often arrive at their counselors with poor self-esteem issues, no sense of control over their lives, a lack of future orientation or goals, drug dependency, and the presence of moderate to severe mental illness (Estes & Weiner, 2001). These children remain at risk for a number of long-term consequences as a result of being prostituted, such as depression, post-traumatic stress disorder, alcohol abuse, drug abuse, and other psychological and physical illnesses (Estes &Weiner, 2001; Willis & Levy, 2002). A quick fix does not exist for these children. The time and resources necessary to accomplish a meaningful, permanent transformation for the lives of these children must be put into place.

Conclusion

Prostituted children are victims, *not* criminals. The criminals are those individuals who supply or demand the children. The criminal justice community must become leaders in recognizing these crimes as forms of child sexual abuse. Cases against all individuals who sexually exploit children, whether for economic gain or their own sexual gratification, must be thoroughly investigated and resolutely prosecuted. A guilty defendant is a sex offender; the penalties for those convicted of prostituting children should reflect the seriousness of this reality.

The realities of the recovered child must also be addressed. Facilities and resources need to be made available to these children to help them transition out of exploitation. Physical and mental health counseling, education, and basic job skills are the types of fundamental, but far-reaching, assistance that must be offered to these children. If these children are to have any realistic hope of successfully reintegrating into a mainstream community, they must have meaningful and genuine access to the tools necessary to permanently rebuild and redirect their lives.

References

Brinkley J. Vast trade in forced labor portrayed in CIA report. *New York Times.* April 2, 2000:A7.

Collins P. Plenary address. Presented at: Internet Crimes Against Children Conference; December 7, 2001; New Orleans, La.

Davidson JO. The sex exploiter. Paper presented at: World Congress Against Commercial Sexual Exploitation of Children; August 28, 1996; Stockholm, Sweden.

ECPAT International. *Child Sex Tourism Action Survey.* New York, NY: ECPAT; 2001.

ECPAT International. Frequently asked questions about commercial sexual exploitation of children. Available at: http://www.ecpat.com/eng/CSEC/faq/faq6.asp. Accessed May 2, 2004.

ECPAT-USA. Child sex tourism. Available at: http://www.ecpatusa.org/travel_tourism.asp. Accessed May 2, 2004.

8 USCS §1101(a)(15)(T)(i).

8 USCS §1184(n)(2).

18 USC §1952.

18 USC §1956(a)(1).

18 USC § 2241.

18 USC § 2242(b).

18 USC § 2243.

18 USC § 2423(b), 1994.

18 USCA § 2422(b).

18 USCA § 2423(a).

18 USCA § 2423(b).

18 USCS § 1591.

Estes RJ, Weiner NA. *The Commercial Sexual Exploitation of Children in the US, Canada and Mexico.* Philadelphia: University of Pennsylvania, School of Social Work; 2001.

Federal Rule of Evidence 412.

Federal Rule of Evidence 803.

Finkelhor D, Ormrod R. *Offenders Incarcerated for Crimes Against Juveniles* . Washington, DC: US Dept of Justice, Office of Justice Programs, Office of Juvenile Justice and Delinquency Prevention; 2001.

Hammer H, Finkelhor D, Sedlak A. *National Incidence Studies of Missing, Abducted, Runaway, and Thrownaway Children. Runaway/Thrownaway Children: National Estimates and Characteristics.* Washington, DC: US Dept of Justice; October 2002. Available at: http://www.ncjrs.org/pdffiles1/ojjdp/196469.pdf. Accessed May 2, 2004.

Klain EV. Prostitution of children and child-sex tourism: an analysis of domestic and international responses. *NCMEC.* 1999; 2.

Kreston SS. Prostituted children: not an innocent image. *The Prosecutor.* 2000;34(6).

Kreston SS. Search and seizure in cases of computers and child pornography. Available at: http://www.ndaa-apri.org/publications/newsletters/apri_update_vol_12_no_9_1999.html. Accessed May 2, 2004.

Lanning KV. *Child Molesters: A Behavioral Analysis.* 4th ed. Alexandria, Va: National Center for Missing & Exploited Children; 2001.

Lanning KV. The compliant and cooperating victim. *APSAC Advisor.* 2002;14(2) (special issue):4-9.

La Rev Stat Ann § 14.42.

La Rev Stat Ann § 14.82.1 (West, 1986; Supp, 1999)

La Rev Stat Ann § 14.86.

Malcolm J. Opening (US) session statement. Presented at: Second World Congress on the Commercial Sexual Exploitation of Children; December 17-20, 2001; Yokohama, Japan.

Marx SP. Victim recantation in child sexual abuse cases: a team approach to prevention, investigation and trial. *J Aggression Maltreatment Trauma.* 1999;2(2)(pt 4).

Minn Stat Ann § 609.322 (West Supp, 2000).

Myers JEB. *Evidence in Child Abuse and Neglect Cases.* 3rd ed. New York, NY: Aspen Law and Business; 1997(suppl 2002):101-121, 557.

NCPCA. State statutes. Available at: http://ndaa-apri.org/apri/programs/ncpca/statutes.html. Accessed May 2, 2004.

NY Penal Code § 230.04-06.

Phipps CA. Children, adults, sex and the criminal law: in search of reason. *Seton Hall Legis J.* 1997;22(1):33-34,119-124.

Spangenberg M. *Prostituted Youth in New York City: An Overview.* New York, NY: ECPAT-USA; 2001.

State v DeCosta, 772 A 2d 340, 343 (NH 2001).

Summit RC. The child sexual abuse accommodation syndrome. *Child Abuse Negl.* 1983;7:177-192.

Tyrangiel J, Bonesteel A. Pinch on the pimps. *Time.* March 19, 2001;157(11):63.

Under plea deal, former NIH scientist will spend up to a year in jail. *Washington Post.* February 19, 1997:A1.

United States v Farner, 251 F3d 510 (5th Cir 2001).

United States v Griffith, 284 F3d 338 (2nd Cir 2002).

United States v Lawrence, 1999 US App LEXIS 16967.

United States v Long, 238 F3d 655 (DC Cir 2003).

United States v Romero, 189 F3d 576 (7th Cir 1999), *cert denied.*

United States v Root, 296 F3d 1222 (11th Cir 2002).

United States v Spruill, 296 F3d 580 (7th Cir 2002).

United States v Taylor, 239 F3d 994 (9th Cir 2001).

22 USCA 7101, et seq.

22 USCS § 7102(2)(A).

22 USCS § 7102(9).

22 USCS § 7105(b)(1)(A).

22 USCS § 7105(b)(1)(E)(i)(I).

US Department of State (USDOS). Trafficking in persons report. US Dept of State. July 2003. Available at: http://www.state.gov/g/tip/rls/tiprpt/2003/21262.htm. Accessed May 2, 2004.

Vieth VI. In my neighbor's house: a proposal to address child abuse in rural America. *Hamline Law Rev* 1998;22:143.

Walsh W, Fassett B. Juvenile prostitution: an overlooked form of child sexual abuse. *The APSAC Advisor.* 1994;7(1):9.

Whitcomb D, Eastin J. *Joining Forces Against Child Sexual Exploitation: Models for a Multijurisdictional Team Approach.* Washington, DC: Office for Victims of Crime, US Dept of Justice; 1998.

Willis BM, Levy BS. Child prostitution: global health burden, research needs, and interventions. *Lancet.* 2002;359:1417-1422.

World Health Organization. *Commercial Sexual Exploitation of Children: The Health and Psychosocial Dimensions.* Stockholm, Sweden: CSEC World Congress; 1996. Available at: http://www.csecworldcongress.org/PDF/en/Stockholm/Background_reading/Theme_papers/Theme%20paper%20Health%201996_EN.pdf. Accessed May 2, 2004.

APPENDIX 32-1: CRIMES INVOLVING THE PROSTITUTION OF CHILDREN

The following lists a synopsis of statutes dealing with the prostitution of children in the United States.* This list is current as of January 14, 2004. Please note that these statutes may change; criminal justice professionals should consult their state's statutes regularly to monitor such changes.

STATE LEGISLATION

Alabama

Ala Code § 13A-12-110. Definitions.
The following definitions are applicable in Sections 13A-12-111 through 13A-12-113:

A person "advances prostitution" if, acting other than as a prostitute or a patron of a prostitute, he knowingly causes or aids a person to commit or engage in prostitution, procures or solicits patrons for prostitution, provides persons or premises for prostitution purposes, operates or assists in the operation of a house of prostitution or a prostitution enterprise.

A person "profits from prostitution" if, acting other than as a prostitute receiving compensation for personally rendered prostitution services, he accepts or receives money or other property pursuant to a prior agreement with any person whereby he participates or is to participate in the proceeds of prostitution activity.

Ala Code § 13A-12-111. Promoting Prostitution in the First Degree.
A person commits the crime of promoting prostitution in the first degree if he knowingly advances or profits from prostitution of a person less than 16 years of age.

Promoting prostitution in the first degree is a Class B felony, *which carries a definite term of imprisonment with hard labor for not more than 20 years or less than 2 years, pursuant to § 13A-5-6. A Class B felony offender is also required to pay a fine fixed by the court of not more than $10 000, pursuant to § 13A-5-11.*

Ala Code § 13A-12-112. Promoting Prostitution in the Second Degree.
A person commits the crime of promoting prostitution in the second degree if he knowingly advances or profits from prostitution of a person less than 18 years of age.

Promoting prostitution in the second degree is a Class C felony, which carries a definite term of imprisonment with hard labor for not more than 10 years or less than 1 year and 1 day. A Class C felony offender is also required to pay a fine fixed by the court of not more than $5000 pursuant to § 13A-5-11.

---

* *Disclaimer: Test provisions in italics are not part of the child prostitution statutes but are sentence provisions that correspond to the enumerated statutory offense levels.*

Alaska

Alaska Stat § 11.66.110. Promoting Prostitution in the First degree.

A person commits the crime of promoting prostitution in the first degree if the person as other than a patron of a prostitute, induces or causes a person under 16 years of age to engage in prostitution. A person convicted under this section is guilty of a Class A felony. A defendant convicted of a Class A felony may be sentenced to a definite term of imprisonment of not more than 20 years and shall be sentenced to presumptive terms that are subject to adjustment pursuant to § 12.55.125.

A person commits the crime of promoting prostitution in the first degree if the person induces or causes a person in that person's legal custody to engage in prostitution. A person convicted under this section is guilty of a Class B felony. *A defendant convicted of a Class B felony may be sentenced to a definite term of imprisonment of not more than 10 years and shall be sentenced to presumptive terms that are subject to adjustment pursuant to § 12.55.125.*

In a prosecution under this section, it is not a defense that the defendant reasonably believed that the person induced or caused to engage in prostitution was 16 years of age or older.

Alaska Stat § 11.66.130. Promoting Prostitution in the Third Degree.

A person commits the crime of promoting prostitution in the third degree if, with intent to promote prostitution, the person as other than a patron of a prostitute, induces or causes a person 16 years of age or older to engage in prostitution. Promoting prostitution in the third degree is a Class A misdemeanor. *A defendant convicted of a Class A misdemeanor may be sentenced to a definite term of imprisonment of not more than 1 year pursuant to § 12.55.135.*

Arizona

Ariz Rev Stat Ann § 13-3206. Taking Child for Purpose of Prostitution; Classification.

A person who takes away any minor from such person's father, mother, guardian, or other person having the legal custody of such person, for the purpose of prostitution, is guilty of a Class 4 felony. If the minor is under 15 years of age, taking a child for prostitution is a Class 2 felony.

Ariz Rev Stat Ann § 13-3212. Child Prostitution; Classification.

A person commits child prostitution by knowingly: causing any minor to engage in prostitution; using any minor for purposes of prostitution; permitting a minor under such person's custody or control to engage in prostitution; receiving any benefit for or on account of procuring or placing a minor in any place or in the charge or custody of any person for the purpose of prostitution; receiving any benefit pursuant to an agreement to participate in the proceeds of prostitution of a minor; financing, managing, supervising, controlling or owning, either alone or in association with others, prostitution activity involving a minor; or transporting or financing the transportation of any minor through or across this state with the intent that such minor engage in prostitution.

Child prostitution is a Class 2 felony, and if the minor is under 15 years of age, it is punishable pursuant to § 13-604.01.

Pursuant to § 13-701, a Class 2 felony carries a term of imprisonment of 5 years, and a Class 4 felony carries a term of imprisonment of 2 years. If the defendant stands convicted of a dangerous crime against children, the provisions of § 13-604.01 apply. A "dangerous crime against children" includes taking a child for the purpose of prostitution and child prostitution when committed against a minor who is under 15 years of age. If the convicted person is at least 18 years of age or was tried as an adult and that person was convicted of a dangerous crime against children in the first degree, that person shall be sentenced to a presumptive term of imprisonment for 20 years.

Arkansas

Ark Code Ann § 5-70-101. Definitions.

A person advances prostitution if, acting other than as a prostitute or a patron of a prostitute, he knowingly: causes or aids a person to commit or engage in prostitution; procures or solicits patrons for prostitution; provides persons or premises for prostitution purposes; operates or assists in the operation of a house of prostitution or a prostitution enterprise; or engages in any other conduct designed to institute, aid, or facilitate an act or enterprise of prostitution.

A person profits from prostitution if, acting other than as a prostitute receiving compensation for personally rendered prostitution services, he accepts or receives money or other property pursuant to an agreement or understanding with any person whereby he participates or is to participate in the proceeds of prostitution.

Ark Code Ann § 5-70-104. Promoting Prostitution in the First Degree.

A person commits the offense of promoting prostitution in the first degree if he knowingly advances prostitution, or profits from prostitution, of a person less than 18 years old.

Promoting prostitution in the first degree is a Class D felony, *which carries a sentence not to exceed 6 years pursuant to § 5-4-401 and a fine not to exceed $10 000 pursuant to § 5-4-201.*

California

Cal Penal Code § 266. Inveiglement or Enticement of Unmarried Female Under 18 for Purposes of Prostitution, etc.; Aiding and Abetting; Procuring Female for Illicit Intercourse by False Pretenses; Punishment.

Every person who inveigles or entices any unmarried female, of previous chaste character, under the age of 18 years, into any house of ill fame, or of assignation, or elsewhere, for the purpose of prostitution, or to have illicit carnal connection with any man; and every person who aids or assists in such inveiglement or enticement; and every person who, by any false pretenses, false representation, or other fraudulent means, procures any female to have illicit carnal connection with any man, is punishable by imprisonment in the state prison, or by imprisonment in a county jail not exceeding 1 year, or by a fine not exceeding $2000 or by both such fine and imprisonment.

Cal Penal Code § 266i. Pandering; Punishment.

(a) Except as provided in subdivision (b), any person who does any of the following is guilty of pandering, a felony, and shall be punished by imprisonment in the state prison for 3, 4, or 6 years:

(1) Procures another person for the purpose of prostitution.

(2) By promises, threats, violence, or by any device or scheme, causes, induces, persuades or encourages another person to become a prostitute.

(3) Procures for another person a place as an inmate in a house of prostitution or as an inmate of any place in which prostitution is encouraged or allowed within this state.

(4) By promises, threats, violence or by any device or scheme, causes, induces, persuades or encourages an inmate of a house of prostitution, or any other place in which prostitution is encouraged or allowed, to remain therein as an inmate.

(5) By fraud or artifice, or by duress of person or goods, or by abuse of any position of confidence or authority, procures another person for the purpose of prostitution, or to enter any place in which prostitution is encouraged or allowed within this state, or to come into this state or leave this state for the purpose of prostitution.

(6) Receives or gives, or agrees to receive or give, any money or thing of value for procuring, or attempting to procure, another person for the purpose of prostitution, or to come into this state or leave this state for the purpose of prostitution.

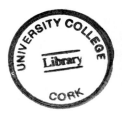

(b) If the other person is a minor over the age of 16 years, the offense is punishable by imprisonment in the state prison for 3, 4, or 6 years. Where the other person is under 16 years of age, the offense is punishable by imprisonment in the state prison for 3, 6, or 8 years.

Cal Penal Code § 267. Abduction; Person Under 18 for Purpose of Prostitution; Punishment.

Every person who takes away any other person under the age of 18 years from the father, mother, guardian, or other person having the legal charge of the other person, without their consent, for the purpose of prostitution, is punishable by imprisonment in the state prison and a fine not exceeding $2000.

Colorado

Colo Rev Stat § 18-7-401. Definitions.

A "child" is a person under 18 years of age.

"Prostitution by a child" means either a child performing or offering or agreeing to perform any act of sexual intercourse, fellatio, cunnilingus, masturbation, or anal intercourse with any person not the child's spouse in exchange for money or other thing of value or any person performing or offering or agreeing to perform any act of sexual intercourse, fellatio, cunnilingus, masturbation, or anal intercourse with any child not the person's spouse in exchange for money or other thing of value.

"Prostitution of a child" means either inducing a child to perform or offer or agree to perform any act of sexual intercourse, fellatio, cunnilingus, masturbation, or anal intercourse with any person not the child's spouse by coercion or by any threat or intimidation or inducing a child, by coercion or by any threat or intimidation or in exchange for money or other thing of value, to allow any person not the child's spouse to perform or offer or agree to perform any act of sexual intercourse, fellatio, cunnilingus, masturbation, or anal intercourse with or upon such child. Such coercion, threat, or intimidation need not constitute an independent criminal offense and shall be determined solely through its intended or its actual effect upon the child.

Colo Rev Stat § 18-7-402. Soliciting for Child Prostitution.

A person commits soliciting for child prostitution if he: solicits another for the purpose of prostitution of a child or by a child; arranges or offers to arrange a meeting of persons for the purpose of prostitution of a child or by a child; or directs another to a place knowing such direction is for the purpose of prostitution of a child or by a child.

Soliciting for child prostitution is a Class 3 felony.

Colo Rev Stat § 18-7-403. Pandering of a Child.

Any person who does any of the following for money or other thing of value commits pandering of a child: inducing a child by menacing or criminal intimidation to commit prostitution, which is a Class 2 felony; or knowingly arranging or offering to arrange a situation in which a child may practice prostitution, which is a Class 3 felony.

Colo Rev Stat § 18-7-403.5. Procurement of a Child.

Any person who intentionally gives, transports, provides, or makes available, or who offers to give, transport, provide, or make available, to another person a child for the purpose of prostitution of the child commits procurement of a child, which is a Class 3 felony.

Colo Rev Stat § 18-7-404. Keeping a Place of Child Prostitution.

Any person who has or exercises control over the use of any place that offers seclusion or shelter for the practice of prostitution and who performs any one or more of the following commits keeping a place of child prostitution if he: knowingly grants or permits the use of such place for the purpose of prostitution of a child or by a child or permits the continued use of such place for the purpose of prostitution of a child or by a child after becoming aware of facts or circumstances from which he should reasonably know that the place is being used for purposes of such prostitution.

Keeping a place of child prostitution is a Class 3 felony.

Colo Rev Stat § 18-7-405. Pimping of a Child.
Any person who knowingly lives on or is supported or maintained in whole or in part by money or other thing of value earned, received, procured, or realized by a child through prostitution commits pimping of a child, which is a Class 3 felony.

Colo Rev Stat § 18-7-405.5. Inducement of Child Prostitution.
Any person who by word or action, other than conduct specified in section 18-7-403(1)(a) *(ie, inducing a child by menacing or criminal intimidation to commit prostitution)*, induces a child to engage in an act that is prostitution by a child, commits inducement of child prostitution.

Inducement of child prostitution is a Class 3 felony.

Colo Rev Stat § 18-7-406. Patronizing a Prostituted Child.
Any person who performs any of the following with a child not his spouse commits patronizing a prostituted child: engages in an act that is prostitution of a child or by a child; or enters or remains in a place of prostitution with intent to engage in an act that is prostitution of a child or by a child.

Patronizing a prostituted child is a Class 3 felony.

Colo Rev Stat § 18-7-407. Criminality of Conduct.
In any criminal prosecution under sections 18-7-402 to 18-7-407, it shall be no defense that the defendant did not know the child's age or that he reasonably believed the child to be 18 years of age or older.

Pursuant to § 18-1.3-401, the presumptive range of penalty for a Class 3 felony is a minimum of 4 years' imprisonment, a maximum of 12 years' imprisonment, and a mandatory parole period of 5 years. A defendant who stands convicted of a Class 3 felony is subject to a fine in addition to, or in lieu of, any sentence of imprisonment in the specified range of $3000 to $750 000.

Connecticut
Conn Gen Stat Ann § 53a-85. Promoting Prostitution: Definitions.
A person "advances prostitution" when, acting other than as a prostitute or as a patron thereof, he knowingly causes or aids a person to commit or engage in prostitution, procures or solicits patrons for prostitution, provides persons or premises for prostitution purposes, operates or assists in the operation of a house of prostitution or a prostitution enterprise, or engages in any other conduct designed to institute, aid, or facilitate an act or enterprise of prostitution.

A person "profits from prostitution" when acting other than as a prostitute receiving compensation for personally rendered prostitution services, he accepts or receives money or other property pursuant to an agreement or understanding with any person whereby he participates or is to participate in the proceeds of prostitution activity.

Conn Gen Stat Ann § 53a-86. Promoting Prostitution in the First Degree: Class B Felony.
A person is guilty of promoting prostitution in the first degree when he knowingly advances or profits from prostitution of a person less than 16 years old.

Promoting prostitution in the first degree is a Class B felony, *which carries a definite sentence of imprisonment fixed by the court of a term not less than 1 year nor more than*

20 years pursuant to § 53a-35a. Pursuant to § 53a-41, the court shall fix a fine following the conviction of a felony offense in an amount not to exceed $15 000.

Conn Gen Stat Ann § 53a-87. Promoting Prostitution in the Second Degree: Class C Felony.
A person is guilty of promoting prostitution in the second degree when he knowingly advances or profits from prostitution of a person less than 18 years old.

Promoting prostitution in the second degree is a Class C felony, *which carries a definite sentence of imprisonment fixed by the court of a term not less than 1 year nor more than 10 years pursuant to § 53a-35a. Pursuant to § 53a-41, the court shall fix a fine following the conviction of a felony offense in an amount not to exceed $10 000.*

Conn Gen Stat Ann § 53a-90a. Enticing a Minor. Penalties.
A person is guilty of enticing a minor when such person uses an interactive computer service to knowingly persuade, induce, entice or coerce any person under 16 years of age to engage in prostitution or sexual activity for which the actor may be charged with a criminal offense. For purposes of this section, "interactive computer service" means any information service, system, or access software provider that provides or enables computer access by multiple users to a computer server, including specifically a service or system that provides access to the Internet and such systems operated or services offered by libraries or educational institutions.

Enticing a minor is a Class A misdemeanor for a first offense, a Class D felony for a second offense and a Class C felony for any subsequent offense.

Pursuant to § 53a-36, a sentence of imprisonment for a Class A misdemeanor shall not exceed 1 year. Pursuant to § 53a-42, a fixed fine for a Class A misdemeanor shall be fixed at an amount not to exceed $2000. Pursuant to § 53a-35a, a Class C felony carries a fixed term of imprisonment not less than 1 year nor more than 10 years. A Class D felony, pursuant to the same, carries a fixed term of imprisonment of not less than 1 year nor more than 5 years. Pursuant to § 53a-41, the court shall fix a fine following the conviction of a felony offense in an amount not to exceed $5000 for a Class D felony and an amount not to exceed $10 000 for a Class C felony.

Delaware
Del Code Ann tit 11, § 1352. Promoting Prostitution in the Second Degree; Class E Felony.
A person is guilty of promoting prostitution in the second degree when the person knowingly advances or profits from prostitution of a person less than 18 years old. *A Class E felony carries a fixed term of incarceration of up to 5 years, pursuant to tit. 11, § 4205.*

Del Code Ann tit 11, § 1353. Promoting Prostitution in the First Degree; Class C Felony.
A person is guilty of promoting prostitution in the first degree when the person knowingly advances or profits from prostitution of a person less than 16 years old. *A Class C felony carries a fixed term of incarceration of up to 15 years pursuant to tit. 11, § 4205.*

Del Code Ann tit 11, § 1356. Definitions Relating to Prostitution.
"Advance prostitution." A person advances prostitution when, acting other than as a prostitute or as a patron thereof, the person knowingly causes or aids a person to commit or engage in prostitution, procures or solicits patrons for prostitution, provides persons or premises for prostitution purposes, operates or assists in the operation of a house of prostitution or a prostitution enterprise, or engages in any other conduct designed to institute, aid, or facilitate an act or enterprise of prostitution.

"Profit from prostitution." A person profits from prostitution when, acting other than as a prostitute receiving compensation for personally rendered prostitution services, the person accepts or receives money or other property pursuant to an agreement or understanding with any person whereby the person participates or is to participate in the proceeds of prostitution activity.

District of Columbia

DC Code Ann § 22-2704. Abducting or Enticing Child From his or her Home for Purposes of Prostitution; Harboring Such Child.

Any person who, for purposes of prostitution, persuades, entices, or forcibly abducts a child under 16 years of age from his or her home or usual abode, or from the custody and control of the child's parents or guardian, shall be punished by imprisonment for not less than 2 years and not more than 20 years; and whoever knowingly secretes or harbors any child so persuaded, enticed, or abducted shall be punished by imprisonment for not more than 8 years.

Florida

Fla Stat Ann ch 796.03. Procuring Person Under Age of 18 for Prostitution.

A person who procures for prostitution, or causes to be prostituted, any person who is under the age of 18 years commits a felony of the second degree, punishable according to § 775.082, § 775.083, and § 775.084.

Pursuant to § 775.082, a felony of the second degree is punishable by a term of imprisonment not exceeding 15 years. A fine not to exceed $10 000 may also be imposed, pursuant to § 775.083.

Georgia

Ga Code Ann § 16-6-13. Punishment for Keeping a Place of Prostitution, Pimping, or Pandering.

A person convicted of keeping a place of prostitution, pimping, or pandering when such offense involves keeping a place of prostitution for, the pimping for, or the solicitation of a person under the age of 18 years to perform an act of prostitution or the assembly of two or more persons under the age of 18 years at a fixed place for the purpose of being solicited by others to perform an act of prostitution shall be guilty of a felony and shall be punished by imprisonment for a period of not less than 5 nor more than 20 years and such convicted person shall be fined not less than $2500 nor more than $10 000. Adjudication of guilt or imposition of a sentence for a conviction of a second or subsequent offense when such offense involves keeping a place of prostitution for, the pimping for, or pandering of a person under the age of 18 years pursuant to this subsection, including a plea of *nolo contendere*, shall not be suspended, probated, deferred, or withheld.

Hawaii

Haw Rev Stat Ann § 712-1200. Prostitution.

A person commits the offense of prostitution if the person engages in, or agrees or offers to engage in, sexual conduct with another person for a fee.

Haw Rev Stat Ann § 712-1201. Promoting Prostitution; Definition of Terms.

A person "advances prostitution" if, acting other than as a prostitute or a patron of a prostitute, he knowingly causes or aids a person to commit or engage in prostitution, procures or solicits patrons for prostitution, provides persons for prostitution purposes, permits premises to be regularly used for prostitution purposes, operates or assists in the operation of a house of prostitution or a prostitution enterprise, or engages in any other conduct designed to institute, aid, or facilitate an act or enterprise of prostitution.

A person "profits from prostitution" if, acting other than as a prostitute receiving compensation for personally rendered prostitution services, he accepts or receives money or other property pursuant to an agreement or understanding with any person whereby he participates or is to participate in the proceeds of prostitution activity.

Haw Rev Stat Ann § 712-1202. Promoting Prostitution in the First Degree.
A person commits the offense of promoting prostitution in the first degree if the person knowingly advances or profits from prostitution of a person less than 16 years old.

Promoting prostitution in the first degree is a Class B felony, *which carries an indeterminate term of imprisonment of up to 10 years pursuant to § 706-660. A person convicted of a Class B felony may also be sentenced to pay a fine not exceeding $25 000 pursuant to § 706-640.*

Haw Rev Stat Ann § 712-1203. Promoting Prostitution in the Second Degree.
A person commits the offense of promoting prostitution in the second degree if the person knowingly advances or profits from prostitution of a person less than 18 years old.

Promoting prostitution in the second degree is a Class C felony, *which carries an indeterminate term of imprisonment of up to 5 years, pursuant to § 706-660. A person convicted of a Class C felony may also be sentenced to pay a fine not exceeding $10 000 pursuant to § 706-640.*

Idaho
Idaho Code § 18-5609. Inducing Person Under 18 Years of Age into Prostitution: Penalties.
Every person who induces or attempts to induce a person under the age of 18 years to engage in prostitution shall be guilty of a felony punishable by imprisonment in the state penitentiary for a period of not less than 2 years, which may be extended to life imprisonment, or by a fine not exceeding $50 000, or by both such fine and imprisonment.

Idaho Code § 18-5611. Inducing Person Under 18 Years of Age to Patronize a Prostitute: Penalties.
Any person who induces or attempts to induce a person under the age of 18 years to patronize a prostitute shall be guilty of a felony *which is punishable by imprisonment in a state prison not exceeding 5 years, or by a fine not exceeding $50 000, or by both pursuant to § 18-112.*

Illinois
720 Ill Comp Stat § 5/11-14. Prostitution.
Any person who performs, offers, or agrees to perform any act of sexual penetration for any money, property, token, object, or article or anything of value, or any touching or fondling of the sex organs of one person by another person, for any money, property, token, object, or article or anything of value, for the purpose of sexual arousal or gratification commits an act of prostitution.

Prostitution is a Class A misdemeanor. A person convicted of a second or subsequent violation of this Section is guilty of a Class 4 felony. When a person has one or more prior convictions, the information or indictment charging that person shall state such prior conviction so as to give notice of the State's intention to treat the charge as a felony. The fact of such prior conviction is not an element of the offense and may not be disclosed to the jury during trial unless otherwise permitted by issues properly raised during such trial.

A person who violates this Section within 1000 feet of real property comprising a school commits a Class 4 felony.

720 Ill Comp Stat § 5/11-15.1. Soliciting for a Juvenile Prostitute.
Any person who violates any of the provisions of this act commits soliciting for a ju-

venile prostitute where the prostitute for whom such person is soliciting is under 16 years of age.

It is an affirmative defense to a charge of soliciting for a juvenile prostitute that the accused reasonably believed the person was of the age of 16 years or over at the time of the act giving rise to the charge.

Soliciting for a juvenile prostitute is a Class 1 felony, *which carries a sentence of imprisonment of not less than 4 years and not more than 15 years and a period of mandatory supervised release of 2 years pursuant to 730 Ill Comp Stat § 5/5-8-1.*

720 Ill Comp Stat § 5/11-17.1. Keeping a Place of Juvenile Prostitution.

Any person who knowingly violates any of the provisions of Section 5/11-17 of this Act commits keeping a place of juvenile prostitution when any prostitute in the place of prostitution is under 16 years of age.

It is an affirmative defense to a charge of keeping a place of juvenile prostitution that the accused reasonably believed the person was of the age of 16 years or over at the time of the act giving rise to the charge.

Keeping a place of juvenile prostitution is a Class 1 felony, *which carries a sentence of imprisonment of not less than 4 years and not more than 15 years, and a period of mandatory supervised release of 2 years, pursuant to 730 Ill Comp Stat § 5/5-8-1. A person convicted of a second or subsequent violation of this Section is guilty of a Class X felony, which carries a sentence of imprisonment of not less than 6 years and not more than 30 years, as well as a period of mandatory supervised release of 3 years pursuant to 730 Ill Comp Stat § 5/5-8-1.*

720 Ill Comp Stat § 5/11-18.1. Patronizing a Juvenile Prostitute.

Any person who engages in an act of sexual penetration as defined in Section 12-12 of this Code with a prostitute under 17 years of age commits the offense of patronizing a juvenile prostitute.

It is an affirmative defense to the charge of patronizing a juvenile prostitute that the accused reasonably believed that the person was of the age of 17 years or over at the time of the act giving rise to the charge.

A person who commits patronizing a juvenile prostitute is guilty of a Class 4 felony *which carries a sentence of imprisonment of not less than 1 year and not more than 3 years, as well as a period of mandatory supervised release of 1 year pursuant to 730 Ill Comp Stat § 5/5-8-1.*

720 Ill Comp Stat § 5/11-19.1. Juvenile Pimping.

Any person who receives any money, property, token, object, or article or anything of value from a prostitute under 16 years of age, not for a lawful consideration, knowing it was earned in whole or in part from the practice of prostitution, commits juvenile pimping.

It is an affirmative defense to a charge of juvenile pimping that the accused reasonably believed the person was of the age of 16 years at the time of the act giving rise to the charge.

Juvenile pimping is a Class 1 felony, *which carries a sentence of imprisonment of not less than 4 years and not more than 15 years, as well as a period of mandatory supervised release of 2 years pursuant to 730 Ill Comp Stat § 5/5-8-1.*

720 Ill Comp Stat § 5/11-19.2. Exploitation of a Child.

A person commits exploitation of a child when he or she confines a child under the age of 16 against his or her will by the infliction or threat of imminent infliction of great bodily harm, permanent disability or disfigurement or by administering to the child without his or her consent or by threat or deception and for other than medical purposes, any alcoholic intoxicant or a drug and: compels the child to become a prostitute; arranges a situation in which the child may practice prostitution; or receives any money, property, token, object, or article or anything of value from the child knowing it was obtained in whole or in part from the practice of prostitution.

Exploitation of a child is a Class X felony, *which carries a sentence of imprisonment of not less than 6 years and not more than 30 years, as well as a period of mandatory supervised release of 3 years pursuant to 730 Ill Comp Stat § 5/5-8-1.*

Indiana
Ind Code § 35-45-4-4. Promoting Prostitution.
A person who knowingly or intentionally entices or compels another person to become a prostitute commits promoting prostitution, a Class B felony, if the person enticed or compelled is under 18 years of age. *Pursuant to § 35-50-2-5, a person who commits a Class B felony shall be imprisoned for a fixed term of 10 years, with not more than 10 years added for aggravating circumstances or not more than 4 years subtracted for mitigating circumstances; in addition, he may be fined not more than $10 000.*

Iowa
Iowa Code § 725.3(2). Pandering.
A person who persuades, arranges, coerces, or otherwise causes a minor to become a prostitute or to return to the practice of prostitution after having abandoned it, or keeps or maintains any premises for the purpose of prostitution involving minors or knowingly shares in the income from such premises knowing the character and content of such income, commits a Class C felony.

The maximum sentence prescribed by statute for a Class C felon, not a habitual offender, shall be for no more than 10 years, and an additional fine of at least $1000, but not more than $10 000, pursuant to § 902.9.

Kansas
Kan Stat Ann § 21-3512. Prostitution.
Prostitution is performing for hire or offering or agreeing to perform for hire where there is an exchange of value, any of the following acts: sexual intercourse, sodomy, or manual or other bodily contact stimulation of the genitals of any person with the intent to arouse or gratify the sexual desires of the offender or another. Prostitution is a Class B nonperson misdemeanor.

Kan Stat Ann § 21-3513. Promoting Prostitution.
Promoting prostitution is: establishing, owning, maintaining, or managing a house of prostitution, or participating in the establishment, ownership, maintenance, or management thereof; permitting any place partially or wholly owned or controlled by the defendant to be used as a house of prostitution; procuring a prostitute for a house of prostitution; inducing another to become a prostitute; soliciting a patron for a prostitute or for a house of prostitution; procuring a prostitute for a patron; procuring transportation for, paying for the transportation of, or transporting a person within this state with the intention of assisting or promoting that person's engaging in prostitution; or being employed to perform any act which is prohibited by this section.

Promoting prostitution is a Class A person misdemeanor when the prostitute is 16 or more years of age.

Promoting prostitution is a severity level 6, person felony when the prostitute is under 16 years of age.

The sentencing grid that provides the penalties for non-drug offenses may be found in § 21-4704.

Kentucky

Ky Rev Stat Ann § 529.030. Promoting Prostitution in the First Degree.
A person is guilty of promoting prostitution in the first degree when he knowingly advances or profits from prostitution of a person less than 18 years old. Promoting prostitution in the first degree is a Class C felony if the minor so used is less than 18 years old at the time the minor engages in the prohibited activity, a Class B felony if the minor so used is less than 16 years old at the time the minor engages in the prohibited activity, and a Class A felony if the minor so used incurs physical injury thereby.

The authorized maximum terms of imprisonment for a Class A felony are not less than 20 years or more than 50 years or life imprisonment; not less than 10 years or more than 20 years for a Class B felony; and not less than 5 years or more than 10 years for a Class C felony pursuant to § 532.060.

In addition to any other punishment imposed, a person convicted of a felony shall be sentenced to pay a fine in an amount not less than $1000 and not more than $10 000, or double his gain from the commission of the offense, whichever is greater. The amount to be paid shall be determined by the court after consideration of enumerated factors, set forth in § 534.030.

Louisiana

La Rev Stat Ann § 14:82. Prostitution; Definition; Penalties; Enhancement.
Prostitution is: (1) the practice by a person of indiscriminate sexual intercourse with others for compensation or (2) the solicitation by one person of another with the intent to engage in indiscriminate sexual intercourse with the latter for compensation.

Whoever commits the crime of prostitution shall be fined not more than $500 or be imprisoned for not more than 6 months or both.

On a second conviction, the offender shall be fined not less than $250 or more than $2000 or be imprisoned, with or without hard labor, for not more than 2 years, or both. On a third and subsequent conviction the offender shall be imprisoned, with or without hard labor, for not less than 2 or more than 4 years and shall be fined not less than $500 or more than $4000.

La Rev Stat Ann § 14:82.1. Prostitution; Persons Under 17; Additional Offenses.
It shall be unlawful: (1) for any person over the age of 17 to engage in sexual intercourse with any person under the age of 17 who is practicing prostitution, and there is an age difference of greater than 2 years between the two persons. Lack of knowledge of the latter person's age shall not be a defense; (2) for any parent or tutor of any person under the age of 17 knowingly to consent to the person's entrance or detention in the practice of prostitution.

Whoever violates the provisions of this section shall be fined not more than $5000 or imprisoned, with or without hard labor, for not less than two years nor more than 10 years or both.

La Rev Stat Ann § 14:86. Enticing Persons Into Prostitution.
Enticing persons into prostitution is committed when any person over the age of 17 entices, places, persuades, encourages, or causes the entrance of any other person under the age of 21 into the practice of prostitution, either by force, threats, promises, or by any other device or scheme. Lack of knowledge of the other person's age shall not be a defense.

Whoever commits the crime of enticing persons into prostitution shall be imprisoned, with or without hard labor, for not less than 2 years nor more than 10 years.

Maine

Me Rev Stat Ann tit 17-A, § 852. Aggravated Promotion of Prostitution.
A person is guilty of aggravated promotion of prostitution if he knowingly promotes

prostitution of a person less than 18 years old. Aggravated promotion of prostitution is a Class B crime.

For a Class B crime, the court may sentence the offender to imprisonment for a definite term to be served at a specified county jail if the term of imprisonment is 9 months or less, or at the Department of Corrections if the term of imprisonment is more than 9 months. The court shall set a definite period not to exceed 10 years (§ 1252).

Me Rev Stat Ann tit 17-A, § 855. Patronizing Prostitution of a Minor.
A person is guilty of patronizing prostitution of a minor if in return for another's prostitution he gives or agrees to give a pecuniary benefit either to the person whose prostitution is sought or to a third person and the person whose prostitution is sought has not yet attained his eighteenth birthday.

Patronizing prostitution of a minor is a Class D crime. *For a Class D crime, the court must specify a county jail as the place of imprisonment, and the court shall set a definite period of imprisonment of less than 1 year (§ 1252).*

Maryland
Md Ann Code § 11-303. Pandering.
A parent, guardian, or person who has permanent or temporary care or custody or responsibility for supervision of another may not consent to the taking or detention of the other for prostitution. A person who violates this section is guilty of the misdemeanor of pandering and on conviction is subject to imprisonment not exceeding 10 years or a fine not exceeding $5000 or both.

Md Ann Code § 11-305. Abduction of Child Under 16.
A person may not: (1) persuade or entice or aid in the persuasion or enticement of an individual under the age of 16 years from the individual's home or from the custody of the individual's parent or guardian; or (2) knowingly secrete or harbor or aid in the secreting or harboring of an individual under the age of 16 years who has been persuaded or enticed in the manner described in item (1) of this subsection.

A person who violates this section is guilty of a misdemeanor and on conviction is subject to imprisonment not exceeding 10 years or a fine not exceeding $5000 or both.

Massachusetts
Mass Gen Laws Ann ch. 272, § 4A. Inducing Minor Into Prostitution.
Whoever induces a minor to become a prostitute, or who knowingly aids and assists in such inducement, shall be punished by imprisonment in the state prison for not more than 5, nor less than 3 years, and by a fine of $5000. The sentence of imprisonment imposed under this section shall not be reduced to less than 3 years, nor suspended, nor shall any person convicted under this section be eligible for probation, parole, or furlough or receive any deduction from his sentence for good conduct or otherwise until he shall have served 3 years of such sentence. Prosecutions commenced under this section shall not be continued without a finding nor placed on file.

Mass Gen Laws Ann ch 272, § 4B. Living off or Sharing Earnings of Minor Prostitute.
Whoever lives or derives support or maintenance, in whole or in part, from the earnings or proceeds of prostitution committed by a minor, knowing the same to be earnings or proceeds of prostitution, or shares in such earnings, proceeds or monies, shall be punished by imprisonment in the state prison for not less than 5 years and by a fine of $5000. The sentence imposed under this section shall not be reduced to less than 5 years, nor suspended, nor shall any person convicted under this section be eligible for probation, parole or furlough or receive any deduction from his sentence for good conduct or otherwise until he shall have served 5 years of such sentence. Prosecutions commenced under this section shall not be continued without a finding nor placed on file.

Michigan

Mich Stat Ann § 750.13. Enticing Away Female Under 16.

Any person who shall take or entice away any female under the age of 16 years, from her father, mother, guardian, or other person having the legal charge of her person, without their consent, either for the purpose of prostitution, concubinage, sexual intercourse or marriage, shall be guilty of a felony, punishable by imprisonment in the state prison not more than 10 years.

Minnesota

Minn Stat Ann § 609.322. Solicitation, Inducement, and Promotion of Prostitution.

Whoever, while acting other than as a prostitute or patron, intentionally does any of the following may be sentenced to imprisonment for not more than 20 years or to payment of a fine of not more than $40 000, or both: (1) solicits or induces an individual under the age of 18 years to practice prostitution; (2) promotes the prostitution of an individual under the age of 18 years; or (3) receives profit, knowing or having reason to know that it is derived from the prostitution, or the promotion of the prostitution, of an individual under the age of 18 years.

Whoever, while acting other than as a prostitute or patron, intentionally does any of the following may be sentenced to imprisonment for not more than 15 years or to payment of a fine of not more than $30 000, or both: (1) solicits or induces an individual to practice prostitution; or (2) promotes the prostitution of an individual; or (3) receives profit, knowing or having reason to know that it is derived from the prostitution, or the promotion of the prostitution, of an individual.

Subdivisions 1, clause (3), and 1a, clause (3), do not apply to: (1) a minor who is dependent on an individual acting as a prostitute and who may have benefited from or been supported by the individual's earnings derived from prostitution; or (2) a parent over the age of 55 who is dependent on an individual acting as a prostitute, who may have benefited from or been supported by the individual's earnings derived from prostitution, and who did not know that the earnings were derived from prostitution; or (3) the sale of goods or services to a prostitute in the ordinary course of a lawful business.

Minn Stat Ann § 609.324. Other Prostitution Crimes; Patrons, Prostitutes, and Individuals Housing Individuals Engaged in Prostitution; Penalties.

Whoever intentionally does any of the following may be sentenced to imprisonment for not more than 20 years or to payment of a fine of not more than $40 000, or both: (1) engages in prostitution with an individual under the age of 13 years; or (2) hires or offers or agrees to hire an individual under the age of 13 years to engage in sexual penetration or sexual contact.

Whoever intentionally does any of the following may be sentenced to imprisonment for not more than 10 years or to payment of a fine of not more than $20 000 or both: (1) engages in prostitution with an individual under the age of 16 years but at least 13 years; or (2) hires or offers or agrees to hire an individual under the age of 16 years but at least 13 years to engage in sexual penetration or sexual contact.

Whoever intentionally does any of the following may be sentenced to imprisonment for not more than 5 years or to payment of a fine of not more than $10 000 or both: (1) engages in prostitution with an individual under the age of 18 years but at least 16 years; or (2) hires or offers or agrees to hire an individual under the age of 18 years but at least 16 years to engage in sexual penetration or sexual contact.

Any person, other than one related by blood, adoption, or marriage to the minor, who permits a minor to reside, temporarily or permanently, in the person's dwelling without the consent of the minor's parents or guardian, knowing or having reason to know that the minor is engaging in prostitution may be sentenced to imprisonment for not more than one year or to payment of a fine of not more than $3000, or both; except that, this subdivision does not apply to residential placements made, sanctioned, or supervised by a public or private social service agency.

Whoever solicits or accepts a solicitation to engage for hire in sexual penetration or sexual contact while in a public place may be sentenced to imprisonment for not more than one year or to payment of a fine of not more than $3000 or both. Except as otherwise provided in subdivision 4, a person who is convicted of violating this subdivision while acting as a patron must, at a minimum, be sentenced to pay a fine of at least $1500.

Whoever intentionally does any of the following may be sentenced to imprisonment for not more than 90 days or to payment of a fine of not more than $700, or both: (1) engages in prostitution with an individual 18 years of age or above; or (2) hires or offers or agrees to hire an individual 18 years of age or above to engage in sexual penetration or sexual contact. Except as otherwise provided in subdivision 4, a person who is convicted of violating clause (1) or (2) while acting as a patron must, at a minimum, be sentenced to pay a fine of at least $500.

Whoever violates the provisions of this subdivision within 2 years of a previous conviction may be sentenced to imprisonment for not more than one year or to payment of a fine of not more than $3000 or both. Except as otherwise provided in subdivision 4, a person who is convicted of a gross misdemeanor violation of this subdivision while acting as a patron, must, at a minimum, be sentenced as follows: (1) to pay a fine of at least $1500; and (2) to serve 20 hours of community work service.

Minn Stat Ann § 609.352. Solicitation of Children to Engage in Sexual Conduct.

"Child" means a person 15 years of age or younger.

"Sexual conduct" means sexual contact of the individual's primary genital area, sexual penetration as defined in section 609.341, or sexual performance as defined in section 617.246.

"Solicit" means commanding, entreating, or attempting to persuade a specific person in person, by telephone, by letter, or by computerized or other electronic means.

A person 18 years of age or older who solicits a child or someone the person reasonably believes is a child to engage in sexual conduct with intent to engage in sexual conduct is guilty of a felony and may be sentenced to imprisonment for not more than three years or to payment of a fine of not more than $5000 or both.

Mistake as to age is not a defense to a prosecution under this section.

Mississippi

Miss Code Ann § 97-5-5. Enticing Child Under Fourteen; Punishment.

Every person who shall maliciously, willfully, or fraudulently lead, take, carry away, decoy or entice away, any child under the age of 14 years, with intent to detain or conceal such child from its parents, guardian, or other person having lawful charge of such child, or for the purpose of prostitution, concubinage, or marriage, shall, on conviction, be imprisoned in the penitentiary not exceeding 10 years, or imprisoned in the county jail not more than 1 year, or fined not more than $1000 or both.

Missouri

Mo Rev Stat § 567.050. Promoting Prostitution in the First Degree.

A person commits the crime of promoting prostitution in the first degree if he knowingly promotes prostitution of a person less than 16 years old. Promoting prostitution in the first degree is a Class B felony. *For a Class B felony, the authorized term of imprisonment is not less than 5 years and not more than 15 years, pursuant to § 558.011.*

Montana

Mont Code Ann § 45-5-603. Aggravated Promotion of Prostitution.

A person commits the offense of aggravated promotion of prostitution if the person purposely or knowingly promotes prostitution of a child under the age of 18 years, whether or not the person is aware of the child's age; or promotes the prostitution of one's spouse, child, ward, or any person for whose care, protection, or support the person is responsible. A person convicted of aggravated promotion of prostitution of a child, who at the time of the offense is under 18 years of age, shall be punished by life imprisonment, or imprisonment in a state prison for a term of not less than 4 years or more than 100 years or a fine in an amount not to exceed $100 000, or both.

Nebraska

Neb Rev Stat § 28-805. Debauching a Minor; Penalty.

Any person not a minor commits the offense of debauching a minor if he or she shall debauch or deprave the morals of any boy or girl under the age of 17 years by lewdly inducing such boy or girl carnally to know any other person; or soliciting any such boy or girl to visit a house of prostitution or other place where prostitution, debauchery, or other immoral practices are permitted or encouraged, for the purpose of prostitution or sexual penetration; or arranging or assisting in arranging any meeting for such purpose between any such boy or girl and any female or male of dissolute character or any inmate of any place where prostitution, debauchery, or other immoral practices are permitted or encouraged; or arranging or aiding or assisting in arranging any meeting between any such boy or girl and any other person for the purpose of sexual penetration.

Debauching a minor is a Class I misdemeanor, and *shall be penalized by a sentence of not more than 1 year's imprisonment or $1000 in fine, pursuant to §28-106.*

Nevada

Nev Rev Stat § 201.300. Pandering: Definition; Punishment; Exception.

A person who: (a) induces, persuades, encourages, inveigles, entices, or compels a person to become a prostitute or to continue to engage in prostitution; (b) by threats, violence or by any device or scheme, causes, induces, persuades, encourages, takes, places, harbors, inveigles or entices a person to become an inmate of a house of prostitution or assignation place, or any place where prostitution is practiced, encouraged, or allowed; (c) by threats, violence, or by any device or scheme, by fraud or artifice, or by duress of person or goods, or by abuse of any position of confidence or authority, or having legal charge, takes, places, harbors, inveigles, entices, persuades, encourages or procures a person to enter any place within this state in which prostitution is practiced, encouraged, or allowed, for the purpose of prostitution; (d) by promises, threats, violence, or by any device or scheme, by fraud or artifice, by duress of person or goods, or abuse of any position of confidence or authority or having legal charge, takes, places, harbors, inveigles, entices, persuades, encourages or procures a person of previous chaste character to enter any place within this state in which prostitution is practiced, encouraged or allowed, for the purpose of sexual intercourse; (e) takes or detains a person with the intent to compel the person by force, threats, menace, or duress to marry him or any other person; or (f) receives, gives, or agrees to receive or give any money or thing of value for procuring or attempting to procure a person to become a prostitute or to come into this state or leave this state for the purpose of prostitution, is guilty of pandering.

A person who is found guilty of pandering of a child, if physical force or the immediate threat of physical force is used upon the child, is guilty of a Category B felony and shall be punished by imprisonment in the state prison for a minimum term of not less than 2 years and a maximum term of not more than 20 years and may be further punished by a fine of not more than $20 000. If no physical force or immediate threat of physical force is used upon the child, is guilty of a Category B felony and shall be punished by imprisonment in the state prison for a minimum term of not less than 1 year and a maximum term of not more than 10 years and may be further punished by a fine of not more than $10 000.

This section does not apply to the customer of a prostitute.

Nev Rev Stat § 201.330. Pandering: Detaining Person in Brothel Because of Debt; Penalties.

A person who attempts to detain another person in a disorderly house or house of prostitution because of any debt or debts the other person has contracted or is said to have contracted while living in the house is guilty of pandering.

A person who is found guilty of pandering of a child: (1) If physical force or the immediate threat of physical force is used upon the child, is guilty of a Category B felony and shall be punished by imprisonment in the state prison for a minimum term of not less than 2 years and a maximum term of not more than 20 years and may be further punished by a fine of not more than $20 000. (2) If no physical force or immediate threat of physical force is used upon the child, is guilty of a Category B felony and shall be punished by imprisonment in the state prison for a minimum term of not less than 1 year and a maximum term of not more than 10 years and may be further punished by a fine of not more than $10 000.

Nev Rev Stat § 201.340. Pandering: Furnishing Transportation; Penalties.

A person who knowingly transports or causes to be transported, by any means of conveyance, into, through or across this state, or who aids or assists in obtaining such transportation for a person with the intent to induce, persuade, encourage, inveigle, entice or compel that person to become a prostitute or to continue to engage in prostitution is guilty of pandering.

A person who is found guilty of pandering of a child: (1) If physical force or the immediate threat of physical force is used upon the child, is guilty of a Category B felony and shall be punished by imprisonment in the state prison for a minimum term of not less than 2 years and a maximum term of not more than 20 years and may be further punished by a fine of not more than $20 000. (2) If no physical force or immediate threat of physical force is used upon the child, is guilty of a Category B felony and shall be punished by imprisonment in the state prison for a minimum term of not less than 1 year and a maximum term of not more than 10 years and may be further punished by a fine of not more than $10 000.

Nev Rev Stat § 201.360. Placing Person in House of Prostitution: Penalties.

A person who is the spouse, parent, guardian or other legal custodian of a person under the age of 18 and permits, connives at or consents to the minor's being or remaining in any house of prostitution; or decoys, entices, procures, or in any manner induces a person, under the age of 21 years, to go into or visit, upon any pretext or for any purpose whatever, any house of ill fame or prostitution, or any room or place inhabited or frequented by any prostitute, or used for purposes of prostitution, is guilty of a felony.

A person who violates the above provisions shall be punished: (a) Where physical force or the immediate threat of physical force is used upon the other person, for a Category C felony; or (b) where no physical force or immediate threat of physical force is used, for a Category D felony. *A Category C felony is a felony for which a court shall sentence a convicted person to imprisonment in the state prison for a minimum term of not less than 1 year and a maximum term of not more than 5 years. In addition to any other penalty, the court may impose a fine of not more than $10 000, unless a greater fine is authorized or required by statute. A Category D felony is a felony for which a court shall sentence a convicted person to imprisonment in the state prison for a minimum term of not less than 1 year and a maximum term of not more than 4 years. In addition to any other penalty, the* *court may impose a fine of not more than $5000, unless a greater fine is authorized or required by statute (§ 193.130).*

New Hampshire

NH Rev Stat Ann § 645:2. Prostitution and Related Offenses.

A person is guilty of a misdemeanor if the person: (a) solicits, agrees to perform, or engages in sexual contact or sexual penetration in return for consideration; or (b) induces or otherwise purposely causes another to violate subparagraph (a); or (c) transports another into or within this state with the purpose of promoting or facilitating such other in engaging in conduct in violation of subparagraph (a); or (d) not being a legal dependent incapable of self support, knowingly is supported in whole or in part by the proceeds of violation of subparagraph (a); or (e) knowingly permits a place under such person's control to be used for violation of subparagraph (a); or (f) pays, agrees to pay, or offers to pay another person to engage in sexual contact or sexual penetration with the payor or with another person.

A person is guilty of a Class B felony if such person violates the provisions of subparagraphs (b), (c), (d), or (e) of paragraph I and the violation involves another person who is under the age of 18. A person is guilty under this section regardless of the sex of the persons involved.

The maximum sentence for a Class B felony is 7 years' imprisonment. A fine may also be imposed in addition to any sentence of imprisonment, the amount of which should not exceed $4000 (§ 651:2).

New Jersey

NJ Stat Ann § 2C:34-1. Prostitution and Related Offenses.

A person commits a crime of the second degree if: the actor knowingly promotes prostitution of a child under 18 whether or not the actor mistakenly believed that the child was 18 years of age or older, even if such mistaken belief was reasonable; or the actor knowingly promotes prostitution of the actor's child, ward, or any other person for whose care the actor is responsible. *In the case of a crime of the second degree, a person may be sentenced to imprisonment for a specific term of years that shall be fixed by the court and shall be between 5 years and 10 years, pursuant to § 2C:43-6. A person who has been convicted of an offense may be sentenced to pay a fine, to make restitution or both, such fine not to exceed $150 000.00 when the conviction is of a crime of the second degree pursuant to § 2C:43-3.*

A person commits a crime of the third degree if the actor knowingly engages in prostitution with a person under the age of 18, or if the actor enters into or remains in a house of prostitution for the purpose of engaging in sexual activity with a child under the age of 18, or if the actor solicits or requests a child under the age of 18 to engage in sexual activity. It shall be no defense to a prosecution under this paragraph that the actor mistakenly believed that the child was 18 years of age or older, even if such mistaken belief was reasonable. *In the case of a crime of the third degree, a person may be sentenced to imprisonment for a specific term of years which shall be fixed by the court and shall be between 3 years and 5 years, pursuant to § 2C:43-6. A person who has been convicted of an offense may be sentenced to pay a fine, to make restitution, or both, such fine not to exceed $15 000.00 when the conviction is of a crime of the third degree pursuant to § 2C:43-3.*

A person, other than the prostitute or the prostitute's minor child or other legal dependent incapable of self-support, who is supported in whole or substantial part by the proceeds of prostitution is presumed to be knowingly promoting prostitution.

New Mexico

NM Stat Ann § 30-6A-4. Sexual Exploitation of Children by Prostitution.

Any person knowingly receiving any pecuniary profit as a result of a child under the age of 16 engaging in a prohibited sexual act with another is guilty of a second-degree felony, unless the child is under the age of 13, in which event the person is guilty of a first-degree felony.

Any person hiring or offering to hire a child over the age of 13 and under the age of 16 to engage in any prohibited sexual act is guilty of a second-degree felony.

Any parent, legal guardian or person having custody or control of a child under 16 years of age who knowingly permits that child to engage in or to assist any other person to engage in any prohibited sexual act or simulation of such an act for the purpose of producing any visual or print medium depicting such an act is guilty of a third-degree felony.

The basic sentence of imprisonment for a first-degree felony is 18 years. The basic sentence for a second-degree felony for a sexual offense against a child is 15 years' imprisonment. For a third-degree felony for a sexual offense against a child, the basic term of imprisonment is 6 years. In addition to the imposition of a sentence of imprisonment, the court may impose a fine not to exceed: $15 000 for a first-degree felony; $12 500 for a second-degree felony for a sexual offense against a child; and $5000 for a third-degree felony. (§ 31-18-15)

New York
NY Penal Law § 230.04. Patronizing a Prostitute in the Third Degree.
A person is guilty of patronizing a prostitute in the third degree when, being over 21 years of age, he patronizes a prostitute and the person patronized is less than 17 years of age.

Patronizing a prostitute in the third degree is a Class A misdemeanor.

An offender shall be sentenced to a definite sentence not to exceed 1 year upon conviction of a Class A misdemeanor, pursuant to § 70.15. An offender may be sentenced to pay a fine in a fixed amount not to exceed $1000 for a Class A misdemeanor, pursuant to § 80.05.

NY Penal Law § 230.05. Patronizing a Prostitute in the Second Degree.
A person is guilty of patronizing a prostitute in the second degree when, being over 18 years of age, he patronizes a prostitute and the person patronized is less than 14 years of age.

Patronizing a prostitute in the second degree is a Class E felony.

NY Penal Law § 230.06. Patronizing a Prostitute in the First Degree.
A person is guilty of patronizing a prostitute in the first degree when he patronizes a prostitute and the person patronized is less than 11 years of age.

Patronizing a prostitute in the first degree is a Class D felony.

NY Penal Law § 230.07. Patronizing a Prostitute; Defense.
In any prosecution for patronizing a prostitute in the first, second, or third degrees, it is a defense that the defendant did not have reasonable grounds to believe that the person was less than the age specified.

NY Penal Law § 230.25. Promoting Prostitution in the Third Degree.
A person is guilty of promoting prostitution in the third degree when he knowingly advances or profits from prostitution of a person less than 19 years old.

Promoting prostitution in the third degree is a Class D felony.

NY Penal Law § 230.30. Promoting Prostitution in the Second Degree.
A person is guilty of promoting prostitution in the second degree when he knowingly advances or profits from prostitution of a person less than 16 years old.

Promoting prostitution in the second degree is a Class C felony.

NY Penal Law § 230.32. Promoting Prostitution in the First Degree.
A person is guilty of promoting prostitution in the first degree when he knowingly advances or profits from prostitution of a person less than 11 years old.

Promoting prostitution in the first degree is a Class B felony.

NY Penal Law § 230.35. Promoting Prostitution; Accomplice.
In a prosecution for promoting prostitution, a person less than 17 years of age from whose prostitution activity another person is alleged to have advanced or attempted to advance or profited or attempted to profit shall not be deemed to be an accomplice.

Pursuant to § 70, the maximum sentence of imprisonment for a person convicted of a felony is an indeterminate sentence and carries a term of imprisonment not exceeding: 25 years for a Class B felony, 15 years for a Class C felony, 7 years for a Class D felony, and 4 years for a Class E felony.

An offender may be sentenced to pay a fine for a felony in an amount fixed by the court, not exceeding the higher of $5000 or double the amount of the defendant's gain from the commission of the crime pursuant to § 80.00.

North Carolina

NC Gen Stat § 14-190.18. Promoting Prostitution of a Minor.
A person commits the offense of promoting prostitution of a minor if he knowingly:

(1) entices, forces, encourages, or otherwise facilitates a minor to participate in prostitution; or

(2) supervises, supports, advises, or protects the prostitution of or by a minor.

Mistake of age is not a defense to a prosecution under this section.

Violation of this section is a Class D felony.

NC Gen Stat § 14-190.19. Participating in Prostitution of a Minor.
A person commits the offense of participating in the prostitution of a minor if he is not a minor and he patronizes a minor prostitute. As used in this section, "patronizing a minor prostitute" means:

(1) soliciting or requesting a minor to participate in prostitution;

(2) paying or agreeing to pay a minor, either directly or through the minor's agent, to participate in prostitution; or

(3) paying a minor, or the minor's agent, for having participated in prostitution, pursuant to a prior agreement.

Mistake of age is not a defense to a prosecution under this section.

Violation of this section is a Class F felony.

Pursuant to § 15A-1340.17, the punishment limit for each class of felony offense is charted according to the prior record level.

North Dakota

ND Cent Code § 12.1-29-02. Facilitating Prostitution.
The offense of facilitating prostitution is a Class C felony if the actor intentionally causes another to remain a prostitute by force or threat, or the prostitute is the actor's spouse, child, or ward, or a person for whose care, protection, or support he is responsible, or the prostitute is, in fact, less than 16 years old.

The maximum penalty for a Class C felony is 5 years' imprisonment and/or a fine of $5000, pursuant to § 12.1-32-01.

Ohio

Ohio Rev Code Ann § 2907.21. Compelling Prostitution.

No person shall knowingly do any of the following: (1) compel another to engage in sexual activity for hire; (2) induce, procure, encourage, solicit, or request, or otherwise facilitate a minor to engage in sexual activity for hire, whether or not the offender knows the age of the minor; (3) pay or agree to pay a minor, either directly or through the minor's agent, so that the minor will engage in sexual activity, whether or not the offender knows the age of the minor; (4) pay a minor, either directly or through the minor's agent, for the minor having engaged in sexual activity, pursuant to a prior agreement, whether or not the offender knows the age of the minor; (5) allow a minor to engage in sexual activity for hire if the person allowing the child to engage in sexual activity for hire is the parent, guardian, custodian, person having custody or control, or person in loco parentis of the minor. Whoever violates this section is guilty of compelling prostitution. Except as otherwise provided in this division, compelling prostitution is a felony of the third degree. If the offender commits a violation of division (1) of this section and the person compelled to engage in sexual activity for hire in violation of that division is less than 16 years of age, compelling prostitution is a felony of the second degree.

The court shall impose a definite term of imprisonment in the range of 2 to 8 years for a felony of the second degree and a term in the range of 1 to 5 years for a felony of the third degree, pursuant to § 2929.14.

Ohio Rev Code Ann § 2907.22. Promoting Prostitution.

No person shall knowingly: (1) establish, maintain, operate, manage, supervise, control, or have an interest in a brothel; (2) supervise, manage, or control the activities of a prostitute in engaging in sexual activity for hire; (3) transport another or cause another to be transported across the boundary of this state or of any county in this state, in order to facilitate the other person's engaging in sexual activity for hire; (4) for the purpose of violating or facilitating a violation of this section, induce or procure another to engage in sexual activity for hire.

Whoever violates this section is guilty of promoting prostitution, a felony of the fourth degree. If any prostitute in the brothel involved in the offense, or the prostitute whose activities are supervised, managed, or controlled by the offender, or the person transported, induced, or procured by the offender to engage in sexual activity for hire, is a minor, whether or not the offender knows the age of the minor, then promoting prostitution is a felony of the third degree.

The court shall impose a definite term of imprisonment in the range of 1 to 5 years for a felony of the third degree and a term in the range of 6 to 18 months for a felony of the fourth degree, pursuant to § 2929.14.

Oklahoma

Okla Stat Ann tit 21, § 1087. Child Under 18 Years of Age—Procuring for Prostitution, Lewdness or Other Indecent Act—Punishment.

No person shall offer, or offer to secure, a child under 18 years of age for the purpose of prostitution, or for any other lewd or indecent act, or procure or offer to procure a child for, or a place for a child as an inmate in, a house of prostitution or other place where prostitution is practiced; receive or to offer or agree to receive any child under 18 years of age into any house, place, building, other structure, vehicle, trailer, or other conveyance for the purpose of prostitution, lewdness, or assignation, or to permit any person to remain there for such purpose; or direct, take, or transport, or to offer or agree to take or transport, or aid or assist in transporting, any child under 18 years of age to any house, place, building, other structure, vehicle, trailer, or other conveyance, or to any other person with knowledge or having reasonable cause to believe that the purpose of such directing, taking, or transporting is prostitution, lewdness, or assignation.

Any person violating the provisions of this section shall, upon conviction, be guilty of a felony punishable by imprisonment of not less than 1 year nor more than 10 years.

Any owner, proprietor, keeper, manager, conductor, or other person who knowingly permits any violation of this section in any house, building, room, or other premises or any conveyances under his control or of which he has possession shall, upon conviction for the first offense, be guilty of a misdemeanor and punishable by imprisonment in the county jail for a period of not less than 6 months nor more than 1 year, and by a fine of not less than $500 nor more than $5000. Upon conviction for a subsequent offense pursuant to this subsection such person shall be guilty of a felony and shall be punished by imprisonment in the state penitentiary for a period of not less than 1 year nor more than 10 years, or by a fine of not less than $5000 nor more than $25 000 or by both such fine and imprisonment.

Okla Stat Ann tit 21, § 1088. Child Under 18 Years of Age—Inducing, Keeping, Detaining or Restraining for Prostitution—Punishment.

No person shall: By promise, threats, violence, or by any device or scheme, including but not limited to the use of any controlled dangerous substance prohibited pursuant to the provisions of the Uniform Controlled Dangerous Substances Act, cause, induce, persuade, or encourage a child under 18 years of age to engage or continue to engage in prostitution or to become or remain an inmate of a house of prostitution or other place where prostitution is practiced; keep, hold, detain, restrain, or compel against his will, any child under 18 years of age to engage in the practice of prostitution or in a house of prostitution or other place where prostitution is practiced or allowed; directly or indirectly keep, hold, detain, restrain, or compel or attempt to keep, hold, detain, restrain, or compel a child under 18 years of age to engage in the practice of prostitution or in a house of prostitution or any place where prostitution is practiced or allowed for the purpose of compelling such child to directly or indirectly pay, liquidate, or cancel any debt, dues, or obligations incurred, or said to have been incurred by such child.

Any person violating the provisions of this section other than paragraph two of this subsection, upon conviction, shall be guilty of a felony punishable by imprisonment for not less than 1 year nor more than 25 years, and by a fine of not less than $5000 nor more than $25 000.

Any owner, proprietor, keeper, manager, conductor, or other person who knowingly permits a violation of this section in any house, building, room, tent, lot or premises under his control or of which he has possession, upon conviction for the first offense, shall be guilty of a misdemeanor punishable by imprisonment in the county jail for a period of not less than 6 months nor more than 1 year, and by a fine of not more than $5000. Upon conviction for a subsequent offense pursuant to the provisions of this subsection such person shall be guilty of a felony punishable by imprisonment for a period of not less than 1 year nor more than 10 years, and by a fine of not less than $5000 nor more than $25 000.

Oregon

Or Rev Stat § 167.017. Compelling Prostitution.

A person commits the crime of compelling prostitution if the person knowingly induces or causes a person under 18 years of age to engage in prostitution; or induces or causes the spouse, child or stepchild of the person to engage in prostitution.

Compelling prostitution is a Class B felony.

A Class B felony carries a maximum term of an indeterminate sentence of 10 years, pursuant to § 161.605. An amount not exceeding $200 000 shall be fixed by the court upon a sentence to pay a fine for a Class B felony, pursuant to § 161.625.

Pennsylvania

18 Pa Cons Stat Ann § 5902. Prostitution and Related Offenses.
An offense under this section constitutes a felony of the third degree if the actor promotes prostitution of a child under the age of 16 years, whether or not he is aware of the age of the child.

A person commits a summary offense if he hires a prostitute or any other person who is 16 years of age or older to engage in sexual activity with him, or if he enters or remains in a house of prostitution for the purpose of engaging in sexual activity. A person commits a misdemeanor of the third degree if the person hires a prostitute or any other person who is under 16 years of age, whether or not the person is aware of the age of child.

A person who has been convicted of a felony of the third degree shall be sentenced to a fixed term of imprisonment not to exceed 7 years pursuant to § 1103. A person who has been convicted of a misdemeanor of the third degree may be sentenced to imprisonment for a definite term that shall be fixed by the court and shall not be more than 1 year pursuant to § 1104.

A person who is convicted of a felony of the third degree may be sentenced to pay a fine not exceeding $15 000; $2500 when the conviction is of a misdemeanor of the third degree, pursuant to § 1101.

Rhode Island

RI Gen Laws § 11-9-1. Exploitation for Commercial or Immoral Purposes.
Every person who shall exhibit, use, employ or shall in any manner or under pretense so exhibit, use, or employ any child under the age of 18 years to any person for the purpose of prostitution or for any other lewd or indecent act shall be imprisoned not exceeding 20 years, or be fined not exceeding $20 000 or both.

South Carolina

SC Code Ann § 16-15-415. Promoting Prostitution of a Minor Defined; Defenses; Penalties.
An individual commits the offense of promoting prostitution of a minor if he knowingly:

(1) entices, forces, encourages, or otherwise facilitates a minor to participate in prostitution; or

(2) supervises, supports, advises, or promotes the prostitution of or by a minor.

Mistake of age is not a defense to a prosecution under this section.

An individual who violates this section is guilty of a felony and, upon conviction, must be imprisoned for not less than three years nor more than ten years. No part of the minimum sentence may be suspended nor is the individual convicted eligible for parole until he has served the minimum sentence. Sentences imposed pursuant to this section shall run consecutively with and shall commence at the expiration of any other sentence being served by the individual sentenced.

SC Code Ann § 16-15-425. Participating in Prostitution of a Minor Defined; Defenses; Penalties.
An individual commits the offense of participating in the prostitution of a minor if he is not a minor and he patronizes a minor prostitute. As used in this section, "patronizing a minor prostitute" means:

(1) soliciting or requesting a minor to participate in prostitution;

(2) paying or agreeing to pay a minor, either directly or through the minor's agent, to participate in prostitution; or

(3) paying a minor, or the minor's agent, for having participated in prostitution, pursuant to a prior agreement.

Mistake of age is not a defense to a prosecution under this section.

A person who violates the provisions of this section is guilty of a felony and, upon conviction, must be imprisoned not less than 2 years nor more than 5 years. No part of the minimum sentence may be suspended nor is the individual convicted eligible for parole until he has served the minimum term. Sentences imposed pursuant to this section shall run consecutively with and shall commence at the expiration of any other sentence being served by the individual sentenced.

South Dakota

SD Codified Laws § 22-23-2. Procuring or Promoting Prostitution as Felony.
Any person who encourages, induces, procures, or otherwise purposely causes another to become or remain a prostitute; or promotes prostitution of a minor; or promotes prostitution of his spouse, child, ward or any person for whose care, protection or support he is responsible, is guilty of a Class 5 felony, *which carries a term of 5 years' imprisonment in the state penitentiary and/or a fine of $5000, pursuant to § 22-6-1.*

Tennessee

Tenn Code Ann § 37-5-103. Definitions.
Tennessee recognizes encouraging or forcing a child (under the age of 18 years) to solicit or engage in prostitution as the sexual exploitation of a child. A child who is or has been allowed, encouraged, or permitted to engage in prostitution also meets the definition of a "dependent and neglected" child for purposes of those statutory sections.

Texas

Tex Penal Code Ann § 43.05. Compelling Prostitution.
A person commits an offense if he knowingly causes by any means a person younger than 17 years to commit prostitution. An offense under this section is a felony of the second degree, and *is punishable by imprisonment for any term of not more than 20 years or less than 2 years in addition to a possible fine not to exceed $10 000, pursuant to § 12.33 of the penal code.*

Utah

Utah Code Ann § 76-10-1306. Aggravated Exploitation of Prostitution.
A person is guilty of aggravated exploitation if the person procured, transported, or persuaded or with whom he shares the proceeds of prostitution is under 18 years of age or is the wife of the actor. Aggravated exploitation of prostitution is a felony of the second degree. *A felony of the second degree is subject to an indeterminate term of imprisonment of not less than 1 year nor more than 15 years, pursuant to § 76-3-203.*

Virginia

Va Code Ann § 18.2-355. Taking, Detaining, etc., Person for Prostitution, etc., or Consenting Thereto.
Any person who: (1) for purposes of prostitution or unlawful sexual intercourse, takes any person into, or persuades, encourages or causes any person to enter, a bawdy place, or takes or causes such person to be taken to any place against his or her will for such purposes; (2) takes or detains a person against his or her will with the intent to compel such person, by force, threats, persuasions, menace or duress, to marry him or her or to marry any other person, or to be defiled; or (3) being parent, guardian, legal custodian or one standing in loco parentis of a person, consents to such person being taken or detained by any person for the purpose of prostitution or unlawful sexual intercourse; is guilty of pandering, and shall be guilty of a Class 4 felony. *The authorized punishment for a conviction of a Class 4 felony is a term of imprisonment not*

less than 2 years nor more than 10 years and a fine of not more than $100 000, pursuant to § 18.2-10.*

Va Code Ann § 18.2-48. Abduction With Intent to Extort Money or for Immoral Purpose.

Abduction (i) with the intent to extort money or pecuniary benefit, (ii) of any person with intent to defile such person, or (iii) of any child under 16 years of age for the purpose of concubinage or prostitution, shall be a Class 2 felony. *The authorized punishment for a conviction of a Class 2 felony is a term of imprisonment not less than 20 years and a fine of not more than $100 000, pursuant to § 18.2-10.*

Va Code Ann § 18.2-49. Threatening, Attempting or Assisting in Such Abduction.

Any person who (1) threatens, or attempts, to abduct any other person with intent to extort money, or pecuniary benefit, or (2) assists or aids in the abduction of, or threatens to abduct, any person with the intent to defile such person, or (3) assists or aids in the abduction of, or threatens to abduct, any female under sixteen years of age for the purpose of concubinage or prostitution, shall be guilty of a Class 5 felony. *The authorized punishment for a conviction of a Class 5 felony is a term of imprisonment not less than 1 year nor more than 10 years and a fine of not more than $2500, either, or both, pursuant to § 18.2-10.*

Washington

Wash Rev Code Ann § 9.68A.100. Patronizing Juvenile Prostitute.

A person is guilty of patronizing a juvenile prostitute if that person engages or agrees or offers to engage in sexual conduct with a minor in return for a fee, and is guilty of a Class C felony, and is subject to the provisions under § 9A.88.130, *which requires that the sentencing court require that the offender refrain from patronizing a prostitute and remain outside of the geographical area in which the person was arrested,* and § 9A.88.140, *which authorizes the sentencing court to impound the offender's vehicle.* (As described in the originating document found at http://www.ndaa-apri.org/pdf/statutes_child_prostitution_2004.pdf, "Text provisions in red [italicized here] are not part of the child prostitution statutes, but are sentence provisions that correspond to the enumerated statutory offense levels.")

Pursuant to § 9A.20.021, the maximum sentence for a Class C felony is confinement in a state correctional institution for 5 years, or by a fine in an amount fixed by the court of $10 000, or by both such confinement and fine.

West Virginia

WVa Code § 61-8-6. Detention of Person in Place of Prostitution; Penalty.

Whoever shall by any means keep, hold, detain, or restrain any person in a house of prostitution or other place where prostitution is practiced or allowed; or whoever shall, directly or indirectly, keep, hold, detain, or restrain, or attempt to keep, hold, detain or restrain, in any house of prostitution or other place where prostitution is practiced or allowed, any person by any means, for the purpose of compelling such person, directly or indirectly, to pay, liquidate, or cancel any debt, dues, or obligations incurred or said to have been incurred by such person shall, upon conviction for the first offense under this section, be punished by imprisonment in the county jail for a period of not less than 6 months nor more than 1 year and by a fine of not less than $100 nor more than $500 and, upon conviction for any subsequent offense under this section, shall be punished by imprisonment in the penitentiary for not less than 1 nor more than 3 years provided that in any offense under this section where the person so kept, held, detained, or restrained is a minor, any person violating the provisions of this section shall be guilty of a felony and, upon conviction, shall be confined in the penitentiary not less than 2 years nor more than 5 years or fined not more than $5000 or both.

WVa Code § 61-8-7. Procuring for House of Prostitution; Penalty; Venue; Competency as Witness; Marriage No Defense.

Any person who shall procure an inmate for a house of prostitution, or who, by promises, threats, violence, or by any device or scheme, shall cause, induce, persuade, or encourage a person to become an inmate of a house of prostitution, or shall procure a place as inmate in a house of prostitution for a person; or any person who shall, by promises, threats, violence, or by any device or scheme cause, induce, persuade, or encourage an inmate of a house of prostitution to remain therein as such inmate; or any person who shall, by fraud or artifice, or by duress of person or goods, or by abuse of any position of confidence or authority, procure any person to become an inmate of a house of ill fame, or to enter any place in which prostitution is encouraged or allowed within this state, or to come into or leave this state for the purpose of prostitution, or who shall procure any person to become an inmate of a house of ill fame within this state or to come into or leave this state for the purpose of prostitution; or shall receive or give or agree to receive or give any money or thing of value for procuring or attempting to procure any person to become an inmate of a house of ill fame within this state, or to come into or leave this state for the purpose of prostitution, shall be guilty of pandering, and, upon a first conviction for an offense under this section, shall be punished by imprisonment in the county jail for a period of not less than 6 months nor more than 1 year, and by a fine of not less than $100 nor more than $500 and, upon conviction for any subsequent offense under this section, shall be punished by imprisonment in the penitentiary for a period of not less than one nor more than 5 years provided that where the inmate referred to in this section is a minor, any person violating the provisions of this section shall be guilty of a felony and, upon conviction, shall be confined in the penitentiary not less than 2 years nor more than 5 years or fined not more than $5000 or both.

WVa Code § 61-8-8. Receiving Support From Prostitution; Pimping; Penalty; Prostitute May Testify.

Any person who, knowing another person to be a prostitute, shall live or derive support or maintenance, in whole or in part, from the earnings or proceeds of the prostitution of such prostitute, or from money loaned or advanced to or charged against such prostitution by any keeper or manager or inmate of a house or other place where prostitution is practiced or allowed, or shall tout or receive compensation for touting for such prostitution, shall be guilty of pimping, and, upon the first conviction for such offense, shall be punished by imprisonment in the county jail for a period of not less than 6 months nor more than 1 year, and by a fine of not less than $100 nor more than $500; and, upon a conviction for any subsequent offense hereunder, shall be punished by imprisonment in the penitentiary for a period of not less than 1 year nor more than 3 years provided that where the prostitute referred to in this section is a minor, any person violating the provisions of this section shall be guilty of a felony and, upon conviction, shall be confined in the penitentiary not less than 2 years or fined not more than $5000 or both. A prostitute shall be a competent witness in any prosecution hereunder to testify for or against the accused as to any transaction or conversation with the accused, or by the accused with another person or persons in the presence of the prostitute, even if the prostitute may have married the accused before or after the violation of any of the provisions of this section, whether called as a witness during the existence of the marriage or after its dissolution.

Wisconsin

Wis Stat Ann § 948.07. Child Enticement.

Whoever, with intent to cause the child to engage in prostitution, causes or attempts to cause any child who has not attained the age of 18 years to go into any vehicle, building, room, or secluded place is guilty of a Class D felony.

Wis Stat Ann § 948.08. Soliciting a Child for Prostitution.
Whoever intentionally solicits or causes any child to practice prostitution or establishes any child in a place of prostitution is guilty of a Class D felony.

The penalty for a Class D felony is a fine not to exceed $100 000 or imprisonment not to exceed 25 years or both pursuant to § 939.50.

Wyoming
Wyo Stat Ann § 6-4-103. Promoting Prostitution; Penalties.
A person commits a felony if he knowingly or intentionally entices or compels another person to become a prostitute. The crime is a felony punishable by imprisonment for not more than 5 years, a fine of not more than $5000 or both, if the person enticed or compelled is under 18 years of age.

FEDERAL LEGISLATION
18 USCA § 2423. Transportation of Minors.
A person who knowingly transports an individual who has not attained the age of 18 years in interstate or foreign commerce, or in any commonwealth, territory, or possession of the United States, with intent that the individual engage in prostitution, or in any sexual activity for which any person can be charged with a criminal offense, shall be fined under this title and imprisoned not less than 5 years and not more than 30 years.

A person who travels in interstate commerce or travels into the United States, or a United States citizen or an alien admitted for permanent residence in the United States who travels in foreign commerce, for the purpose of engaging in any illicit sexual conduct with another person shall be fined under this title or imprisoned not more than 30 years or both.

Any United States citizen or alien admitted for permanent residence who travels in foreign commerce, and engages in any illicit sexual conduct with another person shall be fined under this title or imprisoned not more than 30 years or both.

Whoever, for the purpose of commercial advantage or private financial gain, arranges, induces, procures, or facilitates the travel of a person knowing that such a person is traveling in interstate commerce or foreign commerce for the purpose of engaging in illicit sexual conduct shall be fined under this title, imprisoned not more than 30 years, or both.

Whoever attempts or conspires to violate the above sections shall be punishable in the same manner as a completed violation of that subsection.

As used in this section, the term "illicit sexual conduct" means (1) a sexual act with a person under 18 years of age that would be in violation of chapter 109A if the sexual act occurred in the special maritime and territorial jurisdiction of the United States; or (2) any commercial sex act with a person under 18 years of age.

In a prosecution under this section based on illicit sexual conduct, it is a defense, which the defendant must establish by a preponderance of the evidence that the defendant reasonably believed that the person with whom the defendant engaged in the commercial sex act had attained the age of 18 years.

INTERNET PEDOPHILIA

Terry Jones, BA (Hons), PGCE

INTRODUCTION

Internet pedophile activity is first and foremost a child protection issue, not a computer technology problem. While developing strategies and solutions to manage this complex, challenging, and at times confusing phenomenon, the fundamental goal must be remembered. The politics of institutions and organizations, individual career paths and egos, and other issues including computer technology, can distract people from the most important objective in managing the challenge of Internet pedophilia, protecting children.

This chapter identifies and explores some of the key issues involved in the growth of Internet pedophile activity, particularly those related to the exponential growth in the availability of child abuse images. (The phrase *child abuse images* is increasingly being used to differentiate child-related sexual images from overall adult pornography.) Controlling the potential harm that can result from Internet pedophilia is a significant and daunting prospect. Nonetheless, managed carefully, creatively, and constructively, the control of the Internet presents a significant opportunity to protect children from those who seek to exploit them.

HISTORICAL PERSPECTIVE

Internet pedophilia was first recognized by American law enforcement officials in the early 1990s and landed on the shores of the United Kingdom in 1995. Operation Starburst (Adkeniz, 2003), an international investigation of an Internet pedophile ring, resulted in 6 men from the United Kingdom being convicted of possessing indecent child images and led to more arrests worldwide. The Internet and other technological developments have created an unprecedented platform for pedophiles to communicate, create and share materials, and target new victims. However, the vast majority of child molestation takes place secretly and behind closed doors involving offenders who are closely connected with the victim.

Internet pedophilia raises many unanswered questions:

— Are individuals who download child-abuse images dangerous?

— Does Internet pedophilia create new pedophiles?

— How widespread is Internet pedophilia?

— Internet pedophilia is a global problem, so how can it be addressed at a local level?

— Whose responsibility is it to address the Internet pedophilia problem?

Though identified more than a decade ago, key aspects of Internet pedophile behaviors and risk factors for victims are finally being identified. This process of understanding and assessment is gradual, but technological advancements are rapid and unceasing.

LAW ENFORCEMENT DIFFICULTIES

For society in general and law enforcement officials in particular, the Internet poses unprecedented and myriad opportunities, difficulties, and dilemmas. It neither recognizes nor respects geographical, cultural, commercial, or legal boundaries. At a local or regional level, law enforcement business plans and priorities are almost always focused on relatively small geographical areas. Understandably, they are created to address local issues and concerns.

Law enforcement agencies with national and international responsibilities are preoccupied with conventional concepts of serious and organized crime, concepts usually based on traditional ideas of profit and commercial gain. Other concerns such as terrorism have understandably become higher on the list of priorities.

Locally, nationally, and internationally, the issues of drugs, firearms, antisocial behavior, and violent crimes such as murder and robberies are typically priorities, so support infrastructures such as intelligence and analysis systems have been designed and deployed to address these concerns. These infrastructures are not designed for Internet pedophilia primarily because, until relatively recently, child abuse was almost exclusively considered a local problem that required a local law enforcement response. General research findings, protocols, and best practices are shared, but offender detection and prosecution issues have been solely a local issue. In most cases in which disclosure of abuse from a child in a local neighborhood resulted in apprehension of the offender, the offender was almost always from the same area as the child.

Though rhetoric is vociferous, especially after high-profile events, child protection is not a high priority in UK police business plans at local, regional, or national levels. For example, the UK government 3-year National Policing Plan 2005-2008 (Home Office, 2004) does not list child protection as a primary objective and neither the Internet nor Internet pedophilia is mentioned within the document. The plan merely asks chief officers to "review their force policy and local policing plans to ensure child protection is given the appropriate priority." Resources for child protection are, therefore, in direct competition with many other policing tasks, many of which are the subject of specific government performance measurements.

A major dilemma is that a key component of Internet pedophilia is local, yet the posted images are instantaneously global. Throughout the world, many pedophiles view, collect, and use child abuse images for sexual arousal, creating a global problem. The same individuals who view their downloaded images while masturbating and fantasizing are likely to be a risk to children in the neighborhood, creating a local problem.

In a study of Internet offenders, Quayle & Taylor (2002) comment "[o]ffending fantasies in relation to images were not always confined to looking at the pictures on screen, and within this sample had also acted as a blue print both for abuse and for the production of photographs." From a local perspective, the proactive identification of such individuals is difficult and normally requires national or international police tactics. In one local initiative, SurfControl, an international developer of Web and e-mail filtering software, working with the Greater Manchester Police, developed Chat Monitor, which can identify individuals from specific countries who have been using Internet Relay Chat (IRC). This software was used, for example, during Operation Magenta in 2002, a 6-month investigation of Internet pedophilia leading to the execution of 75 warrants (Numerous arrests, 2002; SurfControl and Greater Manchester Police, 2002).

Conversely, but of paramount importance, is the recovery of evidence and intelligence during the post-arrest examination of computers. Though this takes place within the local police area where the suspect is arrested, it is likely to be valuable nationally and internationally for identifying other unknown offenders and child victims (Holland, 2003). Acquiring evidence and intelligence in this way, for example collecting more images from the same Internet child victim series, is like collecting pieces for a puzzle. However, those individual puzzle pieces are located on the hard drives of seized computers which sit in police forensic units all over the world. For example, in 2003, a victim identification investigation called Operation Defiance required evidence be gathered from local police departments from as far as the United Kingdom, United States, and New Zealand to track down an offender and child victim who, in geographical terms, were relatively close to the police unit in Manchester that set out to identify them.

For practical and political reasons, local law enforcement agencies all over the world find it difficult to respond effectively to Internet pedophilia in such a comprehensive manner, for example by harvesting all the useful intelligence about further possible suspects from seized computers. Examining the increasing quantities of stored pedophilia-related data and media is time consuming, so if the issue is not a local policing priority, it will be overlooked.

Many presume that centralized national units with international briefs (such as the recently described Virtual Global Task Force [Dear, 2004]) are the solution. Though these are important developments because the worldwide exchange of information is critical to investigating Internet pedophilia, the foundation blocks for such a process can only start with the effective examination and analysis of valuable data from seized computers at local and regional levels.

Most successful Internet victim identification investigations have resulted from the collection and sharing of information from local sources (eg, seized computers, offender interviews). In fact, many Internet child abuse images are part of a large set of images that can collectively furnish information about the location and time span of the abuse as well as other clues.

Despite widespread and at times glorified media reports of sophisticated pedophile rings, the vast majority of Internet offenders act alone (as do those who abuse children). Based on personal experience with numerous Internet investigations, including more than 100 suspects from Operation Ore (the United Kingdom arm of Operation Avalanche USA) (see http://www.usps.com/postalinspectors/avalanch.htm for more information on Operation Avalanche), the author has found that some pedophiles loosely network by conversing with others online, but few become part of a hierarchical, formal, structured group. Though worthy of additional investigation, a high level of technical sophistication does not necessarily equate to a greater risk to children. It is a misconception that the most dangerous pedophiles use highly technical methods and form complex, clandestine Internet groups.

Headline news stories about high-tech forms of pedophilia will continue to fuel misunderstandings about child abuse. Perhaps it is a symptom of people's need to distance themselves from the true profile of a child abuser and reinforce the myth that abusers are demonic figures who are not a part of mainstream society. The reality is that approximately 80% of child abuse occurs in the home of the victim or offender, and typically the child knows the offenders (Grubin, 1998).

The sexual abuse of children has always existed, and it may be more prevalent than people choose to acknowledge. The following is a summary of Grubin's (1998) description of child abuse prevalence and offenders:

— Child sexual abuse may be more prevalent than indicated by previous population surveys.

— The consequences of abuse by a person known to the victim can be more serious than those from abuse by strangers because abuse by a known person involves a serious breach of trust.

— The vast majority of offenders abuse in their home or the home of the victim and are family members or people the victim know.

Internet pedophilia is likely the result of a fluctuating mix of many factors including social, psychological, and physical issues. Though members of organized crime groups recently have become interested in the commercial aspects of pedophilia, particularly Web-based pedophilia (National Criminal Intelligence Service, 2003), commercial concerns are not usually a motivation for pedophiles who use the Internet to explore and engage in child abuse.

Collecting illegal, sexually explicit child abuse images is a common practice for many, but the practice of gathering child erotica is underreported. As well as illegal material, suspects will often seek out and save decent images of children. These may depict children in specific poses, wearing certain types of clothing or underwear, or in whatever form appeals to the sexual fantasies of that particular collector. Text-based child abuse accounts or fantasy stories are widely used by suspects to stimulate sexual arousal. Identifying which types of images a pedophile suspect has chosen to save in a collection can provide invaluable insight into the suspect's interests. The recovery and examination of this type of material should form an integral part of any subsequent child protection risk assessment process on that individual, but the sheer volume of seized material and lack of resources often precludes this. If a physical education teacher at a boy's school is arrested in possession of a few illegal indecent images of children but he has material in his collection such as sexual fantasy stories about boys or hundreds of erotic pictures of boys in shorts, it is important to recover and present such material to determine his suitability to work with children in the future.

The scope and nature of Internet pedophilia challenges traditional models of and responses to managing and investigating conventional criminal activity. Original and resourceful ways to combat Internet pedophilia must be developed because it is a unique crime with unique complications. The number of Internet users, and thus presumably suspects, increases daily. Far fewer women than men are pedophiles; in the author's 8 years of experience with Internet pedophile operations that identified more than 450 pedophile suspects, only 2 were women. In addition, attempting to analyze the increasingly large amounts of data on personal computers is an overwhelming task. Roy Williams of the California Institute of Technology has an analogy that puts the enormity of this task into perspective. One gigabyte of data is the equivalent of "a pickup truck filled with books" and 100 gigabytes is "a library floor of academic journals" (Williams, 2005). Computers with 150 gigabytes or more are fairly common for home usage. The sheer number of child abuse images in circulation is overwhelming. Attempting to provide a comprehensive and effective law enforcement response is daunting.

Historically, the detection and prosecution of child sexual abuse has been a complicated challenge. The initial accusation of abuse from a victim typically is delayed (in some instances for decades), so supporting forensic evidence is often nonexistent. In addition, the victim and the offender often know each other, which can make the victim reluctant to disclose the abuse. Unlike many other crimes, child abuse typically does not involve witnesses. Detection of child abuse crimes in progress is almost impossible because it is a hidden crime that takes place behind closed doors and often within the confines of a family.

IMAGES AND THE INTERNET

The actual images being circulated of children are indecent and abusive. The Internet allows pedophiles to effortlessly circulate all types of material, whether it is illegal or offensive. The real faces of abuse victims are available in a wide-open forum—constantly recirculating, continually revictimizing—with no prospect of deletion or closure for the victims.

Though Internet pedophilia is an immense problem, it has provided the world with a unique opportunity to address child sexual abuse. It has brought the issue to the forefront of society and could have an unprecedented impact on international child protection procedures. It is forcing people to develop ways to protect children from abusive situations.

Though the Internet provides a forum for pedophiles to circulate material, it also helps law enforcement officials to identify pedophiles. People who create, distribute, or download indecent images of children and pedophiles who engage in chat room conversations can be investigated, which may help establish their connection with and the type of threat they pose to actual children. In some situations, the child abuse images may help identify children who are currently being abused though this has not yet become a common practice. Because of the global nature of image exchange and the sheer number of images in circulation, many people are understandably reluctant to take on the cumbersome task of tracing the individual children in the images. This situation needs to change immediately.

Until now, primarily because victims have not been routinely asked, little has been known about the relationship between physical child molestation and photographing such abuse. With advancements in technology, especially the increase in digital camera use, such questioning should become routine.

Initially, it was difficult to access pornographic images of children. In some instances, locating and obtaining images required expensive travel, significant risk of discovery by third parties through written correspondence via contact magazines, and risk of detection by customs and border inspections. The pedophiles who were photographing the children had to devise a way to surreptitiously develop or reproduce the illegal pictures. Producing photographs from negatives required special equipment and facilities. The risks of outsourcing this task (eg, through magazine advertisements offering "discreet and confidential photo processing") were high. The Internet and the relatively recent development of digital photography have eliminated those barriers. Child abuse images can be instantaneously recorded, stored, and distributed with ease.

During the early and mid 1990s—before digital photography became mainstream—many of the child abuse images being circulated on the Internet were comparatively dated. Clothing, furniture, hairstyles, and image quality indicated that the images had been taken many years—probably decades—before. Photographs were scanned to produce computerized images, videocassettes were transferred into a digital computer format, and the material was uploaded to Internet bulletin boards, newsgroups, and File Transfer Protocol (FTP) sites. The Internet gave individuals who had existing private collections, however dated, the ability to share and distribute their material worldwide. Anyone anywhere in the world could access and download the images, generally for free. Though we have witnessed large police operations targeting those who access this material using credit card payment Web sites, the vast majority of child abuse material in circulation on the Internet is not commercially driven or controlled, especially the most recent images, which include photos set in domestic surroundings with increasingly younger victims being subjected to more violence (Taylor, 2003). The motivation for offenders to access or distribute child abuse images is seldom commercial.

Other early sources for Internet child abuse material were scanned copies of commercially produced magazines, old videos, and the use of child pictures from medical reference books as child erotica. The photos were converted into the appropriate format and uploaded to the Internet. All forms of pornography, including child pornography, were decriminalized in some European countries during the late 1960s and early 1970s, so they served as sources of child abuse material as well. Pages from magazines were scanned and uploaded, often with their title, issue number, and accompanying text. In some instances, the center paper fold and staples could be seen in the Internet images. The child victims of these early pornographic images were 20 or 30 years older when the images began circulating on the Internet in the 1990s.

The ease of use and widespread availability of digital cameras and increased electronic transfer capabilities provided by faster Internet access has brought a dramatic change in the circulation of pornography. High-quality digital moving images with clear audio recordings have brought the graphic nature of child abuse into real focus. The pornographic images of children are relatively new, meaning that the victims may still be in abusive situations.

VICTIM IDENTIFICATION BY IMAGE ANALYSIS

False images of child abuse (referred to as ***pseudo images***) do exist, but in relativity low numbers. Created by manually or digitally replacing the heads on adult pornographic images with those of children. The adult features can then be altered to present a more childlike body image. More recently, some limited examples of generating fake images using computer software have appeared. Whether the material is old or new, almost all the victims in child abuse images are real children. A research group called Combating Paedophile Information Networks in Europe (COPINE) has monitored some publicly available Internet newsgroups since 1997 and now has an archive of 600 000 child abuse images. At its Victim Identification Project presentation at the European Parliament in December 2003, COPINE estimated that their collection includes approximately 60 000 individual child victims. Images can be found almost anywhere on the Internet, from the World Wide Web to the less well-known public and private areas of newsgroups and IRC rooms.

Because of the nature and scale of Internet activity, ascertaining the number of distinct images in existence or the actual number of individual victims depicted in them is impossible. Whereas 1 victim may appear within 1 unique image, 2 or more child victims may be visible in other images. The more common scenario victim image files are given names, sometimes by the original producer, or are added or changed later by those who copy them. These names may or may not be true, but often they are repeatedly referred to as the title of a particular series of images that may total hundreds or thousands of photos (eg, "the David Series").

Worldwide, hundreds of thousands of child abuse images exist on the Internet, but only 261 victims have been identified and removed from their abusive situation (McCulloch, 2004). There are many reasons why so few have been identified, but one theory is that the law enforcement response to Internet pedophilia has focused more on apprehending the offender than on rescuing the victim (Taylor & Quayle, 2003). For example, seized images are primarily used as evidence to convict suspects for possession and distribution, not as an opportunity to examine the crime scene, which is revealed within each photograph of abuse.

VICTIM IDENTIFICATION PROCESS

How is a child in an abusive image on the Internet located? The photo could have been taken anywhere in the world and at any time in history since the invention of photography in 1839. The following questions, plus many others, must be answered:

— *Who are the children?* Child abuse often takes place within the home of the victim or offender and is committed by someone known to the victim; therefore, identifying the child will almost certainly lead to the offender. On at least 6 known occasions, law enforcement officials have made the somewhat controversial decision to publish an abusive image in the media. This innovative approach has significant risks, but in each instance the victim and offender were quickly identified.

— *Where are the children?* Some images have features that suggest a geographical location. Others provide additional information, such as environmental clues (eg, trees, flora), decor, electrical fittings, and product labels.

— *When was the image created?* The primary objective is to trace children *currently* being abused, but details in photographs can be misleading. For example, black and white images are not necessarily old, and clothing styles or decor that seem dated may be contemporary. For example, some of the interiors of properties in former Eastern Bloc countries look rather dated. Commercially produced goods and products, such as children's toys or soda labels, can be useful date references.

— *Has the child been found?* A prerequisite for any victim identification investigation is an attempt to answer this question. The universal access provided by the Internet makes duplication of effort a real possibility; worldwide coordination and information sharing is essential. In some countries, domestic legislation prohibits sharing material with other countries, and in other countries, child protection is not a priority.

— *Who should investigate the crime?* The world does not have a global police force. Interpol facilitates investigations but does not investigate child abuse crimes. Someone must take charge of an investigation, but what would prompt individual law enforcement agencies in any specific country to initiate an investigation of a crime that is not within their geographical or legislative jurisdiction and does not feature as a high priority on their declared business objectives?

In approximately 1997, a series of child abuse images began circulating on the Internet. The images featured multiple victims as young as 2 years of age, and the backgrounds of the images had a common theme. As the years passed, the abuse continued. The children aged in the photos, and the total number of images in the series reached the thousands. It was not until an academic working in this field discussed the matter at an Interpol conference in 2000 that a country volunteered to undertake an investigation. In 2003, the victims and offender were traced to a quiet residential suburb in Stockholm (Sweden shocked, 2003). Ironically, in 1996, one year before the images were first discovered, "fewer words and more action" was the plea of a young delegate at the First World Congress on the Commercial Sexual Exploitation of Children in Stockholm (Harvey, 2002). Fortunately, albeit belatedly, this plea was realized in this case.

Investigations

Between 1998 and 2003, the Abusive Images Unit (AIU) of the Greater Manchester police in the United Kingdom launched numerous ad hoc investigations to establish the identity of victims from seized child abuse material. As a local unit, the division had no specific remit or resources for such an investigation, which at times conflicted with their own organization's goals and local policing business objectives. Other than staff salaries, the largest expenditure incurred during any of the investigations was a $1400 printing bill to reproduce Internet material for circulation to other UK law enforcement agencies.

The police unit formed a strong working relationship with the nongovernmental organization COPINE, so most investigations were treated as joint ventures. Information, knowledge, and expertise were shared, crossing organizational and geographical divides. The motivation for the investigations stemmed from a mix of individual and collective frustration at the lack of action in the area of child protection. Viewing—and especially listening to—child abuse images and videos were strong motivators. To view child abuse images can be distressing, but when moving images are brought to life with voices and real sounds, the abuse is palpable. During the Manchester investigations, more than 20 children were identified and removed from abusive situations. In some instances, the identification of an individual victim led to the identification of multiple victims.

During one Manchester investigation (Operation Sedan), the COPINE team was routinely monitoring an Internet newsgroup and discovered 269 still images. The images had been posted anonymously through a Web site that hid the technical identity of the person who posted it. The images depicted 2 girls who were approximately

4 years old, one of whom was subjected to abuse that included oral sex and rape. Based on the background room décor and clothing of the abused victim, COPINE predicted that the images had been taken in the United Kingdom (**Figure 33-1**).

COPINE shared their concerns with the AIU, which commenced a low-key, informal investigation. They found that in 1 of the images, a child was watching a television advertisement of an easily identifiable product (**Figure 33-2**). Enquiries to the product's manufacturer and advertising agency revealed that the advertisement had been released during a short time frame and only on certain UK television channels. Thus, the probable year and general geographical region of the abuse were ascertained.

COPINE continued to monitor newsgroups, and the AIU searched for details in the original material and new images found on the Internet. They realized that some of the images were sequential shots taken one after another and were, therefore, likely still images created from a video clip (**Figures 33-3-a** and **b**).

On an FTP site hosted in Japan, the AIU discovered what appeared to be moving image files with the same name of the series they were investigating. Six separate files had been downloaded; the person who posted them had split the original video clip into the 6 parts, which, when combined into the complete video, could only be viewed with a password (which was subsequently posted on the site).

Figure 33-1. The border wallpaper divide is a common feature in British households.

Figure 33-2. The television advertisement in this image helped determine the time and region this image was created.

Figures 33-3-a and b. These images appear to be sequential, making it likely that they are stills from a video.

The color video clip, which included sound, was 9 minutes and 58 seconds long. It provided new details for the investigators and confirmed their suspicions that the 269 still images they initially discovered originated from a video. Other video clips of the same victim were discovered on the Internet. The offender and children could be heard on the videos, and they had British accents. A pediatrician and speech-language development pathologist predicted the probable age of the victims.

Some of the material was circulated among other UK police units. A family was found that had 2 girls who closely resembled the Internet images and were the predicted age of the victims. A social worker and the police viewed the Internet material and visited the household to investigate. One investigator thought that the children at the house were the victims, but the other investigator was not sure. A more detailed physical examination of the children (eg, of their moles and other body marks) revealed they were not the victims.

Because all indications were that the abuse was recent and possibly still ongoing, a decision was made to release certain details about the case on a national UK television program that featured unsolved crimes. The offender's face, voice, clothing, tattoo, and internal house features were going to be shown. Details about the children and the specific nature of the crime were not going to be revealed.

Because the original newsgroup images had been posted to the Internet through an American site, details of the investigation had been provided to the United States

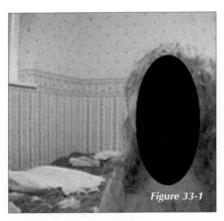

Figure 33-1

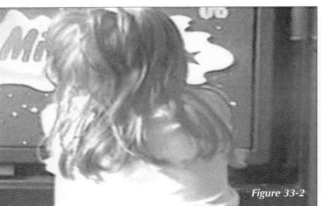

Figure 33-2

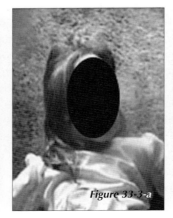

Figure 33-3-a

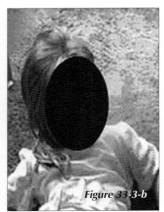

Figure 33-3-b

early in the investigation. A week before the UK television appeal was to be broadcast, an American customs officer working in New York contacted the AIU about an Internet chat room conversation that mentioned the name of the series of images being investigated. The AIU followed up and was able to identify the suspect's UK company e-mail account. Additional investigations with an Internet Service Provider led to the suspect's location. The girls, who were then 5 years of age, were immediately identified, but the abused child did not disclose her abuse. The suspect was arrested but refused to comment on the case. The Internet images were presented to him as evidence, and he plead guilty to all matters including rape, indecent assault, gross indecency, and distributing indecent photographs of children. He was sentenced to 12 years in prison.

CONCLUSION

The Internet and digital photography are providing the world with a unique and realistic view of child sexual abuse. It is an old form of abuse, but until the advent of the Internet, people were only able to imagine what the sexually abused children were enduring. Most knowledge of abuse has come from verbal accounts from offenders and victims, often from victims who are too young to comprehend the events and unable or unwilling to provide explicit details. Internet abuse images, some of which are videos with sound, are giving society a glimpse of the stark reality of sexual abuse.

Pedophiles can be seen and heard as they begin luring and then abusing their victims. They can be seen and heard cajoling, persuading, encouraging, and lying to the children. Adults who see these videos recognize the deceit that goes unnoticed by the children. The wholesale exploitation of the victim can be observed: the breach of trust, the dismantling of innocence, the abuse of power, and, of course, the deplorable physical acts of sexual gratification.

On a more positive note, the details provided by Internet pedophilia images reveal information that can help identify offenders, victims, and the extent of abuse. The clothing, physical appearance of the victim, and environment can be linked with more typical evidence (eg, verbal accounts from the victims and witnesses) to substantiate particular details of a case and reveal long-term abuse.

Professionals, but only those acting in an authorized and controlled legal setting, have an unprecedented source of material with which to study the sexual abuse of children. They can observe offenders, noting their words and body language, to learn about child abuse and perhaps ways to help prevent it. This would be difficult, demanding, but invaluable research; the hopes are that it will increase the world's understanding of child sexual abuse and protect children.

REFERENCES

Akdeniz A. Regulation of child pornography on the Internet: cases and materials. 2003. Available at: http://www.cyber-rights.org/reports/child.htm. Accessed December 29, 2004.

Dear P. Can we really police online chat? *BBC News Online*. June 9, 2004. Available at: http://news.bbc.co.uk/1/hi/uk/3791603.stm. Accessed December 29, 2004.

Grubin D. *Sex Offending Against Children: Understanding the Risk*. London, England: Policing and Reducing Crime Unit; 1998. Police Research Series Paper 99.

Harvey R. Fewer words and more action: evaluating the progress made in ending the commercial sexual exploitation of children. *ChildRIGHT*. 2002;184:16-18. Available at: http://www.essex.ac.uk/armedcon/story_id/000040.doc. Accessed January 5, 2005.

Holland G. Victim identification project. Presented at: COPINE Presentation to European Parliament; December 2003; Brussels, Belgium.

Home Office. *The National Policing Plan 2005-2008*. London, England: Home Office; 2004. Available at: http://www.policereform.gov.uk/nationalpolicingplan05. html. Accessed January 20, 2005.

McCulloch H. Interpol presentation. Presentation at: COPINE Conference; May 24-26, 2004; Cork, Ireland.

National Criminal Intelligence Service (NCIS). Sex offences against children, including online abuse. In: *United Kingdom Threat Assessment of Serious and Organised Crime 2003*. London, England: NCIS; 2003. Available at: http://ncis.gov.uk/ukta/2003/threat09.asp. Accessed January 5, 2005.

Numerous arrests in blitz on Internet paedophiles. *Ananova*. April 24, 2002. Available at: http://www.ananova.com/news/story/sm_574156.html?menu=news. technology.internetcrime%20. Accessed December 17, 2004.

Quayle E, Taylor M. Child pornography and the Internet: perpetuating a cycle of abuse. *Deviant Behav*. 2002;23:331-362.

SurfControl and Greater Manchester Police win international cyber policing award. CyberPatrol Web site. November 18, 2002. Available at: http://www.cyberpatrol. com/about_us/newsitem.aspx?id=490. Accessed December 29, 2004.

Sweden shocked by paedophile case. iafrica.com Web site. May 16, 2003. Available at: http://www.iafrica.com/news/worldnews/237411.htm. Accessed January 5, 2005.

Taylor M. Victim identification project. Presented at: COPINE Presentation to European Parliament; December 2003; Brussels, Belgium.

Taylor M, Quayle E. *Child Pornography: An Internet Crime*. Hove, England: Brunner-Routledge; 2003.

Williams R. Data powers of ten. University of California, Berkley Web site. Available at: http://www.sims.berkeley.edu/research/projects/how-much-info/datapowers.html. Accessed January 21, 2005.

THE MEDICAL EXPERT AND CHILD SEXUAL EXPLOITATION

Sharon W. Cooper, MD, FAAP

Child sexual exploitation (CSE) is thought to be the most underreported form of child abuse. In the great majority of cases, sexual exploitation involves sexual abuse. The exceptions to this rule are seen in cyber-enticement attempts and in certain types of child pornography cases. However, these cases comprise only a small minority, and the overwhelming number of cases of CSE involve sexual abuse. Consequently, the medical expert must have the same knowledge and background as is present in a child sexual abuse case. In addition, however, the expert needs to understand the common critical pathways of seduction for children in sexual exploitation so as to explain how children are lured into child pornography, the prostitution of children and juveniles, cyber-enticement, or, on a more global level, sex tourism and human trafficking. The expert healthcare provider must be well versed in growth and development and sexual maturation norms for different ethnic groups. **Table 34-1** lists scenarios for which a medical expert may be called as a witness in a child sexual exploitation case.

Table 34-1. Scenarios in Which a Medical Expert May Be a Witness	
CHILD PORNOGRAPHY CASE	
The child victim(s) are from within a family	The pornography is being made by family members and no computer is used (eg, photos, videos)
The child victim(s) are from within a family	The pornography is being made with the use of a computer and may include live Web cast transmission
The child victim(s) are known by database information only (eg, Interpol, National Center for Missing & Exploited Children)	The child is not physically available to the medical provider and no computer was used (eg, photos, videos, magazines)
The child victims are known by database information	The child is not physically available to the medical provider and a computer was used (eg, Internet images, saved hard drive images, saved digital photos, CDs, video clips, DVDs, zip disks)
The child victim(s) are unknown to the examiner or others	There are only images available (eg, Internet images, saved hard drive images, CDs, video clips, DVDs, zip disks)
The child victim is unknown, but the images were made in conjunction with child sex tourism, and there is obvious indigence of the victims	The child is not physically available to the medical provider but images have been stored in a digital photo format or videotape and confiscated because of probable cause from international travel

(continued)

Table 34-1. Scenarios in Which a Medical Expert May Be a Witness *(continued)*

PROSTITUTED CHILDREN AND YOUTHS

The child or youth is being marketed from within the home	No computer is used
The child or youth is marketed from within the home and pornographic images have been made and/or have been transmitted via the Internet	A computer is used for the purposes of arranging sexual encounters, advertising the availability of the victim, or collecting pornography involving the child or youth
The child or youth is being commercially marketed from outside the family by nonfamily members	No computer is used
The child or youth is being commercially marketed from outside the family by nonfamily members	A computer is often used through such venues as Internet cafes, escort services, brothels, or other means by which the offender (pimp) contacts the youth or a potential client to arrange illegal encounters
The child or youth is being marketed for an international sex tourism situation	No computer is used
The child or youth is being marketed for an international sex tourism situation and pornography has been made by the perpetrator as a keepsake of the trip	A computer and digital photo technology is often used through the connection of a 'travel agency' that purposefully arranges sex tourism trysts, which may be legally marketing children for prostitution in accordance with their country laws
The child or youth has been coerced into prostitution at the insistence or intimidation of a gang or other form of organized crime	No computer is used
The child or youth has been trafficked across state lines for the purpose of prostitution by an individual or an organized crime group	This may or may not include the use of a computer for the purpose of establishing arrangements or for forging false documents
The child or youth has been trafficked into a country which is foreign to him or her by an individual or an organized crime group	This may or may not include the use of a computer for the purpose of establishing arrangements or for forging false documents.

CYBER-ENTICEMENT OF CHILDREN OR YOUTHS

The child or youth has been enticed to leave the home to meet a potential perpetrator	The child or youth is involved in a case in which there is *prima facie* use of a computer
The child or youth has been enticed to leave his or her home and a perpetrator has already either taken the child or has been caught in the process of taking the child who has become a compliant victim	A computer has been used and many other types of evidence confirm the premeditated nature of the crime
The child or youth is enticed to leave his or her state home of record or even the country	The compliant victim is traveling, possibly into other jurisdictions, causing an increased complexity in the investigation and prosecution

The circumstances in which sexual exploitation cases may not meet the criteria of child sexual abuse are those in which sexual abuse has been averted by discovery of an impending event such as in cyber-enticement cases or when children are advertised over the Internet for prostitution purposes but may not have been sexually abused. Though frank abuse may not have occurred, these children have been placed at great risk for such an event. Occasionally, such events are thwarted because of an undercover investigation.

Child sexual exploitation presents as a diverse type of case in many areas. The medical expert may need to be versed in aspects of computer technology and there may be a need for chat room shorthand information or the ability to interpret emotions from an e-mail cyber-enticement investigation. An expert must have an understanding of the overall physical, sexual, and psychological maturation of children. They may be required to explain the visualization of sexual behaviors, which are well outside the normal developmental level for a certain age range in children. The expert must have a comprehensive knowledge of the long-term effect of child sexual abuse. An understanding is necessary of the close relationship between runaway behavior, thrownaway situations, and street survival sex. That many prostituted children and youth in the United States are introduced to this life by their biological families is an important and illuminating point, which might bring the jury back to the reality of the facts of the case. In a CSE case, the medical expert has to understand the undulant nature of months worth of chat room relationship-building such that the friendship or romance cast from this die is hard to break. Such a relationship may involve a deception between a trusting teen and typically an older man with the intended outcome of at least sexual assault and possibly a far more dangerous and potentially fatal end. The risk for teens leaving their home to pursue a fantasy relationship with total strangers is significant, and a medical expert can play an important role in elevating such cases to a higher level of concern with law enforcement.

The medical expert in sexual exploitation cases may have to explain to the jury reasons why a child victim may have disclosed within the medical evaluation details about sexual abuse but may consistently deny that pornographic images exist. The sexual exploitation case demands a significant understanding of the national and international aspects of the production and distribution of child pornography. As in other forms of abuse, investigation often involves a multidisciplinary group of professionals, some of whom the medical expert may never meet but who may be working on the case from international soil. This form of child sexual abuse involves youth offenders, military personnel, sex offenders with many visible paraphilias, photographic "artists," the wealthy and the poor, and the use of high technology as well as occasionally the high school library computer. Victims are often so young, as is seen in baby and toddler pornography, that long-term victim impact remains unknown. However, the medical expert must be able to draw on the literature of infant and toddler child sexual abuse to educate a jury on the potential harm that is being done. The story of the life of Thea Pumbroek illustrates how extraordinarily destructive CSE may be. Thea died at the age of 6 years from a drug overdose given to her while she was being photographed pornographically at a hotel in the Netherlands (Taylor & Quayle, 2003). The scope of this form of abuse is far-reaching, and each case provides further enlightenment that may often be brought to the witness stand.

The complexity of the seduction traps set for sexual exploitation victims can be so unusual that the medical expert has to be knowledgeable in how to connect the pieces of a puzzle. This often includes a compliant victim voluntarily deserting a nurturing family and home, leading to international lairs for severe and sometimes bizarre forms of sexual abuse. The summary of events will usually be presented on closing arguments. However, the medical expert may be able to play a role in educating a jury about the convoluted nature of the evident victimization and that this can happen to any child who has access to a computer and the Internet. Sexual exploitation cases have the potential of *visibly* hurting a child for decades. As school-aged children mature, anxiety about their images on the Internet has untold impact and contributes to frequent denials of the original events. The medical expert is often the final witness in a child sexual abuse case, providing an explanatory conclusion of all of the presented facts. Conversely, in an exploitation case, the medical expert has to review evidence that may be complex to pull together for the jury the premeditated nature of the crime. Understanding current research regarding why child pornographers collect images helps the medical expert who may be called upon to explain generic offender dynamics. At times, a sexual exploitation case may include a medical expert's testimony about a child whom the expert has never examined and whose diagnosis of "child sexual abuse victim" is drawn only from pictures that have been placed in evidence. This scenario, unfortunately, is common for many medical experts. Review of clinical information is often part of court preparation. In the exploitation case, the evidence is not merely "clinical" but evidentiary. CSE cases are probably the only types of child abuse cases in which the victim may end up as a member of the criminal justice system and the perpetrator is left unscathed.

Consequently, the medical expert must be a person who understands this diagnosis, asks the right questions during an evaluation, assists law enforcement in analysis of Internet images when necessary, recommends appropriate rehabilitation for reintegration of a victim into society, and advocates for the most assertive community response when a child is missing to make a difference in this, one of the most complicated forms of child abuse.

EXPERT WITNESS ROLE IN COMORBID FORMS OF CHILD ABUSE

At times, different forms of abuse exist in the life of a given child. An example would be a child who is physically and psychologically abused. CSE cases are as diverse as other forms of child abuse cases. A medical expert may have to address other forms of abuse in conjunction with that of sexual exploitation in a given child. The comorbid occurrence of sexual abuse and physical abuse, neglect, or emotional abuse has been well described. Consequently, understanding testimony strategy for other types of abuse may be necessary when a medical expert is preparing for trial in a case of sexual exploitation.

It is prudent to consider comorbid diagnoses separately in the charging and prosecution process. If a child has been physically and sexually abused, each crime should be noted. As with sexual exploitation and sexual abuse, characteristic behaviors are seen by perpetrators of physical abuse. For example, in addition to understanding the mechanisms of injury and recognized pathognomonic patterns of injury, the usual physical abuse case requires medical recognition of varying or inconsistent histories, which are given to different care providers. The expert in a physical abuse case must have knowledge of frequent parental attitude misconceptions, which contribute to abusive behaviors, such as a lack of empathy for the child. This often leads to a failure to seek medical care in a timely fashion. Often, parents have a vested belief in the value of punishment or unrealistic expectations for the developmental level of the child, which may frequently lead actively or passively to abusive injuries (Bavolek, 1990).

Physical abuse cases are frequently associated with care provider histories that are inconsistent with the injuries. The expert has an understanding of typical accidental injury patterns and can explain the difference between an accidental and inflicted injury. In addition, children who are abused often present with injuries for which there is no proposed explanation. At the least, this would constitute poor supervision and a probable diagnosis of neglect, but more often the injury is abusive in nature.

Individuals other than the offender often refer physically abused children for medical care. Failure to seek medical care in a timely fashion is characteristic of an inflicted injury. This offender behavior increases the morbidity and mortality rates in child abuse. Closed head injuries in accidents have both a better prognosis in general and less central nervous system impact as compared to abusive head injuries (Ewing-Cobbs et al, 1998). Children studied prospectively with inflicted head injury as compared to accidental head injury demonstrated a mental retardation rate of 45% as compared to the accidentally injured group that had only a 5% rate of mental deficiency. Inconsistent response by the care provider to the injury would support the premise that lack of empathy for the child's injury and a self-protective motive leads to delayed access to medical care in intentionally injured children.

Finally, in every form of abuse, the medical expert should be prepared to discuss the victim impact that the event precipitates. In physical abuse cases, this might include permanent disability, disfigurement, or psychological impact resulting in chronic signs of trauma. There are 3 components to the testimony of an expert that are important to stress in a physical child abuse case:

1. *Inconsistent Renditions.* A physical abuse case often has an inconsistent history when related by the perpetrator to different sources (eg, emergency medical technicians, 911 operators, the emergency department physicians, social workers). Tabulations of these various stories presented as a demonstrative aid are convincing with respect to an expert's review of all medical documents.

2. *Inconsistent Explanations.* A physical abuse case usually involves injuries inconsistent with the offered history (eg, falling from a bed as a cause of death in an otherwise normal infant). Using the literature as the standard for accidental injuries associated with the proposed history assists in making a case that such a history is inconsistent with the extent of the injuries. In addition, use of an "injury inventory" as a demonstrative aid at the close of the medical expert's testimony, with an explanation of the most likely mechanism of each injury, demystifies the inconsistent explanations for the jury.

3. *Inconsistent Responses.* A physical abuse case is commonly associated with a delay in seeking medical care despite the severity of the inflicted injury. This response is inconsistent with what normally happens in an accidental injury. In physical abuse cases, children are often brought to the emergency room without the assistance of emergency medical teams, and the care provider may have a nonchalant affect even though the child is seriously injured or near death. Others who see the child may react immediately even if they have no medical training. A response that is inconsistent with the severity of the injury may be a peculiar affect in the care provider or a failure to seek medical care despite knowledge of the mechanism of the injury.

A child who is being sexually exploited may be a physical abuse victim. Reports from women who were prostituted as adolescents frequently cite a high incidence of beatings by their family "sponsors" or their pimp "sponsors." *Sponsor* is another term for an offender or the individual who is marketing the victim. Documentation by history or physical examination of comorbid physical abuse in youths who may be in juvenile detention by the time medical care is made available is an important aspect of the medical evaluation of a sexual exploitation victim. It reinforces to investigators and the court system the frequent involuntary nature of this form of abuse.

Case Study 34-1

Pornographic images were found via a newsgroup on the Internet. These particular images were of a young, partially clad prepubescent girl, lying prone and talking to an unseen person. The images were transmitted in the form of video clips. During the video, the child began to receive injections in and around her buttocks, which caused her to cry and beg the offender to stop. This physical sadistic treatment preceded visualization of the actual subsequent child sexual abuse images. Information regarding long-term anal trauma was not available, but anal intercourse was videotaped at the time of the pornography production. Intense police investigation located this child in England, and she was rescued from the care of her grandfather, who was the perpetrator and producer of these pornographic images (Jones & Holland, 2003).

Often in the occurrence of sexual exploitation and physical abuse, the physical abuse needs to be addressed separately from the sexual exploitation. At times the physical abuse is manifested by sadistic treatment. Careful testimony regarding sadistic abuse, which falls into the category of physical abuse, is important to assist a jury in understanding the multiple forms of maltreatment, which may be present in certain forms of child pornography. Juries are more comfortable with physical abuse diagnoses, such as shaken baby syndrome or battered child syndrome, because they can more easily grasp the concept. Also, sadism is so "over the edge" that even in the face of photographic or computer evidence, many will disbelieve, thinking that the images are staged for special effects. Once the medical expert has discussed the initial form of abuse, the more complex diagnosis of sexual exploitation can be presented.

Prosecution of neglect cases involves an expert's ability to explain a family's actions or lack thereof that may have contributed to the child's poor quality of life or death. Neglect legal cases are at times more difficult to prove because the jurors have values and traditions difficult to discern on *voir dire* (ie, the process through which potential jurors are questioned to determine their suitability for service) but influence their interpretation of the neglectful family's actions. Nutritional deprivation can be straight forward if removal of the child from a family is associated with rapid weight gain and return to a robust nature. However, if a child is significantly malnourished and environmentally deprived, return to health is often delayed. This natural course of events may cause a jury to feel that this is a "child problem" and not a "parent problem." The expert must explain the long-term impact of deprivation with possible use of examples from the refugee and orphan adoption literature as comparison to make the point most riveting. Neglect within the context of safety disregard or environmental risks that lead to injury are self-evident, but the issue of parental intelligence and understanding often becomes the concern. The injury to the child may take a back seat to the jury's speculations of the parent's intent. Neglect is pertinent, for example, when a child is brought to a crack house with a parent who is addicted. When the child is left unattended for long periods of time, or traded sexually for drugs, there is no question that the child's victimization is real.

Case Study 34-2

A case from Bossier City, Louisiana, illustrates the occurrence of neglect and child sexual exploitation. According to news reporters, Bertha Hill, a 28-year-old mother, traded her 8-year-old daughter to a man in a deal for crack. The child was rescued when police responded to a local motel where the mother was inebriated and making a ruckus. The police cited the fact that they found the child at that point who "said that she was the one who needed help" (Mother traded daughter, 1999).

Presentation of the facts might begin with the neglect component of the case. Demonstrating recidivism despite random drug screens is a good starting point for a prosecutor to illustrate that a child victim has been neglected and sexually abused because of actions and inactions taken by their parents or other caregivers. The sexual exploitation component of the prostitution of the child places the child's body at risk for sexually transmitted diseases (STDs) and HIV/AIDS and places the child's mind at risk for traumatic sequelae. **Case Study 34-2**, which began as a neglect case, transitioned into a child endangerment and sexual exploitation case. Defense strategies may highlight that the parent was "not in her right mind" and now that she is, family restoration rather than punishment is the most important outcome needed for this child. In this case, the medical expert can speak of the literature regarding drug rehabilitation relapse even with the best of program options. In addition, research has shown that when surveying child protective service workers across the United States, the most significant deterrent to rehabilitation for child abuse and neglect is parental substance abuse. Information such as this will provide a background from which the expert can communicate the high level of risk when a comorbid scenario, such as neglect and sexual exploitation, exists.

Psychological abuse cases entail a medical expert's knowledge of mental health cause-and-effect associations and long-term outcomes for victims when psychological damage has occurred. These cases frequently require the input of a counselor, psychologist, or psychiatrist and an understanding of the *Diagnostic and Statistical Manual of Mental Disorders*, 4th Edition, Text Revision. Psychological abuse is often underdiagnosed by medical practitioners. For example, a child is commonly victimized by child sexual abuse and emotionally affected. Even the medical record of a child sexual abuse case may include a mental health diagnosis such as depression or posttraumatic stress disorder (PTSD), but the concomitant diagnosis of emotional abuse is not included among the diagnoses for the patient. If a firm diagnosis has not been established for the child victim before trial, the expert will have to explain on the stand why the child's constellation of symptoms is consistent with a specific "label." It is unfortunate if an expert on the witness stand must make the first diagnostic conclusion, but at times this is necessary to meet the formal definitions of psychological abuse. This form of abuse has a significant victim impact. With and without intervention, children frequently have ongoing problems for years and sometimes for life. Categories of psychological abuse are summarized in **Table 34-2** (Pearl, 1998).

Case Study 34-3

AB was a 14-year-old female who was forced to move in with family friends when her own home was destroyed by fire and her mother became too destitute and overwhelmed to provide for her children. For several months, AB worked in the home helping her "aunt" take care of household chores. She was often reminded of how grateful she needed to be for the charity, which was being provided for her. After a few months, her "uncle" began including AB as part of his barter in his weekly card games. If he lost, he would make arrangements for AB to provide sexual fellatio to the winner later that night or during the week. He also coerced AB to provide fellatio to him, in return for any money that she might need. AB became depressed and felt that there was no escape for her. In addition, her "aunt" began to encourage her to drink alcohol with her, "so that she would feel better." AB made a disclosure to a school guidance counselor, and immediate steps were taken to remove her from the care of this family. Medical history was consistent over several interviews, and AB repeatedly stated that she knew that "it was all my fault because I took the money." Physical examination was normal, but behavioral evaluation revealed major depression with suicidal ideations.

Table 34-2. Categories of Psychological Abuse

Ignoring a child by failing to provide necessary stimulation, responsiveness, and validation of the child's worth in normal family routine.

Terrorizing a child with continued verbal assaults, creating a climate of fear, hostility, and anxiety, thus preventing the child from gaining feelings of safety and security.

Isolating a child from the family and community or denying the child normal human contact.

Corrupting a child by encouraging and reinforcing destructive, antisocial behavior until the child is so impaired in socioemotional development that interaction in normal social environments is impossible.

Rejecting a child's value, needs, and requests for adult validation and nurturance.

Verbally assaulting a child with constant name-calling, harsh threats, and sarcastic put-downs that continually "beat down" the child's self-esteem with humiliation.

Overpressuring a child with subtle but consistent pressure to grow up quickly and achieve too early in the areas of academics, physical/motor skills, and social interaction, which leaves the child feeling that he or she is never good enough.

This case illustrates the occurrence of psychological abuse and sexual exploitation. The victim experienced the trauma of forced sex with strange men and her care provider in exchange for her continued domicile and money. This form of corruption led the victim to see herself as the primary person at fault. She was hesitant to make a disclosure because of her dependence upon the offender for all of her survival needs. Complete dependence is a common familial dynamic when prostitution of children and youths occurs from the home.

THE QUALIFICATION EXAMINATION

The presentation of credentials and qualifications for an expert witness is important. Too often, an attorney will ask the healthcare provider to list his or her professional achievements and experience, usually beginning with undergraduate education. This method frequently results in a continuous sentence, which traverses possibly 2 or more decades of time. This is not the best way to present oneself to a jury or judge as a person whose opinion should be considered in a child abuse case. Instead, a healthcare provider should communicate with the attorney before trial and ask to be allowed to present his or her qualifications in a manner that allows the jury to understand the significance of each highlighted accomplishment. Using a template for qualification questions (**Table 34-3**) helps the attorney as well as the expert witness in providing information in a sequential and meaningful manner. This will afford the "sentence" to be broken into parts that are more easily understood.

Many healthcare providers who testify as experts may not be academics but may have extensive experience with respect to the clinical diagnosis of child sexual abuse and sexual exploitation. In addition, it may be clear that they attend conferences and stay abreast of the literature in this evolving field. Such experience is invaluable and should be quantified for a jury or judge so there is an understanding that final medical opinions or knowledge of the literature are intuitive. If a clinician has evaluated more than a thousand children over a period of years, such information should be provided to clarify the witness' clinical acumen.

On occasion, the training and expertise of an expert are accepted without a verbal challenge. This strategy serves to prevent the jury or judge from hearing the expert's qualifications, allowing the court to accept as a matter of record that the medical witness is acceptable as an expert. This method of shortening the qualification process should be avoided. A jury or judge must understand the breadth of an expert's knowledge and experience to consider the testimony for its substantive value. An expert may offer an attorney a template for a qualifying examination and a copy of his or her curriculum vitae as a working document of suggested questions.

THE MEDICAL DIAGNOSIS OF A CHILD SEXUAL ABUSE ARGUMENT

ICD-9-CM DETERMINATION

A universally accepted standard for documentation of medical diagnoses in the United States is the *International Classification of Diseases*, 9th Revision, Clinical Modification (ICD-9-CM) (American Medical Association, 2003). This classification was provided in October 2002 by the National Center for Health Statistics and the Centers for Medicare and Medicaid Services, 2 departments within the US Department of Health and Human Services. The purpose of the ICD-9-CM codes is to allow a physician and coder to work in a joint fashion to achieve complete and accurate documentation, assignment, and reporting of diagnoses and procedures. The ICD-9-CM assigned a specific section for the diagnoses of child and adult abuse. Published by the American Hospital Association, the classification places child abuse in the "E code" category, with guidelines that state that "E codes for child and adult abuse take priority over all other E codes" (American Medical Association, 2003). The guidelines state that when the cause of an injury or neglect is intentional child or

Table 34-3. Template for Medical Expert Qualifying Examination

QUESTION	EXPECTED RESPONSE
Please tell the jury your name.	Name
What is your profession?	Forensic (or child abuse) pediatrician, sexual assault nurse examiner (SANE), etc
Could you explain what a Forensic Pediatrician/SANE is?	A specialist who has training and experience in the evaluation, evidence gathering and treatment of children and adolescents who have been maltreated
Do you have an office practice?	Explanation
Do you have hospital affiliations?	List of affiliations
Do you provide consultations to agencies?	List of agencies, including law enforcement, nonprofit agencies, and all child abuse prevention programs
Please describe your educational background.	Undergraduate education to the highest degree of formal education, including any fellowship trainings
Please explain your work experience.	Internship until the present time, with a brief description of scope of practice in each site
Please give a summary of your professional experience in the area of child maltreatment.	Beginning in the year of the first case, explanation of child abuse cases seen as a consultant or staff healthcare provider
Do you have areas of specialty training in child maltreatment?	Fellowship training (if applicable); focused continued medical education training with approximately how many hours per year and the number of years of such training
Do you hold licenses or certifications?	List of all such documentation
Are there professional organizations in your field?	Yes, list of specific organizations
What is the purpose of these organizations?	Explanation that they provide ongoing education, peer interaction, and practice guidelines for clinicians in this field.
Do you hold memberships in any of these organizations?	List of specific organizations
Have you ever published any articles in the area of child abuse?	Yes (if works are relevant)
Would you summarize what these articles are about?	Explanation of pertinent works
Is it necessary for other experts to review potential articles in order to determine if they are scientifically based and reflect the opinions of the field?	Yes, and explain the relevance

(continued)

Table 34-3. Template for Medical Expert Qualifying Examination *(continued)*

QUESTION	EXPECTED RESPONSE
Is this review often referred to as a "peer review"?	Yes
Were the articles which you have published submitted for peer review?	Yes
Do you attend regular conferences in this field?	Yes, list of those that are relevant
Why do you attend conferences on a regular basis?	Explanation of the need to stay abreast of changes in practice guidelines
Have you presented lectures at conferences?	Yes, statement of whether local, national, and/or international
In how many conferences have you presented?	Number
Is your practice of medicine limited to child abuse?	Yes or no; if the answer is no, give percentage of time that is devoted to child maltreatment cases as compared to the remainder of the practice
How many child maltreatment cases have you evaluated?	Number
Have you been asked to evaluate children who did not have a diagnosis of child maltreatment?	Yes, statement of general circumstances
Have you testified in court before today?	Yes
In what types of court proceedings have you testified?	Explanation
Have you been qualified as an expert witness before?	Yes
In what types of courts have you been qualified as an expert?	List of courts
Have you had the opportunity to work with defense attorneys in the past in child abuse cases?	Yes; if relationship has been consultative, citation of such
Do you always testify as a witness for the prosecution in child abuse cases?	Yes or no; explanation of what percentage of cases as prosecution or defense witness

adult abuse, the first listed E code should be assigned from categories E960-968, which define the nature of the abuse. Perpetrator information falls into the following E categories: E967.0, which indicates abuse by a father or stepfather; E967.2, which indicates abuse by a mother or stepmother; and E967.3, which indicates abuse by spouse or partner. The specific ICD-9-CM codes for the various forms of child maltreatment are listed in **Table 34-4**.

This information will assist in refuting the argument that child sexual abuse or sexual exploitation is not a diagnosis but a preceding event, which leads to a more mental health-related diagnosis. A medical expert could certainly argue that hospitals, insurance companies, and other health care providers accept ICD-9-CM codes. If such a

Table 34-4. ICD-9-CM Codes for Child Maltreatment	
995.5	Child maltreatment syndrome
995.50	Child abuse, unspecified
995.51	Child emotional/psychological abuse
995.52	Child neglect (nutritional)
995.53	Child sexual abuse
995.54	Child physical abuse (battered baby or child syndrome, excluding shaken infant syndrome)
995.55	Shaken infant syndrome (with instructions to use additional codes to identify other associated injuries)
995.59	Other child abuse and neglect

Adapted from American Medical Association. International Classification of Diseases, 9th Revision, Clinical Modification. *Chicago, Ill: American Medical Association; 2003.*

standard is acceptable in the medical community, which is responsible for the establishment of the concept of "diagnosis," there should be no justification for a legal challenge.

DSM-IV-TR CRITERIA DETERMINATION

An additional accepted standard for the recognized medical diagnosis of child abuse and child sexual abuse is the *Diagnostic and Statistical Manual of Mental Disorders*, 4th Edition, Text Revision (DSM-IV-TR) (American Psychiatric Association, 2000). Devised by the American Psychiatric Association, this diagnostic instrument assists clinicians in categorizing patient symptoms into brief criteria sets with clarity of language and explicit statements, which assist in the establishment of a mental health diagnosis. The DSM-IV-TR criteria for mental health diagnoses have been widely accepted internationally to include input from the World Health Organization so as to increase diagnostic compatibility.

The diagnostic code for child maltreatment in the DSM-IV-TR is referred to as a "V code." The original maltreatment "V code" applied if the focus of attention was on the perpetrator of the abuse or neglect or on the relational unit in which it had occurred. Consequently, if the diagnosis of an offender of sexual abuse exists, why would the diagnosis of a victim be excluded? This would constitute the first phase of argument for the expert witness. When the individual being evaluated or treated is the victim of the abuse or neglect, the code 995.5 is used for a child and 995.81 is used for an adult (American Psychiatric Association, 2000). These codes consequently coincide with that in the ICD-9-CM and constitute 2 different recognized international agencies, which accept the diagnosis of child sexual abuse.

The presence of diagnostic codes for child abuse, including sexual abuse, assists in rebutting the argument by some that there is no such diagnosis as that of "child sexual abuse." These proponents argue that if no illness or injury is present, no medical diagnosis is appropriate. They would argue, therefore, that a medical expert is not qualified for this testimony, since a "diagnosis" is not in question. Diagnoses, which are recognized by the American Hospital Association, are one way in which physicians and healthcare systems are able to bill for services. It is illogical that a condition that is recognized as a billable diagnosis would not be seen as a true diagnosis in a court of law. The counter argument to this line of thought is that physical abuse has long been recognized as a diagnosis. Battered child syndrome and shaken baby syndrome are diagnoses readily accepted by the judicial system. Child sexual abuse is a similarly recognized form of abuse, and it would be seen as a frivolous argument to attempt to separate this form of child abuse from the diagnostic criteria as compared to the other forms of abuse. Since the majority of CSE cases involve sexual abuse, the standard diagnosis is appropriate.

PRACTICE GUIDELINES FROM NATIONAL ORGANIZATIONS

A final justification for the recognition of a diagnosis of child sexual abuse would be as has been established by national organizations, which provide practice guidelines for clinicians who care for children. The American Academy of Pediatrics (AAP) and the American Professional Society on the Abuse of Children (APSAC) have agreed upon and published guidelines for making the decision to report sexual abuse in children. These guidelines exist because all healthcare providers have a duty to identify sexually abused children and ensure their safety (Finkel & Giardino, 2002; Reece, 2000; Reece & Ludwig, 2001).

When establishing the diagnosis of child sexual abuse and CSE, it is important to be able to verbalize that other diagnoses were considered. For this reason, a careful history from the parent or care provider is as essential as is the child's own medical history (Myers et al, 2002). Information should include the following:

— Inquiries about past sexual abuse

— Determination of family relationships; a ***genogram***, or an organizational chart showing genetic history, can be used

— Screens for other history of abuse and neglect, as well as a history of family violence or inappropriate sexuality

— Developmental history including function in school and peer relationships

— Genitourinary and menstrual history to include vaginal and anal pain, bleeding, enuresis, encopresis, STDs, and pregnancy

— Family history of physical and mental illness

— Screens for risk factors in the perpetrator (eg, drug use, sexual preference, etc.)

Table 34-5 summarizes guidelines to follow when formulating a diagnosis of sexual abuse or sexual exploitation.

TYPES OF MEDICAL EXPERT TESTIMONY

At times, a medical expert is called upon to testify in the form of "a dissertation or exposition of the scientific or other principles relevant to the case, leaving the [jury] to apply them to the facts" (Federal Rules of Evidence 702). This type of testimony is primarily to educate a jury or judge. The expert must keep the information relevant to the specific case. A common application of this testimony is seen in child sexual abuse cases in which an expert must explain delayed disclosure, recantation, or the complexity of a multiple victim child sexual abuse scenario (Myers et al, 2002).

Sexual exploitation cases may be more difficult because of the diverse dynamics present beyond those seen in sexual abuse without exploitation. Unlike physical abuse, where a judge must determine the most likely etiology of an injury which is present, or a neglect case, where a child might be able to testify regarding supervision or parental expectations, CSE cases may have a victim who has never disclosed or who at trial refuses to admit that he or she has been victimized. In cases of prostituted children and youths, for example, one of the key deterrents to prosecution is the unwillingness of the victim to testify against her "pimp," who has often established a romantic control relationship with the juvenile. The victim is intimidated regarding exposing details about her pimp and may be fearful about her fate if the person who represents her sole support is incarcerated. Though he or she is providing the sex work, he or she often sees the pimp as the person who protects him or her and provides well-

Table 34-5. Guidelines for Making the Decision to Report Sexual Abuse of Children

DATA AVAILABLE			RESPONSE	
History	Physical Examination	Laboratory Findings	Level of Concern About Abuse	Report Decision
None	Normal	None	None	No report
Behavioral changes*	Normal	None	Variable depending upon behavior	Possible report†; follow closely (possible mental health referral)
None	Nonspecific findings	None	Low (worry)	Possible report†; follow closely
Nonspecific history by child or history by parent only	Nonspecific findings	None	Intermediate	Possible report†; follow closely
None	Specific Findings‡	None	High	Report
Clear Statement	Normal	None	High	Report
Clear Statement	Specific Findings	None	High	Report
None	Normal, nonspecific or specific findings	Positive culture for gonorrhea; positive serologic test for HIV; syphilis; presence of semen, sperm acid phosphatase	Very high	Report
Behavior changes	Nonspecific findings	Other sexually transmitted diseases	High	Report

* Some behavioral changes are nonspecific, and others are more worrisome (Krugman, 1986).

† A report may or may not be indicated. The decision to report should be based on discussion with local or regional experts and/or child protective services agencies.

‡ Other reasons for findings ruled out (Bays & Jenny, 1990).

Reprinted from American Academy of Pediatrics Committee on Child Abuse and Neglect. Reproduced with permission from Pediatrics, Vol. 103, Pages 186-191, Copyright © 1999 by the AAP.

being. CSE cases often require advanced technical and psychological testimony to explain the investigation of the crime and the dynamics of victimology. This portion of the case may be confusing to the judge, jury, and the attorneys.

The medical expert who is testifying regarding child behavior in a sexual exploitation case may provide substantive evidence or may serve to rehabilitate a child's damaged credibility after it has been attacked by a defense attorney (Myers & Stern, 2002).

SUBSTANTIVE TESTIMONY

Substantive expert testimony regarding a child's behavior or mental health status has at least the following 3 forms:

1. The expert offers an opinion that the child has a diagnosis of child sexual abuse and/or CSE.

2. The medical expert may avoid the statement that the child has a diagnosis of sexual abuse or CSE and opt instead for the use of the phrase "consistent with" a

specific diagnosis. In other words, the expert states that the child's history and behaviors are consistent with those seen in children who have been sexually abused and or exploited. A medical expert may state in an analysis of child pornography that the images are consistent with a child less than 18 years of age.

3. The expert may avoid mention whatsoever of the specific child in the case at hand and confine testimony to a description of methods of seduction or symptoms frequently observed in sexually abused or exploited children as a group.

REHABILITATIVE TESTIMONY

Rehabilitative testimony is uncontroversial and is offered solely to provide rehabilitation to a child's credibility after it is attacked by the defense attorney. When expert testimony is offered for this purpose, it is not offered as substantive evidence. Specific issues that a defense attorney may emphasize to discredit a child would include the child's delayed disclosure as an example of a fictitious report; abnormal behaviors being compatible with other life circumstances that the child is experiencing; or recantation, which often occurs in child sexual abuse and is misinterpreted as "finally telling the truth" but reflects family pressure on a child. In a CSE case, a defense attorney might cite that increased sexual knowledge in a child might be secondary to the child having accessed pornography on the Internet. There may be the inference that sexual abuse images of the child were digitally derived, are virtual in nature, and are not true reproductions of the child. This is particularly relevant because children often will not admit that Internet pornographic images are self-portraits. In the circumstance of home-based prostitution, the defense might state that the adolescent is consensually sexually available to the various perpetrators. The incidence of behavioral dysfunction in sexually abused adolescents in particular makes them especially vulnerable to castigation. Such behaviors as drug or alcohol abuse, runaway behavior, or indiscriminate sexual activity make them easy prey for damaging cross-examination by a defense attorney. When a teen develops a romantic relationship with the pimp and denies that he or she has experienced sexual assault, but, instead, willingly had sexual relationships with others, rehabilitative testimony is essential.

When the medical expert must respond with rehabilitative testimony, the scope will be limited to the specific points highlighted by the defense attorney. For example, in home-based prostitution, sexual cooperation presented as consensual and volitional behaviors must be explained within the context of accommodation and resignation to the dependent nature of the child's survival. In the circumstance of child pornography, where the child is smiling and appearing to have willingly posed for images that could therefore be seen as "self-made," the expert would need to testify regarding evidence from previous investigations that reveal the "director" behavior of child pornographers.

In the majority of cases, expert rehabilitation testimony is limited to a general review of the literature and the expert's experience of children as a group who have manifested specific behaviors. The testimony should not be case-specific. If it is necessary to refer to the particular child, the expert should avoid the use of the term "victim" because this sends a message to the jury that the expert believes that the child has been abused; this conclusion is for the jury to decide (Myers & Stern, 2002).

Expert testimony in general and rehabilitative testimony in particular should avoid the use of the term "syndrome," such as the child abuse accommodation syndrome (Summit, 1983) or the parental alienation syndrome (Gardner, 1992). The use of the word syndrome, specifically by a medical expert, infers that a specific diagnosis has been determined and causes the jury to feel no other option is available for their consideration (Myers & Stern, 2002). The parental alienation syndrome is frequently suggested by the defense, and the medical expert may be called upon to educate the jury regarding its controversial stance in the literature (Faller, 1998; Myers, 1993, 1997, 1998).

TYPES OF EXPERT WITNESSES

Expert witnesses can function in 1 of 3 ways: as a background witness, a case witness, or an evaluating witness (Stern, 1997). Although the jobs of each of these types of witnesses are different, one can visualize the process on a continuum (**Figure 34-1**).

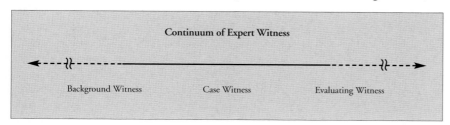

Continuum of Expert Witness

Background Witness   Case Witness   Evaluating Witness

Figure 34-1. The 3 types of expert witnesses can be placed on a continuum because of their varying degrees of involvement in a case.

BACKGROUND WITNESS

The background witness educates the judge or jury regarding the general scientific information regarding relevant information about the abuse case. Child sexual abuse and CSE require more jury education than any other type of maltreatment because of numerous jury biases and stereotypes (eg, the belief that juvenile prostitution is usually a voluntary form of sexual activity). The background witness can explain the development of the field of forensic pediatrics, and the need for knowledge in multiple areas when evaluating abuse. Medical information without investigative data would often yield an inappropriate diagnosis. Background witnesses do not have to render a medical opinion about the case since their task is to provide general scientific information (Stern, 1997). For example, such a witness might testify regarding the relationship between being a runaway or thrownaway child and succumbing to survival sex after a period of time of being homeless. The background witness could cite specifics in the literature regarding the number of children who are involved in prostitution, the related difficulties in medical problems, and the high incidence of depression and posttraumatic stress disorder (PTSD) as the mental health impact of child and juvenile prostitution.

CASE WITNESS

A case witness is further along the continuum in that this expert would review information specific to the case, including clinical medical records, videotaped interviews, mental health records, investigative reports, and child protection evaluations. This expert would be responsible for interpreting this information based upon knowledge of the literature and his or her experience. Such an expert could draw further conclusions that are case-specific and allow for testimony, which might reinforce the information provided by the victim (Stern, 1997). For example, if a child gives the history of having been thrownaway, resulting in the child becoming homeless and having to resort to survival sex, child protection reports and social service interviews of family members might indeed substantiate this history. Family and care provider interviews might indicate the complete lack of support for the child, and if the child had disclosed neglect and sexual abuse while still at home, there may be evidence of these matters.

The provision of case information can be important in that many child and juvenile witnesses may be ineffective in their courtroom testimony. Young children may not even be deemed competent to testify. Delay in the timing of a trial may contribute to a young child's inability to recall important details, which he or she may have already disclosed in previous records of the investigation. Furthermore, detecting underlying jury bias may be very difficult, especially in the adolescent victim. Allowing the jury or judge to hear the collateral circumstances from a professional who is experienced in explaining the cause and effect phenomenon of family disintegration may provide a more convincing stance for the victim status of the juvenile. The case witness provides more information than just background and makes the record relevant to the specific trial. Despite this degree of applicability, a case witness does not evaluate the child or juvenile. His or her testimony can, however, include an opinion, which is directly related to the facts of the case.

EVALUATING WITNESS

The evaluating witness has knowledge of the background science and literature, has reviewed the medical records, videotaped interview, investigative reports, and other information, and has personally evaluated the child or juvenile. The evaluating witness can, therefore, draw his or her conclusion based upon access to the greatest amount of information. This type of witness is likely to have significant credibility and his or her opinions can be made with the highest degree of confidence (Stern, 1997). This witness's function is at the end of the continuum of expert witness testimony. Using the original example of the runaway or thrownaway youth, whose plight results in homelessness and survival sex, this witness would have had the opportunity to review all available records regarding a prostituted juvenile and could then testify about an interview with the young man or woman, describing his or her degree of depression and sense of hopelessness after having been on the streets for 3 years.

Child sexual abuse cases require that a medical expert be able to lay a foundation in a substantive manner about the pertinent aspects of child sexual abuse present in the specific case. The testimony must explore that 3 elements are usually required to diagnose this type of case: the history, the child's behaviors, and the physical examination. After these specifics have been discussed in a generic fashion, the expert may then begin to testify regarding the specific facts of the case, making correlations as they become apparent.

TESTIMONY IN CHILD SEXUAL ABUSE

To testify effectively in a CSE case, even one that is specifically that of child pornography, the medical expert needs to be prepared to discuss child sexual abuse. Whether a victim has been pornographically photographed, solicited online by a stranger who presents himself or herself as someone that he or she is not, or is a child who is being sold with or without the use of a computer for money or other tangible favors for the sole purpose of sex, the medical expert needs to be versed in the important elements in confirming the diagnosis of child sexual abuse.

ELEMENT I: THE MEDICAL HISTORY

The medical history is a standard part of every medical evaluation. In general pediatrics, the history may be obtained from 2 sources: a care provider such as a parent and/or the child. An expert must explain this is a normal procedure, and that getting information from a parent or other care provider does not constitute hearsay but is an acceptable standard of care in medical practice. Another aspect of the medical history as taken from a child or adolescent involves instructing a child as to the medical provider's role so the child will understand that the encounter is indeed for a medical "check up." Specific states require this information be shared with the child at the beginning of the medical interview so no confusion occurs that the questions are being asked to obtain a medical diagnosis and provide treatment.

Obtaining the medical history is important since trials often occur months to years after a child has had a medical evaluation, and the child's ability to recall minute details may become impaired due to the time lapse. In child sexual abuse cases, there is frequently information from an investigative source, such as a child protection social worker or a law enforcement agent. The collateral and circumstantial information is then considered within the context of the care provider and the child victim interview so as to collect all of the pieces and come to the most complete medical opinion possible. At times, the medical evaluation may include the gathering of outside information, such as school records, therapist's reports, or foster care provider interviews. If the medical expert witness is the child's healthcare provider for the sexual abuse evaluation, these ancillary items of information afford a more thorough medical record. If not, the medical expert should request this information when preparing to testify.

The medical expert may establish a foundation of testimony regarding the 3 elements of a child sexual abuse and sexual exploitation case: the history, the child's behaviors, and the physical examination. Using this template, the expert can educate the jury and judge regarding the complex and diverse details, which are taken into consideration before a healthcare provider can arrive at the diagnosis of child sexual abuse and CSE.

Historical information includes the following factors:

— *Method of disclosure.* Spontaneous, an excited utterance, coerced

— *Content of the child's disclosure.* Who, what happened, when, where, how long in the child's life, what did the abuser say would happen if the child ever told

— *Consistency of the child's information.* Consistent with explicit sexual knowledge (eg, fellatio, forced masturbation techniques), consistent core elements over time

— *Sensory memory of the child.* What the child felt, saw, heard, tasted, and smelled

The method of disclosure is always important. In sexual exploitation, this may occur when a child is shown pictures that were discovered showing the child in a sexually explicit pose or being sexually abused. Such pictures may be of such an explicit nature that the child may acknowledge that sexual abuse has occurred.

At times, a child's disclosure is described as "accidental." This refers to the child who makes a spontaneous utterance, which might be during a moment of anger or fright. It might occur as information shared in confidence with a best friend or another adult other than a family member. Another motivation for disclosure is that of altruism. A child commonly verbalizes the choice of disclosing sexual abuse or exploitation to save another child or sibling from suffering the same abusive dynamics that the victim has experienced. Because of the complex feelings and emotions that surround child sexual abuse and the fact that many victims feel responsible for their abuse and have significant self-blame, denigration by the perpetrator as a frequent motivator for disclosure is uncommon. Occasionally in the circumstance when an adolescent wants the abuse to stop or wants to seek revenge for abuse or other perceived infringements upon his or her independence, a disclosure may be made that might cause questions regarding veracity. The circumstance does not necessarily negate the truthfulness of the disclosure.

Case Study 34-4

RH was a 12-year-old female who was seen in a child sexual abuse clinic because of sexual abuse and exploitation. Her mother related that a female coworker found several Polaroid pictures taken of RH by the coworker's 2 sons, who were ages 19 and 20 years. The young men resided near the victim's neighborhood. The photos were in the possession of the sheriff's deputies at the time of the RH's medical evaluation, and the accompanying law enforcement officer shared these photos with the physician. All of the photos had the child in a nude position, with her legs widely abducted as she was seated on a bed. In some photos, she was separating her labia with her fingers, and relatively close-up photos were taken, though her entire body, including her face, was in all of the photos. While obtaining a history of the episode(s), RH admitted to the examiner that the young men had given her wine coolers before taking the photos. She was subsequently told that the photos would be circulated to her family and friends unless she agreed to have sexual intercourse with each man, separately. She acquiesced to the extortion. She reported that both men hurt her since this was her first sexual experience. She spoke of bleeding vaginally after these events had occurred. This took place on one occasion at the home of the young men. Later, she felt guilty about having ever gone to the men's home. She had made no disclosure of this sexual abuse and exploitation until her mother confronted her with the photos.

RH was an average student at school but had begun to show a decline in her school performance. Her review of systems and past medical history was unremarkable. She had

If pornographic pictures have been discovered as part of the crime scene investigation or as part of the beginning of the investigation and the child insists that no images were ever taken, the medical professional should not force the child to admit cul-

onset of her menses at 11 years and she was regular. She had begun to get poor grades particularly in physical education because of refusal to "dress out" for class. She used to have

Table 34-7. Questions Pertinent to Sexual Exploitation

CHILD PORNOGRAPHY

— Were pornographic images shown to the child?

— In what format were these images (photos, videos, computer images, etc)?

— Were these images inclusive of adults only, or did they include children?

— Did the perpetrator take any pictures of the child?

— If yes, in what format (eg, photos, videos, Web cam)?

— What did the perpetrator say would happen to the pictures?

— Was the child alone or were other children involved in the image production?

— Was the child offered or coerced to use drugs or alcohol before being sexually abused?

— Was the child instructed to do certain things to himself or herself, to another child, or with the perpetrator while images were taken?

— Was the child told to pose and smile?

— Was the child hit, slapped, kicked, beaten, or physically abused as a means of coercion for the production of the pornography or as a method to assure secrecy?

— Was the child offered any incentives for the sexual abuse and exploitation (eg, money, gifts, excursions)?

— Did the child witness any incentives being given to a family member or caregiver (eg, money, drugs) in exchange for the child's sexual abuse and exploitation?

— Has the child ever seen these sexual images since the abuse, and if so, where?

PROSTITUTED CHILDREN AND YOUTHS

— Did the offender* ask the child to engage in sexual activity with someone else?

— Did the offender offer the child money, survival needs, or safety from abandonment if the child would comply with sexual requests?

— Was the child related in any way to the offender?

— Was the child encouraged or coerced to commit crimes (eg, stealing from the perpetrator[†])?

— Was the child offered or coerced to use drugs or alcohol before or after being sexually abused and exploited?

— At what age did sexual abuse occur if indeed this preceded the sexual exploitation?

— At what age was the child forced into prostitution?

— Was the child or juvenile's survival (food, clothing, or shelter) linked to providing sexual favors for a primary offender or others at his or her direction?

— Was the child hit, slapped, kicked, beaten, or otherwise sexually injured by the perpetrator to whom he or she was sold for sexual purposes?

— Was the child or juvenile hit, slapped, punched, beaten, kicked, or otherwise battered by an offender before or during coercion to perform sexual acts for money or other collateral?

— Was the child threatened with injury or death if he or she was not compliant with either the desires of the perpetrator or the offender who was marketing the child for gain?

— Has the child ever been arrested for prostitution and if so, at what age?

(continued)

Table 34-7. *(continued)*

CYBER-ENTICEMENT OF CHILDREN AND YOUTHS

— Was the child in contact with the perpetrator through use of the Internet in any way?

— How was the child contacted by this perpetrator?

— Did the child have an Internet identity that was different from his or her true identity and if so, in what ways (eg, age, profile)?

— Was the child advised to keep his or her relationship secret from family and friends?

— How long did the child have an online relationship with the perpetrator?

— Is the child a compliant victim in this case?

— Was the child given any gifts during the online "friendship" (eg, money, camera, cell phone)?

— Was the child encouraged to leave his or her home to meet or runaway with the perpetrator?

— Did the child leave home, and what consequences occurred upon meeting his or her "online friend"?

— How was the child recovered?

— Was the child hit, slapped, punched, beaten, kicked, or otherwise battered during the commission of the crimes of enticement, sexual abuse, and exploitation?

— Was the child pornographically photographed by the perpetrator or others?

— Was there evidence of any specific sexual fetish evidenced in the manner of the sexual abuse and exploitation (eg, bondage, sadomasochism)?

* *Offender refers to the individual selling a victim for sexual abuse and exploitation*

† *Perpetrator refers to the individual who buys the child for sexual abuse and exploitation.*

pability. The denial on the part of the child constitutes a defense mechanism, and even if the child does not admit to pictures being taken but acknowledges sexual abuse, the sexual abuse images are self-evident. The child may not recall the production of sexual abuse images, or intensive therapy may need to take place before the child can admit to what may constitute clear evidence of complicity in the perception of the child victim. Though this perception on the part of the child is erroneous, one can not underestimate the impact of photographic evidence of the child's victimization.

Children who are being sold for sexual abuse as a condition of residence in this country or at their current domicile, such as adolescent domestic workers, may have a strong motive to deny exploitation because their survival may rest upon keeping this a secret. A medical expert must be able to explain the need for a child to keep the prostitution a secret. The medical expert should seek to establish that the child's health history is credible. Collateral witnesses discovered by law enforcement may be necessary to confirm the situation. When the child prostitution victim is young, recollection of sexual abuse may encompass the reality of multiple unknown perpetrators who are often brought to the child's room at night by their parent or custodial caregiver. On the other hand, they may be transported to a client by a care provider with minimal ability to recall matters related to perpetrator identification. An additional factor that can impact a court hearing is the possible presence of a dissociative disorder affecting the child. This psychiatric diagnosis has symptoms of a flat affect, associated with recounts of sexual trauma verbally delivered in such an unemotional manner that a victim's testimony often requires significant expert witness rehabilitation. The child may have no knowledge of the sex-for-money arrangement that is often present.

A common defense strategy is to castigate the child or adolescent victim for the delay in disclosure. A stereotypical response to a sexual assault, erroneously felt, is that a victim will immediately relate the details to anyone that he or she can. A jury needs to be advised that nothing could be further from the truth. Children often feel responsible for what happens to them, and consequently, sexual abuse will make them feel they have been particularly bad. They have no desire for anyone to know how bad they have been, so they often tuck this secret away, frequently waiting until adulthood before making a disclosure. The typical delayed disclosure has been discussed at length in the child maltreatment literature (Finklehor et al, 1990; Gomes-Schwartz et al, 1990; Hanson et al, 1999; Mullen et al, 1993; Paine & Hansen, 2002; Smith et al, 2000).

When a child or juvenile has been forced into a prostitution scenario, intimidation is so common that these victims are often exceedingly reluctant to give important and relevant details. Often the entry for these victims into the justice system is through the juvenile criminal justice route, and they are personally charged as culprits. They may have been arrested because of the commission of other crimes out of the necessity for survival. Nevertheless, these children and juveniles present as perpetrators of crime rather than the victims that they are. The public holds a common bias that prostitutes readily participate in sexual work and that it is a choice for which the client should not be held culpable. Even when children are marketed from within their own biological or custodial family, sexual abuse through prostitution is mistakenly perceived to be a volitional action. Often it is not recognized that children and youths acquiesce at best. Disclosure of such abuse is typically delayed. In one sample, 76% of children did not disclose sexual abuse of any sort within a week of the last event (Gomes-Schwartz et al, 1990). Often the child makes a disclosure to a friend or other family member in what is sometimes referred to as an ***accidental disclosure***. Such a disclosure appears to have been made without prior thought or planning, and if spoken while the child is in a state of excitation, is referred to as an ***excited utterance***. Other manners in which disclosure occurs is when there is an eyewitness discovery of a sexual event; if there are pornographic pictures, videos, or other evidence found; if the child has suspicious behaviors; or if medical evaluations reveal evidence supportive of sexual abuse. In the circumstance of intrafamilial sexual exploitation with either prostitution or pornography, a nonoffending family member may discover "sexual props" such as provocative clothing, sexual toys, or photographic items not recognized as belonging to the family in general.

Children who have been sexually abused in an exploitative manner from within the family may be in a similar circumstance as that described by Dr. Roland Summit in the Child Sexual Abuse Accommodation Syndrome (CSAAS), a compilation of behaviors that explain delayed disclosure and the risk for recantation (**Table 34-8**) (Summit, 1983, 1994). Summit described the psychological state of a child or adolescent who is in a sexually abusive home as one in which the child must accommodate to the abuse. He explains the 5 aspects of this adjustment as first entailing secrecy such that the child is unable to disclose or share with family members or others the details of the sexual abuse that is happening to them. Once secrecy has been engrained into the child's thoughts and behaviors, a sense of helplessness takes place, followed by the realization that he or she is trapped and must consequently accommodate. At a certain point, the child does make an effort to escape from victimization by making a delayed and often unconvincing disclosure. Because the outcry is often met with disbelief or an immense family endorsement of the perpetrator, the child frequently feels that the problem rests within himself or herself and the child recants the original information.

Table 34-8. The Child Sexual Abuse Accommodation Syndrome (CSAAS)
— Secrecy
— Helplessness
— Entrapment and accommodation
— Delayed and often unconvincing disclosure
— Retraction

Many courts restrict testimony regarding the CSAAS because it does not meet the formal definition within the medical and mental health community of a syndrome. However, Summit has been clear that the purpose of this clinical observation is to explain this constellation of behaviors so commonly seen in intrafamilial child sexual abuse. It has relevance when pressure is placed upon a child by nonsupportive family members that recantation is the best option, even if the family partially believes the child's disclosure. An expert may need to educate a jury regarding these well-accepted behaviors though the term may have to be omitted. In addition, since child pornography production and child prostitution often begins in the home (Estes & Weiner, 2001), the CSAAS has significant relevance.

ELEMENT II: BEHAVIOR

The second major element in a child sexual abuse and exploitation case would be the child's behavior. Changes in behavior are important because at times, one can establish a timeline that could correlate the onset of the abuse with the changes in the child's behavior. This behavioral history requires that the observer of the child is supportive, accurate, and able to provide significant details. Behavior, though included as a historical parameter, deserves its own categorization because the examiner will often observe abnormalities during the encounter. This places the significance of behavior somewhere between the history and the physical examination since there is an overlap between the 2 (**Figure 34-2**).

Behavior is often the most compelling of the 3 elements in child sexual abuse. It is compelling because it is least likely to be contrived. Depending upon the age of the child, realization of actual vaginal or anal penetration can at times be confusing. But even if in court a child is described as being "mistaken about having been raped," it is unlikely that the child can fabricate recurrent nightmares, fearfulness of males or females, sudden behavioral changes associated with increased sexual interest, or being self-conscious about his or her body. The child would not have knowledge of the association of intrusive thoughts of abuse, and he or she would not know that sexually explicit play (in a younger child) would have significance and relevance to his or her "fabricated" victimization.

An important body of evidence in the child sexual abuse literature confirms that abnormal behaviors are often seen in child sexual abuse victims during and after the abuse (**Table 34-9**). Frequent effects of sexual abuse include reports of higher rates of emotional and behavioral problems in victims as compared to nonabused peers (Boney-McKoy & Finkelhor, 1995; Kilpatrick & Saunders, 1999), more depressive symptoms and low self-esteem (Mannarino & Cohen, 1996; McLeer et al, 1998; Stern et al, 1995), and a wide range of interpersonal problems as compared to children with no history of sexual abuse (Boney-McCoy & Finkelhor, 1995; Friedrich, 1993; Friedrich et al, 1992; Gomes-Schwartz et al, 1990; Hibbard et al, 1990;

Figure 34-2. *There is overlap between the reported (medical history) and the observed behavior (physical examination).*

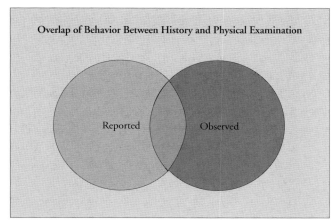

Overlap of Behavior Between History and Physical Examination

Reported   Observed

Table 34-9. Modified Clinical Encounter Form for Child Sexual Abuse

Headaches	Anger outbursts
Stomachaches	Sexual acting out
Sleep disturbances	Inappropriate masturbation
Eating disorders	Unusual fearfulness
School problems	Withdrawn behavior
Intrusive thoughts of the abuse	Easy crying
Signs of depression	Sexually explicit play

Adapted from Clinical Encounter Form. North Carolina Child Medical Evaluation Program, University of North Carolina at Chapel Hill; 2001.

Lindblad et al, 1995; Mannarino & Cohen, 1996; Wolfe & Birt, 1995). Suicidal behavior (Lanktree et al, 1991), posttraumatic behaviors (Boney-McCoy & Finkelhor, 1995; Briere, 1996; McLeer, 1998; Ruggiero et al, 2000), substance abuse problems (Kilpatrick & Saunders, 1999), and increased sexualized behaviors especially associated with genital sexual activity, such as mimicking intercourse and inserting objects in the vagina and anus (Friedrich et al, 2001) have been reported. The sexual abuse victim has been noted to have more sexualized behaviors than clinical comparisons of victims of neglect, physical abuse, and psychiatrically disturbed children (Friedrich et al, 1997; Adams et al 1995). In older children, sexualized behaviors may be seen with girls demonstrating provocative dressing and poor stranger interpersonal boundaries. Boys may often engage in genital exposure and sexual coercion (Adams et al, 1995).

School performance declines and cognitive distortions have been noted in sexually abused children (Rust & Troupe, 1991) as well as a heightened degree of self-blame and reduced interpersonal trust (Mannarino et al, 1994). Documentation of such school decline usually entails review of report cards and midterm reports. When considering offering information regarding school performance as a demonstrative aid, a graph reflecting the child's grades per subject over several school years should be presented. An example is shown in **Figure 34-3**. An indication of preexisting academic performance, followed by a marker indicating the onset of abuse as per the child's disclosure would then be presented. A decline in grades is better understood when visualized in this manner.

In a study surveying experienced forensic professionals regarding behaviors that they felt were indicators of sexual abuse (Conte et al, 1991), more than 90% ranked the following to be important:

—Age-inappropriate sexual knowledge

—Sexualized play during the interview

—Precocious or seductive behavior

—Excessive masturbation

—Consistency in the child's description of the abuse over time

—The child's report of pressure or coercion

—Medical evidence of abuse

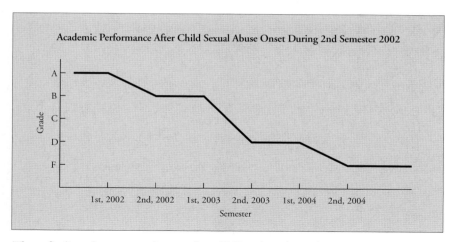

Academic Performance After Child Sexual Abuse Onset During 2nd Semester 2002

These findings have some degree of credibility though professional judgment based upon clinical experience alone, without knowledge of the literature to augment decision making, can at times lead to erroneous decisions (Conte et al, 1991; Myers et al, 2002).

Though the majority of children do not disclose at the time of their victimization (Palmer et al, 1999), an equal number of children deteriorate behaviorally over time as those who improve behaviorally (Tebbutt et al, 1997). Between 10% and 24% of child victims deteriorate or do not improve over time. Interestingly, children who seemed highly symptomatic at their first presentation did better 1½ years later, compared to those children who were initially least symptomatic. These data assist in explaining that some children are resilient, and their behaviors may be minimal in quantity. Regardless, the long-term sequelae of child sexual abuse have been well researched (Finklehor et al, 1990; Smith et al, 1993). Their impact upon the quality of a person's adult life is significant. No matter whether symptoms are mild or severe, those found in adults usually represent an extension of those found in children (Neumann et al, 1996). This information is important for the members of the jury to hear as they begin to recognize the life-changing impact that sexual abuse can cause.

It is a common defense strategy to attribute behavioral changes in a victim to other family and social circumstances in a child's life, such as intimate partner violence or separation and divorce. The medical expert may need to reinforce the fact more than once in the testimony that specifically intrusive thoughts of sexual abuse have never been attributed to any untoward family circumstance.

A recent study in families with twins where only 1 child has been a victim of sexual abuse found compelling results in the victimized child: "In this large twin study, we found that individuals reporting a history of [childhood sexual abuse] had increased risk for subsequently occurring adverse outcomes of depression, suicide attempts, conduct disorder, alcohol and/or nicotine dependence, social anxiety, rape after the age of 18 years old, and divorce" (Nelson et al, 2002).

The most common mental health diagnoses seen in child sexual abuse cases are some form of depression and/or PTSD (**Table 34-10**). Symptoms of PTSD are observed in more than half of sexually abused children (Kendall-Tackett et al, 1993). "Although most child sexual abuse victims do not meet the full diagnostic criteria for PTSD, more than 80% are reported to have some posttraumatic symptoms" (Briere & Elliott, 1994). Other researchers add that "the type, duration, and frequency of trauma determines the likelihood of PTSD development, and as such [PTSD] may result from a single or repeated traumatic event exposure" (Famularo et al, 1996).

Flashbacks of sexual abuse are often reported by children suffering from PTSD. This constitutes a reexperiencing of the traumatic event. It is often caused by distract-

Table 34-10. Posttraumatic Stress Disorder (PTSD)
— Life changing experience causing intense fear, helplessness, or horror (disorganized or agitated behavior)
— Reexperiencing the trauma events by intrusive thoughts, dreams, or trauma-specific reenactment
— Persistent avoidance of stimuli associated with the trauma
— Symptoms of increased arousal not present before the trauma (eg, insomnia, anger outbursts, inattentiveness, hypervigilance)
— Impairment of social, occupational, or other important areas of functioning
— Duration of symptoms for greater than 1 month

ibility in the classroom, which is sometimes alluded to by school-aged children. In addition, children frequently describe rising anxiety as they are returning home. The school bus ride represents for many a fearful experience, not because of the ride, but because of what awaits at its conclusion. This desire to avoid the site of abuse is another component of PTSD and present when the offender is no longer in the home. Children and youth may have trouble sleeping in the same room as the site of their abuse. When a child's symptoms meet the criteria for PTSD, the medical expert should explain the significance of this most important aspect of behavior. Posttraumatic stress with intrusive thoughts of sexual abuse must be scientifically attributed to sexual abuse unless others have victimized the child before this particular case.

An additional defense stance is to accuse the medical expert of being a zealot regarding sexual abuse, finding that the majority of children whom they evaluate indeed have the diagnosis of sexual abuse. There are 2 important distinctions to be made in light of these assertions. First, most children who receive a forensic evaluation are being seen in a specialty clinic. Referrals to specialized clinics usually require a previous medical assessment to determine if enough index of suspicion exists for a secondary level evaluation. It would, consequently, stand to reason that an assessment by a professional social worker and a healthcare provider leading to the decision that a specialty consultation was needed would screen out those children whose presenting complaints did not fit any criteria for the diagnosis of child sexual abuse. Therefore, the forensic specialist is likely to see children who have findings that are consistent with the diagnosis of sexual abuse.

A second response to the argument that forensic experts overdiagnose sexual abuse by behaviors alone is found in the research of Heiman et al (1998). In this comparative study, the question was addressed as to whether professionals "overpathologize sexual behaviors." The research found that there was little evidence to support the assertion that experts in the field of child sexual abuse gave excess credence to the sexual behaviors of children.

Case Study 34-5

CO was 6 years old when a close family friend, Uncle Billy, began inviting her and her 3 other cousins to his house to swim and occasionally spend the night. The 4 girls were rapidly groomed and sexually abused, followed shortly thereafter by coerced videotaping of each other's victimization. Their abuse involved sexual intercourse, oral copulation, and exposure to adult pornography. The abuse continued for 2 years and then ended as the girls began to become more sexually mature. Discovery of Polaroid photos 7 years later by other relatives visiting Uncle Billy's house led to multiple charges. Videotapes were discovered by law enforcement as well as a computer storing child pornography.

At the time of discovery of the homemade pornography, neither CO nor any of her cousins had disclosed the child sexual abuse or sexual exploitation. Over the ensuing 7 years after the onset of her abuse, she had become obese, a progressively poor student, and was thought to be depressed. Her parents divorced in this interim but remained close to their daughter, as they all resided in a closely knit neighborhood. At the time of the discovery of the videotape, CO initially denied the abuse. During a medical interview, she broke down and related as many details that she could recall. Her self-guilt was evident, and she was upset because she was the oldest child to be abused, and felt that she should have protected her younger cousins. Furthermore, Uncle Billy had always been "such a nice guy," frequently rewarding the children with gifts and excursions. CO had always had trouble sleeping, experienced a return of significant nightmares after the discovery, spoke of wishing to run away so no one would know her, had anger outbursts, and had exacerbation of her depressive symptoms.

CO's physical examination revealed significant obesity, but no vaginal abnormalities, even though the videotape showed long episodes of vigorous penile-vaginal penetration.

Evaluation of the other children who were pornographically videotaped revealed no disclosure until the discovery of the photos and tape. All of the victims revealed psychological pathology.

This case illustrates the expected delay in disclosure even when there has been a multiple victim scenario. Pretrial preparation was difficult because of a continued conviction that the offender had not been at fault, but that the victims had been "bad girls." The undulant psychological impact on this specific victim illustrates how long the effects can last, even when abuse has occurred fairly early in life. The comorbid diagnoses for this victim should be included in the evidence at trial (ie, child sexual abuse, psychological abuse, and sexual exploitation).

ELEMENT III: PHYSICAL EXAMINATION

The third element in a child sexual abuse and exploitation case is the physical examination. This is the least reliable of the elements for 2 reasons. First, only a small percentage of children are found to have positive findings. The probability of normal findings in child sexual abuse has been revealed in numerous studies for girls and boys (Adams et al, 1994; Berenson et al, 2000; Finkel, 1989; Holmes & Slap, 1998; Jenny, 1997; Muram, 1989; Pokorny et al, 1992). Second, experience in the examination and interpretation of physical findings is necessary as inexperience is associated with a higher false positive rate of physical examination interpretation. Despite these limitations, this element is the most important to the jury though it carries the least amount of weight in the determination of a diagnosis of child sexual abuse. For this reason, a great deal of education is needed, particularly if the victim does have a normal or nonspecific examination. Explanations for normal findings include the following:

— *Method of abuse would not leave physical findings.* Oral copulation, forced fellatio, forced masturbation, fondling, coerced exhibitionism, or sucking of the breasts

— *Findings if initially present would heal and disappear with time.* Digital molestation, digital vaginal penetration, digital anal penetration, penetration of the anus with a small foreign body, and, even at times, penile vaginal penetration; highest yield of findings would be if the child were examined within hours to just a few days after the abuse

— *Onset of puberty.* Tissues of the hymen change during this time, and a small tear, scar, or defect may no longer be detectable

Explanation of this information as well as the previously mentioned aspects of diagnostic steps helps lay a foundation for a child sexual abuse and exploitation case before presenting the specific facts in the case.

Case Study 34-6

LM was a 7-year-old Native American child who was referred to the clinic because of genital herpes. The history obtained from her child protective service worker was that LM's biological mother was incarcerated and, before being committed, had given custody of her only child to her next-door neighbor, a woman whom she did not know well. The child related to the social worker that shortly after coming to live with her "aunt," men began to come into her bedroom at night when she was asleep and hurt her in her private parts. She could not recall the identity of any of these men, and to her recollection, at times, there were more than one who came during the night.

LM described having been forced to put something in her mouth during these nights though her room was usually kept dark, and she was not sure of what was happening. She did mime, however, forced fellatio. She also spoke of the fact that she did not go to school often since her "aunt" often "smoked a pipe" during the day and would fall asleep.

LM's affect while relating the history that many men had sexually assaulted her over an unknown period of time was one of ***la belle indifference***, or a well-described affect of indifference to the severity of the circumstances. She smiled somewhat constantly, had fleeting eye contact, and seemed detached from the details she was relating. She spoke of missing her mother and that sometimes her "aunt" beat her if she did not cooperate. She related recurrent stomachaches, poor sleeping, intrusive thoughts of sexual abuse, feelings of sadness, and fearfulness whenever she was around adult men. Though she has been placed in foster care, she often requires that her lights be left on all night in her room or will attempt to sleep with someone else in the family. Her school performance is poor, and she is expected to have to repeat her school grade.

On physical examination, there was evidence of loss of hymenal tissue and ulcerative painful lesions, which were culture positive for herpes simplex, type 2.

This case illustrates that a child who is being prostituted may not be able to give a detailed history of the sexual abuse events because of multiple offenders, lack of explanation of what is experienced, and a degree of dissociation or detachment that may have developed as a means of coping with the abuse. Bodily injury, genital trauma, or a serious STD can motivate a care provider to seek medical care for the prostituted child. In addition, an unwanted pregnancy may be the immediate cause for an ER or clinic visit, with a vague history of how the child may have been sexually abused. Inadequate supervision may be a façade for what actually represents the prostitution of a child or juvenile. It is important for the medical history to be as detailed as possible.

In the circumstance of child pornography, actual sexual abuse images may suggest that physical findings would be present. However, the literature shows that most patients have a normal examination even when there is a perpetrator confession or a conviction in a court of law. So, these physical findings have been noted even when there is pornographic evidence of vaginal or anal penetration in prepubescent children (Adams et al, 1994; K. St. Clair, oral communication, April 2004).

At times, a child will have been examined without colposcopy in a primary care site or in an ER setting. Justification for referral to a clinic that specializes in child maltreatment may have to be presented to a jury carefully. A forensic pediatric examination is medically indicated, as compared to legally so because many times primary care physicians do not have the experience to interpret the history, the child's behaviors, and physical examination findings. Just as a secondary level evaluation is indicated in many childhood diseases and conditions, child abuse is no different. Referral to a forensic specialist is indicated to gain an evaluation from a specially trained healthcare provider and not to obtain a second opinion. There are at least 5 medical reasons to justify this type of referral (**Table 34-11**). A medical expert should be versed in these justifications as their entire evaluation may be challenged as a defense strategy to exclude important hearsay exception information.

In summary, when the medical expert is preparing to testify in a child sexual abuse or exploitation case, 3 elements of information are of critical importance in establishing a diagnosis: the medical history, the child's behavior, and the physical examination. The latter is least important, since the majority of victims will have a normal examination. The history often constitutes a compilation of information from a parent, social worker, possibly a law enforcement investigator, and the information provided by the child to the healthcare provider on that clinic visit. Though most children never disclose sexual abuse in childhood, a disclosure may represent courage and a need to protect others even when the child may feel that he or she is the cause of his

Table 34-11. Medical Justifications for a Forensic Pediatric or Forensic Nurse Examination in Child Sexual Abuse and Exploitation

1   To assure that the correct diagnosis has been made and the child will be discharged to a safe environment

2   To assure that there are no acute sexually transmitted infections, and if so, that appropriate medical management is instituted

3   To assure that there is no evidence of acute genital trauma that might have long-term chronic consequences (eg, anal trauma leading to anal fistula in ano)

4   To assure that no chronic sexually transmitted infections exist (eg, syphilis, human immunodeficiency virus), and if so, appropriate medical management is instituted

5   To assure that mental health diagnoses are preliminarily established and appropriate referrals are made

or her own victimization. The presence of a consistent history, a physical examination, and characteristic behaviors with particular attention to depression and PTSD offer a clinical presentation, which is consistent with that seen in children who have been sexually abused. Should a judicial ruling be made that forbids the use of the term "diagnosis," the determination of "a constellation of factors which are consistent with child sexual abuse and exploitation," is generally accepted.

Though jurors have an expectation that genital and anal penetration should result in significant physical findings, the medical expert should have a well-defined list of explanations for normal findings in children who have been sexual abused.

Concerns in **Case Study 34-4** (cited earlier) would include delayed disclosure, the significance of the victim's behavioral changes, whether the child's history is consistent over time and in details and the significance of the physical findings. These matters are common in child sexual abuse prosecutions. The difference in these more mainstream dynamics and those of sexual exploitation is that the "normal" points for testimony must now include the link between the existence of the photos and the proof that the men in question were the photographers, and that the pornographic evidence constitutes "abuse." Information regarding the execution of a thorough crime scene is noted elsewhere. Information of this type would be the primary aspect of the substantive medical expert testimony. However, there would be the following additional factors, which are specific to CSE and which have different dynamics as compared solely to child sexual abuse.

Though children may frequently be coerced to have sex with an offender and, therefore, experience physical abuse, it has been reported by investigators that children and teens may be forced to pose for nude photos, which would be used for blackmail. Extortion is an important component of maintaining the secret of an exploitation case. Sexual exploitation is often presented to the child as something he or she would want to keep secret. This joint pact brings the perpetrator and the victim to one accord, and the child develops a strong sense of denial regarding any production of pornography. When provided with the proof of the abuse, a promise of exposure is often sufficient to keep the child from sharing information about his or her abuse with another.

VICTIM IMPACT TESTIMONY

The medical expert is qualified to testify regarding long-term sequelae in CSE. As the information is embedded in the child sexual abuse literature, an expert can draw upon a wealth of knowledge. Victim impact testimony is often included at the end of the prosecution's presentation of facts, with the medical expert representing the summarizing witness. In this case, the expert is providing background information regarding potential ramifications. The victim is generic, and the facts of the case are typified when taken into consideration during the conclusive testimony. The expert is able to render, in essence, a prognosis for long-term outcome based upon the expert's experience and knowledge of the literature.

In contrast, impact testimony, which is often provided by the victim and/or the family, may be preceded and augmented by medical expert testimony at the time of sentencing. When the expert testifies at this juncture in the trial, the victim is no longer generic, but specific, and the predictions are made based upon the circumstances cited most particularly in this case. Review of therapy records, family interviews, and direct victim interview is often allowed during this testimony. Issues of pain and suffering can be addressed, as well as mitigating and aggravating circumstances. The child abuse expert may testify regarding recidivism of the specific form of abuse as based upon the literature since this has relevance to a criminal justice decision regarding the occurrence and/or length of incarceration. For example, in the circumstance of commercial sexual exploitation by an offender with numerous prostituted juveniles, monetary gain and commodification of the victims would be an important point of testimony.

An additional point of testimony by a medical expert would include the psychological impact of a prostituted child or youth who has been trafficked from one state to another. Such circumstances would increase victims' anxiety level as they realize that they have no idea of their location, and the possibility of seeking supportive family members decreases. The medical expert should address the emotional impact of this scenario or one associated with prostituted youths who have been trafficked into the US from foreign countries.

At times, the forensic expert assists the prosecution in determining if a child victim is psychologically able to testify on sentencing. Some researchers believe that children benefit from facing their abusers at such times and that a potential for a positive therapeutic outcome exists by allowing the child to make his or her own statement (Runyan et al, 1998). On the other hand, many children experience ambivalence regarding the positive attachment in a family relationship and the negative experience of sexual abuse and may be a less effective witness. The National Institute of Child Justice reviewed the literature regarding this quandary and found no agreement as to whether the effect of testimony on children is positive or negative. All of the children had high levels of anxiety and concern before testimony. The presence of a non-offending parent who provided support to the child was associated with the best mental health outcome. Reassuringly, the review of studies revealed that the psychological health of most children improved over time, regardless of a positive or negative court experience (Whitcomb et al, 1994).

The prostitution of children and juveniles has a high association with multiple perpetrators and physical abuse before or during the sexual assaults. These experiences have a significant association with chronic PTSD. Though the presence of PTSD does not directly prove sexual abuse, the disorder does mean that some life-changing and trauma-related event has occurred and sexual abuse should be considered as a possibility (Myers et al, 2002). One helpful detail in establishing this mental health relationship within the context of child sexual abuse and CSE would be to stress the component of PTSD that included intrusive thoughts of the event. It is logical that if a child has PTSD and the child's specific intrusive thoughts were of a sexual abuse encounter, the connection would be self-explanatory. Pornography and prostitution share a significant link, and the expert can testify regarding the "normalizing" effect of frequent photography in sexual poses or during sexual abuse.

Exploring the mental health diagnoses as well as the extreme medical risk of prostitution at the time of sentencing is an important contribution that can best be made by the forensic expert. It is important to discuss the resulting self-image that a child or adolescent may develop when their lives have been molded into a sex-for-gain pattern.

Case Study 34-7

MH was an 11-year-old girl who had been in foster care between the ages of 4 and 6 years old. She had been a sexual abuse victim of her mother's boyfriend before being placed. She was returned to the care of her 24-year-old mother at 7 years of age and after her mother's fourth marriage in 5 years, MH made a new disclosure of sexual exploitation. This disclosure came after a local drugstore photo development lab called the police department because a newly developed roll of film had an apparent minor posing in several shots with breast exposure and with adult lingerie. In one shot, the child was depicted as an Easter bunny, with her breasts painted as the eyes of a rabbit. Her new 67-year-old stepfather was a professional photographer who specialized in topless wedding photos. The roll of film accompanied many others, which had adult women in wedding gowns first fully clothed and then with their gowns pulled down to the waist.

The investigation revealed a full confession of the new stepfather, who continued to stress that he did not know that there might be any laws broken by photographing his 11-year-old stepdaughter in this fashion. He readily revealed his collection of hundreds of photos in his home and stored in a storage facility of women who were posing in topless positions. There were no other pictures of children.

The history obtained from the child and her mother confirmed that the stepfather was anxious to take pictures of MH even before the marriage. There was no disclosure of any sexual behaviors other than the posing. There was, however, a past history of child sexual abuse for which MH had been released from counseling about 2 years before.

MH related sexually explicit knowledge in her interview as she continued to compare this experience to the sexual abuse with a former maternal boyfriend, which began when she was 5 years old. It was difficult for her to separate the details of this event, it seemed, from the former events. It was apparent that this form of exploitation had vividly brought back memories of her previous sexual abuse. She displayed regressive behaviors, such as playing with dolls that she had discarded more than 2 years before, and was afraid to sleep alone. She had tried to sleep with her new foster care mother at night. She described intrusive thoughts of the former abuse though, before the photographic events, she had not mentioned the abuse for more than a year.

Testimony in Internet Child Pornography Analysis

Child pornography investigations often involve a collection of sexual abuse images, which have been discovered on a computer or in some other information storage capacity (eg, disks, CD-ROMs, videotapes). The medical expert may be asked to analyze some or all of these images for the purpose of determining if they represent images of children younger than a specific age.

Testimony regarding the review of images is important. At times, a medical expert may have produced a specific document regarding the pornographic data, and this document will suffice for the purposes of the court, with respect to an expert's assessment. However, there may be times when testimony is required during the presentation of facts or possibly to facilitate education regarding victim impact during a sentencing hearing.

An important point in testimony regarding analysis is that unless the actual child is known, by discovery and formal investigation or by access to birth certificate, an expert can only approximate the child's age. The question to be answered is not the exact age of the child but if the image is consistent with a child who is less than a specific age (so-called age of consent, or legal definition of child pornography). In the United States, federal statute cites this to be 18 years of age.

Many factors influence the expert's ability to make the determination whether images are consistent with children, not the least of which is sexual maturation. Information regarding likely ethnic origin of the children depicted pornographically can help in some cases as well as a thorough knowledge of all parameters of growth and development. Some images will depict sexual and physical abuse, such as is seen in sadism or bestiality images, and the expert would be prepared to elaborate regarding such forms of abuse.

Determination of whether the images appear to be digitally altered usually requires the assistance of a forensic computer analyst who can provide evidence to a reasonable degree of certainty that computer alterations have not taken place. When images are determined to be vintage (having been produced before 1985), analysts will be able to infer that the original sources were from older pornographic publications, and computer manipulation is not possible for such images.

The medical expert should avoid the use of Tanner stage language in reports and testimony except to explain the role of this well-known and accepted method of determining the sequence of sexual maturation. Though a firm disclaimer regarding the use of the Tanner stages in child pornography analysis and litigation exists, an expert would want to explain how the use of other parameters of growth and development assist in determining if the images are consistent with children (Rosenbloom & Tanner, 1998).

A summary statement by the medical expert may reflect the amount of pornographic images consistent with children less than a certain age, those images that are of particularly young children (less than 12 years of age), and those images that would constitute particularly egregious content (suggesting extreme harm to victims).

At any time, a medical expert may be called upon to testify upon sentencing for the purpose of providing victim impact information. The basis of such testimony has been established in the child sexual abuse literature and should be provided to prognosticate potential mental health, physical health, and social, family, and academic achievement problems that might result.

SUMMARY OPINION IN CHILD SEXUAL EXPLOITATION

If allowed, many medical experts are asked if they have a final medical opinion regarding a diagnosis of child sexual abuse. This opinion is more commonly provided when the expert has functioned as a case witness or an evaluating witness. The final statement by the medical expert regarding an opinion should succinctly stated as a summary of all prior background and case review testimony. An example of such an opinion pertinent to child sexual abuse and CSE would be the following:

Based upon my knowledge of the literature and my years of clinical experience, it is my opinion that the history provided by this child, the behaviors that were described by both her mother and herself, and the physical examination are consistent with those seen in children who have the diagnosis of child sexual abuse and exploitation.

In the circumstance of child pornographic image analysis, the summary opinion would explain the numbers of images analyzed, the number of images consistent with children less than the legal age of consent or that met the legal definition of child pornography, and whether there existed egregious images worthy of special mention due to the significant impact upon the child depicted.

These statements give a complete synopsis of the decision-making process the expert has used to arrive at the opinion that child sexual abuse and sexual exploitation is the most likely diagnosis. A medical expert must speak of his or her role in making a medical diagnosis and prescribing treatment in a child sexual abuse or CSE case when the child is indeed available. Subsequent clinical treatments made after a child has been evaluated are therefore to be expected after the expert states agreement that the healthcare provider in fact made appropriate therapeutic recommendations. In the circumstance of child sexual abuse images, without the presence of the actual child, other collaborating information may be necessary to confirm the actual identity of the child. If this detail is not required, determination of the numbers of victims and statements regarding such abuse are well within the scope of the medical expert witness.

REFERENCES

Adams J, McClellan J, Douglass D, McCurry C, Storck M. Sexually inappropriate behaviors in seriously mentally ill children and adolescents. *Child Abuse Negl.* 1995; 19:555-568.

Adams JA, Harper K, Revilla J. Examination findings in legally confirmed child sexual abuse: it's normal to be normal. *Pediatrics.* 1994;94:310-317.

American Academy of Pediatrics Committee on Child Abuse and Neglect. Guidelines for the evaluation of sexual abuse of children: subject review. *Pediatrics.* 1999; 103:186-191.

American Medical Association. *International Classification of Diseases, 9th revision, Clinical Modification.* Chicago, Ill: American Medical Association; 2003.

American Psychiatric Association. *Diagnostic and Statistical Manual of Mental Disorders.* 4th ed. Text Revision. Washington, DC: American Psychiatric Association; 2000.

Bavolek S. *A Handbook for Understanding Child Abuse and Neglect.* Park City, Utah: Family Development Resources Inc; 1990.

Bays J, Jenny C. Genital and anal conditions confused with child sexual abuse trauma. *Am J Dis Child.* 1990;144:1319-1322.

Berenson AB, Chacko MR, Wiemann CM, Mishaw CO, Friedrich WN, Grady JJ. A case-control study of anatomic changes resulting from sexual abuse. *Am J Obstet Gynecol.* 2000;182:820-831.

Boney-McCoy S, Finkelhor D. Psychosocial sequelae of violent victimization in a national youth sample. *J Consult Clin Psychol.* 1995;63:726-736.

Briere JN. A self-trauma model for treating adult survivors of severe child abuse. In: Briere JN, Berliner L, Bulkley J, Jenny C, Reid T, eds. *APSAC Handbook on Child Maltreatment.* Thousand Oaks, Calif: Sage Publications; 1996:140-157.

Briere JN, Elliott DM. Immediate and long-term impacts of child sexual abuse. *Future Child.* 1994;4:54-59.

Conte JR, Sorenson E, Fogarty L, Dalla Rosa J. Evaluating children's reports of sexual abuse: results from a survey of professionals. *Am J Orthopsychiatry.* 1991;61:428-437.

Estes RJ, Weiner NA. The commercial sexual exploitation of children in the US, Canada and Mexico. September 2001. Available at: http://caster.ssw.upenn.edu/~restes/CSEC.htm. Accessed December 27, 2004.

Ewing-Cobbs L, Kramer L, Prasad M, et al. Neuroimaging, physical, and developmental findings after inflicted and non-inflicted traumatic brain injury in children. *Pediatrics.* 1998;102:300-307.

Faller KC. The parental alienation syndrome: what is it and what data support it? *Child Maltreat.* 1998;3:100-115.

Famularo R, Fenton T, Augustyn M, Zuckerman B. Persistence of pediatric post traumatic stress disorder after 2 years. *Child Abuse Negl.* 1996;20:1245-1248.

Fed R Evidence 702.

Finkel MA. Anogenital trauma in sexually abused children. *Pediatrics.* 1989;84:317-322.

Finkel MA, Giardino AP. *Medical Evaluation of Child Sexual Abuse: A Practical Guide.* Thousand Oaks, Calif: Sage Publications; 2002

Finkelhor D, Hotaling G, Lewis IA, Smith G. Sexual abuse in a national survey of adult men and women: prevalence, characteristics, and risk factors. *Child Abuse Negl.* 1990;14:19-28.

Friedrich WN. Sexual victimization and sexual behavior in children: a review of recent literature. *Child Abuse Negl.* 1993;17:59-66.

Friedrich WN, Grambsch P, Damon L, et al. The child sexual behavior inventory: normative and clinical findings. *Psychol Assess.* 1992;4:303-311.

Friedrich WN, Jaworski TM, Huxsahl JE, Bengtson BS. Dissociative and sexual behaviors in children and adolescents with sexual abuse and psychiatric histories. *J Interpers Violence.* 1997;12:155-171.

Friedrich WN, Dittner CA, Action R, et al. Child sexual behavior inventory: normative, psychiatric and sexual abuse comparisons. *Child Maltreat.* 2001;6:37-49.

Gardner RA. *The Parental Alienation Syndrome and the Differentiation Between Fabricated and Genuine Child Sex Abuse.* Cresskill, NJ: Creative Therapeutics; 1992.

Gomes-Schwartz B, Horowitz JM, Cardarelli AP. *Child Sexual Abuse: The Initial Effects.* Thousand Oaks, Calif: Sage Publications; 1990.

Hanson RF, Resnick HS, Sanders BE, Kilpatrick DG, Best C. Factors related to the reporting of childhood rape. *Child Abuse Negl.* 1999;23:559-569.

Heiman ML, Leiblum S, Esquilin SC, Patillo LM. A comparative study of beliefs about "normal" childhood sexual behaviors. *Child Abuse Negl.* 1998;22:298-304.

Hibbard RA, Ingersoll GM, Orr DP. Behavior risk, emotional risk, and child abuse among adolescents in a nonclinical setting. *Pediatrics.* 1990;86:896-901.

Holmes WC, Slap GB. Sexual abuse of boys: definitions, prevalence, correlates, sequelae, and management. *JAMA.* 1998;280:1855-1862.

Jenny C. Pediatric fellowships in child abuse and neglect: the development of a new subspecialty. *Child Maltreat.* 1997;2:356-361.

Jones T, Holland G. Victim identification. Speech presented at: Colloquium: Victimisation with Child Pornography; March 31, 2003; Cork, Ireland.

Kendall-Tackett KA, Williams LM, Finkelhor D. Impact of sexual abuse on children: a review and synthesis of recent empirical studies. *Psychol Bull.* 1993;113:164-180.

Kilpatrick DG, Saunders BE. *Prevalence and Consequences of Child Victimization: Results From the National Survey of Adolescents.* Charleston: National Crime Victims Research & Treatment Center, Department of Psychiatry & Behavioral Sciences, Medical University of South Carolina; 1999. No 93-IJ-CX-0023.

Krugman RD. Recognition of sexual abuse in children. *Pediatr Rev.* 1986;8:25-30.

Lanktree CB, Briere J, Zaidi L. Incidence and impact of sexual abuse in a child outpatient sample: the role of direct inquiry. *Child Abuse Negl.* 1991;15:447-453.

Lindblad F, Gustafsson PA, Larsson I, Lundin B. Preschoolers' sexual behavior at daycare centers: an epidemiological study. *Child Abuse Negl.* 1995;19:569-577.

Mannarino AP, Cohen JA. Abuse-related attributions and perceptions, general attributions, and locus of control in sexually abused girls. *J Interpers Violence.* 1996;11: 162-180.

Mannarino AP, Cohen JA, Berman SR. The Children's Attributions and Perceptions Scale: a new measure of sexual abuse-related factors. *J Clin Child Psychol.* 1994;23: 204-211.

McLeer SV, Dixon JF, Henry D, et al. Psychopathology in non-clinically referred sexually abused children. *J Am Acad Child Adolesc Psychiatry.* 1998;47:1326-1333.

Mother traded daughter, 8, for crack. *The Fayetteville Observer Times.* May 15, 1999; National Briefs section.

Mullen PE, Martin JL, Anderson JC, Romans SE, Herbison GP. Childhood sexual abuse and mental health in adult life. *Br J Psychiatry.* 1993;163:721-732.

Muram D. Child sexual abuse: relationship between sexual acts and genital findings. *Child Abuse Negl.* 1989;13:211-216.

Myers JEB. Expert testimony regarding psychological syndromes. *Pac Law J.* 1993; 24:1449-1464.

Myers JEB. *A Mother's Nightmare: Incest: A Practical Legal Guide for Parents and Professionals.* Thousand Oaks, Calif: Sage Publications; 1997.

Myers JEB. *Legal Issues in Child Abuse and Neglect.* Thousand Oaks, Calif: Sage Publications; 1998.

Myers JEB, Berliner L, Briere J, Hendrix CT, Jenny C, Reid TA, eds. *The APSAC Handbook on Child Maltreatment.* 2nd ed. Thousand Oaks, Calif: Sage Publications; 2002.

Myers JEB, Stern P. Expert testimony. In: Myers JEB, Berliner L, Briere J, Hendrix CT, Jenny C, Reid TA, eds. *The APSAC Handbook on Child Maltreatment.* 2nd ed. Thousand Oaks, Calif: Sage Publications; 2002:386-395.

Nelson EC, Heath AC, Madden PAF, et al. Association between self-reported childhood sexual abuse and adverse psychosocial outcomes: results from a twin study. *Arch Gen Psychiatry.* 2002;59:139-145.

Neumann DA, Houskamp BM, Pollock VE, Briere J. The long-term sequelae of childhood sexual abuse in women: a meta-analytic review. *Child Maltreat.* 1996;1:6-16.

Paine ML, Hansen DJ. Factors influencing children to self-disclose sexual abuse. *Clin Psychol Rev.* 2002;22:271-295.

Palmer SE, Brown RA, Rae-Grant NI, Loughlin J. Responding to children's disclosure of familial abuse: what survivors tell us. *Child Welfare.* 1999;78:259-282.

Pearl PS. Psychological abuse. In: Monteleone J. *Child Maltreatment.* 2nd ed. St. Louis, Mo: GW Medical Publishing; 1998:371-396.

Pokorny SF, Pokornoy WJ, Kramer W. Acute genital injury in the prepubertal girl. *Am J Obstet Gynecol.* 1992;166:1461-1466.

Reece RM. *Treatment of Child Abuse: Common Ground for Mental Health, Medical, and Legal Practitioners.* Baltimore, Md: Johns Hopkins University Press; 2000.

Reece RM, Ludwig S. *Child Abuse: Medical Diagnosis and Management.* Philadelphia, Pa: Lippincott Williams & Wilkins; 2001.

Rosenbloom AL, Tanner JM. Misuse of Tanner puberty stages to estimate chronologic age. *Pediatrics.* 1998;102:1494.

Ruggiero KJ, McLeer SV, Dixon JF. Sexual abuse characteristics associated with survivor psychopathology. *Child Abuse Negl.* 2000;24:951-964.

Runyan DK, Everson MD, Edelsohn GA, Hunter WM, Coulter ML. Impact of legal intervention on sexually abused children. *J Pediatr.* 1998;113:647-653.

Rust JO, Troupe PA. Relationships of treatment of child sexual abuse with school achievement and self-concept. *J Early Adolesc.* 1991;11:420-429.

Smith BE, Elstein SG, Trost T, Bulkley J. *The Prosecution of Child Sexual and Physical Abuse Cases.* Washington, DC: American Bar Association Center on Children & the Law; 1993.

Smith DW, Letourneau EJ, Sanders BE, Kilpatrick DG, Resnick HS, Best CL. Delay in disclosure of childhood rape: results of a national survey. *Child Abuse Negl.* 2000; 24:273-287.

Stern P. *Preparing and Presenting Expert Testimony in Child Abuse Litigation: A Guide for Expert Witnesses and Attorneys.* Thousand Oaks, Calif: Sage Publications; 1997.

Stern AE, Lynch DL, Oates RK, O'Toole BI, Cooney G. Self esteem, depression, behaviour and family functioning in sexually abused children. *J Child Psychol Psychiatr.* 1995;36:1077-1089.

Summit RC. The child sexual abuse accommodation syndrome. *Child Abuse Negl.* 1983;7:177-192.

Summit RC. The dark tunnels of McMartin. *J Psychohist.* 1994;21:397-416.

Taylor M, Quayle E. *Child Pornography: An Internet Crime.* Hove, England: Brunner-Routledge; 2003.

Tebbutt J, Swanston H, Oates RK, O'Toole BI. Five years after child sexual abuse: persisting dysfunction and problems of prediction. *Child Adolesc Psychiatry.* 1997;36: 330-339.

Thoennes N, Tjaden PG. The extent, nature, and validity of sexual abuse allegations in custody/visitation disputes. *Child Abuse Negl.* 1990;14:151-163.

Whitcomb D, Goodman GS, Runyan DK, Hoak S. *The Emotional Effects of Testifying on Sexually Abused Children.* Washington, DC: The National Institute of Child Justice; 1994.

Wolfe VV, Birt J. The psychological sequelae of child sexual abuse. *Adv Clin Child Psychol.* 1995;17:233 Testifying263.

COMPUTER FORENSIC SOFTWARE AND ITS LEGAL VALIDATION

John Patzakis, Esq*

Computer forensics is a discipline dedicated to the collection, analysis, and presentation of computer evidence for judicial purposes. Computer forensics is particularly important in the field of child exploitation because nearly all child pornography cases involve digital images. Unfortunately, the Internet serves as a means for sex offenders to stalk and attempt to lure minors. In such cases, the seizure and analysis of the computers used by the perpetrator and any victims is essential to investigate and prosecute such cases. Those who practice computer forensics need to be familiar with the laws of evidence in their relevant jurisdictions so they may use the proper procedures, tools, and methodologies to collect and process computer evidence.

EnCase is one example of a computer forensics software program used by thousands of computer crime investigators worldwide in many computer crime cases, including those involving the exploitation of minors. The software is a fully integrated, Windows-based application that performs all stages of the computer forensics investigation from the imaging of seized computer media to the analysis and recovery of relevant information to the verification and reporting of the recovered evidence.

This chapter reports on recent trial court developments involving EnCase, as well as notable court decisions and cases studies involving computer evidence in general. Additionally, this chapter addresses the way EnCase facilitates the authentication and admission of electronic evidence in light of past industry practices and the current status of the law, and it provides investigators and their counsel with an added resource when addressing questions involving computer forensics.

AUTHENTICATION OF RECOVERED DATA FOR ACCURACY

AUTHENTICATION OF COMPUTER EVIDENCE

Documents and writings must be authenticated before they may be introduced into evidence. The United States Federal Rules of Evidence, as well as the laws of other jurisdictions, define computer data as documents. Electronic evidence presents particular challenges for authentication since such data can be easily altered without proper handling. The proponent of evidence normally carries the burden of offering sufficient evidence to authenticate documents or writings, and electronic evidence is no exception.

This section addresses some of the questions that face computer investigators and counsel when seeking to introduce electronic evidence. These include the following:

— What testimony is required to authenticate computer data?

* © 2003 Guidance Software, Inc. Mr. Pazakis is President and CEO of Guidance Software, Inc.

— How does a witness establish that the data he or she recovered from a hard drive are not only genuine but completely accurate?

— Are there guidelines or checklists that should be followed?

— How familiar with the software used in the investigation must the examiner be to establish a proper foundation for the recovered data?

Often, the admission of computer evidence, typically in the form of active (ie, "non-deleted") text or graphical image files, is accomplished without the use of specialized computer forensic software. Federal Rule of Evidence 901(a) provides that the authentication of a document is "satisfied by evidence sufficient to support a finding that the matter in question is what the proponent claims." The Canada Evidence Act specifically addresses the authentication of computer evidence in chapter C-5, providing that an electronic document can be authenticated "by evidence capable of supporting a finding that the electronic document is that which it is purported to be" (section 31.1). Under these statutes, a printout of an e-mail message can often be authenticated through direct testimony from the recipient or the author (*Laughner v State*, 2002; *United States v Siddiqui*, 2000).

The US federal courts have addressed the authentication of computer-generated evidence based on Rule 901(a), much in the same manner as statutes that have existed before computer usage became widespread (Kurzban, 1995). *United States v Tank* (2000), which involves evidence of Internet chat room conversation logs, is an important illustration.

In *Tank*, the defendant appealed his conviction for conspiring to engage in the receipt and distribution of sexually explicit images of children and other offenses. Among the issues addressed on appeal was whether the government made an adequate foundational showing of the relevance and the authenticity of a coconspirator's Internet chat room log printouts. A search of a computer belonging to one of Tank's coconspirators, Riva, revealed computer text files containing "recorded" online chat room discussions that took place among members of the Orchid Club, an Internet chat room group to which Tank and Riva belonged (*United States v Tank*, 2000). Riva's computer was programmed to save all of the conversations among Orchid Club members as text files whenever he was online.

At an evidentiary hearing, Tank argued that the district court should not admit the chat room logs into evidence since the government failed to establish a sufficient foundation. Tank contended that the chat room log printouts should not be entered into evidence because of the following (*United States v Tank*, 2000):

1. They were not complete documents.

2. Undetectable "material alterations," such as changes in either the substance or the names appearing in the chat room logs, could have been made by Riva before the government's seizure of his computer.

The district court ruled that Tank's objection went to the evidentiary weight of the logs rather than to their admissibility and allowed the logs into evidence. Tank appealed, and the appellate court addressed the issue of whether the government established a sufficient foundation for the chat room logs.

The appellate court considered the issue in the context of Federal Rule of Evidence 901(a), noting that "[t]he rule requires only that the court admit evidence if sufficient proof has been introduced so that a reasonable juror could find in favor of authenticity or identification ... The government must also establish a connection between the proffered evidence and the defendant" (*United States v Black*, 1985; *United States v Tank*, 2000).

In authenticating the chat room text files, the prosecution presented testimony from Riva, who explained how he created the logs with his computer and stated that the printouts appeared to be an accurate representation of the chat room conversations among members of the Orchid Club. The government established a connection between Tank and the chat room log printouts. Tank admitted that he used the screen name "Cessna" when he participated in one of the conversations recorded in the chat room log printouts. Additionally, several coconspirators testified that Tank used the chat room screen name "Cessna" that appeared throughout the printouts. They further testified that when they arranged a meeting with the person who used the screen name "Cessna," it was Tank who met them (*United States v Tank*, 2000).

Based on these facts, the court found that the government made an adequate foundational showing of the authenticity of the chat room log printouts under Rule 901(a). Specifically, the government "presented evidence sufficient to allow a reasonable juror to find that the chat room log printouts were authenticated" (*United States v Tank*, 2000).

The *Tank* decision is consistent with other cases that have addressed the issue of the authenticity of computer evidence in the general context of Federal Rule of Evidence 901(a). (See *United States v Whitaker* (1997) for more information.) *Tank* illustrates that there are no specific requirements or set procedures for the authentication of chat room conversation logs but that the approach generally favored by the courts is that the facts and circumstances of the creation and recovery of the evidence is applied to Rule 901(a). (See also *United States v Scott-Emuakpor* (2000), which concluded that the government properly authenticated documents recovered from a computer forensic examination under Rule 901(a).) In *State (Ohio) v Cook* (2002) an Ohio Appellate Court upheld the validity of the EnCase® Software under Ohio Rule of Evidence 901(a), which is nearly identical to the corresponding federal rule.

AUTHENTICATION OF THE RECOVERY PROCESS

Whenever direct testimony is unavailable, a document may be authenticated through circumstantial evidence. A computer forensic examination is often an effective means to authenticate electronic evidence through circumstantial evidence. The examiner must be able to provide competent and sufficient testimony to connect the recovered data to the matter in question.

Courts have recognized the importance of computer forensic investigations to authenticate computer evidence. *Gates Rubber Company v Bando Chemical Industries, Ltd* (1996) is an important published decision involving competing computer forensic expert testimony in which the court defines a mandatory legal duty on the part of litigants or potential litigants to perform computer forensic investigations. In this case, one party's examiner failed to make a mirror-image copy of the target hard drive and instead performed a "file-by-file" copy in an invasive manner, which resulted in lost information. The opposing expert noted that the technology needed for a mirror-image backup was available at the time (February 1992) even though such technology was not widely used. The court's ruling issued harsh evidentiary sanctions by criticizing the errant examiner for failing to make an image copy of the target drive and finding that when processing evidence for judicial purposes a party has "a duty to utilize the method which would yield the most complete and accurate results" (*Gates Rubber Company v Bando Chemical Industries, Ltd*, 1996).

Some courts have required only minimal testimony concerning the recovery process, particularly when the defense fails to raise significant or adequate objections to the admission of the computer evidence. In *United Sates v Whitaker* (1997), a Federal Bureau of Investigation (FBI) agent obtained a printout of business records from a suspect's computer by operating the computer, installing Microsoft Money, and printing the records. The court affirmed the admission of the printouts, finding that testimony of the agent with personal knowledge of the process used to retrieve and print the data provided sufficient authentication of the records; however, in an apparent admonition to the defense bar, the court noted that the defense conspicuously failed to question the FBI agent "about how the disks were formatted, what type of computer was used, or any other questions of a technical nature" (*United States v Whitaker*, 1997).

In a similar decision, *Bone v State* (2002), the defendant contended that the trial court erred when it admitted pictorial images recovered from a hard drive without proper authentication. The appellate court noted that the computer investigator testified about the process he used to recover the data: He "remove[d] the hard drive" from Bone's computers and "made an image of it" then he "write protected" the various floppy diskettes before viewing them, and testified about the software program he used to recover deleted files (*Bone v State*, 2002). The detective further testified about the way he exported images found on the image of Bone's computer media. He testified that he printed copies of images in Bone's computer files "exactly" as he found them and further stated that the copies "fairly and accurately" showed the images that he had seen "on the computer that [he was] using to examine Mr. Bone's computer" (*Bone v State*, 2002). In reviewing Indiana Evidence Rule 901(a), which is identical to the federal rule, and citing *United States v Whitaker* (1997), the appellate court determined that the trial court testimony was sufficient to establish the authenticity of the images contained in Bone's computer (*Bone v State*, 2002).

People v Lugashi (1988) is another notable case involving a detailed analysis by the court on this subject. Though not involving a computer forensic investigation per se, the court addressed issues concerning the authentication of computer-based evidence challenged by the defense in a criminal prosecution. *Lugashi* involved a credit card fraud investigation in which a bank's internal computer system recorded and stored relevant data related to a series of transactions in question. Each night the bank's computer systems ran a program known as a "data dump," which retrieved and organized the daily credit card transactions reported to the bank. Shortly thereafter, a backup tape was made of the "dump" from which a microfiche record was prepared and maintained (*People v Lugashi*, 1988).

The prosecution sought to introduce the computer-generated evidence generated by this process largely through the testimony of one of the bank's systems administrators, who conceded that she was not a computer expert. She did, however, work with those who ran the "data dumps" and maintained the microfiche records, and she was familiar with the system. She personally produced the data in question from the microfiche records and knew how to interpret the data (*People v Lugashi*, 1988). The defense contended that since the systems administrator was not a computer expert, she was incompetent to authenticate the data in question and that, essentially, only the computer programmers involved in the design and operation of the bank's computer systems could establish that the systems and programs in question were reliable and error-free. The defense asserted that because the systems administrator's understanding of the way the system worked came from her discussions with the bank's programmers and other technical staff members, her testimony constituted hearsay and should not be allowed (*People v Lugashi*, 1988).

The court rejected the defense's argument, noting that the defense's position incorrectly assumed that only a computer expert "who could personally perform the programming, inspect and maintain the software and hardware, and compare competing products, could supply the required testimony" (*People v Lugashi*, 1988). Instead the court ruled that "a person who generally understands the system's operation and possesses sufficient knowledge and skill to properly use the system and explain the resultant data, even if unable to perform every task from initial design and programming to final printout, is a 'qualified witness'" for purposes of establishing a foundation for the computer evidence (*People v Lugashi*, 1988). The court noted that if the defense's proposed test were applied to conventional, hand-entered accounting records, for example, the proposal "would require not only the testimony of the bookkeeper records custodian, but that of an expert in accounting theory that the particular system employed, if properly applied, would yield accurate and relevant information" (*People v Lugashi*, 1988). Further, if the defense's position were correct, "only the original hardware and software designers could testify, since everyone else necessarily could understand the system only through hearsay" (*People v Lugashi*, 1988). The *Lugashi* court commented that the defense's proposed test would require production of "hordes" of technical witnesses that would unduly burden the crowded trial courts and the business employing such technical witnesses "to no real benefit" (*People v Lugashi*, 1988).

Some factors and aspects of the *Lugashi* decision may not be completely applicable to computer forensics. For instance, *Lugashi* deals with records created in the normal course of business, which courts in the United States generally presume to be authentic, subject to the presentation of any direct evidence to the contrary. Further, a disinterested third party to the litigation generated the computer records in *Lugashi*, and courts would likely scrutinize the records generated by a law enforcement investigator or retained party expert. However, certain aspects of the *Lugashi* decision seem applicable to questions regarding what is required to establish a proper foundation for evidence obtained from a computer forensic examination. (See also *Federal Deposit Insurance Corporation v Carabetta* [1999], which is similar in facts and holding to *People v Lugashi* [1988]; *Hahnemann University Hospital v Dudnick* [1996]; and *Garden State Bank v Graef* [2001].)

AUTHENTICATION OF THE ENCASE RECOVERY PROCESS

Under the standard articulated under *Lugashi* and several other similar cases, the examiner need not be able to detail the way each function of a cloning software works to provide sufficient testimony regarding the process. There are no known authorities requiring otherwise for commercially available and generally accepted software. A skilled and trained examiner who is familiar with the process should be able to present evidence obtained through a forensic examination.

An examiner should possess a strong working familiarity of the way the program is used and what the cloning process involves when seeking to introduce evidence recovered by the program. This means that the examiner should ideally have received computer forensic training though such training should not be required, especially when the witness is an experienced computer forensic investigator and has received computer forensic training on computer systems. Examiners should conduct their own software testing and validation to confirm that the program functions as advertised. However, a "strong working familiarity" does not mean that an examiner must obtain and be able to decipher all 300 000 lines of the program source code or be able to reverse-engineer the program on the witness stand.

CHALLENGES TO FOUNDATION MUST HAVE FOUNDATION

In the event that the initial evidentiary foundation established by the computer forensic examiner's testimony is sufficiently rebutted so as to challenge the admissibility or the weight of the evidence, expert testimony to rebut such contentions may be required. However, courts will normally disallow challenges to the authenticity of computer-based evidence absent a specific showing that the computer data in question may not be accurate or genuine—mere speculation and unsupported theories generally will not suffice (*United States v Tank*, 2000; *Wisconsin v Schroeder*, 2000). Ample precedent shows that unsupported claims of possible tampering or overlooked exculpatory data are common and met with considerable skepticism by the courts. One federal court refused to consider allegations of tampering that was "almost wild-eyed speculation … [without] evidence to support such a scenario" (*United States v Whitaker*, 1997). Another court noted that the mere possibility that computer data could have been altered is "plainly insufficient to establish untrustworthiness" (*United States v Bonallo*, 1988). (See also *United States v Glasser*, (1985) for more information.)

One court suggests that the defense should perform its own credible computer forensic examination to support any allegation of overlooked exculpatory evidence or tampering (*United States v Tank*, 2000). Another court noted that though some unidentified data may have been inadvertently altered during the course of an exam, the defendant failed to establish how such alteration, even if true, affected the relevant data (*Wisconsin v Schroeder*, 2000). As such, for a court to allow a challenge based on alleged tampering or alteration of the computer data, the defense should be required to establish specific evidence of alteration or tampering and evidence that such alteration affected relevant data. Further, if there is some basis to allegations that relevant computer records have been altered, such evidence would go to the weight of the evidence not to its admissibility (*United States v Bonallo*, 1988).

VALIDATION OF COMPUTER FORENSIC TOOLS

The previous section addressed authenticating computer evidence through direct or circumstantial evidence to establish that the recovered data are genuine and accurate. Another form of an objection to authenticity may involve questioning the reliability of the computer program that generated or processed the computer evidence in question. In such cases the proponent of the evidence must testify to the validity of the program or programs utilized in the process. This section discusses the standards the courts apply in such challenges and the testimony the examiner may need to provide to validate computer forensic tools.

DAUBERT/FRYE STANDARD

Daubert v Merrell Dow Pharmaceuticals, Inc (1993) is an important federal court decision that sets forth a legal test to determine the validity of scientific evidence and its relevance to the case at issue. Many state court jurisdictions in the United States follow the *Frye v United States* (1923) test, which is similar to *Daubert*. The introduction of deoxyribonucleic acid (DNA) evidence is a typical scenario in which a court may require a *Daubert/Frye* analysis though many courts now take judicial notice of the accuracy of DNA typing procedures since the science is no longer considered "novel" (*United States v Beasley*, 1996).

Daubert/Frye has been raised in most concerted challenges to EnCase; however, a corporate defendant advocating the EnCase-based evidence in *Matthew Dickey v Steris Corporation* (2000) asserted that the software constituted an automated process that produces accurate results, and thus, evidence obtained from that process would be subject to a presumption of authenticity under Rule 901(b)(9). Rule 901(b)(9) provides that evidence produced by an automated process, including computer-generated evidence, may be authenticated if such an automated process is shown to produce accurate results. The court addressed the *Daubert* factors however. Though EnCase meets the standards under both Rule 901 and *Daubert* (*Kumho Tire Company, Ltd v Carmichael*, 1999), the recent trend of the courts is to include "non-scientific" technical evidence within the purview of *Daubert/ Frye*, in addition to the purely scientific forms of evidence (eg, DNA analysis) that are more traditionally subject to *Daubert*. The judicial analysis applied in recent, notable challenges to EnCase is consistent with this trend. As such, a computer forensic examiner should be familiar with the basic elements of the *Daubert* analysis, which are as follows (*Daubert v Merrell Dow Pharmaceuticals, Inc*, 1993):

1. Whether a "theory or technique … can be (and has been) tested"

2. Whether it "has been subjected to peer review and publication"

3. Whether, in respect to a particular technique, there is a high "known or potential rate of error"

4. Whether the theory or technique enjoys "general acceptance" within the "relevant scientific community"

Under the first prong of the test, courts have expressly noted that EnCase is a commercially available program that can easily be tested and validated. This is in contrast to tools that are not commercially available to the general public or custom tools with arcane command line functionality that are not easily tested by third parties unfamiliar with those processes. The law clarifies that in the context of computer-generated evidence, the courts favor commercially available and standard software. Further, many agencies have tested EnCase in their laboratories before standardizing their agents with the software. The widespread adoption of the software by the computer forensics community serves as a crucial factor for authentication because the community generally knows the capabilities and accuracy of the program through such extensive usage.

The National Institute of Standards & Technology (NIST) has conducted important testing of computer forensics tools, in which EnCase has fared well. The NIST, under its Computer Forensics Tools Testing Project, conducts independent testing and validation of disk imaging tools. The comprehensive nature of this testing may involve more than 50 separate test scenarios of Internet Drive Electronics (IDE) and Small Computer System Interface (SCSI) hard drives. An excellent computer forensics tool should image all sectors and verify the imaged media and should report and log input and output errors during the imaging process as well as detect and report verification errors when the image files are altered with a disk editor.

These reviews are among several industry publications featuring EnCase and are relevant to the second prong of the *Daubert* test. Peer review and publication in the relevant industry is an important factor looked to by the courts in considering the validity of a technical process under *Daubert/Frye*. Computer forensic examiners must remain abreast of peer review of computer forensic tools in industry publications. Examiners should be cognizant of whether developers decline invitations from respected industry publications to participate in testing and peer review opportunities because such refusals could raise questions regarding the tools' validity.

An important peer review article that appeared in *The Computer Paper*, Canada's leading IT publication, illustrates how peer review is an important source to establish general acceptance and industry trends.

Because courts around the world have accepted EnCase as a standard, [a] commercially available forensic software application, defense attorneys have switched from attacking the accuracy of the software to attacking the methodology of the operator, or forensic technician. This makes training important (Chappelle, 2002).

Investigators are commonly asked to testify to specific examples of peer review and publication of technical or scientific processes. For instance, in *People v Rodriguez* (2001), a recent case in Sonoma County, California, in which EnCase was subjected to a *Frye* analysis, the district attorney investigator referenced in his testimony several available articles regarding the software. Often, testifying experts will bring copies of relevant articles from industry publications to court for admission into evidence as part of the validation process.

Courts have referred to the need for a body of data from "meaningful testing" efforts to guide them in their *Daubert* analysis. There is no requirement for a regimented and universal standard for such testing agreed on by all the experts in the field. However, any testing should be meaningful and objective, as well as subject to the same peer review as the tools and processes being analyzed. Further, professional testing ideally culminates in the preparation of a detailed report or "white paper," thereby allowing for proper analysis and comment. In *United States v Saelee* (2001), the court noted that peer review should be conducted by "disinterested parties, such as academics."

Because computer forensics remains a new field, no ideal amount of published testing exists. Many large agencies have conducted tests with industry standard software but have not published their results. Additionally, determining if a particular tool has a high rate of error is difficult unless the testing process and methodologies are disclosed and documented in full. Defining a "high rate of error" is difficult when many developers of popular forensic tools decline to allow testing on their tools, which deprives the analysis of a wider field of comparison. As this industry matures, however, the amount of documented and objective testing should increase.

The final prong, whether a process enjoys "general acceptance" within the "relevant scientific community," is an important factor strongly considered by the courts in validating scientific tools and processes. "'[A] known technique that has been able to attract only minimal support within the community' ... may properly be viewed with skepticism" (*Daubert v Merrell Dow Pharmaceuticals, Inc*, 1993). More than 3000 law enforcement agencies and companies worldwide employ EnCase for their computer investigations. The widespread, general acceptance of a process is often considered to be the most important prong in a *Daubert/Frye* analysis.

In the case of many other technical processes, counsel will often struggle to establish that all the *Daubert* factors are sufficiently met. However, it is difficult to imagine any other computer forensic process that could better qualify under the *Daubert/Frye* analysis. In fact, at least one trial court has taken official judicial notice that EnCase is a commercially available tool with widespread general acceptance (*State of Washington v Leavell*, 2001). If possible, counsel should consider seeking judicial notice* from the court of several of the *Daubert* factors as applied to forensic software, including its general acceptance and the fact that it is commercially available and subject to widespread peer review.

Computer Forensics as an Automated Process

Federal Rule of Evidence 901(b)(9) provides a presumption of authenticity to evidence generated by or resulting from a largely automated process or system shown to produce an accurate result. (For more information, see *People v Lugashi* (1988) in which data collection software program was presumed accurate and *People v Mormon* (1981) in which data retrieval program was presumed accurate.)

This rule is often cited in the context of computer-processed evidence. There is some debate as to whether testimony from computer forensic examiners should be considered expert scientific testimony and subject to an analysis under *Daubert*, or nonscientific technical testimony regarding the recovery of data through a technical investigation process, and subject to Federal Rule of Evidence 901(a), 901(b)(9). The United States Supreme Court blurred this distinction between scientific versus nonscientific expert testimony in *Kumho Tire Company, Ltd v Carmichael* (1999), which extended the *Daubert* test to cover technical processes and scientific opinion evidence. However, many courts still draw a general distinction between scientific and nonscientific expert testimony.

At least one federal appeals case has referred to this issue in dicta, hypothesizing that in light of Rule 901(b)(9), computer or x-ray evidence resulting from a process or system would not fall under a *Frye* analysis since "[t]he underlying principles behind x-ray and computers are well understood; as to these technologies, serious questions of accuracy and reliability arise, if at all, only in connection with their application in a particular instance" (*United States v Downing*, 1985). The court in *United States v Whitaker* (1997) held that, without addressing *Daubert*, a foundation for forensically recovered computer evidence could be established by the investigating agent with personal knowledge of the process used to retrieve and print the data.

In *United States v Quinn* (1994), the prosecution sought to introduce "photogrammetry" evidence through expert testimony to determine the height of a suspect

---

* Judicial Notice is the act of a court recognizing the existence and truth of certain facts relevant to the case at bar. Such notice excuses a party from having the burden of establishing fact from necessity of producing formal proof.

from surveillance photographs. The trial court allowed the testimony after a simple proffer from the government as to the basis of a photogrammetry process, which the court found to be "nothing more than a series of computer-assisted calculations that did not involve any novel or questionable scientific technique" (*United States v Quinn*, 1994). The court of appeal rejected the defendant's contention that the photogrammetric evidence required an evidentiary hearing under *Daubert*, finding that the trial court acted within its discretion (*United States v Quinn*, 1994). In *Burleson v State* (1991), the court held that expert testimony resulting from a complicated computer-generated display showing deleted records was admissible because the software and computer systems creating the output relied upon by the expert were shown to be standard, accurate, and reliable. The court noted the computer system technology did not have to be authenticated under a *Frye* test, thereby finding that the showing of an accurate and reliable system producing the display was sufficient (*Burleson v State*, 1991).

In *State (Ohio) v Cook* (2002), an Ohio appellate court upheld the validity of the EnCase® Software. The court cited, in part, Ohio Rule of Evidence 901(b)(9), which is nearly identical to the corresponding federal rule.

The best cloning software packages have proven to provide a more accurate, objective, and complete search and recovery process through a substantially automated process. In more complex computer forensic cases, evidence concerning the search and recovery function with its resulting visual outputs and printed reports is often as important as the recovered data itself. Some tools exclusively employed by a minority of computer forensics examiners are little more than basic single-function DOS disk utilities that, when combined as a nonintegrated suite, are manipulated to perform computer forensic applications. This formerly common practice presents the following 3 fundamental problems:

1. Results from the examiner's search and recovery process are often subjective, incomplete, and variant.

2. The data restoration process can improperly alter the evidence on the evidentiary image copy or provide a visual output that is an incomplete and inaccurate reflection of the data contained on the target media.

3. The lack of integration of all essential forensic functions within a single software application presents potential challenges to the authenticity of the processed computer evidence.

Applying Rule 901(b)(9) to the context of electronic data discovery, computer forensic software should ideally provide an objective and automated search and data restoration process that facilitates consistency and accuracy. To provide a hypothetical illustration, a group of 10 qualified and independently operating forensic examiners who analyze the same evidentiary image should achieve almost the same search results when entering identical text search keywords or seek to recover all specified file types on the image, such as all graphical images or spreadsheet files. If not, the process used can not be considered automated or accurate and, therefore, would not be considered a process qualifying for a presumption of authenticity under Rule 901(b)(9). Further, search processing results often need to be duplicated before or during trial; therefore, if a colleague or, worse, an opposing expert obtains significantly differing search results from the same media, the impact or the foundation of the evidence may be weakened. Though the court in *Gates Rubber Company v Bando Chemical Industries, Ltd* (1996) did not expressly cite Rule 901(b)(9), its holding that a computer examiner has "a duty to utilize the method which would yield the most complete and accurate results" is consistent with the statute.

Results from search and recovery procedures that use DOS utilities will significantly vary depending on the type and sequence of the nonintegrated utilities used, the amount of media to be searched, and the examiner's skill, biases, and time available. Further, each piece of acquired media must be searched separately, using the same tedious and time-consuming protocol for each hard drive, floppy disk, compact disk (CD), or other media involved in the case. As a result, the likelihood of different, independently operating examiners duplicating the search and restoration process on the same evidentiary image is remote, if not impossible.

As a result of the inordinate burden of searching a Windows image with DOS utilities, some investigators resort to operating Windows Explorer on the evidentiary image disk. In addition to being unable to view temporary and fragmented data such as file slack, swap files, and all other types of unallocated data, Windows Explorer will corrupt the data in such a situation by altering file date stamps, temporary files, and other transient information. Better practice requires specially designed Windows-based computer forensic software that uses a noninvasive and largely automated search process. A more objective search process facilitates more accurate and consistent results, thereby enabling duplication of the process at trial and by independently operating examiners. For example, when using EnCase, clicking a request to display all graphical image files contained on an evidentiary image disk will instantly list all such files in a graphical interface, including files renamed or hidden in obscure directories by a suspect to conceal these files and even previously deleted files. EnCase duplicates the Windows Explorer interface and viewing functions with the critical added benefits of viewing deleted files and all other unallocated data in a noninvasive manner. Most importantly, an examiner can present the discovered evidence in court with confidence that the search and recovery process provided more complete, consistent, and objective results than other search processes.

The line of cases that applied Rule 901(a)(b) previously discussed preceded *Kumho Tire* (1999), which extended the *Daubert* test to technical processes and scientific opinion evidence. EnCase has been authenticated at trial under *Daubert/Frye* and Rule 901(b)(9), and it is advisable that both approaches be considered in authenticating the software.

COMMERCIAL VERSUS CUSTOM FORENSIC SOFTWARE AND AUTHENTICATION ISSUES

Some computer forensic investigations use custom software tools developed by the investigating agency or a private company that are not commercially available to the general public. Courts have addressed issues concerning the type of software involved when computer-generated evidence is at issue. Such cases provide a presumption of authenticity for evidence resulting from or processed by commercially available computer systems and software over customized systems and software. One respected treatise on the subject (71 Am Jur Trials 111, 1999) noted the following:

Evidence generated through the use of standard, generally available software is easier to admit than evidence generated with custom software. The reason lies in the fact that the capabilities of commercially marketed software packages are well known and cannot normally be manipulated to produce aberrant results. Custom software, on the other hand, must be carefully analyzed by an expert programmer to ensure that the evidence being generated by the computer is in reality what it appears to be. Nonstandard or custom software can be made to do a host of things that would be undetectable to anyone except the most highly trained programmer who can break down the program using source codes and verify that the program operates as represented.

In fact, courts in many jurisdictions require that any computer-generated evidence be a product of a "standard" computer program or system in order to admit such evidence (*Burleson v State*, 1991; *People v Bovio*, 1983; *People v Lombardi*, 1999; *Weisman v Hopf-Himsel, Inc*, 1989). This body of authority would seem especially relevant to software used by law enforcement for computer forensic purposes, given the sensitive function of such software. A law enforcement agency that used customized proprietary software for computer forensic investigations could face various complications when seeking to introduce evidence processed with such software. Such actual or potential pitfalls could include the following:

— The defense could seek to exclude the results of any computer investigation that used tools inaccessible to all non-law enforcement agencies. Federal courts are unanimous in holding that computer evidence generated by or resulting from a process is only admissible if the defense has access to such software to independently duplicate the results of that process and thus "is given the same opportunity to inquire into the accuracy of the computer system involved in producing such evidence" (*United States v Liebert*, 1975; *United States v Weatherspoon*, 1978).

— If the defense is provided with a copy of the proprietary software and all evidentiary images, an expert retained by the defense will require substantial time to learn the software and recreate the process, thereby resulting in substantial cost to the government in cases involving indigent defendants. The government will incur further costs if the purchase of supporting operating systems and file servers is required to support the custom software.

— Though the source code for commercially available software is not required to be introduced into evidence to establish the authenticity of computer processed evidence, as previously noted, such presumptions of authenticity would not be afforded to customized software. Thus, the defense would seek to exclude the results of any computer investigation that uses custom software tools unless the source code was made available to the defense for testing and analysis. This would be true for computer forensic software given the sensitive nature of presenting evidence of deleted files and other transient electronic information.

Conversely, when questioned in court regarding the reliability of a commercially available software application, the proponent of the evidence could testify that it is a widely used and commercially available software program; as a result, any member of the public can purchase, use, and test the program. The defense could not claim prejudice by the use of the software since any reasonably skilled computer examiner could examine the discovery copy of the evidence, and the government would not be subject to questions regarding access to the source code of the program.

EXPERT WITNESS TESTIMONY

Are computer forensic investigators considered experts? Many courts outside of the United States (eg, Great Britain) use a higher (and perhaps wiser) threshold to determine who is qualified to provide expert testimony regarding a technical subject. This section discusses the threshold for qualifying a computer investigator as an expert and some cases in which the court addressed this issue. Also presented are 2 fictional transcripts of sample direct examinations. The first example is a transcript from a mock pretrial evidentiary hearing under Federal Rules of Evidence 104 and 702 and/or *Daubert v Merrell Dow Pharmaceuticals* (1993). A court may schedule such an evidentiary hearing to consider any foundational questions regarding the forensic software process. The second example is a direct examination in the context of a jury trial presenting evidence obtained from a computer forensic examination.

Though these examples are fictional, they are based upon actual investigation procedures and techniques taught in Guidance Software's training program and are used in the field daily by hundreds of agencies and organizations. These examples should provide a general reference for prosecutors in preparing direct examinations of their computer examiners in the context of either an evidentiary hearing or a jury trial.

THRESHOLD UNDER RULE 702

In the United States, Federal Rule of Evidence 702 provides that for a witness to be qualified as an expert, the expert must be shown to have "knowledge, skill, experience, training, or education" regarding the subject matter involved. Under this threshold, trained computer forensic experts have qualified as experts in US courts; however, prosecutors oftentimes opt not to offer the examiner as an expert, especially when the records in question can be authenticated under Federal Rule of Evidence 901(b)(9) or a corresponding state statute or if the examiner can be offered as a percipient witness presenting more objective and empirical findings of their investigation. This approach tends to be more common in many state courts.

This question was directly addressed in *United States v Scott-Emuakpor* (2000) (*United States v Liebert*, 1975; *United States v Weatherspoon*, 1978), during which the court considered whether the US Secret Service (USSS) agents who conducted the computer forensic examination needed to be qualified experts in computer science to present their findings.

The defendant in *Scott-Emuakpor* brought a motion *in limine* contending that the USSS agents should be precluded from providing testimony regarding the results of their computer examinations since one of the agents admitted that he was not an expert in the area of computer science. However, the court opined that

there is no reason why either witness may not testify about what they did in examining the computer equipment and the results of their examinations. The question before the Court at this time is not whether these witnesses have the expertise, for example, to develop sophisticated software programs. The question is whether they have the skill to find out what is on a hard drive or a zip drive. Apparently, they have this skill because they determined what was on the drives. By analogy, a person need not be an expert on English literature in order to know how to read. ... The fact that [the USSS agent] admitted that he is not an expert in the area of computer science is not binding on the Court (*United States v Scott-Emuakpor*, 2000).

However, an examiner can commonly be asked to interpret the recovered data. The recent case of *United States v Hilton* (2001) provides a strong example of a computer forensic examiner offering expert witness testimony to interpret the data gleaned from his examination. Among the issues in *Hilton* was whether the defendant had used interstate commerce (ie, the Internet) in the process of distributing child pornography, which satisfied a key element and requirement of the statute. The computer investigator from the US Customs Service testified that the images in question were located in a subdirectory named "MIRC," which contained software and files related to Internet Relay Chat (IRC). The special agent testified that, in his expert opinion, because the contraband was located in the MIRC subdirectory that contained Internet chat-related files, the images were likely associated with the Internet.

The special agent testified that the file time and date stamps reflecting the creation time of each subject image indicated that the defendant downloaded the images from the Internet via a modem. The special agent made this conclusion because the images were created on the defendant's computer at intervals of time consistent with downloading the images via a modem. The special agent's expert testimony, among other factors, convinced the court that the subject images were transmitted to the defendant's computer via the Internet, thereby satisfying the interstate commerce requirement of section 18 USC § 2252A(a)(5)(B).

ILLUSTRATIONS OF TESTIMONY

Direct Examination: Pretrial Evidentiary Hearing

If any challenge is raised to the qualifications of the computer examiner or the foundation of the evidence concerning the tools or methodologies used in the course of a computer forensic investigation, many prosecutors prefer to address such objections outside the presence of the jury through a hearing under Federal Rule of Evidence 702, Rule 104, or *Daubert*. Judges are typically more receptive to technical evidence, and this evidence avoids presenting complex testimony on contested technical issues before a jury by resolving such foundational issues in a separate hearing beforehand. The following fictional "mock-trial" direct examination is designed to illustrate the way a proper foundation could be established for the cloning software process under

Rule 901(b)(9) and *Daubert*, using EnCase as an example. For illustration purposes, the following example contains more detail than what would normally be presented on direct examination, even in the context of a court trial or hearing; however, much of the information may be useful for redirect examination.

Background
[After stating name for the record]

Q: Sir, are you a senior special agent for the US Customs Service?

A: Yes, I am.

Q: Do you have any specialized duties as a customs agent?

A: I am a computer evidence examiner certified as a Seized Computer Evidence Recovery Specialist by the United States Department of the Treasury.

Q: Please tell us how long you have been a computer evidence examiner.

A: I have been a Seized Computer Evidence Recovery Specialist with Customs for 8 years.

Q: Tell us about your educational background.

A: I received a bachelor of science degree in electrical engineering from the University of _____ in 19__.

Q: Could you briefly describe your training for the handling and examination of computer evidence?

A: In 19__, I received 3 weeks of intensive training, known as Seized Computer Evidence Recovery Specialist training, at the Federal Law Enforcement Training Center. In 19__, I obtained Computer Forensic Examiner Certification from the International Association of Computer Investigative Specialists, known as IACIS, after receiving 2 weeks of intensive training. That next year, I received Advanced Course Certification from IACIS after taking a 2-week advanced training course. I have also received computer forensic training from the National Consortium for Justice Information and Statistics, known as SEARCH.

Q: Are you a member of any professional organizations?

A: Yes, I am.

Q: Which ones?

A: I am a member of the International Association of Computer Investigative Specialists (IACIS) and the High Technology Crime Investigation Association (HTCIA).

Overview of Computer Forensics

Q: You mentioned the subject of computer forensics. Can you provide an overview of what computer forensics is?

A: Computer forensics is the acquisition, authentication, and reconstruction of electronic information stored on computer media, such as hard drives, floppy disks, or zip drives. A computer forensics technician is needed whenever evidence is stored in a computer.

Q: Can you briefly tell us how a computer forensic specialist such as yourself conducts a typical investigation?

A: First, the electronic information contained on computer storage media must be acquired by making a complete physical copy of every bit of data located on computer media in a manner that does not alter that information. Then the information must be authenticated in a special process that establishes that the acquired electronic information remained completely unaltered from the time the examiner acquired it. Finally, the examiner must use special software and processes to recover and reconstruct the information in its forensic state even if such information is found in files that have been deleted by the user.

The Acquisition Process

Q: You described 3 basic steps. I want to discuss them one at a time beginning with the acquisition process. How is digital information copied from computer media in a proper forensic manner?

A: Specialized computer forensic software uses a special boot process that ensures that the data on the subject computer are not changed. After the boot procedure is initiated, the examiner utilizes the forensic software to create a complete forensic image copy, or "exact snapshot," of a targeted piece of computer media, such as a hard drive, or external media, such as floppy or zip disks. This forensic image is a sector-by-sector copy of all data contained on the target media and, thus, all information, including available information from deleted files, is included in the forensic image created by the examiner.

The Authentication Process

Q: The second step you mentioned was the authentication process. Please briefly describe how the acquired electronic information is authenticated and verified.

A: Computer forensic examiners rely on software that generates a mathematical value based on the exact content of the information contained in the forensic image copy of the seized computer media. This value is known as an MD5 hash value and is often referred to as a special type of digital signature. The same software verifies that this value remains the same from the time it is generated. If one bit of data on the forensic image copy is altered, meaning that if a single character is changed or one space of text is added, this value changes. So, if the hash value of the information contained on seized media remains the same, then it is established that the electronic data have not been altered.

Q: What are the odds of 2 forensic images with different contents having the same hash value?

A: The odds of 2 computer files, including a forensic image file, with different contents having the same hash value is roughly 1 in 10 raised to the 38th power.

The Recovery Process

Q: Because the third step of data recovery is complex, I am going to first ask you a few basic questions about how a computer works. First, and without being too technical, could you give us a description of how information on a hard drive is stored by the computer?

A: Yes. Basically, computer disks are storage media divided into concentric circles or tracks. This can be thought of as a small version of the old 78 rpm records people played on phonographs. The tracks are divided into sectors. Each sector has its own address, a number that is unique to that part of the disk. The operating system assigns and stores the address so that it may retrieve all information constituting a computer file stored in a specific sector when requested by the user.

Q: How is the information recorded on the hard disk?

A: The disk is covered with a thin coat of magnetic material. When information is written to the disk, the data are recorded by magnetizing specific parts of the disk coating. The information resides there until it is overwritten.

Q: Thank you. I am interested in how a computer technician can recover electronic information that has been deleted or automatically purged. Please tell us what is involved in this process.

A: When the computer user deletes electronic information, it is often assumed that the information is removed from the computer forever; however, that is not necessarily true. The information is still in the computer, but now the information is marked by the computer to allow it to be overwritten. A general analogy would be a library card catalog system in which books represent files and the card catalog represents the file directory with information as to where the files are located on the disk. When a file is deleted, its location information is removed from the card catalog index, but the book remains on the shelf until another book randomly replaces it.

Q: To what extent can this deleted information be retrieved?

A: If the information has not been overwritten by other data, it is still there and can be retrieved using specialized software.

Authenticating the EnCase Process Under Rule 901

Q: What specialized software did you use for this investigation?

A: I used the computer forensic software known as EnCase.

Q: Tell us a little about this software.

A: EnCase is a standard, commercially available software program specifically designed for computer forensic investigations. It is a fully integrated tool, which means it performs all essential functions of a computer forensic investigation, including the imaging of a target drive, the generation of an MD5 hash of the evidentiary forensic image, and the analysis of the subject evidence. The software allows for a completely noninvasive investigation to view all information on a computer drive, whether it is in the form of a deleted file, a nondeleted file, file fragments, or temporary or buffer files.

Q: How does the investigator use EnCase to recover deleted files?

A: First, it creates a complete forensic image copy, or exact snapshot, of a targeted computer drive. All existing information on that forensic image will be read, regardless of whether the information is in the form of a deleted file marked by the operating system to be overwritten. Any information that has not been overwritten will be recovered for analysis. EnCase will organize all the files, deleted files, and blocks of physical data (known as ***unallocated clusters***) in a convenient graphical user interface (GUI) to allow the evidence to be viewed and sorted by the examiner.

Q: Does the same software perform these functions?

A: Yes. EnCase is a fully integrated program in which all the required computer forensic investigation functions are integrated into a single application in a Windows-based GUI.

Q: How is this process more automated than other tools?

A: To a large extent, EnCase duplicates the Windows Explorer interface and file viewing functions, with the critical added benefits of viewing deleted files and all other information on the disk that the user can not normally see or detect without specialized software. Just as Windows Explorer presents the entire file directory and folder structure on a computer to the user in an organized manner, EnCase presents that information and other data on the target drive, in a similar manner.

Addressing Daubert Factors

Q: To your knowledge, is the EnCase® Software generally accepted in the computer forensic investigation community?

A: Yes. It is widely used in the computer forensics industry and, in my experience, it is the tool of choice for most computer forensic investigators in law enforcement.

It is the primary computer forensic tool used by the US Customs Agency, which is my agency, and I am aware that it is the primary tool of other federal agencies, including the US Secret Service. EnCase is a major part of the Seized Computer Evidence Recovery Specialist training curriculum for federal agents and is part of the curriculum in many computer forensic training courses offered by professional organizations, most notably the annual IACIS training conference.

Q: How would one go about testing computer forensic software?

A: There are 3 main steps in testing computer forensic software. The first step is to generate an MD5 hash value for an image of a targeted computer drive using the forensic tool being tested and then using another standard tool to repeat the process for the same drive. The MD5 hash values generated by both tools for the same drive should be the same. The second step is to verify that whatever evidence is recovered from an evidentiary forensic image can be independently confirmed by a standard disk utility. With EnCase, for instance, the program will identify the precise location on the original drive for each bit of data recovered by the examiner. With that information, the examiner can then use a disk utility, such as Norton DiskEdit, to independently confirm the existence and precise location of that data. The third step is to confirm that throughout the examination process, the content on the forensic image has been unaltered by repeating the MD5 hash analysis of the forensic image to verify the MD5 hash has not changed since acquisition. These tests should be performed several times with different pieces of computer media.

Q: To what extent can EnCase be tested by a third party?

A: This is a commercially available software, so all examiners can purchase, use, and test the program on their own. One of the advantages of the program is that all the required forensic functions are integrated into a single program with a Windows-based GUI. Thus, compared to other computer forensic software, the program is easy to use.

Q: Has your agency tested the software?

A: Yes.

Q: How was it tested?

A: Before we purchased the software on a large scale, there were 2 computer investigation agents in my agency who conducted an extensive evaluation of the software by using the 3 steps I just described. I am aware that the Secret Service conducted a similar testing procedure as well. Since our agency's adoption of the software, we have had nearly 100 computer examination agents using the program on a daily basis in the field.

Q: What were the results of those tests?

A: By all accounts, the software has met the 3 standards I described.

Q: Are you aware of whether EnCase has been subjected to any publication in the industry?

A: Yes. I have read various published articles in the information security and high-tech crime investigation industries that favorably review the product or mention the product favorably. An article in the April 2001 issue of *SC Magazine* featured the most detailed and documented published testing results to date.

Q: At this time, your Honor, I would like to submit as the government's exhibit __, which are copies of published articles in the industry discussing the EnCase® Software.

THE COURT: So received.

Q: Thank you, your Honor, nothing further.

Direct Examination for the Presentation of Computer Evidence

Many prosecutors maintain that when presenting computer evidence before a jury, the testimony should be as simple and straightforward as possible. Burdening the jury with overly technical information could prove counter-productive and may open the door to areas of cross-examination that the court would normally have disallowed. As such, the following direct examination is more detailed than is likely needed but should provide a general resource in preparing direct examinations or for responding on redirect.

When presenting EnCase-based evidence, the proponent should take full advantage of the software process and GUI by presenting screen shots and other views to show the full context of the electronic evidence. This technique may be required to comply with Best Evidence Rule considerations in computer evidence. Federal Rule of Evidence 1001(3) provides that "[if] data are stored in a computer or similar device, any printout or other output readable by sight, shown to reflect the data accurately, is an 'original.'" When presenting evidence contained within a computer file, a screen shot may be the best means to present a visual output that is "shown to reflect the data accurately," thereby constituting an "original" under Rule 1001(3). (For a more detailed discussion see the section titled *The Best Evidence Rule*.)

When seeking to establish a defendant's state of mind by presenting an electronic audit trail or connecting file date stamps, the ability to display a visual output showing various file attributes and other metadata provides a tremendous advantage to the advocate of such evidence. The best software packages display all physical and logical data contained on the target drive, while showing the context of such files by displaying file metadata and other means. When providing testimony, many examiners present evidence through screenshots in a PowerPoint presentations format or take the cloning sofware with them into court for a live demonstration. In *United States v Dean*, the opinion reflects that the prosecution presented results of its computer forensic examination through PowerPoint (*United States v Dean*, 2001). This case is discussed in the section titled *Presenting Electronic Evidence at Trial*.

For sake of brevity, many of the foundational portions of the direct examination are incorporated by reference from the previous section.

Background
[After stating name for the record]

Q: Sir, what is your current occupation?

A: I am a Senior Special Agent for the US Customs Service.

Q: Do you have any specialized duties as a Customs agent?

A: I am a computer evidence examiner certified as a Seized Computer Evidence Recovery Specialist by the US Department of the Treasury.

Q: What was your involvement in the investigation of this case?

A: I conducted a computer forensic investigation of the defendant's computer to recover relevant evidence.

Q: OK, before we discuss the results of your investigation, please tell us how long you been a computer evidence examiner.

[Please refer to the previous section, which is incorporated herein by reference, for foundation testimony.]

Q: Turning to the computer forensic investigation you conducted in this case, please tell when you first came into contact with the defendant's computer and computer disks.

A: Pursuant to a search warrant, on May 18, 2000, I seized the defendant's computer at his home, along with 7 CD-ROMs and 16 floppy disks that were in his desk or in the vicinity of his computer.

Q: What did you do with the defendant's computer equipment and disks after you seized them?

A: After leaving receipts for the computer and disks, I transported the items back to our laboratory, where I immediately proceeded to make forensic image copies of the hard drive found in the defendant's computer. I made forensic images of each of the CD-ROMs and floppy disks. Using the EnCase® Software, I generated MD5 hash values for the hard drive and for each floppy disk and CD-ROM at the same time the forensic images were made. Then, I logged the defendant's computer and the floppy and CD-ROM disks as evidence and secured them in our evidence storage room.

Q: Did you then analyze the forensic images you made?

A: Yes, I did.

Q: Please describe your analysis on the forensic image of the defendant's hard drive.

Recovery of Hidden Files With Renamed File Extensions
A: In my analysis of the forensic image of the hard drive, I first used an automated function of the Forensic Software that analyzes all the computer files on an image of a computer drive and identifies any file signature mismatches.

Q: What are file signature mismatches?

A: A file signature mismatch is a situation in which the file name extension that normally identifies the file type has been renamed, which is usually done to hide the true contents of a file.

Q: What is a file name extension?

A: A file name extension is an optional addition to the file name that allows a file's format to be described as part of its name so users can quickly understand the file type without opening files on a trial-and-error basis. For instance, a text file will usually have a ".txt" extension, and the most common type of picture file has a ".jpg" extension.

Q: How does EnCase identify file signature mismatches?

A: Most computer files containing text or graphical images have a well-defined signature of electronic data unique to that file type. This allows file viewers to recognize the type of file regardless of the file extension. EnCase uses the same process as file viewers to identify files that have renamed file extensions.

Q: What was the result of the file mismatch analysis that you conducted in this case?

A: The file signature mismatch analysis revealed 16 files that were renamed as text files with a ".txt" extension but were graphical image files that originally had a ".jpg" extension until they were renamed manually. I viewed those files and, upon determining that those images appeared to be child pornography, I printed out those images.

Q: Showing to you what have been pre-marked as United States exhibits 1 through 16, can you identify these exhibits?

A: Yes. These are the printouts I made of the 16 images in question that I recovered from the defendant's hard drive.

[Exhibits are introduced into evidence.]

Recovery of Deleted Files.

Q: Did you examine the images you made of the defendant's floppy disks?

A: Yes, I did.

Q: What did you find?

A: I found that one of the floppy disks had 5 files with a ".jpg" extension that had been deleted, meaning that the computer had marked the data of those files to be overwritten; however, we recovered those deleted graphical image files because the data had not been overwritten by the computer.

Q: How did you identify those deleted files?

A: The EnCase® Software automatically identifies any files that are marked by the computer to be overwritten. I located and viewed those 5 graphical image files and, upon determining that those images appeared to be child pornography, I printed out those images.

Q: Showing to you what have been pre-marked as United States exhibits 17 through 21, can you identify these exhibits?

A: Yes. These are the printouts I made of the 5 images that I recovered from the defendant's reformatted floppy drive.

[Exhibits are introduced into evidence.]

Recovery of Files "Deleted" From Multiple CD-ROM Sessions.

Q: Special Agent _____, did you examine the images you made of the defendant's CD-ROM disks?

A: Yes, I did.

Q: What did you find?

A: I found that the CD-ROM disks were writeable, which means that data can be written to this type of compact disc to store computer files. A special CD-writing software program, such as CD Creator, is needed to write data to a writeable compact disc. One of the writeable CDs we seized from the defendant's home had multiple sessions on it. A CD session is created when the user writes any number of files to the CD. When this is done, the CD writing software creates a table of contents for that session that points the operating system to the location of the files on the CD within the session.

Q: Can files on a writeable CD be deleted?

A: Not really. Unlike a hard drive or floppy disk, data written to a CD are burned to the media by a small optical laser instead of being magnetized. Once data are burned to a CD, they can not be overwritten. However, if a new session is created on the CD, the user can omit existing files from the new table of contents created for the new session. A computer operating system will read only the table of contents from the latest created session on a CD. Thus, by omitting existing files from the table of contents of a new session, those files will normally be hidden from the view of a user. Specialized software will see all the sessions on a writeable compact disc and allow the user to compare any differences in the file contents of each session.

Q: You mentioned that one of the CDs you examined had multiple sessions. What did your analysis of the multiple session CD reveal?

A: The CD actually had 2 sessions on it. Using EnCase, we discovered that the second session contained 7 files with ".jpg" extensions that were not included in the table of contents of the first session. I examined those 7 files, which turned out to be graphical images appearing to be child pornography, and printed out those images.

Q: Showing to you what have been pre-marked as United States exhibits 22 through 28, can you identify these exhibits?

A: Yes. These are the printouts I made of the 7 images that I recovered from the first session of the defendant's writeable compact disc.

[Exhibits are introduced into evidence.]

Evidence From Swap Files
Q: What else did you find in your examination of the defendant's computer?

A: I conducted a text string search of the forensic image of the defendant's hard drive. In the course of our investigation, we received information that the defendant had contacted a minor over the Internet who had an America Online account under the screen name "Jenny86." I ran a text search by entering the keyword "Jenny86. The search registered several hits in an area of unallocated clusters identified as a swap file.

Q: What is a swap file?

A: A swap file is a random area on a hard disk used by the computer's operating system to store data temporarily as a means to manage the available operating memory of a computer. The operating system will swap information as needed between the memory chips and the hard disk to process that information. As a result, temporary data are placed on the computer that can not be viewed without special software designed for that purpose.

Q: What type of data are typically written to the swap file?

A: Any data that appears on the computer screen, even in the form of an unsaved word processing document or a Web page being viewed by the user, are often written to the swap file by the operating system.

Q: What did you do after you identified search hits for the keyword "Jenny86" in the swap file area?

A: I retrieved the full text of the information contained in the swap file and printed it.

Q: I am now handing you what has been previously marked as exhibit 29, and ask if you can identify it.

A: Yes. This is the printout I made of the data contained in the swap file in which my keyword search registered hits for the keyword "Jenny86."

Q: If you would, please read the text as it appears on this printout.

A: The text appears in transcript form and reads, "Welcome to Yahoo Young Teen Chat … [full text is read]."

[Exhibit is introduced into evidence.]

Evidence Found in File Slack
Q: What else did you find in your examination of the defendant's computer?

A: I conducted a separate text string search of the forensic image of the defendant's hard drive. In our investigation, we received additional information that the defendant had corresponded approximately 1 to 2 years ago with another individual on more than one occasion. That person has since been convicted of possession of child pornography and sexual assault with a minor. This person's name is John Doe; he commonly went by the nickname "Lolita's Man." We conducted a text string search with the keyword "Lolita's Man" and registered a hit in an area of data known as file slack, which contained remnants of a deleted file.

Q: What is file slack?

A: Data storage areas on a hard disk are segmented into clusters. All the data constituting a file may occupy an entire cluster, or the file data may not take up all of the space in the physical cluster. The space between the end of a file and the physical end of a cluster is called the file slack. After the point in the cluster at which the file ends, there may be preexisting bytes in a cluster that are remnants of previous files or folders.

*[NOTE: A projected PowerPoint slide or other form of demonstrative graphic illustrating this issue would be effective during this part of the examination (**Figure 35-1**).]*

Q: What did you do after you identified search hits for the keyword "Lolita's Man" in the area of file slack?

A: I retrieved the full text of the remainder of the document contained in the file slack and printed it.

Q: Could you determine what kind of document the remnant text in file slack was originally a part of?

A: Based on my observation of the format of the 2 remaining paragraphs in the document and the signature block at the end of the document, it appears that the text recovered from file slack was the remnants of a correspondence of some type.

Q: I am now handing you what has been previously marked as exhibit 30, and ask if you can identify it.

A: Yes. This is the printout I made of the data contained in the file slack area where my text search registered a hit for the text string search "Lolita's Man."

Q: If you would, please read the text as it appears on this printout.

A: *[The text is read into the record.]*

[NOTE: Because oral testimony of the recovery of file slack may seem too abstract to the jury and the court and because of best evidence rule considerations, it is recommended that a full screen shot from a forensic software with the highlighted text hid in file slack be projected to show the full context of the relevant text.]

Q: Showing what has been pre-marked as exhibit 31 on the projection screen, does this look familiar to you?

A: Yes, that is a screen shot of the File View of EnCase I created, showing the search hit for "Lolita's Man" in file slack.

Q: Part of the text on the screen is in red, while the text before it is in normal black font. Does the text coloring have any significance?

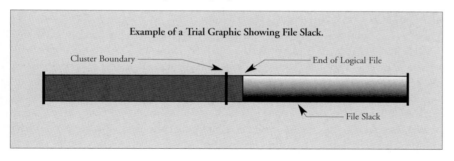

Figure 35-1. *Remnants of previous files may be found in the file slack. This is sometimes best shown with a representative figure.*

A: The black text is the active, or nondeleted, file that occupies the point from the beginning of the cluster to the end of that file. The red text represents the file slack in the area from the end of the nondeleted file to the end of the cluster.

[Exhibits are introduced into evidence.]

Evidence of Windows Metafiles Recovered From Unallocated Clusters

Q: What else did you find in your examination of the defendant's computer?

A: As part of my routine practice, I recovered all Windows metafiles that were located on the hard drive.

Q: What are Windows metafiles?

A: When a user sends a command to print a file, the Windows operating system makes a copy of that file and sends the copy to the printer. After the file is sent to the printer, Windows deletes that file. Windows does not inform the user that the copy, or metafile, has been made, nor can the user usually detect the existence of the metafiles without special software.

Q: How did you recover the metafiles in this case?

A: The EnCase® Software has an automated function that locates all the metafiles residing in normally unseen areas on a hard drive, decodes them, and outputs them to a separate folder allowing them to be viewed.

Q: What did you do after you used this software function that located the metafiles and outputted them to a folder?

A: I opened the folder and viewed each of the recovered metafiles.

Q: What did you find?

A: I found a text document in an e-mail format addressed to the defendant's e-mail account. According to the e-mail header information, the message was sent from the account of "Jenny86@_____.com."

Q: What does the fact that this e-mail document existed in the form of a metafile mean to you?

A: This recovered metafile means that this e-mail message was printed out from the defendant's computer.

Q: I am now handing you what has been previously marked as Exhibit 32, and ask if you can identify it.

A: Yes. This is the printout I made of the metafile of the e-mail document from "Jenny86@_____.com" to the e-mail account of the defendant.

Q: If you would, please read the text as it appears on this printout.

A: *[The text is read into the record.]*

[Exhibit 32 is introduced into evidence.]

THE BEST EVIDENCE RULE

Probably the most misunderstood rule of evidence among many computer forensic investigators is the "Best Evidence Rule." The Best Evidence Rule is a doctrine of evidentiary law in the United States and Canada requiring that, absent some exceptions, the original of a writing must be admitted to prove its contents. As one might imagine, significant questions arise when applying this evidentiary doctrine to computer data. Among the issues raised by this rule are the ways to present computer evidence at trial, what constitutes a valid image of a computer drive, and what constitutes data compression. This section provides the law and addresses some myths as well.

"Original" Electronic Evidence

The Best Evidence Rule under the US Federal Rules provides that "[t]o prove the content of a writing, recording or photograph, the original writing, recording or photograph is required." Notably, electronic evidence falls under the Federal Rules definition of "documents." However, with electronic evidence, the concept of an "original" is difficult to define. For example, when seeking to reproduce an original photographic image, a negative of that photograph, while containing all the "data" of the original, must be processed to provide an accurate visual replication of the original photograph. Fortunately, the Federal Rules of Evidence have expressly addressed this concern. Rule 1001(3) provides "[if] data are stored in a computer or similar device, any printout or other output readable by sight, shown to reflect the data accurately, is an 'original.'" Under this rule and similar rules in state jurisdictions, multiple or even an infinite number of copies of electronic files may each constitute an "original."

The operative language in Rule 1001(3) is "accurate reflection." It is a mistake to analogize computer files to hard copy documents for purposes of the Best Evidence Rule. A mere bit-stream copy of a graphical image file does not provide a completely accurate "printout or other output readable by sight" unless Windows-supported forensic tools or other viewers are used noninvasively to create an accurate visual output of the recovered data, without changing any of the data. Conversely, if a computer file is compressed, encrypted, and transmitted as an e-mail attachment (thereby sending a copy of that decrypted, compressed file in a different file format and even divided into many packets), and then received, decompressed, decrypted, and opened, then the file in possession of the recipient would be another "original" of that file under the Federal Rules. Printing that file converts it to another file format. However, as long as the printout is an accurate reflection of the original data, it is irrelevant what the operating system or the network does to that file during the printing process.

The important concept here is the accuracy of the visual output once the image is mounted. If an examiner were to extract key data from slack space and export that data to a text file, will a printout of that text file always constitute an accurate reflection of the original data? Many prosecutors do not think so because the context of computer data is often as important as the data. Congress, by enacting Rule 1001(3), placed the emphasis on the accuracy of the visual output of computer data (ie, printout or otherwise) once the image or file is mounted, not on the stored state of that file or image. Obviously, if the original data are compromised, the visual output will be inaccurate. The original data must remain unchanged, but whether those data are compressed, encrypted, or converted to a different file format in a stored state is immaterial as long as the data are uncompromised. This is one of the reasons the MD5 hash and verification processes are so important. Though the file format of the data in question may change, the integrity of those data must remain intact.

The Best Evidence Rule has been raised in the context of an entire drive image and an individual file. A Texas Appellate Court recently ruled that an image copy of a hard drive qualifies as an "original" for the purposes of the Best Evidence Rule (*Broderick v State*, 2000). The issue of whether an EnCase Evidence File suffices as an "original" under the Best Evidence Rule was recently litigated successfully in a pending federal criminal prosecution in New Hampshire (*United States v Naparst*).

In situations in which computer evidence is collected from a business, a drive image copy is often the only "original" available to the examiner since the company often requires immediate return of the original drives to remain in business. However, though there is strong legal support for a drive image copy satisfying the Best Evidence Rule, it is always advisable to retain physical custody of the seized drive whenever possible. An ideal compromise is to retain custody of the original drives while providing restored or cloned drives to the business.

PRESENTING ELECTRONIC EVIDENCE AT TRIAL

The US Department of Justice (USDOJ) Guidelines for Searching and Seizing Computers state that "an accurate printout of computer data always satisfies the Best Evidence Rule" (*Doe v United States*, 1992). This is true in general; however, in *Armstrong v Executive Office of the President* (1993), the court correctly ruled that a "hard copy" paper printout of an electronic document would not "necessarily include all the information held in the computer memory as part of the electronic document." The court further noted that without the retention of a complete digital copy of an electronic document (eg, an e-mail message), "essential transmittal relevant to a fuller understanding of the *context and import* of an electronic communication will simply vanish" [emphasis added] (*Armstrong v Executive Office of the President*, 1993). Monique Leahy writes in "Recovery and reconstruction of electronic mail as evidence," "[i]f the document is a computer printout of an e-mail message, the proponent is required to prove that the printout accurately reflects what is in the computer" (1997).

As illustrated by the *Armstrong* case, the presentation of electronic evidence often requires the visual display of the logical data structure of a file, its context, and its associated metadata, in addition to the physical data of that file. When seeking to establish a defendant's state of mind by presenting an electronic audit trail, the ability to display a visual output showing various file attributes and other metadata and when demonstrating the logical connection to various data files (instead of relying upon dry and technical expert testimony) provides a tremendous advantage to the advocate of such evidence. The best software packages display all physical and logical data contained on the target drive while showing the context of such files by displaying file metadata and other means. When providing testimony, many examiners present evidence through screenshots in a PowerPoint presentation format or take a cloning software with them into court for a live demonstration. In *United States v Dean*, the opinion reflects that the prosecution presented results of its computer forensic examination through PowerPoint slides (*United States v Dean*, 2001). Such a presentation, which is quickly becoming common if not mandatory in modern trial practice, is almost impossible using the available command-line utilities.

In *Dean*, the prosecution sought to establish that the defendant accessed and viewed files on a series of floppy disks. Though the defendant denied ever accessing and viewing those files, his computer operating system created temporary link files when he accessed the files on the floppy disk. A forensic investigator from the US Customs Service recovered those temporary link files from the defendant's hard drive. To show the context and metadata associated with the link files, including file-created dates, full-path location, and other information, the prosecution presented software screen shots as evidentiary exhibits. These screen capture exhibits provided the most accurate display of the data as they existed on the defendant's computer at the time of seizure. The court allowed the screenshots into evidence, and Dean was convicted on all counts (**Figure 35-2**).

Figure 35-2. A screen shot exhibit offered by the prosecution and entered into evidence in United States v Dean *(2001). The court ordered the redaction of certain file names on the grounds that their probative value was outweighed by their prejudicial nature.*

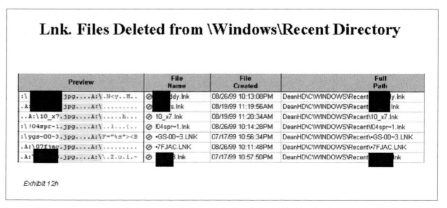

Lnk. Files Deleted from \Windows\Recent Directory

	Preview		File Name	File Created	Full Path
:\	jpg....A:\.N<y..M..	⊘	ddy.lnk	08/26/99 10:13:08PM	DeanHD\C\WINDOWS\Recent y.lnk
.A:\	jpg....A:\........	⊘	s.lnk	08/19/99 11:19:56AM	DeanHD\C\WINDOWS\Recent lnk
..A:\10_x7.jpg....A:\.....h..		⊘	10_x7.lnk	08/19/99 11:20:34AM	DeanHD\C\WINDOWS\Recent\10_x7.lnk
:\ l04spr~1.jpg....A:\..1...{..		⊘	l04spr~1.lnk	08/26/99 10:14:28PM	DeanHD\C\WINDOWS\Recent\l04spr~1.lnk
:\ygs-00-3.jpg....A:\F="%s"><B		⊘	-GS-00-3.LNK	07/17/99 10:56:34PM	DeanHD\C\WINDOWS\Recent\-GS-00-3.LNK
.A:\07Fjac.jpg....A:\........		⊘	-7FJAC.LNK	08/26/99 10:11:48PM	DeanHD\C\WINDOWS\Recent\-7FJAC.LNK
.A:\ .jpg....A:\\.Z.o.l.~		⊘	B.lnk	07/17/99 10:57:50PM	DeanHD\C\WINDOWS\Recent lnk

Exhibit 12h

Dean is an important illustration that the context of computer evidence is often as important as the data. If portions of relevant data are recovered in unallocated or slack space areas of a drive, how is that evidence presented? For example, if those data recovered from slack space are exported to a text file and then printed, a proponent will likely face significant difficulty in admitting that evidence without establishing its context. What file partially overwrote the first section of the cluster where the slack data still reside? When was the file currently occupying that cluster created and last modified? What is the precise address (eg, physical cluster, sector offset, and so on) of the data recovered from slack space? **Figure 35-3** shows the way such data should be presented for demonstrative purposes and to comply with the Best Evidence Rule.

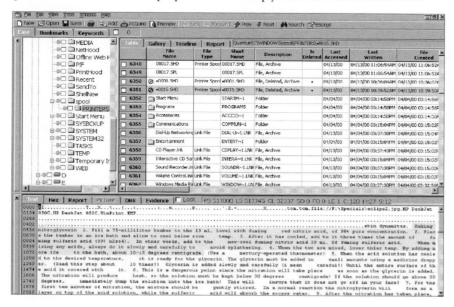

Figure 35-3. *Key evidence of bomb-making instructions found in the slack area of a cluster occupied (at the beginning) by a deleted printer spool file. Screen shot presentation enables full contextual presentation of the data.*

UNITED STATES V NAPARST

The issue of whether EnCase Evidence Files constituted the best evidence of the computer data contained therein was litigated in a pending federal criminal prosecution in New Hampshire, *United States v Naparst*. The prosecution offered to allow the defense access to a copy of the evidence file for discovery purposes. However, the defense contended that it required access to the original computer systems in question so the defense could operate those computers and examine them in their native environment. The defense then filed a formal, written request for a court order allowing such unfettered access to the "original" computer evidence. The government filed a successful objection to the request, asserting that the "mirror image" created by the Special Agent is the proper way to preserve the original evidence since turning on the computer, as the defense requested, would change the state of the evidence by altering critical date stamps and potentially overwriting existing files and information.

The court ruled that the EnCase Evidence File qualified as the Best Evidence and that a discovery copy of the Evidence File would be sufficient discovery disclosure. Alternatively, the court ruled that the defense could have access to the original computer systems only if its expert created another proper forensic image under the supervision of the Special Agent. The defense was barred from booting the original computer systems to its native operating systems. A copy of the brief filed by the government in support of its successful objection is reprinted in **Figure 35-4**.

LEGAL ANALYSIS OF THE EVIDENCE FILE

The central component of the EnCase methodology is the Evidence File, which contains the forensic bit-stream image backup made from a seized piece of computer media. The Evidence File consists of 3 basic parts: the file header, checksums, and

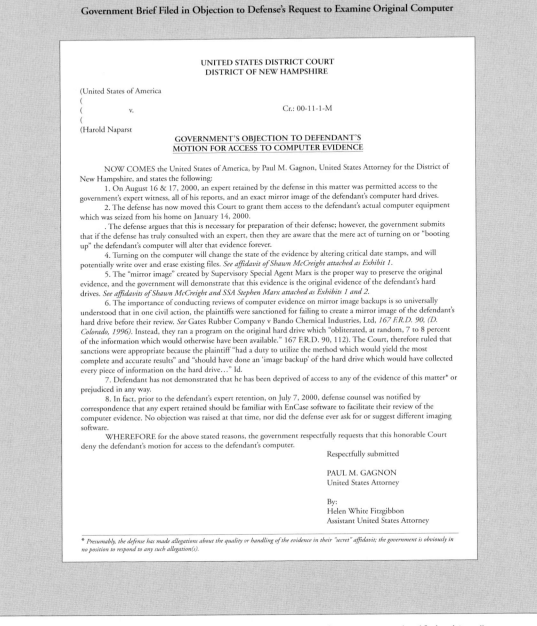

Government Brief Filed in Objection to Defense's Request to Examine Original Computer

UNITED STATES DISTRICT COURT
DISTRICT OF NEW HAMPSHIRE

(United States of America
(
(v.   Cr.: 00-11-1-M
(
(Harold Naparst

**GOVERNMENT'S OBJECTION TO DEFENDANT'S
MOTION FOR ACCESS TO COMPUTER EVIDENCE**

NOW COMES the United States of America, by Paul M. Gagnon, United States Attorney for the District of New Hampshire, and states the following:

1. On August 16 & 17, 2000, an expert retained by the defense in this matter was permitted access to the government's expert witness, all of his reports, and an exact mirror image of the defendant's computer hard drives.

2. The defense has now moved this Court to grant them access to the defendant's actual computer equipment which was seized from his home on January 14, 2000.

. The defense argues that this is necessary for preparation of their defense; however, the government submits that if the defense has truly consulted with an expert, then they are aware that the mere act of turning on or "booting up" the defendant's computer will alter that evidence forever.

4. Turning on the computer will change the state of the evidence by altering critical date stamps, and will potentially write over and erase existing files. *See affidavit of Shawn McCreight attached as Exhibit 1.*

5. The "mirror image" created by Supervisory Special Agent Marx is the proper way to preserve the original evidence, and the government will demonstrate that this evidence is the original evidence of the defendant's hard drives. *See affidavits of Shawn McCreight and SSA Stephen Marx attached as Exhibits 1 and 2.*

6. The importance of conducting reviews of computer evidence on mirror image backups is so universally understood that in one civil action, the plaintiffs were sanctioned for failing to create a mirror image of the defendant's hard drive before their review. *See* Gates Rubber Company v Bando Chemical Industries, Ltd, *167 F.R.D. 90, (D. Colorado, 1996).* Instead, they ran a program on the original hard drive which "obliterated, at random, 7 to 8 percent of the information which would otherwise have been available." 167 F.R.D. 90, 112). The Court, therefore ruled that sanctions were appropriate because the plaintiff "had a duty to utilize the method which would yield the most complete and accurate results" and "should have done an 'image backup' of the hard drive which would have collected every piece of information on the hard drive..." Id.

7. Defendant has not demonstrated that he has been deprived of access to any of the evidence of this matter* or prejudiced in any way.

8. In fact, prior to the defendant's expert retention, on July 7, 2000, defense counsel was notified by correspondence that any expert retained should be familiar with EnCase software to facilitate their review of the computer evidence. No objection was raised at that time, nor did the defense ever ask for or suggest different imaging software.

WHEREFORE for the above stated reasons, the government respectfully requests that this honorable Court deny the defendant's motion for access to the defendant's computer.

Respectfully submitted

PAUL M. GAGNON
United States Attorney

By:
Helen White Fitzgibbon
Assistant United States Attorney

---

* Presumably, the defense has made allegations about the quality or handling of the evidence in their "secret" affidavit; the government is obviously in no position to respond to any such allegation(s).

Figure 35-4. *This brief stopped the defense from fully accessing the original computer. The defense was allowed only to make a forensic image so as not alter the evidence.*

data blocks. They work together to provide a secure and self-checking "exact snapshot" of the computer disk at the time of analysis.

This section discusses in detail the major components and functions of the EnCase Evidence File that may be relevant for purposes of authenticating the Evidence File in a court of law.

EVIDENCE FILE FORMAT

The EnCase process begins with the creation of a complete physical bit-stream forensic image of a target drive in a completely noninvasive manner. With the exception of floppy disks and CD-ROMs, evidence is acquired by the software in a DOS or Windows environment in which a specially designed, hardware write-blocking device is used. The ability of EnCase to image in Windows in conjunction with a write-blocking device presents several advantages to the examiner and provides increased speed, more flexibility, and superior drive recognition.

The acquired bit-stream forensic image is mounted as a read-only "virtual drive" from which EnCase proceeds to reconstruct the file structure by reading the logical data in the bit-stream image. This allows the examiner to search and examine the contents of the drive in a Windows GUI in a completely noninvasive manner. In addition, the integrated process enables the software to identify the original location of all evidence recovered from a targeted drive without using invasive disk utilities.

Every byte of the Evidence File is verified using a 32-bit Cyclical Redundancy Check (CRC), which is generated concurrent to acquisition. Rather than compute a CRC value for the entire disk image, EnCase computes a CRC for every block of 64 sectors (ie, 32KB) that it writes to the Evidence File. A typical disk image contains many tens of thousands of CRC checks. This means that an investigator can determine the location of any error in the forensic image and disregard that group of sectors if necessary. The CRC is a variation of the checksum and works in much the same way. The advantage of the CRC is that it is order-sensitive; that is, the string "1234" and "4321" will produce the same checksum but not the same CRC. In fact, the odds that 2 sectors containing different data will produce the same CRC is roughly 1 in a billion. The CRC function allows the investigators and legal team to stand by the evidence in court.

In addition to the CRC blocks, an MD5 hash is calculated for all the data contained in the evidentiary bit-stream forensic image. As with the CRC blocks, the MD5 hash of the bit-stream image is generated and recorded concurrent to the acquisition of a physical drive or logical volume. The MD5 hash is calculated through a publicly available algorithm developed at RSA Security. The odds of 2 computer files with different contents having the same MD5 hash value are roughly 1 in 10 raised to the 38th power. The MD5 hash value generated is stored in a footer to the Evidence File and becomes part of the documentation of the evidence.

Throughout the examination process, EnCase verifies the integrity of the evidence by recalculating the CRC and MD5 hash values and comparing them with the values recorded at the time of acquisition. This verification process is documented within an automatically generated report. Writing to the Evidence File is impossible once that file is created. As with any file, altering an Evidence File is possible with a disk utility such as Norton Disk Edit. However, if one bit of data on the acquired evidentiary bit-stream image is altered after acquisition, even by adding a single space of text or by changing the case of a single character, EnCase will report a verification error in the report and identify the location where the error registers.

CRC and MD5 Hash Value Storage and Case Information Header

The CRC and MD5 hash values are stored in separate blocks in the EnCase Evidence File, which are external to the evidentiary forensic image. Those blocks containing the CRC and MD5 hash values are separately authenticated with separate CRC blocks, thereby verifying that the recordings have not been corrupted. If any information is tampered with, a verification error will be reported. Conversely, merely generating an MD5 hash value with another tool and recording it manually or in an unsecured file in which that file may be altered without detection may not fully insulate the examiner from questions of evidence tampering (**Figure 35-5**). For this reason, the CRC and MD5 hash value calculations generated with EnCase are secure and tamper-proof.

The Case Info header contains important information about the case created at the time of the file's acquisition. This

Figure 35-5. *CRC and MD5 hash values are separated from the forensic image. This can be represented at trial with a graphical representation such as this one.*

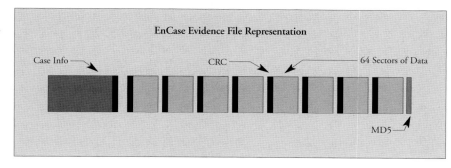

EnCase Evidence File Representation

Case Info   CRC   64 Sectors of Data

MD5

information includes system time, actual date, and time of acquisition; the examiner name; notes regarding the acquisition, including case or search warrant identification numbers; and any password entered by the examiner before the acquisition of the computer evidence. There is no "backdoor" to the password protection. The information contained in the Case Info file header, with the exception of the examiner password, is documented in an integrated written reporting feature. The Case Info file header is authenticated with a separate CRC, thereby making it impossible to alter the file without registering a verification error.

CHAIN-OF-CUSTODY DOCUMENTATION

A distinct advantage of the EnCase process is the documented chain-of-custody information that is generated at the time of acquisition and continually self-verified thereafter. The time and date of acquisition, the system clock readings of the examiner's computer, the acquisition MD5 hash value, the examiner's name, and other information are stored in the header to the Evidence File. This important chain-of-custody information can not be modified or altered; in addition, EnCase will report a verification error if the Case Info file is tampered with or altered (**Figure 35-6**).

Figure 35-6. Chain-of-custody information is documented in an automatically generated report.

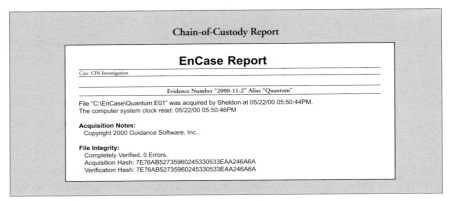

Chain-of-Custody Report

EnCase Report

Case: CIN Investigation

Evidence Number "2000-11-2" Alias "Quantum"

File "C:\EnCase\Quantum.E01" was acquired by Sheldon at 05/22/00 05:50:44PM.
The computer system clock read: 05/22/00 05:50:46PM

Acquisition Notes:
 Copyright 2000 Guidance Software, Inc..

File Integrity:
 Completely Verified, 0 Errors.
 Acquisition Hash: 7E76AB52735960245330533EAA246A6A
 Verification Hash: 7E76AB52735960245330533EAA246A6A

CHALLENGES TO ENCASE AND OTHER LITIGATED ISSUES

Computer forensic investigators throughout the world use EnCase for the seizure, analysis, and court presentation of computer evidence. In only 2 instances, an appellate court addressed the validity of the EnCase process in a published decision. Appellate court rulings are important since they stand as binding law in their subject jurisdiction while providing compelling "persuasive authority" everywhere else.

The following provide summaries of notable appellate and trial court decisions that address the EnCase® Software in detail.

STATE (OHIO) V COOK

State (Ohio) v Cook (2002) represents the first appellate decision that validates and addresses the EnCase® Software. In *Cook*, the defendant appealed his conviction on 20 separate counts of possessing child pornography and his designation as a sexual predator, thereby challenging what he claimed to be "the lack of reliability of processes used to create two mirror images of the hard drive" (*State [Ohio] v Cook*, 2002). The Ohio appellate court addressed this argument by providing a detailed description of the process taken by the law enforcement investigator in that case to make a forensic "mirror image" of the target drive. The court then noted that "[u]sing EnCase with the mirror-image hard drive, [the investigator] generated a report hundreds of pages long, containing a complete history of everything on the computer's hard drive. Among the contents were over 14 000 pornographic pictures, covering a wide range of dates" (*State [Ohio] v Cook*, 2002). The court specifically noted that the investigator was trained in the use of the EnCase® Software. In upholding the validity of the software, the court stated that "[i]n the present case, there is no doubt that the mirror image was an authentic copy of what was present on the computer's hard drive" (*State [Ohio] v Cook*, 2002).

The court cited Ohio Rules of Evidence 901(a) and 901(b), which are nearly identical to the corresponding federal rules. (See the sections titled *Authentication of Recovered Data for Accuracy* and *Validation of Computer Forensic Tools* for more information.) The court found that Rule 901(a), which provides that authentication "as a condition precedent to admissibility is satisfied by evidence sufficient to support a finding that the matter in question is what its proponent claims," governed the issue of authentication of the computer evidence. The court further noted that Rule 901(B)(9), which provides that "[e]vidence describing a process or system used to produce a result and showing that the process or system produces an accurate result," is one example of authentication being established under 901(A). The court concluded that the EnCase® Software was such a process or system that produced an accurate result, thereby satisfying authentication under Rule 901(A).

TAYLOR V STATE

Taylor v State (2002) is another appellate decision, though not to the same degree as *Cook*. *Taylor* involved several issues on appeal, most of which did not involve EnCase. The issue that did address the software centered on whether the acquisition and verification MD5 hash readings constituted hearsay. The court determined that, because the acquisition and verification hash readings are generated by a computer analysis independent of any data inputted by a human, the information is not hearsay (*Taylor v State*, 2002). As a result, the court rejected the defendant's contention that the drive image was not authentic.

This ruling is significant since it provides that Evidence Files can potentially be authenticated at trial even if the examiner who created the image is unavailable to testify. EnCase generates an MD5 hash value of an acquired drive concurrent with acquisition in a secure, integrated, and automated manner, which means that these critical authentication data are computer-generated and automatically documented. Other processes used to generate and record an MD5 hash are not integrated or secure, so they require the manual recording and documentation of the readings. Under *Taylor*, processes requiring manual recording or documentation of the readings would be inadmissible hearsay if the examiner who acquired the drive was unavailable at trial; even if the examiner were available, the examiner would be subjected to additional scrutiny.

MATTHEW DICKEY V STERIS CORPORATION

The first known instance of a "serious" challenge to the use of EnCase occurred in a civil litigation matter before the US Federal District Court in Kansas. In *Matthew Dickey v Steris Corporation* (2000), the trial court overruled evidentiary objections to the introduction of EnCase-based evidence at an April 14, 2000, pretrial hearing. Plaintiff Dickey brought a motion *in limine* seeking to exclude the testimony of an Ernst & Young expert regarding the results of his computer forensic investigation based on the use of the software. The plaintiff's motion was based on the report of his own expert, which consisted of a critique of the Ernst & Young report. The court ruled that the testimony of the Ernst & Young expert would be allowed, thereby overruling objections from the plaintiff.

Steris Corporation ("Steris") successfully opposed Dickey's motion, thereby clearing the way for the expert testimony based on EnCase. Steris brought its own motion to exclude the testimony of the plaintiff's expert. Among Steris' arguments was the contention that the plaintiff's expert was unqualified to provide an expert opinion about computer forensics since, among other reasons, she was admittedly unfamiliar with the EnCase® Software. The court denied both motions and found that (1) the challenge to the software process used by the Ernst & Young expert was without merit and (2) the testimony of the plaintiff's expert would be included though she could be questioned at trial regarding her unfamiliarity with the software, which would be relevant to her credibility as a computer forensics expert.

UNITED STATES V HABERSHAW

In *United States v Habershaw* (2002), the court upheld the legality of a computer search by a computer forensic expert, David Papargiris, over the defendant's objections. While not reflected in the court's published opinion, EnCase was used by the experts for the prosecution and the defense. The expert report submitted to the court by David Papargiris is included in full in **Appendix 35-1**.

Habershaw involved a prosecution for possession of child pornography in which the defendant orally agreed to have his computer searched. The first responder agents briefly (and, as contended by the defense, improperly) reviewed the defendant's computer and found child pornography. The defendant subsequently signed a written consent form providing the police consent to search his computer and take "from the premises any property which they desired as evidence for criminal prosecution." The police then took the defendant's computer and some floppy disks into police custody. A few days later, the police obtained a search warrant to search the computer, which was in police custody, for any material and information related to child pornography that may be stored in the computer. Papargiris then conducted a computer forensics analysis of the hard drive and found a great deal of incriminating evidence.

There are several compelling rulings and lessons in *Habershaw*, including the following:

— The court rejected the defense's claims that a "sector by sector" search with computer forensic software exceeded the scope of the warrant. The court relied on the *United States v Upham* (1999) decision, which upheld a search in which the government retrieved "deleted" computer files, and thus determined that the government could use any means to retrieve information from a computer so long as the information was within the scope of the warrant.

— The EnCase Timeline feature proved to be important in this case. The opinion reflects intensive testimony regarding file time and date stamps (eg, which files were accessed by the case agent, which files were accessed by the suspect before the case agent arrived, and the time and date when the computer was shut down for imaging and Papargiris arrived on the scene). The expert report submitted to the court by Papargiris (**Appendix 35-1**) reflects that screen captures from the Timeline view were instrumental in providing important context to the sequence of events described at length in the opinion. Papargiris' report features effective use of screen captures from the software.

— The actions of the case agent, who operated the target computer and accessed files in a live environment, were called into question by the defense's computer forensic expert, who claimed that evidence may have been planted by the case agent. Papargiris showed that, though files were accessed during the time when the case agent was on the scene and before he arrived, no files on the computer were created or modified during that time. Further, the Timeline showed no additional activity from the point when the computer was shut down for imaging by Papargiris. The Evidence File's integrated chain-of-custody feature helped correlate the imaging of the computer to the cessation in activity on the Timeline.

— This case reflects the growing trend toward increasingly computer-savvy defense experts. Defense experts are not challenging accepted computer forensics software but rather are using the software itself to gather information regarding the steps software users have taken. In turn, this information can be used as supporting evidence in their case. For example, in this case, the defense expert managed to establish that the computer was searched by the case agent before a written consent form was signed; however, the court determined that the suspect had previously given oral consent, and Papagaris demonstrated the files in question were accessed during this "oral consent" period. Though the end result was favorable, this is an important example of the way defense experts can impeach case agents who mishandle computer evidence.

REFERENCES

Armstrong v Executive Office of the President, 1 F3d 1274,1280 (DC Cir 1993).

Bone v State, 771 NE2d 710,716-717 (Ind App 2002).

Broderick v State, 35 SW3d 67 (2000).

Burleson v State, 802 WW2d 429,441 (Tex Ct App 1991).

Canada Evidence Act, chapter C-5, section 31.1.

Chappelle D. Sherlock Holmes meets data. HUB Canada Web site. December 5, 2002. Available at: http://www.hubcanada.com/story_9638_27. Accessed December 8, 2004.

Daubert v Merrell Dow Pharmaceuticals, Inc, 509 US 579,592-594, 113 S Ct 2786, 125 L Ed 2d 469 (1993).

Doe v United States, 805 F Supp 1513,1517 (D Hawaii, 1992).

Frye v United States, 293 F 1013 (DC Cir 1923).

Federal Deposit Insurance Corporation v Carabetta, 55 Conn App 384, 739 A2d 311 (1999).

Fed R Evidence 104.

Fed R Evidence 702.

Fed R Evidence 901.

Fed R Evidence 1001.

Garden State Bank v Graef, 775 A2d 189, 191, 341 NJ Super 241, 245 (2001).

Gates Rubber Company v Bando Chemical Industries, Ltd, 167 FRD 90,112 (DC Colo 1996).

Hahnemann University Hospital v Dudnick, 678 A2d 266, 292 NJ Super 11 (1996).

Kumho Tire Company, Ltd v Carmichael, 526 US 137, 119 S Ct 1167 (1999).

Kurzban SA. Authentication of computer-generated evidence in the United States Federal Courts. *IDEA: J Law Technol*. 1995;35(4):437-460.

Laughner v State, 769 NE2d 1147 (Ind App 2002).

Leahy MCM. Recovery and reconstruction of electronic mail as evidence. In: Lawyers Cooperative Publishing. *American Jurisprudence Proof of Fact*. 3rd series. Vol 41. St. Paul, Minn: West Group; 1997:1 § 19.

Matthew Dickey v Steris Corporation, No 99-2362-KHV (D Kansas 2000).

People v Bovio, 455 NE2d 829,833 (Ill App 1983).

People v Lombardi, 711 NE2d 426 (Ill App 1999).

People v Lugashi, 205 Cal App 3d 632,636,640,641 (1988).

People v Merken, No 1815448 (Cal Super Ct May 1999).

People v Mormon, 97 Ill App 3d 556, 422 NE2d 1065,1073 (1981).

People v Rodriguez, no SR28424 (Calif Super Ct January 2001).

71 Am Jur Trials 111 (1999).

State (Ohio) v Cook, 777 NE2d 882,886,887 (Ohio App 2002).

State of Washington v Leavell, No 00-1-0026-8 (Wash Super Ct 2001).

Taylor v State, 93 SW3d 487,507-508 (Tex App Texarkana 2002).

United States v Beasley, 102 F3d 1440,1448 (8th Cir 1996).

United States v Black, 767 F2d 1334,1342 (9th Cir 1985).

United States v Bonallo, 858 F2d 1427,1436 (9th Cir 1988).

United States v Dean, 135 F Supp 207, fn 1 (D Me 2001).

United States v Downing, 753 F2d 1224,1240, fn 21 (3rd Cir 1985).

United States v Glasser, 773 F2d 1533 (11th Cir 1985).

United States v Habershaw, 2001 WL 1867803 (D Mass 2002).

United States v Hilton, 257 F3d 50 (1st Cir 2001).

United States v Liebert, 519 F2d 542,547 (3rd Cir 1975).

United States v Quinn, 18 F3d 1461,1465 (9th Cir 1994).

United States v Saelee, 162 F Supp 2d 1097,1103 (D Alaska 2001).

United States v Scott-Emaukpor, 2000 WL 288443 (WD Mich. 2000).

United States v Siddiqui, 235 F3d 1318 (11th Cir 2000).

United States v Tank, 200 F3d 627,629-632 (9th Cir 2000).

United States v Upham, 168 F3d 532,537 (1st Cir 1999).

United States v Weatherspoon, 581 F2d 595,598 (7th Cir 1978).

United States v Whitaker, 127 F3d 595,600-602 (7th Cir 1997).

Weisman v Hopf-Himsel, Inc, 535 NE2d 1222,1226 (Ind Ct App 1st Dist 1989).

Wisconsin v Schroeder, 2000 WL 675942 (Wis App 2000).

APPENDIX 35-1: EXPERT REPORT SUBMITTED TO THE COURT IN *UNITED STATES V HABERSHAW*, 2001 WL 1867803

UNITED STATES DISTRICT COURT
DISTRICT OF MASSACHUSETTS

UNITED STATES OF AMERICA

Criminal No. 01-10195-PBS

KEVIN HABERSHAW

<u>**REPORT OF GOVERNMENT EXPERT WITNESS**</u>
<u>**DETECTIVE DAVID C. PAPARGIRIS**</u>

I, David C. Papargiris do hereby state:

I am a detective with the Norwood Police Department in Norwood Massachusetts. I have been employed with the Norwood Police for 17 Years and have been assigned to the Bureau of Criminal Investigations for 4 years. I conduct all investigations into computer crime, Internet investigations as well as being a computer forensics examiner.

I have been working with personal computers for (8) years. I am a member of the United States Secret Service Electronic Crimes Task Force Boston Region, the High Technology Crime Investigation Association (HTCIA) and the Regional Electronic and Computer Crime Task Force located in Raynham, Massachusetts. I have received formal training on the processing of computer evidence and the science of computer forensics from HTCIA, United States Attorney Generals Office and the Internet Crimes Inc. I have also successfully completed the National White Collar Crime Centers Basic Data Recovery four and a half day school in Portland, Maine. I have completed the four day training course on Guidance Software Corporation's computer forensics software program, "Encase". I have attended the Boston University's weeklong training on Windows NT titled Network Essentials. I have safely recovered evidentiary data from personal computers, during investigations involving fraud, identity fraud, hacking cases and crimes against children. I have testified in district court, grand juries and federal court on computer issues, along with the proper means of securing and processing computer evidence.

In preparing this brief, I conferred with court certified computer forensic expert, William C. Siebert, the Director of Technical Services for Guidance Software, maker of the computer forensic software, EnCase. A copy of his CV is attached at the end of this report.

I. Newsgroups:

USENET is a world-wide distributed discussion system. It consists of a set of "newsgroups" with names that are classified hierarchically by subject. "Articles" or "messages" are "posted" to these newsgroups by people on computers with the appropriate software—these articles are then broadcast to other interconnected computer systems via a wide variety of networks. Usenet is available on a wide variety of computer systems and networks, but the bulk of modern Usenet traffic is transported over either the Internet or UUCP [UNIX-to-UNIX Copy Protocol].

USENET newsgroups consist of some 15,000+ topical entities which constitute an immense worldwide forum for discussion and discourse. These newsgroups actually pre-date the existence of the World Wide Web and are now an integral part of the "Internet experience". These forums for discussion range in subject from Ancient Art to Zen Buddhism, and within the "threaded" structure of each group emerges the true spirit of debate and a poignant example of freedom of speech. Though a few newsgroups are moderated (having a designated member of the group with oversight powers to keep the discussion on track), most newsgroups are free forums, and may seem at times like free-for-alls, but taken as a whole, they provide a noble service in giving each and every user an equal voice.

Newsgroups can be compared to a bulletin board that you might see at a grocery store or on the wall at any college campus, except that imagine if after pinning a postcard to the bulletin board a duplicate postcard appeared on every bulletin board in every grocery store or college campus in the world within one hour.

It is true that Usenet originated in the United States, and the fastest growth in Usenet sites has been there. Nowadays, however, Usenet extends worldwide. The heaviest concentrations of Usenet sites outside the US seem to be in Canada, Europe, Australia and Japan.

No person or group has authority over Usenet as a whole. No one controls who gets a news feed, which articles are propagated where, who can post articles, or anything else. There is no "Usenet Incorporated," nor is there a "Usenet User's Group." You're on your own.

Despite its most noble intent, the darkest side of the Internet will be found within a number of newsgroups. These are the pedophile newsgroups. Perhaps at one time, these forums functioned as discussion groups for people of similar, though no less frightening interests, that being the exploitation of children for the sexual gratification of the adults who control them. These newsgroups, as most pornographic newsgroups, are not moderated.

Granted, there are various activities organized by means of Usenet newsgroups. The newsgroup creation process is one such activity. But it would be a mistake to equate Usenet with the organized activities it makes possible. If they were to stop tomorrow, Usenet would go on without them.

Newsgroups are an area of the Internet that are accessed through a mail program such as Outlook Express. You have to set up your news account using information supplied to you by an Internet Service Provider (ISP); ie Mediaone.net, AT&T Roadrunner, Earthlink.net, etc. Your newsgroup section is different from your mail program that is also managed by your ISP. Your ISP has numerous servers one is a mail server and one is a news server, many customers never set up there news server and never go onto newsgroups at all.

This technology allows for the instantaneous electronic transmission of pictures over the Internet. These pictures are converted or encoded to a binary format and sent in a similar manner as a text message. The process is as simple as sending an email. Once uploaded, the encoded binary message appears within the newsgroup where it can be downloaded by any user and decoded back into its original form, and when this decoded format is accessed through an image viewer, it becomes a photograph. I have witnessed for myself some of the images that have emerged from the pedophilia newsgroups. The computer picture format most often found on the newsgroup [are] JPEGs.

II. What is a JPEG?

JPEG (pronounced "jay-peg") is a standardized image compression mechanism. JPEG stands for Joint Photographic Experts Group, the original name of the committee that wrote the standard.

JPEG is designed for compressing full-color or gray-scale images of natural, real-world scenes. It works well on photographs, naturalistic artwork, and similar material; not so well on lettering, simple cartoons, or line drawings. JPEG handles only still images, but there is a related standard called MPEG for motion pictures.

JPEG is "lossy," meaning that the decompressed image isn't quite the same as the one you started with. (There are lossless image compression algorithms, but JPEG achieves much greater compression than is possible with lossless methods.) JPEG is designed to exploit known limitations of the human eye, notably the fact that small color changes are perceived less accurately than small changes in brightness. Thus, JPEG is intended for compressing images that will be looked at by humans. If you plan to machine-analyze your images, the small errors introduced by JPEG may be a problem for you, even if they are invisible to the eye.

III. Continued Review of Kevin Habershaw's Computer

On February 15, 2002, as part of my research, I signed on to a news server on a computer which never had one assigned to it before. After setting up the account the first thing you are told is that the news server is going to get a list of newsgroups that are available on your ISP's news server. I received a list of 67,019 newsgroups. There are newsgroups available for just about any subject, as described above. After the list comes down into the window you can scroll through the list or type in a keyword of what type of newsgroup you are looking for.

There are two ways to go to a newsgroup one way is to highlight the newsgroup and select GOTO and the other way is to select SUBSCRIBE. If you select GOTO, you are brought to that newsgroup and as much as three hundred messages could appear in the news window. If you double click on a message it could bring you to text or to a hyperlink to go to a web page or show you a graphic (photo) file. Once you exit the newsgroup it will ask you if you would like to SUBSCRIBE to the newsgroup.

If you select GOTO, or SUBSCRIBE to, in the newsgroup box a reference to that newsgroup is placed in your Outlook Express Folder [**Appendix Figure 35-1**]. As you can see from this graphic the left side of the windows indicates that I am in the Outlook Express folder. The right side of the window shows the items in that folder. The right side lists the newsgroups that were visited.

When an individual configures up their newsreader and either selects GOTO or SUBSCRIBE to a newsgroup, that information is stored on their hard drive. The computer forensic software, Encase, allows an examiner to review the contents of a hard drive under investigation.

IV: Newsgroups on Kevin Habershaw's Computer

A review of the contents of Kevin Habershaw's Outlook Express folder shows those newgroups of interest to him. The newsgroups included:

Alt.argentina.adolescents	Alt.bainaries.pictures.erotica.pre-teen
Alt.binaries.adolescents.off-topic	Alt.binaries.britney-spears
Alt.binaries.celebrities.fake.moderated	Alt.binaries.nude.celebrities.female
Alt.binaries.pictures.babies	Alt.binaries.pictures.celebrities
Alt.binaries.pictures.child.starlets	Alt.binaries.pictures.erotica.babies
Alt.binaries.pictures.erotica.bondage.ped	Alt.binaries.pictures.erotica.female.young
Alt.binaries.pictures.erotica.gymnasts-girl	Alt.binaries.pictures.erotica.nude.runaway
Alt.binaries.pictures.erotica.pre-teen.chatter	Alt.binaries.pictures.erotica.sara-young
Alt.binaries.pictures.girls	Alt.binaries.pictures.humor.babies
Alt.binaries.pictures.kids	Alt.binaries.pictures.olsen.twins
Alt.binaries.pictures.spice-girls	Alt.binaries.stories.sex
Alt.disgusting.stories.my-imagination	Alt.fan.britney-spears
Alt.fan.emma-bunton	Alt.fan.Melissa.j-hart
Alt.fan.olsen.twins	Alt.hipclone.kids.sexual-abstinence
Alt.idiot.pedophile.reb-ruster	Alt.idiot.pedophile.snoopy
Alt.no.advertising.files.images.sex.preteens	Alt.no.advertising.files.images.nude.preteens

Alt.Pedophiles	Alt.sex.children
Alt.sex.girls	Alt.sex.incest
Alt.sex.pedo.moderated	Alt.sex.pedophilia
Alt.sex.pedophilia.girls	Alt.sex.pedophilia.glen.webb
Alt.sex.pedophilia.Linda-and-kuibob	Alt.sex.pedophilia.pictures
Alt.sex.preteens	Alt.sex.stories.babies
Alt.sex.stories	Alt.sex.stories.incest
Alt.sex.stories.moderated	Alt.sex.stories.tg
Alt.sex.young	Alt.stories.erotic
Alt.stories.incest	Alt.Transformation.stories
Alt.transgendered	Alt.transgendered.Jeffrey-boyd
Alt.binaries.nude.celebrities.female	Pedo.binaries.pictures.erotica.children

Once you click on a newsgroup name, you can see the database of messages for the newsgroup, alt.sex.pre-teens for March 31 at 10:33:58 AM. These titles could lead you to text or a graphic file or a hyperlink (text that once clicked brings you to a web page) that had shown up in the newsgroup box. These references are left on a person's hard drive only if they have selected GOTO or SUBSCRIBE in their newsreader. Habershaw's Outlook Express folder showed that there were 61 references to newsgroups that he had visited. Alt.Sex.Pre-Teens, showed references to the terms like *lolita*, *alt.sex* and *preteen*, as did other newsgroups that had been accessed at 10:34 AM on the 31 of March. It was said that the term "preteen" did not come up during the keyword search under EnCase. The reason for this was because of the spelling in the newsgroup showed it as P=R=E=T=E=E=N [**Appendix Figure 35-2**].

Looking within the lower box in EnCase it shows references to the newsgroup alt.sex.pre-teens. On the first line you can see a reference to underage51.jpg, which is an attached computer picture file available for downloading.

I also checked the timeline to see that the newsgroups were being updated every 30 minutes.

After checking the timeline I could see that at 0930 hours on the 31 of March, two newsgroups were accessed. At 1002 Hours, four newsgroups were accessed, and starting at 1033 hours forty-five different newsgroups were accessed. At 1101 hours 1 newsgroup was accessed. If the newsgroup were being checked automatically every thirty minutes, there would be the same amount of newsgroups accessed every thirty minutes, and this would show up in the timeline within Encase. Because different numbers of the newsgroups appear at different time intervals on the timeline, I do not believe that Habershaw's computer was automatically updating newsgroups every thirty minutes.

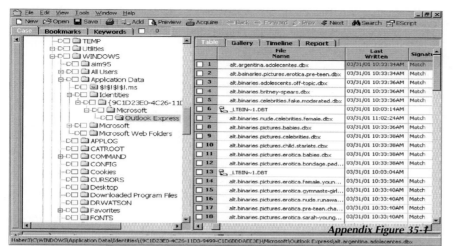

Appendix Figure 35-1. *Screenshot showing a newsgroup reference in Outlook Express.*

Appendix Figure 35-2. *This screenshot shows the newsgroups that had been accessed on the computer.*

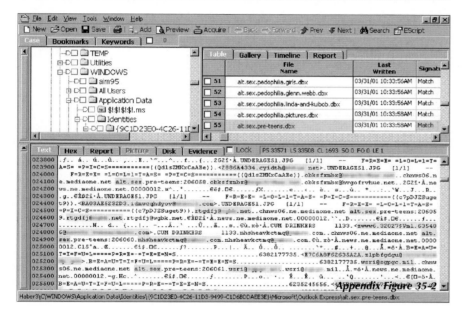

Chapter 36

INTERNET TRAVELERS

Jeffrey A. Dort, Esq

"Police arrest 'traveler' in local sting case" alerts the morning headline. What is a traveler? What is a sting? Why did the man fly from South Korea to Arkansas to have sex with an underage girl? These questions were answered by police officers in Little Rock, Arkansas, when they arrested Robert Combs because he allegedly traveled to have sex with a minor (Robson, 2004). Combs was presumed innocent; however, he had traveled 6800 miles from his US Army job in South Korea to visit the United States, and the e-mail he wrote before this visit disclosed his intentions of photographing and having sexual relations with a young girl. Combs, a 48-year-old grandfather, thought he had been in contact with the mother of the child to arrange the meeting when, in fact, he was communicating with an undercover police officer posing as the mother. Combs had mailed the "mother" a compact disc containing sexually explicit images of children (McLarty, 2004; Robson, 2004). Acquaintances of Combs in South Korea were surprised to hear of his arrest. One woman said the arrest was a "complete shock" because he seemed like a "really nice guy. He seemed genuinely enthusiastic about playing Santa" (Robson, 2004).

Unfortunately, international travelers are common. In Internet sexual exploitation cases, the term *traveler* refers to a person who contacts a person under the age of 18 on the Internet and then attempts to meet the child to engage in sexual activities (Freeh, 1998). These scenarios can lead to violent sexual crimes and murder (Freeh, 1998). The dawn of the digital era (ie, from 1980 to the present) has opened the door to a new brand of evil: sex offenders that can use their computers to find new victims.

EVOLUTION OF THE TRAVELER PHENOMENON

Child abuse is old, and various forms of child abuse (sexual and otherwise) have occurred throughout history. Recently, people have realized the extent to which some children suffer when in the hands of their caretakers (de Mause, 1997). If sexual abuse has always existed, why does the phenomenon of travelers pique the interest of so many people? The use of the Internet to establish the traveler-child relationship remains shocking. The news stories ensure high ratings, and viewers express disbelief as they learn that a crime was committed in their own town. Unfortunately, people are becoming immune. It is becoming more common to hear these stories on the evening news and is no longer as shocking to learn that the crimes were caught on tape (Miami valley crime, 2003).

Ken Lanning (2001), a retired Federal Bureau of Investigation (FBI) agent, has studied sex crimes for more than 25 years and has drawn the following conclusion: "In the United States, society's historical attitude about sexual victimization of children can generally be summed up in one word: *denial*. Most people do not want to hear about it and would prefer to pretend that such victimization just does not occur." Though people may not want be educated about child abuse, they are still curious about travelers. Would a man really fly across the country to have sex with a 13-year-old? Did a girl really meet with a man she had only previously "met" in an online chat room?

THE INTERNET AS A HUNTING GROUND

Before the development of the Internet, *pedophiles* (ie, adults who are sexually attracted to children) had trouble searching for or communicating with other pedophiles without risking arrest. The Internet is a communication conduit that allows like-minded people worldwide to meet and share their ideas. Previously isolated people can find others with similar interests, however deviant, and gain a sense of belonging, which seems to validate their thoughts. Socially shunned people are gathering online and creating virtual support networks (Lanning, 2001). In addition, wireless fidelity (WiFi) technology has made Internet usage commonplace at public places such as local coffee houses and restaurants. People can access the Internet with various portable devices other than computers (Baig, 2003). Wireless Internet access is handy for college students and is becoming common among businesses because it improves productivity (Wireless e-mail use, 2003). Unfortunately, this explosion in Internet access has opened up the lines of communication between child molesters and children.

In the past, without the use of the Internet, abusers had trouble targeting children without first knowing them. The Internet provides anonymity that benefits the abuser, creating a virtual hunting ground of victims. "Some of the great virtues of the Internet—its flexibility, universal accessibility, and privacy—also make it an especially potent venue for sexual predators to communicate with minors regarding illicit sexual encounters" (*United States v Robertson*, 2003). Approximately 78% of US families have Internet access at home, but the average parent is unaware of how dangerous the Internet can be (Corporation for Public Broadcasting, 2003).

Children: Vulnerable Internet Targets

Children have an innate sense of curiosity. Abusers have learned to capitalize on that curiosity and on the rebellious nature typical of many teenagers (Lanning, 2001). According to the *Office of Victims of Crime Bulletin*, approximately 77 million children will be using the Internet in 2005 (Internet crimes against children, 2001). If this number proves to be correct, it will be a 30% increase from 1999 (Corporation for Public Broadcasting, 2003). Child molesters who are trying to find new victims can use their computers to search for unsuspecting children and continue to have more girls and boys from which to choose (Medaris & Girouard, 2002).

Online, molesters attempt to blend into the background, and the Internet provides a safe feeling of anonymity. As darkness protects auto thieves, allowing them to investigate a parking lot safely at night for the right car to steal, abusers hide in the Internet's darkness of anonymity. They explore the Internet, hoping to find an unsuspecting and a gullible youngster who wants some friendly conversation (Lanning, 2001).

Many children who begin online relationships with abusers fit a particular profile. Many reported cases involve children searching for anyone who will listen to them. In a study by Wolak et al (2003a), a pattern was discovered among youth who developed online relationships. Though some characteristics are common among all teenagers, children in contact with online molesters may have a greater tendency for conflict or lack of communication with their parents; high levels of delinquency including committing assault, vandalism, and theft; or a troubled personality due to depression, peer victimization, or a distressing life event.

Many teenagers are more computer savvy than their parents, which opens the lid to a modern Pandora's box. Children tell their parents about half the time when they receive an online solicitation for sex or are harassed online by a stranger (Finkelhor et al, 2000). Thirty-five percent of teenagers report that an adult is in the room or nearby when they use the Internet at home; in comparison, 76% of children between the ages of 6 and 12 years old report having an adult nearby when they go online at home (Lanning, 2001). In addition, fewer than 10% of sexual solicitations are reported to law enforcement officers or a hotline (Finkelhor et al, 2000), leaving the majority unreported. The numbers are disturbing, and the news accounts are more alarming.

Why do parents allow children to have unmonitored Internet access in the face of such danger? No simple answer exists, but education is the remedy. Parents must take control of and supervise their children. More Web sites and software are being developed to allow parents to monitor what their children are doing on the Internet and block access to certain sites and particular content. Each week, children spend 6 hours or more online, so parents need to warn their children about its inherent dangers (Corporation for Public Broadcasting, 2003). Parents have realized their children have enough computer knowledge to create password-protected areas on their family computer and reload software programs with ease (Goodale, 2001). Perhaps it is the fear of the unknown that makes 21st-century parents shy away from addressing Internet dangers (How to overcome fear, 2004). However, the safety of their children is at risk; parents can not claim ignorance to the problem. The following true story shows how dangerous the situation has become.

Denial and disbelief were the first reactions to the news headline, "Teen murdered by a man she met in a chat room" (Loftus, 2002). A California man, David Fuller, met 13-year-old Kacie Woody online, traveled to Arkansas, and abducted her. He brought her to a rented storage garage and sexually assaulted her. Officers traced Fuller to the storage yard, but minutes after they arrived in the area, they heard gunshots as Fuller shot Kacie and then himself (Dead girl had told, 2002; Repard, 2002).

Shocking stories such as these are highlighted in warnings on an interactive, educational Web site created by the National Center for Missing & Exploited Children (NCMEC) and the Boys & Girls Clubs of America (BGCA). The site for NetSmartz, http://www.netsmartz.org, is intended for children ages 5 to 17 years, parents, guardians, educators, and law enforcement officials. This is one of the most effective Web sites available for teaching children safe Internet skills and offering information to parents about the dangers of the Internet.

INTERNET SEX CRIME STUDIES

Few statistics exist regarding Internet sex crimes involving children, but the statistics that have been published are frightening. At the forefront of this research is the Crimes Against Children Research Center located at the University of New Hampshire. Two studies in particular from this center offer insight into the ways law enforcement officials react to the crime and the profiles of the perpetrators.

INTERNET SEX CRIMES AGAINST MINORS: THE RESPONSE OF LAW ENFORCEMENT

Arrest statistics

Wolak et al (2003b) conducted a study of 2577 arrests that occurred between July 2000 and June 2001. The 2577 arrests studied were not the total number of arrests but the total number the authors were able to study during the 1-year research period because of the cooperation level of agencies responding throughout the United States. The researchers focused on the following 3 mutually exclusive types of crimes:

1. *Internet crimes committed against identified victims.* These involve Internet-related sexual assaults and other sex crimes, including production of child pornography (39% of the arrests studied).

2. *Internet solicitations to undercover law enforcement officers.* These involve law enforcement officers who posed as minors but did not involve an identified victim (25% of the arrests studied).

3. *Internet-related possession, distribution, or trading of child pornography.* These include offenders who did not fit into 1 of the other 2 listed categories (36% of the arrests studied).

Of the offenders involved in the cases studied, 67% had child pornography on their computers when arrested. No agreement has been reached on the definition of child pornography in this study, but for clarity, descriptions of the pictures found on the suspects' computers are the following:

— 92% had images of children between the ages of 6 and 12 years.

— 80% had images showing children being penetrated.

— 71% had images showing sexual contact between an adult and a child.

This study used a ***proactive*** approach to isolate and study the traveler. Law enforcement officials consider an investigation to be proactive when the officers initiate an investigation of a problem area (eg, illegal drug sales), rather than of a specific crime, and then wait for a perpetrator to contact them. The Wolak et al (2003b) study suggested that having law enforcement officers pose as minors in Internet chat rooms and then having these officers wait to be contacted by offenders was effective. In contrast, ***reactive*** cases are cases in which victims report crimes to the police and the officers respond to the information provided before an investigation is initiated; these cases are more typical in police work.

Internet Sex Crimes Versus Conventional Sex Crimes

Whether proactive or reactive, monitoring Internet sex crime cases as they went to court and tracking convictions was another facet of the Wolak et al (2003b) study. The authors of the study examined the case outcomes throughout the United States in state and federal courts. In 94% of the cases involving Internet sex crimes against children, the defendants pled guilty before the trial or were convicted at trial. Some defendants may plead guilty before trial because the evidence is overwhelming as many have hundreds or thousands of child pornographic pictures on their personal computer. Combined with accusations of molesting children, many defendants believe the jury will convict them and are able to ask the court for a lesser sentence because they have pled guilty at an early stage of the prosecution. Fewer than 1% of defendants studied won their cases after a trial. The remaining 5% of cases were dismissed by the prosecutor.

In contrast, about 22% of conventional sex crime cases (ie, non–Internet-related cases) that involve child victims are dismissed before trial, and 6% of the cases are acquitted (Cross et al, 2003). In other words, conventional sex crime cases involving child victims have a 71% conviction rate, 23% lower than the conviction rate for Internet sex crimes against children. Though sometimes highly technical, Internet-related crimes are being successfully prosecuted across the country.

Offender Profile

Wolak et al (2003b) created a profile that held true for the majority of offenders. These could be helpful statistics for parents and guardians, law enforcement officials, and institutions or organizations involved with children. The profile includes the following:

— 99% were male.

— 92% were white (non-Hispanic).

— 85% were 26 years or older.

— 97% acted alone.

— 90% had no prior arrests for sex crimes against children.

ONLINE VICTIMIZATION: A REPORT ON THE NATION'S YOUTH

In a 2000 study, *Online Victimization: A Report on the Nation's Youth*, Finkelhor et al (2000) broke new ground when they interviewed 1501 children between the ages of 10 and 17 who used the Internet regularly (ie, had used it at least once a month in the previous 6 months). The following conclusions drawn by the authors of the study are alarming:

— 20% of the children had received an online sexual solicitation.

— 1 in 33 children had received an "aggressive sexual solicitation" in which the suspect asked the child to meet somewhere, called the child on the telephone, or sent the child regular mail, money, or gifts.

— 25% of the children told their parents when they had been sexually solicited.

— 25% of the children had unwanted exposures to Internet images of nude people or people having sex.

Alarming is that 97% of the sexual solicitations were made by people the child victims had originally met online (Finkelhor et al, 2000). However, the authors specifically stated that they knew little about the incidence of traveler cases.

Many of the children in this study who received sexual solicitations online reported that the people wanted them to engage in *cybersex*, a form of fantasy sex that typically occurs while both participants are conversing online in a chat room (Finkelhor et al, 2000). Through instant messages or e-mail, the participants have detailed conversations about sexual acts. The participants may masturbate during the online encounter (Finklehor et al, 2000).

TRAVELER VARIATIONS

Not all travelers can have sex with a child. A local police undercover operation (or sting) can lead to a criminal being captured before a child is sexually abused. Criminal investigations involving travelers may be divided into the following 6 types:

1. Local traveler

2. Interstate or intrastate traveler

3. Global traveler

4. Victim traveler

5. Traveler no-show

6. Sting operation

LOCAL TRAVELERS

Local travelers stay in the town or area in which they reside and travel a short distance (ie, fewer than 50 miles) to meet their intended child victims (Wolak et al, 2003b). These travelers may limit their victim search to a specific state or region or only target chat rooms that have a location as part of their name (eg, *SoCalGirls* for Southern California girls, *RckfrdChx* for girls from Rockford, or *EVLBBoys* for East Village League Basketball Boys). By staying near home, these travelers may feel more in control because they are in a comfortable location and familiar surroundings.

INTERSTATE AND INTRASTATE TRAVELERS

The *interstate* and *intrastate traveler* (ie, a traveler who journeys more than 50 miles out of or within a state) (M. Harmony, oral communication, March 2004) risks more, travels farther, and breaks more laws than the local traveler. Federal law prohibits interstate travel (ie, crossing state lines) with the intent of engaging in a sexual act with a minor (eg, *United States v Root*, 2002). The Mann Act (18 USC §2421 (2003)) indicates that if a person

knowingly transports any individual in interstate or foreign commerce, or in any Territory or Possession of the United States, with intent that such individual engage in prostitution, or in any sexual activity for which any person can be charged with a criminal offense, or attempts to do so, shall be fined under this title or imprisoned not more than 10 years, or both.

In addition, the fact that someone traveled more than 50 miles to commit a crime could be used by prosecutors to argue the crime was premeditated and deliberate, and it solidifies the intent element required by the statute. A cross-town trip of 15 miles could be spontaneous and may only take 15 to 20 minutes; however, for example, a

500-mile drive spanning 2 states and involving 7 hours of driving involves more planning and deliberation, thereby providing more chances for the person to abort the crime. In *Ohio v Moller* (2002), the defendant traveled more than 200 miles to meet his victim, and that fact was used in the legal opinion to help prove that he had violated a state law.

GLOBAL TRAVELERS

Global travelers go to other countries to engage in sexual acts with children. The media refers to these travelers as *sex tourists*. Global travelers plan and prepare more than any other type of traveler. They are sometimes part of tour groups that are centered around sex (Sex "tourist" gets seven years, 2000; Robson, 2004).

The US media has begun reporting stories about adults from the United States who travel abroad for sex (eg, Man charged in US, 2003). The media quickly spotlighted a change in law stating that American citizens can be arrested for sex crimes they have committed while traveling overseas.

VICTIM TRAVELERS

Victim travelers, which are rare, are offenders who set up sex meetings and who convince and pay for children to travel to the offenders' location (eg, Levesque, 2000). Unfortunately, at first glance these situations appear to have a "willing participant" where the victim is the one who travels to the suspect's location for a sexual encounter. However, in these victim traveler cases, it is the offender who has used the lure of sex or money to convince the child to travel to them. The law clearly defines these children as victims. Investigations of crimes involving victim travelers can be more complicated. The travelers can argue they did nothing wrong because the child made the effort to get to the suspect. Most federal and state laws do not distinguish between *who* is doing the actual traveling; they concentrate on whether the purpose of the travel is to bring 2 parties together for sexual purposes (eg, 18 USC § 2423(b) (2003)).

TRAVELER NO-SHOWS

Like a victim traveler, the *traveler no-show* is also atypical but occurs when, even after months of communications between a traveler and a victim (whether with a true child victim or an undercover officer), travelers do not show up at the selected meeting location. This occurs for various reasons, including the following possibilities:

— The traveler got worried and frightened of being caught.

— The traveler discovered the meeting was a sting operation.

— The traveler realized the meeting was illegal.

— The traveler never intended on showing up at all.

Regardless of the motive and though no travel has taken place, traveler no-show incidents remain important. Travelers can take months and even years to coordinate a successful meeting, so some failed meetings must be expected (Nurenberg, 2002).

STING OPERATIONS

A sting operation involves some travel, but a child is not involved. A *sting operation* is an undercover operation in which police officers pose as children online. They let adults strike up conversations with them. In some instances, the adult then propositions or entices the "child" to meet for sex. The officer sets up a meeting and arranges a location. When the adult arrives at the location, no child is there. Officers arrest the suspect for attempting to meet a child for sexual purposes. Any of the previously mentioned 5 categories of travelers can be involved in a sting case.

ADDRESSING THE PROBLEM: LAW ENFORCEMENT

LAW ENFORCEMENT STRUGGLES

Large police departments are organized into area divisions and specialized units. Members of specialized units are specifically trained to handle particular types of

countries should work to end the sex trade and sex tourism industry and noted that "some nations make it a crime to sexually abuse children abroad. Such conduct should be a crime in all nations. Governments should inform travelers of the harm this industry does, and the severe punishments that will fall on its patrons" (Bush, 2003). According to former Secretary of State Colin Powell, sex tourism is "the worst kind of human exploitation imaginable. … It is a sin against humanity, and it is a horrendous crime" (Children for sale, 2004).

Internet Crimes Against Children Task Forces

In 1998, the US federal government realized the problem of Internet sex crimes involving children was growing, so the US Department of Justice (USDOJ) established the ICAC task forces. Law enforcement officials and prosecutors from state and local levels were chosen to run this group to respond to the growing number of Internet child sexual exploitation cases (Program Summary: ICAC, 2004). A nationwide network has been created to provide training, forensic hardware, and ongoing education for the officers working on the Internet investigations. Federal grant money has been allocated to help raise parental awareness of Internet dangers. The grants were awarded to 45 specific agencies nationwide to combat child exploitation on the Internet (NCMEC, 2004; NCMEC & OJJDP, 2003/2004). **Figure 36-1** shows a map of the ICAC task force locations.

Statistics

According to ICAC Program Manager C. Holloway, Office of Juvenile Justice and Delinquency Prevention (OJJDP), since 1998, more than 14 000 cases involving Internet-related crimes against children have been investigated by the various ICAC task forces across the United States (oral communication, February 2004). Of those cases, 2400 involved travelers. These statistics do not include the **online enticement** cases, in which no traveling occurs but adults are sexually soliciting children online.

Figure 36-1. *ICAC task forces have 45 locations throughout the United States, creating a strong network for officer and parent education.* Reprinted with permission from ICAC Board of Director's President, Sgt. Scott Christensen, Program Director for the Nebraska ICAC, Nebraska State Patrol.

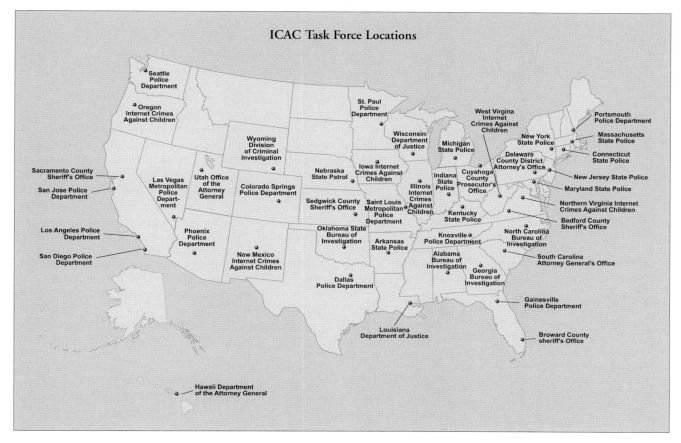

For statistical purposes, ICAC and the NCMEC distinguish suspects who *travel* from those who *entice* online but do not travel. The NCMEC uses the term *pretravel* for cases in which traveling is not part of the enticement (NCMEC, 2004). The job of detection, identification, enforcement, and prosecution of these cases is difficult because of the privacy and anonymity provided by the Internet.

Federal Partners

Part of the reason the ICAC task forces have been successful is that each location on the map shown in **Figure 36-1** is not just a satellite location of the federal entity; it is a unique and an independent task force, such as the previously mentioned Bedford County, Virginia, task force. The federal grant to the local agencies to create the ICAC task force system was written in a way that allows the local and state agencies to make decisions rather than being forced to abide by decisions of a far-removed federal agency. Since 1998, ICAC task forces have facilitated the arrests of more than 1600 suspects who have used the Internet to exploit children (Holloway, oral communication, February 2004).

The backbone of each ICAC task force comprises the local officers, detectives, and agents who work Internet child abuse cases. Federal agencies offer assistance with investigations, technological issues, and manpower and most importantly, provide national and international contacts that local officers do not have. The following list includes some of the agencies with agents assigned to the ICAC task forces:

— *Immigration and Customs Enforcement (ICE) and the Department of Homeland Security (DHS).* Cyber Crimes Center (C3) and Operation Predator (United States ICE, 2004)

— *FBI.* Innocent Images National Initiative (IINI)

— *US Postal Inspection Services (USPIS).* Operation Avalanche with Dallas Police Department

— *Naval Criminal Investigative Service (NCIS).*

As these agencies team up with the local ICAC task forces, more is learned each day about how to locate, track, and prosecute criminals who harm children.

NATIONAL CENTER FOR MISSING & EXPLOITED CHILDREN

Background

In 1984, Congress mandated that the NCMEC be the national clearinghouse for information relating to children who are missing or have been exploited (**Table 36-1**). As a private, nonprofit organization, NCMEC provides technical assistance to the public sector (eg, police officers, prosecutors) and the private sector (eg, parents of missing or exploited children). In addition to child abuse involving travelers, NCMEC handles all types of cases involving missing and exploited children. It has been involved in more than 183 000 cases involving exploited children (NCMEC, 2004).

Web Site Success

The NCMEC maintains a Web site, http://www.missingkids.com, which offers information in a wide range of areas, including tips to help parents keep their children safe and assistance with generating age-progressed photographs of missing children (NCMEC, 2004). The NCMEC Web site is visited by Internet users more than 3 million times each a day and has proven to be an efficient information clearinghouse (Finkelhor et al, 2000). NCMEC has helped recover more than 95 000 missing children (NCMEC, 2004).

The CyberTipline

NCMEC operates nationally and internationally, distributing information to contacts in states and law enforcement agencies throughout the world (M. Collins, ECU program manager, oral communication, February 2004). Central to NCMEC's suc-

Table 36-1. Congressional Findings Regarding Missing and Exploited Children (42 USC § 5771)

— Each year, thousands of children are abducted or removed from the control of a parent having legal custody without the parent's consent and under circumstances that immediately place the child in grave danger.

— Many missing children are at great risk of physical harm and sexual exploitation.

— In many cases, parents and local law enforcement officials have neither the resources nor the expertise to mount expansive search efforts for missing children.

— Abducted children are frequently moved from one locality to another, thereby requiring the cooperation and coordination of local, state, and federal law enforcement efforts.

— The NCMEC has several functions:

    — Serving as the national resource center and clearinghouse for missing and exploited children

    — Working in partnership with the USDOJ, FBI, Department of the Treasury, USDOS, and many other agencies to find missing children and prevent child victimization

    — Operating a national and increasingly worldwide network by linking its own organization online with each of the missing children clearinghouses in the 50 states, the District of Columbia, and Puerto Rico, as well as with Scotland Yard in the United Kingdom; the Royal Canadian Mounted Police in Canada; Interpol headquarters in Lyon, France; and other organizations, enabling NCMEC to transmit images and information regarding missing children to law enforcement officials across the United States and around the world instantly

cess in finding missing children is an online Internet hotline: http://www.cybertipline.com. The hotline handles reports and tips from citizens about Internet-related child sexual exploitation. Visitors to this Web site fill in as much information as they know about the online incident, whether it involves child pornography or online sexual solicitations involving children. NCMEC passes along this information to law enforcement officials in a wide range of cases.

A team of experts from the NCMEC's Exploited Child Unit (ECU), which has its headquarters in Alexandria, Virginia, reviews the reports generated by the Web site. The team members are trained to identify child abuse victims and have the ability to dispatch people to assist local law enforcement officials. The team attempts to identify the origin of the illegal material, find the suspect, and pass on the information to the law enforcement agency closest to the source of the problem.

Statistics from the NCMEC highlight just how dangerous the Internet can be for children. In 2003, the NCMEC received more than 81 000 cybertips (M. Collins, oral communication, February 2004). An average of more than 2000 tips are provided to the NCMEC and CyberTipline Web sites each week (NCMEC, 2004). In addition, legislation (ie, 42 USC § 13032 (1998)) has been passed that requires Internet Service Providers (ISPs) to report all illegal child pornography found on their Web sites to the NCMEC; the passage of this law will likely increase the number of weekly reports to the Web sites. Failing to report known child pornography sites can result in a fine of up to $50 000 for the first offense.

Internet crimes that focus on children are not going away, in fact the numbers are increasing. For example, Sgt. Dave Jones of the San Diego Police Department and project director of the San Diego ICAC task force reported that in 2003, his unit investigated 149 cases involving child-related Internet crimes (oral communication, February and March 2004). Amazingly, 2004 was far busier, and the numbers of open investigations jumped by 400% to 509 cases being investigated by his unit (D. Jones, oral communication, January 2005).

NATIONAL AND INTERNATIONAL COOPERATION

Approximately 79% of Internet child sexual abuse cases involve more than one law enforcement agency (Wolak et al, 2003b). Therefore, it is beneficial to have cooperation among the NCMEC, ICAC task forces, federal law enforcement agencies (eg, FBI, ICE, USPIS, NCIS), and local and state agencies nationwide (eg, the California State Department of Justice, Sexual Assault and Felony Enforcement [SAFE], Sexual Predators Apprehension Team [SPAT]). Law enforcement officials who work in this area previously compared the job of combating Internet sex crimes against children to digging a hole in quicksand. The more recent team approach has given a renewed sense of energy to the most seasoned police officer. Teamwork can not be overemphasized. Travelers come from every nation and walk of life, and they commonly violate federal, state, and local laws on their way to meet a child. Many cases being solved today could not have been solved 10 years ago.

Wolak et al (2003b) noted that 85% of traveler cases were investigated by local law enforcement officials. This statistic may not seem surprising; however, the dynamics of a "typical" traveler case are complex. For example, a mother in Salt Lake City, Utah, reported to the police department that her 12-year-old daughter told her she had been offered money by a Nevada man to meet him for sex. The mother brought in relevant e-mail from the home computer. The police officers quickly did a check and found that the suspect's ISP, and thus digital information, was located in Virginia.

At this point, several different law enforcement agencies became involved: (1) Utah officials got involved because Utah was the victim's home, (2) Nevada officials got involved because the suspect may have had a criminal record in Nevada, and (3) Virginia officials got involved because the digital information resided in Virginia. Federal officials may get involved if federal laws are violated. Which state controls the investigation? Should federal authorities become involved? How do the authorities obtain e-mail from the suspect's computer?

LEGAL ISSUES

JURISDICTION

Theoretical Issues

Jurisdiction, or the territorial authority of the government to prosecute, rarely is at issue in a criminal prosecution. For example, if a robbery is committed at a gas station in Los Angeles, California, California Penal Code section 211 applies, and the Los Angeles Police Department investigates the case. In contrast, when we venture into cyberspace, the jurisdiction question becomes more complicated. Internet crimes may involve numerous physical locations: the location of the perpetrator, the location of the victim, the location of the crime (if the victim and perpetrator meet in person), and the location of the perpetrator's computer.

Consequently, the national ICAC task force network is important. Just as law enforcement officials from various organizations must work together when pursuing a suspect in various jurisdictions, law enforcement agencies must combine their efforts to track the pedophiles who are running loose on the Internet.

State Law

Every state has laws that describe its physical boundaries and jurisdictional authority. Jurisdiction is determined by the geographic location of the court with the authority to hear and decide the case and the subject matter of the case. Unfortunately, jurisdictional laws conflict when the victim and the criminal are in different states. The issue becomes determining which state (ie, the victim's or suspect's) should investigate and prosecute the case. Another issue to address is whether the federal authorities should become involved and coordinate the investigation and the prosecution.

Long-arm statutes (ie, laws that allow a state to extend its jurisdiction to individuals or organizations not currently residing in that state) are used to coordinate investigations beyond a state's physical borders (Berg, 2000). The US Supreme Court uses the following guideline, which is known as the ***detrimental effects test***, to determine whether a state has criminal jurisdiction over criminal acts that do not occur within its borders: "Acts done outside a jurisdiction, but intended to produce and producing detrimental effects within it, justify a State in punishing the cause of the harm as if he had been present at the effect" (*Strassheim v Daily*, 1911). Therefore, states can pursue, investigate, and prosecute a person who harms their citizens even if the perpetrator has never entered the victim's state. Some states take responsibility for crimes that were partially planned or partially carried out within the state boundaries, even if they were not completed within those boundaries (*Strassheim v Daily*, 1911; *Rios v State*, 1987). A few states (ie, Alabama, California, Michigan, Minnesota, Mississippi, Ohio, South Dakota, and Wisconsin) allow law enforcement officials to investigate and prosecute crimes regardless of where the victim or suspect resides, as long as the crime has some material connection to the state (Zeviar-Geese, 1998).

Federal Law

For years, federal courts have wrestled with the complicated issues associated with Internet crimes (*United States v Henriques*, 2000). The issues coalesce when a suspect is charged with a crime, found guilty by a jury, and then appeals the conviction on constitutional grounds. The most basic legal challenge to any court is a claim that it lacks jurisdiction, meaning that the government does not have the right to try the case in a particular court. Though many of these jurisdictional issues have been settled, defendants continually attempt to use the same defense.

Federal law applies to interstate, intrastate, and international traveler cases (eg, 18 USC § 2421-2424) because individuals have physically crossed state lines and/or sent e-mail messages or child pornography images across state lines using the Internet (eg, 18 USC § 2252). The laws that are used to prosecute travelers (ie, the Mann Act, which was first enacted in 1910, and later codified and amended at 18 USC 2421-2424) were originally established to prohibit certain sex acts, specifically to combat forced prostitution and prohibit selling women into prostitution. Amended over the years, the Protection of Children from Sexual Predators Act of 1998 (Pub L No 105-314, 112 Stat 2974 (1998)) helped increase the severity of the punishments and clarify the language of the law.

Today, federal courts use 18 USC § 2421 when a suspect crosses a state line with the intent to engage in an illegal sex act. This law reads as follows:

Whoever knowingly transports any individual in interstate or foreign commerce, or in any Territory or Possession of the United States, with intent that such individual engage in prostitution, or in any sexual activity for which any person can be charged with a criminal offense, or attempts to do so, shall be fined under this title or imprisoned not more than 10 years, or both (18 USC § 2421(1998)).

This section of the law applies regardless of the age of the participants. This law can be used to prosecute a kidnapper in a sex case or an interstate prostitution ring. Because this law does not specifically mention sex acts involving children, 2 other code sections were enacted. Punishments have become more severe for criminals who prey on children and use the Internet to arrange meetings to do so, as seen with the following:

— *18 USC § 2422(b).* "Whoever, using the mail or any facility or means of interstate or foreign commerce, or within the special maritime and territorial jurisdiction of the United States knowingly persuades, induces, entices, or coerces any individual who has not attained the age of 18 years, to engage in prostitution or any sexual activity for which any person can be charged with a criminal offense, or attempts to do so, shall be fined under this title, imprisoned not more than 15 years, or both."

— *18 USC § 2423(b).* "A person who travels in interstate commerce, or conspires to do so, or a United States citizen or an alien admitted for permanent residence in the United States who travels in foreign commerce, or conspires to do so, for the purpose of engaging in any sexual act (as defined in section 2246) with a person under 18 years of age that would be in violation of chapter 109A if the sexual act occurred in the special maritime and territorial jurisdiction of the United States shall be fined under this title, imprisoned not more than 15 years, or both."

— *18 USC § 2246.* "[T]he term 'sexual act' means contact between the penis and the vulva or the penis and the anus, and for purposes of this subparagraph contact involving the penis that occurs upon penetration, however slight; contact between the mouth and the penis, the mouth and the vulva, or the mouth and the anus; the penetration, however slight, of the anal or genital opening of another by a hand or finger or by any object, with an intent to abuse, humiliate, harass, degrade, or arouse or gratify the sexual desire of any person; or the intentional touching, not through the clothing, of the genitalia of another person who has not attained the age of 16 years with an intent to abuse, humiliate, harass, degrade, or arouse or gratify the sexual desire of any person."

An example of the way these laws have been used in court is exemplified in the case of *United States v Byrne* (1999). The defendant, Byrne, was prosecuted for meeting a minor online and enticing the child to engage in sexual acts with him. Byrne met his victim in an online chat room, conversed with the child for several months, then traveled from Texas to New Mexico for a sex meeting. In New Mexico, Byrne was arrested; he was prosecuted and sent to prison for 21 months.

TRAVELERS AND THE COURTS
Lawyers who represent travelers in court tend to use 1 of the following 5 legal theories to build their defense:

1. Impossibility: factual, legal, or both

2. Outrageous government conduct and manufactured jurisdiction

3. Entrapment

4. Constitutional attack

5. Fantasy

Impossibility Defense
Factual Impossibility
Factual impossibility is a defense based on the facts of the crime and focuses on the criminal act *intended* even if the crime could never be completed. For example, consider a woman who shoots a man and believes he is alive when she shoots him. It is later discovered that he was dead when she shot him. Her lawyer could argue that a crime was not committed because the man was already dead. Likewise, the prosecuting lawyer could argue that the woman should be punished for a crime because she *thought* the victim was alive when she shot him and, therefore, thought she was indeed committing a crime. In this case, the woman could not be charged with murder because, by law, **murder** is defined as the killing of a human being. A person who is dead can not be killed. A defense of factual impossibility may keep this woman from being accused of murder, but she may be convicted of attempted murder.

In other words, the factual impossibility defense allows a defendant to be prosecuted for an attempted crime. A prosecutor must jump the following 2 legal hurdles to charge a person with an attempted crime:

1. The prosecutor must prove that had the defendant's plan been carried out according to the defendant's understanding of the facts, a crime would have occurred. For example, had the woman from the previous example shot and killed a man who had been alive (as she thought he was), she could have been charged with murder.

2. The criminal must have taken substantial steps toward committing that crime.

If both criteria are met (and even if the criminal's understanding of the facts were not the actual facts), then the defendant may be charged with an attempted crime.

Legal Impossibility

A *legal impossibility* defense can be used when the actions of the defendant, even if the defendant thought the actions constituted a crime, would not be considered a crime (*United States v Oviedo*, 1976). Legal impossibility differs from factual impossibility in that legal impossibility can be used as a complete defense (*In re Sealed Case*, 2000). The distinction is slight but significant. Factual impossibility focuses on what a defendant *thinks* are the facts of the crime and whether the defendant would have committed a crime had those facts been a reality; legal impossibility does not involve the defendant's thoughts or plans because even if they had been acted on or had been a reality, the defendant's completed actions would not have constituted a crime.

For example, consider a man who thinks that shooting a deer is illegal but shoots it anyway. If according to his state law, shooting a deer is legal, no crime occurred, and it would be legally impossible for his actions to be considered criminal though he *thought* he committed a crime and *intended* to commit a crime. His *understanding of the facts* was that he was committing a crime, but it is irrelevant because shooting a deer is legal. This is a complete defense (*United States v Hsu*, 1998).

Distinguishing Between Factual and Legal Impossibility

The doctrine of impossibility has a complicated history, and courts have noted that "[t]he distinction between factual and legal impossibility is elusive at best" (*United States v Farner*, 2001). Though the difference between factual and legal impossibility may seem minor, the ramifications in traveler prosecutions are significant. For example, in *United States v Farner* (2001), Farner met a 14-year-old girl named Cindy online and corresponded with her via the Internet for 3 months. However, Cindy did not exist; she was an undercover FBI agent named Kathy Crawford. During their online relationship, he attempted to "persuade, induce, entice, and coerce" "Cindy" into having sexual relations with him. He sent her 4 pornographic pictures before he decided to drive from his home in Dallas to meet her in Houston where they had agreed to meet at a restaurant. He never made it inside because he was arrested by the FBI.

Farner tried to use the *legal* impossibility defense, declaring that the fictional Cindy turned out to be an adult, and sex between 2 adults (ie, he and the FBI agent) was completely legal. However, the court ruled that he could only use a *factual* impossibility defense. Like the situation involving the woman who shot a man who was already dead, Farner intended to commit a criminal act, one he knew was illegal. He did not know that he was about to meet an adult. Regardless, he could use the *factual* impossibility defense because had he engaged in sexual relations with "Cindy" (a grown woman), he would have been engaging in sex with an adult, which is completely legal. He could not use the *legal* impossibility defense (which would have resulted in dismissal of his case) because, had Cindy been a young girl (as he believed her to be) and he had engaged in sex with her, he would have committed a crime: "the defendant unquestionably intended to engage in the conduct proscribed by law but failed only because of circumstances unknown to him" (*United States v Farner*, 2001). Farner was sentenced to serve 15 months in prison.

Outrageous Government Conduct and Manufactured Jurisdiction Defense

The *outrageous governmental conduct* defense is used when the nature and extent of the government's involvement in the crime prevents prosecution as a matter of due process of law (*United States v Musslyn*, 1989). Though many attempt to use this defense, it is commonly denied by courts (eg, *Barber v Municipal Court*, 1979; *People v Shaw*, 1989). However, it was applicable in *United States v Lamb* (1996).

In traveler cases, defendants may claim the investigators' conduct was outrageous because they ***manufactured jurisdiction***, or purposefully manipulated the case to affect the relevant jurisdiction. For federal authorities to become involved and claim jurisdiction, more than one state must be involved (eg, 18 USC § 2422(b), and 18 USC § 2423(b)). Defendants occasionally claim that the government authorities purposefully created a scenario requiring federal involvement.

A federal appeals court in New York addressed this situation well before the computer age (*United States v Archer*, 1973). The court agreed with the defense, ruling that jurisdiction was manufactured because agents had placed out-of-state calls to the defendant to create a federal case. Today, federal agents working on a local case are prohibited from creating or furnishing details of the case solely to force federal involvement.

Defendants commonly claim the defense of manufactured jurisdiction when they unwittingly drive across state lines to meet a "child" for sex who turns out to be a federal agent posing as a "child." For example, in *United States v Peters* (1992), Peters drove a stolen truck from Chicago to Indiana to have a sex meeting with a "child" he had been communicating with, though the "child" turned out to be a federal officer. The court ruled that because Peters drove the truck of his own free will from Illinois to Indiana, the jurisdiction had not been manufactured. The defendant was convicted but appealed the conviction for transportation and conspiracy to transport a stolen vehicle across state lines. Peters alleged that the federal agents were involved in manufacturing the jurisdiction because they "tempted" him to drive the truck over state lines. Peters argument failed because the agents did not force him do anything, he freely chatted with the agent who was posing as a child, freely decided to meet that person for sex, and freely stole the truck to travel to the meeting location.

Based on constitutional guarantees of due process and basic fairness, federal agents are not allowed to be the sole federal link in a local prosecution case (*United States v Peters*, 1992); however, courts have ruled in favor of the prosecution when federal agents have "merely provided an opportunity" for a suspect to commit a crime. Courts are reluctant to reverse these types of decisions. Courts attempt to determine whether the suspect seized on the chance to commit a crime or the crime was atypical of the defendant's character and habit (*United States v Gardner*, 1975).

Courts continue to formulate relevant laws for undercover operations and jurisdiction. The courts have tended to rule in favor of undercover operations and continue to allow agents to use deception as long as the fraud does not implant the criminal plan in the defendant's mind. If the deception directly results in the creation of a criminal plan, then the entrapment defense becomes relevant (*Lewis v United States*, 1966).

Entrapment Defense

Sting operations always raise the issue of entrapment. The ***entrapment*** defense applies when law enforcement officers or other government agents induce a person to commit a crime. In *Jacobsen v United States* (1992) the US Supreme Court stated that "government agents may not originate a criminal design, implant in an innocent person's mind the disposition to commit a criminal act, and then induce commission of the crime so that the Government may prosecute." Of all the possible defenses, this is the most litigated claim raised by defendants. If a case involving the entrapment defense proceeds to a jury trial, the jury must answer the following 2 questions during deliberations:

1. Did government agents induce the defendant to commit the crime?

2. Was the defendant predisposed to commit this crime?

United States v Hollingsworth (1994) defined predisposition for criminal ventures as the "willingness to commit the offense before the agents of the government contact the person, in combination with the means to do the crime." The second issue is a federal standard, and though many states follow this law, state standards differ.

Because a defendant says he was tricked and, therefore, entrapped does not mean the case will go before a jury. The defendant must prove he was *not* predisposed to commit the crime. If he is unable to prove this to the court, the defense is precluded from arguing entrapment to the jury (*United States v Osbourse*, 1991).

Law in this area has been shaped by the adage "bad facts make bad law" (*Jacobo v Binur*, 2002). *United States v Poehlman* (2000) is a classic example. Mark Poehlman, a cross-dressing man who had a foot fetish, openly sought contact with other like-minded adults online. One of those contacts was with "Sharon," a woman who supposedly had 3 underage girls and was seeking a "special teacher" for them. "Sharon" was a government agent, posing as a mother online. During 6 months of communication via e-mail, the lurid details of the defendant's foot fetish became clear, but so did Sharon's requests of what she wanted Poehlman to provide for her daughters. Eventually, Poehlman proposed marriage to Sharon. She refused and then revisited the subject of plans for her daughters, which he agreed to. Poehlman traveled from his Florida home to California where Sharon lived. He went directly to a hotel room to meet her and her children. When he entered a room to meet the children, he was arrested by agents from the FBI, NCIS, and the Los Angeles County Sheriff's Office.

Poehlman was charged with crossing state lines for the purpose of engaging in sex acts with a minor and was convicted in state and federal courts and served prison time for both convictions. He appealed his convictions on the grounds of entrapment. The Federal Ninth Circuit Court of Appeals agreed with Poehlman and reversed his conviction. The court paid particular attention to the e-mail correspondence between Sharon and Poehlman, and concluded the following:

> There is no doubt that the government induced Poehlman to commit the crime here. … Sharon made it clear that she had made a firm decision about her children's sexual education, and that she believed that having Poehlman serve as their sexual mentor would be in their best interest. … Through its aggressive intervention, the government materially affected the normal balance between risks and rewards from the commission of the crime, and thereby induced Poehlman to commit the offense (*United States v Poehlman*, 2000).

This case helps delineate the limits of undercover investigations.

Constitutional Attack Defense

"If the law is against you, talk about the evidence … If the evidence is against you, talk about the law, and since you ask me, if the law and the evidence are both against you, then pound on the table and yell like hell" (*Sandburg, 1936*).

In *United States v Bailey* (2000), the defense decided to argue the legal side of the case citing the First Amendment right to free speech and that this protected online communications. Bailey was using the Internet to entice minors into illegal sexual activities and was convicted according to statute 18 USC § 2422(b), which makes it a criminal offense to use any form of communication to entice minors to perform sexual activities. Bailey appealed his conviction on the grounds that the statute was unconstitutional, claiming it was vague, overbroad, and infringed on his right to communicate. The Sixth Circuit Court of Appeals tersely decided that Bailey was wrong, declaring the following:

> The statute only applies to those who "knowingly" persuade or entice, or attempt to persuade or entice, minors. Thus, it only affects those who intend to target minors: it does not punish those who inadvertently speak with minors. … Put another way, the Defendant simply does not have a First Amendment right to attempt to persuade minors to engage in illegal sex acts. Defendant's constitutional challenge is without merit (*United States v Bailey*, 2000).

Though the court quickly dealt with the constitutional challenge in this case, the related facts of the case were chilling. It was *not* a sting case. Bailey had contacted 3 underage girls and urged them to have sex with him. The e-mail exchanges rapidly became terrifying when the girls realized he knew where they were. One girl testified that after school one day, she received a message on her pager that described her hair color, the clothes she had worn to school that day, and the exact time at which she had eaten her lunch. Though officers of the court continue to contemplate the constitutional challenges raised in these types of cases, people should not forget that more people like Bailey exist and at this moment are attempting to contact children for sex.

Fantasy Defense

A fantasy is a fiction of your own mind; however, when you start to act upon your desires, real world criminal law dictates what you may and may not do. Some people have claimed that the surreal nature of the Internet has motivated them to do things they would not normally do. This so-called **fantasy defense** received widespread media attention in 1999 when Patrick Naughton, a happily married man who was the vice president of Infoseek and monitored e-mail and chat rooms for the company, was arrested and charged with attempted "use of the Internet to induce a minor to engage in sexual activity" (McNichol, 2000). He traveled to Los Angeles to meet a 13-year-old girl, "Kris" (the identity assumed by an undercover FBI agent), with whom he had been chatting online for 9 months (McNichol, 2000). Naughton's plan had been to take Kris to a hotel room alone and have her remove all her clothes in front of him, but it never happened (Yamagami, 2001). Much to Naughton's surprise, USDOJ and FBI agents met him when he arrived.

In court, Naughton (who was known online as *HotSeattle*) presented a fantasy defense, claiming that he never intended to have sex with a 13-year-old girl. He claimed that he was planning to meet a grown woman who shared a "daddy-daughter" fantasy, in which the woman, who was part of this fantasy, would pose as a girl who wanted to have sex with her daddy (McNichol, 2000). His legal defense addressed his state of mind when he committed the alleged crime. Generally, an act must involve mental and physical intentions before a court will determine the act to be criminal. Legally, if Naughton had not intended to commit a crime and was flying all the way down from Seattle to meet a woman, not a girl, he was not guilty. All the male jurors believed the defense and voted to acquit Naughton; all the female jurors thought the fantasy defense was a lie and voted to convict. The case resulted in a hung jury, but Naughton later pled guilty to having traveled to Los Angeles with the intent of having sex with a 13-year-old girl, not with a grown woman fantasizing that she was a girl.

It is possible that the novelty of the fantasy defense has worn off and jurors see through it (Yamagami, 2001). Since Naughton's case in 1999, the fantasy defense has been used several times but with little success. For example, in *Commonwealth (Pennsylvania) v Zingarelli* (2003), the defendant testified that he was interested in fantasy. This case originated in a "father/daughter sex" chat room, where Zingarelli contacted the undercover officer who was posing as "Kathy," a 15-year-old girl. Over many conversations (online and via telephone), a date was arranged so Zingarelli could teach "Kathy" how to perform oral sex on him. By the time of the trial, the defendant had concocted a fantasy defense stating his actions did not amount to a criminal offense, as he was arrested outside of an ice cream stand, prior to his arranged "date," and had thus not committed any crime. He claimed everything was just a fantasy that involved Kathy playing the part of his daughter. However, evidence was produced at trial that rebuffed this defense, in that he had rented a hotel room and had purchased condoms and a bottle wine. He was convicted by the trial court of "criminal attempt to commit statutory sexual assault and criminal attempt to commit involuntary deviate sexual intercourse" (*Commonwealth (Pennsylvania) v Zingarelli*, 2003).

Likewise, in *People v Weston* (2003), the 30-year-old defendant testified that he was pursuing a fantasy and thought the voice of the officer posing as the little girl sounded older. Here, the initial meeting between the undercover officer and the defendant occurred in a chat room entitled, "Little Girls Sex Chat." The officer, a Riverside

County Sheriff's officer posed as "Sheila13," a 13-year-old girl. The defendant related in many conversations that he was worried about getting caught as he was "over twice [her] age." The defendant flew from Colorado to California and purchased sexual items in preparation for their meeting. The defendant at trial claimed that he knew she was not 13 based on Internet research of the phone number he had used to call her, and that voice on the phone sounded older than a 13-year-old would sound. The jury found the defendant guilty.

CONCLUSION

The Internet has become a fundamental part of life and forever changed the way people work, play, and interact with one another. Many children today can not conceive of life without the Internet. The Internet has been a remarkable addition to modern life, but it has inherent dangers. Computer-savvy felons are using technology to prey on children. People who are not satisfied with online fantasies are turning their dreams into realities.

Law enforcement officials are dedicated to using available resources to track down these felons, but they can not do it alone. Public awareness and parent involvement are essential components of the struggle against Internet child exploitation. Recognizing the problem and becoming educated about how to prevent it will make the Internet safer for all children.

REFERENCES

Baig EC. Buying a handheld is in your grasp. *USA Today*. December 2, 2003:D10.

Barber v Municipal Court, 24 Cal3d 742 (1979).

Berg T. State criminal jurisdiction in cyberspace: is there a sheriff on the electronic frontier? *Mich Bar J* [serial online]. 2000;79(6):659. Available at: http://www.michbar.org/journal/article.cfm?articleID=94&volumeID=8. Accessed February 16, 2004.

Bush GW. Address to the UN General Assembly. Speech presented at: UN General Assembly; September 23, 2003; New York, NY. Available at: http://www.whitehouse.gov/news/releases/2003/09/20030923-4.html. Accessed December 31, 2004.

Child Sex Crimes Wiretapping Act of 2001. *Hearing Before the Subcommittee on Crime of the Committee on the Judiciary*, 107th Cong, 1st Sess (2001) (statement of Lamar Smith, Texas congressman and chairman of the Subcommittee on Crime).

Children for sale [transcript]. *Dateline*. NBC television. January 30, 2004. Available at: http://msnbc.msn.com/id/4038249. Accessed February 2, 2004.

Commonwealth (Pennsylvania) v Zingarelli, 839 A2d 1064 (2003).

Corporation for Public Broadcasting. Connected to the future: a report on children's Internet use from the Corporation for Public Broadcasting. 2003. Available at: http://www.cpb.org/pdfs/ed/resources/connected/03_connect_report.pdf. Accessed February 2, 2004.

Cross T, Walsh W, Simone M, Jones L. Prosecution of Child Abuse: A Meta-Analysis of Rates of Criminal Justice Decisions. *Trauma Violence Abuse*. 2003;4(4):323-340. Cited by Wolak J, Mitchell KJ, Finkelhor D. *Internet Sex Crimes Against Minors: The Response of Law Enforcement*. Alexandria, Va: National Center for Missing & Exploited Children; 2003.

Dead girl had told online pal she was followed, La Mesa man, 47 also found shot. *San Diego Union*. December 8, 2002:A14.

18 USC § 2421 (2003).

18 USC § 2422 (b).

18 USC § 2423(b) (2003).

18 USC § 2246.

18 USC § 2252 (1998).

Finkelhor D, Mitchell KJ, Wolak J. *Online Victimization: A Report on the Nation's Youth.* University of New Hampshire Crimes Against Children Research Center. Alexandria, Va: National Center for Missing & Exploited Children; 2000.

42 USC § 5771.

42 USC § 13032 (1998).

Freeh L. Child pornography on the Internet and the sexual exploitation of children. Speech presented at: Senate Appropriations Subcommittee for the Departments of Commerce, Justice, and State, the Judiciary, and Related Agencies; March 10, 1998; Washington, DC. Available at: http://www.eff.org/Censorship/Internet_censorship_bills/1998/19980310_freeh_allen_sen_cjs_app.testimony. Accessed November 29, 2004.

Goodale G. Parents out of e-loop. *The Christian Science Monitor.* September 20, 2001. Available at: http://www.csmonitor.com/2001/0920/p11s1-stin.html. Accessed February 2, 2004.

How to overcome fear of the unknown. Stress Management Web site. Available at: http://www.stresstips.com/conquer_fear.htm. Accessed February 20, 2004.

In re Sealed Case, 223 F3d 775,779 (DC Cir 2000).

Internet crimes against children. *OVC Bull.* Washington, DC: US Department of Justice, Office of Justice Programs, Office for Victims of Crime; 2001. NCJ 184931.

Internet stings. A Resource Center to Help the Falsely-Accused Web site. Available at: http://www.accused.com/overview/stings.html. Accessed February 8, 2004.

Jacobo v Binur, dissenting opinion, 70 SW3d 330,339 (2002).

Jacobsen v United States, 503 US 540,548 (1992).

Lanning KV. *Child Molesters: A Behavioral Analysis.* 4th ed. Alexandria, Va: National Center for Missing & Exploited Children; 2001.

Levesque WR. 71 years to punish man's affair with teen. *St. Petersburg Times.* May 27, 2000. Available at: http://www.sptimes.com/News/052700/TampaBay/71_years_to_punish_ma.shtml. Accessed February 1, 2004.

Lewis v United States, 385 US 206,208-209 (1966).

Loftus C. Teen murdered by man she met in chatroom. NetSmartz Web site. December 2, 2002. Available at: http://www.netsmartz.org/news/Dec02-02.htm. Accessed February 20, 2004.

Man charged in US for child sex crimes abroad. CNN Web site. September 25, 2003. Available at: http://www.cnn.com/2003/LAW/09/24/sex.indictment/. Accessed February 1, 2004.

de Mause L. The history of child abuse. Speech presented at: National Parenting Conference; September 25, 1997; Boulder, Col. Available at: http://www.psychohistory.com/htm/05_history.html. Accessed February 8, 2004.

McAuliffe W. Government turnaround on paedophile entrapment. *ZDNet UK* [serial online]. January 30, 2001. Available at: http://news.zdnet.co.uk/internet/0,3902036 9,2084043,00.htm. Accessed February 22, 2004.

McLarty C. NLR police arrest two alleged Internet predators [transcript]. *Channel 7 News*. KATV. January 5, 2004. Available at: http://www.katv.com/news/stories/0104/116783.html. Accessed February 1, 2004.

McNichol T. Naughton pleads guilty. June 2000. Available at: http://www.wired.com/wired/archive/8.06/mustread.html. Accessed January 26, 2005.

Medaris M, Girouard C. *Protecting Children in Cyberspace: The ICAC Task Force Program: The Internet Crimes Against Children Program*. Washington, DC: Office of Juvenile Justice and Delinquency Programs; January 2002. NCJ 191213.

Miami valley crime caught on tape [transcript]. *NewsCenter*. WHIO-TV. February 4, 2003. Available at: http://www.whiotv.com/news/1955175/detail.html. Accessed February 28, 2004.

National Center for Missing & Exploited Children (NCMEC) Web site. Available at: http://www.missingkids.com/. Accessed February 2, 2004.

National Center for Missing & Exploited Children (NCMEC), Office of Juvenile Justice and Dependency Program (OJJDP). Frontline [newsletter]. Winter 2003/2004;51.

Nurenberg G. Cracking down on online predators. G4techTV Web site. August 22, 2002. Available at: http://www.techtv.com/news/internet/story/0,24195,3397013,00.html. Accessed January 27, 2004.

Oconomowoc man charged with attempted sexual assault of a child. *Waukesha Freeman*. January 29, 2004. Available at: http://www.gmtoday.com/news/local_stories/2004/January_04/01292004_05.asp. Accessed February 8, 2004.

Ohio v Moller, 2002 Ohio 1890 (2002).

People v Shaw, 210 Cal App 3d 859 (1989).

People v Weston, 2003 WL 22251409 (2003) (RIF 90871, October 2, 2003), *unpublished decision*.

Program Summary: Internet Crimes Against Children (ICAC) Task Force Program. Office of Juvenile Justice and Delinquency Prevention (OJJDP) Web site. Available at: http://ojjdp.ncjrs.org/Programs/ProgSummary.asp?pi=3. Accessed February 22, 2004.

PROTECT Act of 2003. Pub L No. 108-21, 117 Stat 650.

Pub L No. 105-314, 112 Stat 2974 (1998).

Repard P. SWAT team finds bodies of girl, S.D. man. *The San Diego Union-Tribune*. December 6, 2002. Available at: http://www.signonsandiego.com/news/metro/20021206-9999_2m6arkgirl.html. Accessed December 30, 2004.

Rios v State, 733 P2d 242,246-247 (Wyo 1987).

Robson S. S. Korea base museum director arrested in Arkansas porn sting. *Stars and Stripes*. European ed. January 10, 2004. Available at: http://www.estripes.com/article.asp?section=104&article=18977&archive=true. Accessed February 1, 2004.

Sandburg C. *The People, Yes*. New York, NY: Harcourt Brace & Co; 1936.

Sex "tourist" gets seven years. BBC News Web site. October 20, 2000. Available at: http://news.bbc.co.uk/1/hi/world/europe/980337.stm. Accessed February 1, 2004.

Sherman v United States, 356 US 369,377 (1958), note 7.

Strassheim v Daily, 221 US 280,285 (1911).

28 USC § 2246.

United States Immigrations and Customs Enforcement (ICE) Web site. Available at: http://www.ice.gov/graphics/index.htm. Accessed February 2, 2004.

United States v Archer, 486 F2d 670 (2d Cir 1973).

United States v Bailey, 228 F3d 637 (6th Cir 2000), *cert denied*, 532 US 1009 (2001).

United States v Byrne, 171 F3d 1231,1233 (10th Cir 1999).

United States v Farner, 251 F3d 510,512 (5th Cir 2001), citing *United States v Everett*, 700 F2d 900,905 (3rd Cir 1983).

United States v Gardner, 516 F2d 334,344-345 (7th Cir 1975).

United States v Henriques, 234 F3d 263,267 (5th Cir 2000), citing *United States v Carroll*, 105 F3d 740 (1st Cir 1997), ACLU v Johnson, 194 F3d 1149 (10th Cir 1999), *ACLU v Reno*, 217 F3d 162 (3rd Cir 2000).

United States v Hollingsworth, 27 F3d 1196,1200 (7th Cir 1994).

United States v Hsu, 155 F3d 189,198-200 (3rd Cir 1998).

United States v Lamb, 945 F Supp 441 (NDNY 1996).

United States v Musslyn, 865 F2d 945 (8th Cir 1989).

United States v Osbourse, 935 F2d 32 (4th Cir 1991)

United States v Oviedo, 525 F2d 881,883 (5th Cir 1976).

United States v Peters, 952 F2d 960 (7th Cir 1992).

United States v Poehlman, 217 F3d 692 (9th Cir 2000).

United States v Robertson, 350 F3d 1109,1110 (10th Cir 2003).

United States v Root, 296 F3d 1222 (11th Cir 2002).

United States v Sherman, 200 F2d 880,882 (2d Cir 1952).

Wireless e-mail use increases corporate productivity significantly [press release]. Palo Alto, Calif: Radicati Group Inc; October 13, 2003. Available at: http://www.gii.co.jp/press/rd16677_en.shtml. Accessed February 8, 2004.

Wolak J, Mitchell KJ, Finkelhor D. Escaping or connecting? Characteristics of youth who form close online relationships. *J Adolesc*. 2003a;26:105-119.

Wolak J, Mitchell KJ, Finkelhor D. *Internet Sex Crimes Against Minors: The Response of Law Enforcement*. Alexandria, Va: National Center for Missing & Exploited Children; 2003b.

Yamagami DS. Comment: prosecuting cyber-pedophiles: how can intent be shown in a virtual world in light of the fantasy defense? *Santa Clara Law Rev*. 2001;41:547-579.

Zeviar-Geese G. The state of the law on cyberjurisdiction and cybercrime on the Internet. *Across Borders Gonzaga Int Law J* [serial online]. 1998;1. Available at: http://law.gonzaga.edu/borders/documents/cyberlaw.htm. Accessed February 16, 2004.

Establishing Criminal Conspiracy and Aider and Abettor Liability for Groups That Promote Sexual Exploitation of Children

Duncan T. Brown, JD

Introduction

The Internet has made the world a smaller place, and lines of communication have been strengthened with the advent of the World Wide Web. Information can speed from computer to computer in moments. What once were geographic or temporal boundaries have been shortened, flattened, and altogether distorted. With this new-found access to information and enlightenment, computer users have done great things: science has made geometric progress, and the ability to communicate and transfer ideas has capitalized upon previously untapped reservoirs of creativity and intellect in society. However, with the benefits of increased lines of communication come some negative consequences. In many areas of the Internet, people interested only in their purient sexual appetites have hijacked the Internet's potential for the exchange of ideas.

Most notably, and shockingly, is the explosion of chat rooms, bulletin boards, and newsgroups dedicated solely to the creation, distribution and promotion of child pornography and other materials that sexually exploit children (**Table 37-1**). The speed and anonymity of the Internet has fostered a more aggressive and pervasive breed of online child-oriented sex offender. One recent study found that of 1501 teenagers between the ages of 10 and 17, almost 20% had been propositioned over the Internet (Mitchell et al, 2001). However, despite studies such as this one, and the pervasiveness of sites advertising "Lolita pics," "chickenhawk files," or other forms of child sexual exploitation (**Table 37-2**), the disturbing truth is that child pornography and groups

Table 37-1. Online Messages Terms: Chat Rooms and Bulletin Boards
The Ninth Circuit has defined a **chat room** as "a public or private Internet site that allows people to send messages to one another in 'real time'" (*United States v Laney*, 1999). **Bulletin boards** and **newsgroups** are sites where members can post messages for other members; however, members cannot talk in real time as in chat rooms. Bulletin boards fell out of favor with the advent of chat rooms; however, they are still used.

Table 37-2. Underage Victim Terms: Lolita and Chickenhawk
Lolita, in the parlance of child sexual exploitation, denotes a female who is, or appears to be, a minor. It functions as a code word alerting consumers of child pornography with underage females without otherwise drawing the attention of the public with explicit or graphic terms. This term was derived from the book of the same name by Vladimir Nabokov in which the adult character is sexually attracted to a 13-year-old girl named Lolita.
Chickenhawk is a slang term for underage male victims of sexual exploitation.

dedicated to the sexual exploitation of children are nothing new. What is new, however, is that groups who sexually exploit children have capitalized on the Internet to provide fast, seemingly ubiquitous means of communication and distribution.

To combat this rising wave of exploitation, law enforcement must be able to adapt old methods to new media. Though crimes on the Internet masquerade under the banner of "cyber crime," they essentially resemble many less technologically advanced crimes in one important way: speech. Because the Internet is a tool of communication, the author of the speech rarely physically commits crimes. Rather, the Internet as a communication device lends itself to inchoate crimes such as conspiracy to commit a crime or aiding those actively committing illegal acts. Those engaged in criminal activity rely heavily on the transfer of information and advice before, during, and after a crime is committed. And though the Internet has created a new level of high-tech communication, communication on the Internet is the same as communication printed on a broadsheet, spoken at a rally, or published in a book.

Essentially, the Internet is merely a new forum for speech. Therefore, agencies fighting crime over the Internet should refocus attention on tracing coconspirators or aiders and abettors over the same lines of communication that the defendants used to commit the crime. Prosecution of exploitation crimes such as distribution of child pornography lends itself well to computer crimes because computers leave detailed, precise trails of evidence linking defendants to each other. Likewise, crimes involving conspiracies are easier to establish because the predicates for a conspiracy, an agreement and an act, are aided by the ease of communication provided by the Internet. The crime of conspiracy, once relegated exclusively to letters, phone calls, meetings, and the provision of materials, can be accomplished quickly and conveniently between 2 people using e-mail. While the transfer of information via the Internet makes it easier to engage in a conspiracy, the transfer of illegal information can just as easily be traced or recorded for use as evidence in a prosecution.

In this chapter, the author will examine how conspiracy and aider and abettor liability can be used by law enforcement to broaden the scope of investigations and increase the efficiency of prosecuting participants engaged in the sexual exploitation of children. This chapter will establish how groups such as the North American Man/Boy Love Association (NAMBLA) and online sex rings may create conspiracy or aider and abettor liability through their newsletters, publications, and chat room activities. The speech engaged in by groups such as NAMBLA and Internet sex rings is not speech protected by the First Amendment and rises to the level of criminal activity. Because their speech is not legally protected, these groups are liable for the actions of their members who act upon that speech. This chapter's analysis is divided into 3 parts: (1) why there is no First Amendment protection for the type of speech used by groups engaged in the sexual exploitation of children; (2) the criminal conspiracy liability of groups like NAMBLA and sex rings; and (3) the aider and abettor liability of members of NAMBLA and online sex rings.

The 2 types of groups that will be focused on are structured groups such as NAMBLA, and online sex rings such as the Wonderland Club and the Orchid Club.

NAMBLA has been in existence since 1978. Its officers and members are dedicated to promoting and advocating adult men and minor children to engage in sexual relationships. Groups like NAMBLA tend to be organized, often with an internal structure of officers and national and local chapters. They solicit membership dues and hold national conferences. With the exception of their goal to legalize and promote sexual relationships between adult men and boys under the age of majority, they resemble many legal and legitimate organizations. However, they are secretive and are currently named in a suit alleging that they are civilly liable for 2 members brutally sodomizing and murdering an 11-year-old boy in Massachusetts (Amended Complaint and Jury Demand at Docket No.00c.10956). Conversely, online sex rings are less organized. They are usually groups of people who are members of password-protected chat rooms. In these chat rooms, the members trade child pornography, discuss strategies for molesting children, and talk about previous sexual assaults on children. While they require a membership fee, usually the dues are in the form of child pornography posted to the groups' chat room. For example, the Wonderland Club was a notorious international group that required its members to post 10 000 images of child pornography in order to join. Once a member, an individual had access to the other members' collections of child pornography. The sex rings usually do not have an internal structure like NAMBLA, and often the members contact each other online only.

The crimes involved for the purposes of this chapter are what would be considered the sexual exploitation of minors, (ie, any physical act of sexual abuse committed against a child). Before the Wonderland Club ring was broken up and its members arrested, it became infamous for one of its members sodomizing a victim live on the Internet while taking requests for specific types of abuse typed in by other members (Porn ring was real child abuse, 2001). The Orchid Club was a similar type of group in the United States that also engaged in the live sexual assault of children on the Internet for its members (*United States v Laney*, 1999; *United States v Tank*, 2000). Also included are the crimes of production, distribution, and promotion of child pornography. Although these crimes may cover many different statutes among the states, at the federal level they are summarized in 2 statutes, 18 USC § 2251 (2001) and 18 USC § 2252 (2001) (**Table 37-3**). The statutes criminalize the possession, production, and distribution of any pornographic material depicting a child in a sexually explicit manner (18 USC § 2252 [2001]). Furthermore, the laws prohibit any images created by any means that combine elements of actual children with computer-generated images (18 USC § 2256(8)(C) [2001]). Thus, federal law extends the definition of prohibited child pornography to include images that are not solely composed of actual children. For example, an image of a child in a swimsuit that has been altered to appear as if the swimsuit were removed and the child were completely naked would be prohibited under the law (for a complete discussion of the protections afforded computer-generated versus actual child pornography, see *Ashcroft v Free Speech Coalition*, 2002). Although the language of the Child Pornography Protection Act (CPPA) addressing computer generated child pornography was struck down for vagueness and overbreadth, images of actual children altered or enhanced to become pornographic remain prohibited (**Table 37-4**). This continued prohibition is because the harm to children recognized in *New York v Ferber* (1982) can be directly applied to the cases involving children in altered and enhanced images.

LANGUAGE THAT CREATES CONSPIRACIES OR AIDS AND ABETS CRIMES OF CHILD SEXUAL EXPLOITATION IS NOT PROTECTED UNDER THE FIRST AMENDMENT

The First Amendment does not protect language that creates a conspiracy or assists in the commission of a crime (*Rice v Paladin Enterprises*, 1997). This is a well-accepted proposition because the nature of inchoate crimes emphasizes the intent of the parties

Table 37-3. Federal Statues Regarding Sexual Exploitation of Minors

18 USC § 2251 (2001) and 18 USC § 2252 (2001). Select sections of the 2 statutes read as follows:

18 USC § 2251. Sexual exploitation of children

(a) Any person who employs, uses, persuades, induces, entices, or coerces any minor to engage in, or who has a minor assist any other person to engage in or who transports any minor in interstate or foreign commerce, or in any Territory or Possession of the United States, with the intent that such minor engage in, any sexually explicit conduct for the purpose of producing any visual depiction of such conduct, shall be punished as provided under subsection (d), if such person knows or has reason to know that such visual depiction will be transported in interstate or foreign commerce or mailed, if that visual depiction was produced using materials that have been mailed, shipped, or transported in interstate or foreign commerce by any means, including by computer, or if such visual depiction has actually been transported in interstate or foreign commerce or mailed.

(c) (1) Any person who, in a circumstance described in paragraph (2), knowingly makes, prints, or publishes, or causes to be made, printed, or published, any notice or advertisement seeking or offering—

(A) to receive, exchange, buy, produce, display, distribute, or reproduce, any visual depiction, if the production of such visual depiction involves the use of a minor engaging in sexually explicit conduct and such visual depiction is of such conduct; or

(B) participation in any act of sexually explicit conduct by or with any minor for the purpose of producing a visual depiction of such conduct;

shall be punished as provided under subsection (d).

(2) The circumstance referred to in paragraph (1) is that—

(A) such person knows or has reason to know that such notice or advertisement will be transported in interstate or foreign commerce by any means including by computer or mailed; or

(B) such notice or advertisement is transported in interstate or foreign commerce by any means including by computer or mailed.

18 USC § 2252. Certain activities relating to material involving the sexual exploitation of minors

(a) Any person who—

(1) knowingly transports or ships in interstate or foreign commerce by any means including by computer or mails, any visual depiction, if—

(A) the producing of such visual depiction involves the use of a minor engaging in sexually explicit conduct; and

(B) such visual depiction is of such conduct;

(2) knowingly receives, or distributes any visual depiction that has been mailed, or has been shipped or transported in interstate or foreign commerce, or which contains materials which have been mailed or so shipped or transported, by any means including by computer, or knowingly reproduces any visual depiction for distribution in interstate or foreign commerce by any means including by computer or through the mails, if—

(A) the producing of such visual depiction involves the use of a minor engaging in sexually explicit conduct; and

(B) such visual depiction is of such conduct;

(3) either—

(A) in the special maritime and territorial jurisdiction of the United States, or on any land or building owned by, leased to, or otherwise used by or under the control of the Government of the United States, or in the Indian country as defined in section 1151 of this title, knowingly sells or possesses with intent to sell any visual depiction; or

(B) knowingly sells or possesses with intent to sell any visual depiction that has been mailed, or has been shipped or transported in interstate or foreign commerce, or which was produced using materials which have been mailed or so shipped or transported, by any means, including by computer, if—

(continued)

Table 37-3. *(continued)*

(i) the producing of such visual depiction involves the use of a minor engaging in sexually explicit conduct; and

(ii) such visual depiction is of such conduct; or

(4) either—

(A) in the special maritime and territorial jurisdiction of the United States, or on any land or building owned by, leased to, or otherwise used by or under the control of the Government of the United States, or in the Indian country as defined in section 1151 of this title, knowingly possesses 1 or more books, magazines, periodicals, films, video tapes, or other matter which contain any visual depiction; or

(B) knowingly possesses 1 or more books, magazines, periodicals, films, video tapes, or other matter which contain any visual depiction that has been mailed, or has been shipped or transported in interstate or foreign commerce, or which was produced using materials which have been mailed or so shipped or transported, by any means including by computer, if—

(i) the producing of such visual depiction involves the use of a minor engaging in sexually explicit conduct; and

(ii) such visual depiction is of such conduct; shall be punished as provided in subsection (b) of this section.

Table 37-4. Morphing Images

While the term "morphed image" is commonly applied to computer-generated child pornography photographs, it is a misnomer. Because these images are still images that are altered or enhanced using other still images, they are more properly described as "cut and paste." Morphing, on the other hand, is a technical term of art used in the field of animation.

Morphing is an image processing technique typically used as an animation tool for the metamorphosis from one image to another. The idea is to specify a warp that distorts the first image into the second. Its inverse will distort the second image into the first. As the metamorphosis proceeds, the first image is gradually distorted and is faded out, while the second image starts out totally distorted toward the first and is faded in. Thus, the early images in the sequence are much like the first source image. The middle image of the sequence is the average of the first source image distorted halfway toward the second one and the second source image distorted halfway back toward the first one. The last images in the sequence are similar to the second source image. The middle image is key; if it looks good then the entire animated sequence will look good. For morphs between faces, the middle image often looks strikingly life-like, like a real person, but clearly it is neither the person in the first nor the second source images.

Adapted from: Beier T, Neely S. Feature-based image metamorphosis. SIGGRAPH 1992 Proceedings. Available at: http://www.hammerhead.com/thad/morph. html. Accessed June 12, 2003.

---

to commit a crime rather than focusing on the criminal act itself. The lack of protection afforded crimes that depend upon language as evidence of intent has been justified because

speech that is an integral part of a transaction involving conduct the government otherwise is empowered to prohibit; such "speech acts"—for instance, many cases of inchoate crimes such as aiding and abetting and conspiracy—may be proscribed without much, if any, concern about the First Amendment, since it is merely incidental that such "conduct" takes the form of speech (*Rice v Paladin Enterprises*, 1997, qtd. in Department of Justice, 1997 Report on the availability of bombmaking information).

Unfortunately, this brightline distinction between protected and unprotected speech does little to explain how unprotected speech can be used to prosecute conspiracies or aiders and abettors in crimes involving child sexual exploitation. Merely stating that inchoate crimes are not subject to the same type of First Amendment analysis as other types of crimes or speech inadequately describes why one type of speech is protected while another creates criminal liability for the speaker and listener. Because this chapter will focus on how the speech of groups like NAMBLA and online sex rings create conspiracies and aid and abet crimes of sexual exploitation of children, a more detailed analysis of why the speech used in these crimes is not protected follows.

IMAGES OF CHILD PORNOGRAPHY AND SPEECH INCITING CRIMINAL ACTIVITY ARE NOT AFFORDED FIRST AMENDMENT PROTECTION

There are 2 general types of speech at issue in cases involving child pornography. The first type of speech includes graphic images or descriptions of children engaged in sexually explicit conduct. Photographs, computer images, magazines, books, or other materials that portray, illustrate, or depict children engaged in sexually explicit conduct fall in this category. These images are generally those found stored on a defendant's hard drive or in print media and are the object of countless Web sites and chat rooms dedicated to distributing, producing, and amassing child pornography.

The second type of speech that will be discussed is the type of speech used by defendants incidental to their criminal activities. This type of speech is the speech that creates conspiracies and aiders and abettors. The language is used by organized and centralized groups, such as NAMBLA, to plan strategies for seducing victims (NAMBLA, 1991) or to build structured networks of pedophiles and molesters to trade or distribute pornography among less organized groups, such as the Wonderland Club (Wickedness in Wonderland, 2001). It is the type of language that groups of defendants use to trade or produce pornography casually in chat rooms or on Web sites.

The Supreme Court has long recognized the principle that "the protection of speech often depends on the content of the speech" (*New York v Ferber*, 1982). Simply stated, neither of the 2 types of speech discussed in this chapter are protected by the First Amendment's guarantee of freedom of speech. Images of child pornography included in the first group of speech are not protected under the Constitution for reasons established in *New York v Ferber* (1982) and *Osborne v Ohio* (1990). The second category of speech is likewise unprotected by the First Amendment because it is speech that goes beyond mere advocacy of a position and instructs and encourages the listener to commit illegal acts immediately as explained in *Giboney v Empire Storage & Ice* (1949) and *Brandenburg v Ohio* (1969).

PORNOGRAPHIC IMAGES OF CHILDREN ARE NOT PROTECTED BY THE FIRST AMENDMENT

Child pornography differs from adult obscenity in that it is clearly defined by statute and is not subject to nebulous or vague tests based on community standards of what is impermissibly obscene. The Supreme Court has held that the normal test for adult obscenity outlined in *Miller v California* (1973) (ie, whether the item, when taken as a whole, has any artistic, educational, literary, political, or scientific value, or is designed only to satisfy the purient interests as defined by community standards) does not apply to judging child pornography because there are compelling state interests that make the strict regulation of child pornography permissible (*Miller v California*, 1973). The *Ferber* (1982) court held that

[w]e consider it unlikely that visual depictions of children performing sexual acts or lewdly exhibiting their genitals would often constitute an important and necessary part of a literary performance or scientific or educational work. As a state judge in this case observed, if it were necessary for literary or artistic value, a person over the statutory age who perhaps looked younger could be utilized.

By establishing that child pornography is not protected by the First Amendment, the Supreme Court recognized that there must be a compelling state interest to justify prohibiting child pornography and that the definition of child pornography must be narrowly worded to prohibit only the proscribed conduct. The 2 major legal influences in child pornography cases for courts traditionally have been *New York v Ferber* (1982), and the recently overturned CPPA (18 USCS §§ 2251, 2256).

Compelling State Interest

The regulation of child pornography requires a compelling state interest because laws regulating child pornography are not content-neutral. Therefore, the laws must be narrowly tailored to serve a compelling state interest (*New York v Ferber*, 1982). In *New York v Ferber*, the court was able to find not just 1, but 4 compelling state interests in support of making child pornography unprotected speech. The first interest is in "safeguarding the physical and psychological well-being of a minor" (*Globe Newspaper Co v Superior Court*, 1982). The court recognized that child pornography can harm children who are either used as subjects of the pornography or subjected to it later on. The harm presented to the victim-subject of the pornography and to the victim exposed to the pornography is the physical and emotional harm of being sexually exploited. The right of the government to assume a greater duty to protect children from potential harm is a long-standing, legitimate right, and the Supreme Court has consistently recognized it in cases involving exposure of children to obscenity and lewd material (**Table 37-5**).

The second compelling state interest the court found was to prevent future sexual abuse of children. The court held that the "distribution of photographs and films depicting sexual activity by juveniles is intrinsically related to the sexual abuse of children" (*New York v Ferber*, 1982). The court found that this harm was continued by child pornography in 2 ways: first by making a permanent record of the victim's exploitation that can serve as a reminder of their participation and, second, by creating new items for distribution, making control of the images difficult. The damage that child pornography can inflict on the victim is significant. The Court recognized that

[pornography] poses an even greater threat to the child victim than does sexual abuse or prostitution. Because the child's actions are reduced to a recording, the pornography may haunt him in future years, long after the original misdeed took place. A child who has posed for a camera must go through life knowing that the recording is circulating within the mass distribution system for child pornography (Shouvlin, 1981).

Table 37-5. Cases Establishing the Right of the Government to Assume a Greater Duty to Protect Children from Potential Harm

CASE	RULING
Prince v Massachusetts, 321 US 158 (1944)	"The state's authority over children's activities is broader than over like actions of adults. This is particularly true of public activities and in matters of employment."
Ginsberg v New York, 390 US 629 (1968)	The government's interest in the "well-being of its youth" justified the regulation of otherwise protected expression.
FCC v Pacifica Foundation, 438 US 726 (1978)	Due to the ease that children may obtain access to broadcast material and the government's interest in the well-being of its youth, the government is justified in regulating indecent material.
Globe Newspaper Co v Superior Court, 457 US 596 (1982)	A statute mandating non-disclosure of child sexual abuse witness names and a closed courtroom in child sexual abuse cases when a child testifies was declared unconstitutional. This is because the statute was not narrowly tailored to ensure that denial of right to criminal trial to newspaper serves a compelling state interest.

The second prong of this harm is that once new child pornography enters the distribution chain, regulation becomes more difficult. The more pornography is produced, the harder it is to control. Therefore, the court held that harm is present in that every piece of new pornography represents a new victim and feeds a hard-to-control market for child pornography (*New York v Ferber*, 1982).

The third compelling state interest recognized by the *Ferber* (1982) court was that the production and distribution of child pornography creates an economic motive for producing and distributing more pornography. Thus, like the harm to potential victims created when child pornography is produced and distributed, the need to stop the cycle of satisfying a constantly increasing demand for child pornography created by the constant production of child pornography is grounds for regulation. This interest, however, is not aimed at the harm caused to the victims but at the economic gain pornographers and consumers of pornography reap from their exploitation. Therefore, the compelling state interest is in vitiating the economic benefit of producing and distributing child pornography in an attempt to control and destroy the market.

The fourth, and final, compelling state interest is that child pornography has no redeeming social value beyond its illegal purpose. The court found that the social or artistic value of child pornography has an "exceedingly modest, if not *de minimis*" (*New York v Ferber*, 1982) value. The court found that few instances exist where artistic, scientific, political, or educational expression would be hampered by using alternatives to what would amount to child pornography as a means of expression. In the instances where the use of children in situations considered pornographic would be necessary, the court found that the overall value of that expression would, at most, be of minimally more value than the legal alternative.

Though the Supreme Court partially overturned the CPPA, lower courts supporting it recognized 2 additional concerns created by the use of actual child pornography, morphed images, and computer-generated child pornography. Though the law was partially repealed, these factors are still relevant to how child molesters behave and target victims. In examining the CPPA (18 USCS § 2256), courts developed 2 additional compelling state interests. The first new interest was that child molesters use child pornography as part of the grooming process (*United States v Acheson*, 1999). Grooming is the process through which child molesters lower the inhibitions of their victims. Grooming often begins fairly innocuously, the defendant merely appearing to befriend the victim. However, the friendship or trust offered by the molester is so the victim will feel comfortable around the molester. Once the victim believes he or she can trust the molester, the molester discusses sex with the victim to arouse the victim's curiosity about the subject. The molester often will show the victim child pornography, as well as adult pornography, in an attempt to get the victim to feel comfortable looking at naked people. Child pornography is used to suggest to the victim that certain sexual acts are commonly engaged in by children and are enjoyable and normal. (For a detailed discussion about various forms that grooming may take, see Lanning, 1987.)

The second new state interest recognized by courts is that child pornography serves to "whet the appetite of child molesters" and embolden them to commit actual acts of sexual assault on children. *United States v Acheson* (1999) held that virtual child pornography "whets the appetite" as much as pornography created using real children. Similar to the cycle of demand for pornography created by the production of it, the *Acheson* court, as well as Congress (CPPA, PL 104-208, 1996), recognized that images of children engaged in sexually explicit conduct only nurtures the desire of a child molester to commit an actual physical act of sexual violence.

These concerns echoed the stated intent of Congress for creating the law. In the committee report during the passage of the bill, Senator Orrin Hatch argued that

[c]omputer-imaging technology permits creation of pornographic depictions designed to satisfy the preferences of individual sexual predators. ... The ability to alter or "morph" images via computer to produce any desired child pornographic depiction enables pedophiles and pornographers to create "custom-tailored" pornography which will heighten the material effect on the viewer and thus increase the threat this material poses to children. ... The computer-produced depictions could be shown to the child in an effort to seduce or blackmail the child into submitting to sexual abuse or exploitation, or to other children who know the depicted child in order to seduce them (Committee Reports, 1996).

Thus, despite the Supreme Court's concerns of overbreadth and improper application (*Ashcroft v Free Speech Coalition*, 2002), the courts actually and properly realized the intent of the bill and tried to fulfill it by extending the legacy of the *Ferber* court into new, more technologically advanced, generations.

Narrow Construction and Child Pornography

Regulating child pornography is possible because, unlike adult obscenity, the definition of child pornography is specific and narrowly tailored by law. Because child pornography is a form of speech permissibly proscribed by law because of the compelling state interest its regulation serves (*R.A.V. v City of St. Paul*, 1992; *New York v Ferber*, 1982), the statute defining child pornography must be narrowly tailored to satisfy those interests (*R.A.V. v City of St. Paul*, 1992). To minimize the chance that a state or federal statute unconstitutionally overreaches its permitted grasp and criminalizes protected speech, the Supreme Court decides whether the challenged language's alleged overbreadth or vagueness is not only "real, but substantial as well, judged in relation to the statute's plainly legitimate sweep" (*Broadrick v Oklahoma*, 1973). Though this standard appears to create the expectation of little tolerance for statutes that are not sufficiently narrow in scope or definition, some leeway is granted to child pornography laws.

Traditionally, the court has interpreted the standard of narrow construction liberally, giving states great discretion in passing laws to address the issue of child pornography (*New York v Ferber*, 1982; *Osborne v Ohio*, 1990). Generally, the court's focus has not been on the content of new laws developed to combat new forms of crimes involving child pornography, but rather on whether those new laws are narrowly tailored enough (*Osborne v Ohio*, 1990). To allow states to develop and implement innovative new laws against child pornography, the court has been willing to recognize that a compelling state interest can remain, or increase in scope, as the underlying criminal activity evolves in breadth (*United States v Mento*, 2000; *United States v Ferber*, 1997; *Osborne v Ohio*, 1990).

As demonstrated in *Osborne v Ohio* (1990), a case in which Ohio adapted its distribution and production laws to outlaw the possession of child pornography, the court responded to, and ultimately encouraged, the evolution of law to meet the needs of society identified in earlier decisions:

Given the importance of the State's interest in protecting the victims of child pornography, we cannot fault Ohio for attempting to stamp out this vice at all levels in the distribution chain. According to the State, since the time of our decision in Ferber, much of the child pornography market has been driven underground; as a result, it is now difficult, if not impossible, to solve the child pornography problem by only attacking production and distribution. ... Ferber recognized the materials produced by child pornographers permanently record the victim's abuse. The pornography's continued existence causes the child victims continuing harm by haunting the children in years to come. The State's ban on possession and viewing encourages the possessors of these materials to destroy them. Second, encouraging the destruction of these materials is also desirable because evidence suggests that pedophiles use child pornography to seduce other children into sexual activity.

The Court's discussion of the difficulty of preventing the problem of producing and distributing child pornography, and the state's compelling interest to stop such crimes, provides support for the holding that states "may constitutionally proscribe the possession and viewing of child pornography" (*Osborne v Ohio*, 1990). Furthermore, this holding supports the court's focus on the distinctions between overbroad statutes and those that are narrowly tailored. The court integrates this discussion citing its 2-part constitutional test for the scope of overbreadth: "to be overbroad and unconstitutional, a statute's overbreadth must not only be real, but substantial as well, judged in relation to the statute's plainly legitimate sweep" (*Osborne v Ohio*, 1990). In applying this test to statutes involving child pornography, the court has been careful to examine the entire language and effect of the statute to understand the possibility of overbreadth, "even where a statute at its margins infringes on protected expression, facial invalidation is inappropriate if the remainder of the statute … covers a whole range of easily identifiable and constitutionally proscribable … conduct." Therefore, the court is generally willing to allow a definition of child pornography as broad as needed to meet the compelling state interests already discussed.

THE FIRST AMENDMENT DOES NOT OFFER PROTECTION TO SPEECH USED BY GROUPS THAT PROMOTE AND DISTRIBUTE CHILD SEXUAL EXPLOITATION

Like images, speech (ie, spoken and written words) is usually protected under the First Amendment. Generally, the government has no power to restrict expression because of message, idea, subject matter, or content of the expression (*New York Times Co v Sullivan*, 1964). There are certain exceptions to this protection, such as malicious libel and obscenity. However, the one most relevant to this chapter is speech that incites criminal behavior (*Young v American Mini Theatres*, 1976). Because freedom of speech is so fundamental to the rights of citizens, the government can abridge this form of expression only in circumstances where the speech intentionally and purposefully incites the listener to immediate criminal activity (*Brandenburg v Ohio*, 1969). This standard was initially, yet vaguely, first established in *Brandenburg v Ohio* (1969) and further defined in a string of cases that established clearer standards for judging unprotected speech (**Table 37-6**). Some of those additional guidelines are whether the speech merely advocates or educates the reader on a position or teaches a skill or method for action (*Brandenburg v Ohio*, 1969; *Yates v United States*, 1956; *Central Hudson Gas and Electric v Public Service Commission of New York*, 1980; *Braun v Soldier of Fortune*, 1992; *Rice v Paladin Enterprises*, 1997); what the specific content of the remark was (*Young v American Mini Theatres*, 1976); what the known uses of the materials or information mentioned in the speech were (*Giboney v Empire Storage & Ice*, 1949; *United States v Mendelsohn*, 1990); to whom the remarks were addressed (*Hess v Indiana*, 1973); what sort of marketing accompanied the remarks (*Direct Sales v United States*, 1943); and how close in time or proximity were the remarks to the illegal action (*Watts v United States*, 1969; *United States v Fleschner*, 1996; *United States v Mendelsohn*, 1990). In certain situations, the Supreme Court has described balancing these factors on a sliding scale holding that the more that are present, the less protection the speech is afforded (*Direct Sales v United States*, 1943). Rulings referring to these additional guidelines are summarized in **Table 37-7**.

The first distinction courts look to when deciding whether speech is unprotected by the First Amendment is whether it merely advocates a position or if it describes or encourages specific ways to achieve an illegal end (*Brandenburg v Ohio*, 1969; *Yates v United States*, 1956). For example, *Yates v United States* (1956) provided that the "essential distinction is that those to whom the advocacy is addressed must be urged to do something, now or in the future, rather than merely to believe in something." The Supreme Court has extended protection to speech that rises only to the level of advocacy or education about a certain theory because advocacy in the abstract lacks the intention to generate immediate or foreseeable action to achieve that theory (*Yates v United States*, 1956). This standard was vaguely explained by the *Brandenburg (1969)* court and has been broadly interpreted by later courts. Examples of acceptable

Table 37-6. Cases Establishing Standards for Judging Unprotected Speech

CASE	RULING
Bradenburg v Ohio, 395 US 444,447-449 (1969)	Provided that "the mere abstract teaching of the moral propriety or even moral necessity for a resort to force and violence is not the same as preparing a group for violent action and steeling it to such action."
Yates v United States, 354 US 298,321-322 (1956)	"[I]ndoctrination of a group in preparation for future violent action, as well as exhortation to immediate action, by advocacy found to be directed to 'actions for the accomplishment' of forcible overthrow to violence as 'a rule or principle of action,' and employing 'language of incitement,' is not constitutionally protected when the group is of sufficient size and cohesiveness."
Young v American Mini Theatre, 427 US 50,66 (1979)	Stated that "the line between permissible advocacy and impermissible incitation to crime or violence depends not merely on the setting in which the speech occurs, but also on exactly what the speaker had to say."
McCollum v CBS, 202 Cal App 3d 989 (1988)	"Thus, to justify a claim that speech should be restrained or punished because it is (or was) an incitement to lawless action, the court must be satisfied that the speech (1) was directed or intended toward the goal of producing imminent lawless conduct and (2) was likely to produce such conduct. Speech directed to action at some indefinite time in the future will not satisfy this test."

Table 37-7. Additional Guidelines for Judging Unprotected Speech

CATEGORY	CASE	RULING
Whether the speech merely advocates or educates the reader on a position or teaches a skill or method for action	*Brandenburg v Ohio,* 395 US 444,447-449 (1969)	Distinguished "mere advocacy from incitement to imminent lawless action."
	Yates v United States, 354 US 298,321-322 (1956)	Stated that "advocacy, even though uttered with the hope that it may ultimately lead to violent revolution, is too remote from concrete action to be regarded as the indoctrination preparatory to action which was condemned in *Dennis.*"
	Central Hudson Gas and Electric v Public Service Commission of New York, 447 US 537, 561-571 (1980)	Held that suppression of all advertisements by electric company, including advertisements, which serve state interest of conservation, violates First and Fourteenth Amendments.
	Braun v Soldier of Fortune, 968 F2d 1110,1119 (11th Cir 1992)	Limited tort liability for publishers in order to "ensure that the burden imposed on publishers will have only a minimal impact on their advertising revenue."
	Rice v Paladin Enterprises, 128 F3d 233,248 (4th Cir 1997)	Speech is not protected if it "methodically and comprehensively prepares and steels its audience to specific criminal conduct through exhaustively detailed instuctions on planning, commision, and concealment of criminal conduct."
The specific content of the remark	*Young v American Mini Theatres,* 427 US 50,66 (1976)	"The question of whether speech is or is not protected by the First Amendment often depends on the content of the speech. Thus, the line between permissible advocacy and impermissible incitation to crime or violence depends, not merely on the setting in which the speech occurs, but also on exactly what the speaker had to say."

(continued)

Table 37-7. Additional Guidelines for Judging Unprotected Speech *(continued)*

CATEGORY	CASE	RULING
The known use of the materials or information mentioned in the speech	*Giboney v Empire Storage & Ice*, 336 US 490,498 (1949)	Held that "speech or writing used as an integral part of conduct in violation of a valid criminal statute," such as picketing in order to effect an illegal restraint of trade and prevent wholesalers from selling to non-union ice peddlers, is not protected by the First Amendment.
	United States v Mendelsohn, 896 F2d 1183,1185 (9th Cir 1990)	Held that a computer bookmaking program "is too instrumental in and intertwined with the performance of criminal activity to retrain First Amendment protection ... [because it is] so close in time and purpose to a substantial evil as to become part of the crime itself."
To whom the remarks were addressed	*Hess v Indiana*, 414 US 105,108 (1973)	Held that a student's statement, "[w]e'll take the f**king street later," in response to police action was protected speech because remarks not specifically targeted to a specific group of people enjoy greater protection under the First Amendment.
What sort of marketing accompanied the remarks	*Direct Sales v United States*, 319 US 703,712 (1943)	Stated that "where not only the speaker's dissemination or marketing strategy, but the nature of the speech itself, strongly suggests that the audience both targeted and actually reached is, in actuality, very narrowly confined."
How close in time or proximity were the remarks to the illegal action	*Watts v United States*, 394 US 705,707-708 (1969)	Ordered judgment of acquittal for defendant who threatened the president of the United States due to conditional nature of statement and laughter of listeners.
	United States v Fleschner, 98 F3d 155,158-160 (1996)	Found defendant's instruction on claiming unlawful exemptions and other means of avoiding taxes were proximate in time to the crime and were sufficient to convict the defendants of conspiracy for violations of US tax code.
The more factors that are present, the less protection is afforded	*Direct Sales v United States*, 319 US 703,712 (1943)	Stated that the "inherent capacity for harm" when dealing with commodities such as machine guns and narcotics "makes a difference in the gravity of proof required to show knowledge that the buyer will utilize the article unlawfully. Additional facts, such as quantity sales, high pressure sales methods, abnormal increases in the size of the buyer's purchase, etc, which would be wholly innocuous if not more than grounds for suspicion in relation to unrestricted goods, may furnish conclusive evidence in respect to restricted articles, that the seller knows the buyer has an illegal object and enterprise."

speech include an individual stating during a draft protest, "[i]f they ever make me carry a rifle, the first man I want to get in my sights is LBJ" (*Watts v United States*, 1969); a KKK speaker stating, "[w]e're not a revengent [*sic*] organization, but if our President, our Congress, our Supreme Court, continues to suppress the white, Caucasian race, it's possible that there might have to be some revengance [*sic*] taken" (*Brandenburg v Ohio*, 1969); a student during a rally after being pushed back onto a sidewalk by police, shouting, "We'll take the f***ing street later" (*Hess v Indiana*, 1973); a song about alcohol addiction that ends with, "Suicide is the only way out/ Don't you know what it's really about" (*McCollum v CBS*, 1988); and a magazine article describing auto-erotic asphyxiation, which was followed by a teenager who subsequently suffocated himself (*Herceg v Hustler Magazine, Inc*, 1987).

In order to aid in interpreting the *Brandenburg* standard of advocacy versus teaching, the Supreme Court has outlined several other factors. The court has recognized that it is "the content of the utterance that determines whether it is a protected epithet or an unprotected 'fighting word'" (*Young v American Mini Theatres*, 1976). Somewhat akin to the difference between advocacy and teaching, the court further refined this point by stating that at different times, content might be more properly unprotected than at other points in time (*Young v American Mini Theatres*, 1976). The court used as an example the publication of sailing dates of military fleets. Normally, this speech is protected; however, during times of war, the content is properly regulated because of state interests in maintaining security. This factor recognizes that certain situations call for greater regulation than do others. When this second factor is used in conjunction with the following factors, the *Brandenburg* standard becomes clearer.

The next factor the court has considered is whether the speech teaches the use of, or gives information about, theories or practices that have few legitimate uses. The court has described this type of speech as "speech or writing used as an integral part of conduct in violation of a valid criminal statute" (*Giboney v Empire State Storage & Ice*, 1949). The theory behind this factor is that if a person is teaching a process or advocating the use of tools which are most likely only used for illegal purposes, then that speech should be regulated because of its limited and likely criminal content. A good example of restriction of speech based on this factor is that of a bookmaking program that was not afforded protection under the First Amendment. (Bookmaking is a term of art used to describe the process in which a person [the bookie] determines odds, usually on sporting events, takes bets from gamblers, and pays off on those bets.) In *United States v Mendelsohn* (1990), the defendants sought protection under the Constitution, arguing that their bookmaking software qualified as protected expression. The reviewing court refused to grant an illegal bookmaking program protection, stating that while the program is a form of expression that can be protected, the content is almost only applicable in a criminal setting and, thus, can not be protected:

Although a computer program under other circumstances might warrant First Amendment protection, SOAP [Sports Office Accounting Program] does not. SOAP is too instrumental in and intertwined with the performance of criminal activity to retain First Amendment protection. No First Amendment defense need be permitted when words are more than mere advocacy ... the SOAP computer program was just such an integral and essential part of ongoing criminal activity (*United States v Mendelsohn*, 1990).

Likewise, courts have denied protection to language that "methodically and comprehensively prepares and steels its audience to specific criminal conduct through exhaustively detailed instructions on planning, commission, and concealment of criminal conduct" (*Rice v Paladin Enterprises*, 1997).

Additionally, to whom the speech is made and what sort of marketing accompanied the speech are important factors to consider. The courts have held that First Amendment protection is less likely to be granted when the remarks were intentionally directed at a specific or targeted audience (*Hess v Indiana*, 1973; *Direct Sales v United*

States, 1943; *Watts v United States*, 1969; *Rice v Paladin Enterprises*, 1997). The Supreme Court has held that comments not made to a specific group or individual are more likely to remain protected because the speaker's intent to incite immediate action is not as obvious (*Hess v Indiana*, 1973). Accordingly, the court has held that when a comment or form of speech is directly marketed or targeted at a specific group of listeners, the intent to incite that group into action is more readily identifiable. For example, in *Direct Sales v United States* (1943), the court found that a wholesaler is not allowed First Amendment protections when he knowingly uses high pressure sales techniques and marketing strategies to sell narcotics to customers known to be drug users and distributors. Therefore, "where not only the speaker's dissemination or marketing strategy, but the nature of the speech itself, strongly suggests that the audience both targeted and actually reached is, in actuality, very narrowly confined," the courts have been more willing to restrict the speech aimed at them (*Rice v Paladin Enterprises*, 1997).

Finally, the courts have often looked to the immediacy and proximity that the ultimate crime had to the challenged speech. Generally,

[t]he First Amendment is quite irrelevant if the intent of the actor and the objective meaning of the words used are so close in time and purpose to a substantive evil as to become part of the ultimate crime itself. In those instances, where speech becomes an integral part of the crime, a First Amendment defense is foreclosed even if the prosecution rests on words alone (*United States v Freeman*, 1985).

The closer in time or opportunity that the speech and action in question occur, the more likely a court will be to find an improper connection between the speech and the act. It is important to note one usage of language by the court: When judging the immediacy of an act, imminence is not solely defined by time. Action can be considered immediate in performance despite it being remote in chronological time (*United States v Fleschner*, 1996). Courts have expanded the term "imminent" to include considering the likelihood of an act happening based on speech given the first opportunity to act versus speech as a mere idle threat (*Watts v United States*, 1969).

Therefore, if the speech incites a person to act in the foreseeable future, it will likely be unprotected. The best example of how the courts understand this concept of immediacy is by comparing the incitement of speech with an idle threat. In a string of similar cases, courts have held that people instructing classes on how to falsify tax returns are not protected by the First Amendment (*United States v Kelley*, 1985; *United States v Moss*, 1979; *United States v Freeman*, 1985). Though the classes were removed in time from the actual act of filing false tax returns by many months, the courts found that the speech was imminent enough because "[i]t was no theoretical discussion of non-compliance with laws; action was urged, the advice was heeded, and false forms were filed" (*United States v Kelley*, 1985). Conversely, the Supreme Court held that speech threatening the life of a president contingent on the speaker being drafted was so unlikely to happen that it was only a mere threat (*Watts v United States*, 1969). Thus, immediacy must be measured in chronological time and as a consideration of the likelihood that the speech will be, and is intended to be, acted upon.

Courts have restricted speech that is intended for a specific audience but not made directly to them. Essentially, courts have held that some speech is so intentionally violent and so devoid of social value that it should be prohibited before it can be heard. In *Rice v Paladin Enterprises* (1997), the court limited the protection afforded speech that incites, even if not immediately, a specific, even unknown, listener to violate the law. The speech at issue in *Paladin* is most analogous to the type of speech used by groups and individuals that trade, produce, and distribute child pornography and promote child sexual exploitation.

In *Paladin* (1997), a person purchased a book titled *Hitman: A Technical Manual for Independent Contractors* from Paladin Press. The book provided a detailed and descriptive outline of what to do to kill someone. The book described the weapons to use, methods to bring about death, how to conceal evidence at the crime scene, how to find jobs killing people, and almost every other conceivable step a person could take before, during, and after the commission of a murder for hire. In the underlying criminal case, the purchaser was hired to kill a man's ex-wife and disabled child to collect the child's trust fund. Although the killer was quickly arrested after murdering both victims, the estate of the family brought a civil action against Paladin Press for publishing a book that so methodically and completely described the process of committing murder.

The court found that the language in *Hitman* could not be protected by the First Amendment because it unequivocally and unmistakably meant to instruct and educate the reader on how to commit a murder. The court held that

[t]he First Amendment is quite irrelevant if the intent of the actor and the objective meaning of the words used are so close in time and purpose to a substantive evil as to become part of the ultimate crime itself. In those instances, where speech becomes an integral part of the crime, a First Amendment defense is foreclosed even if the prosecution rests on words alone (*Rice v Paladin Enterprises*, 1997).

The court also held that in addition to the book's language being so closely tied to the encouraged crime, the publisher further created criminal liability by the manner in which it published and distributed the book.

Building on the holdings in *Direct Sales* (1943) (where the court found that the nature of high volume narcotics distribution to a physician in a rural area provided the inference of knowledge and cooperation on behalf of the drug company and a finding of conspiracy to distribute narcotics illegally), the *Paladin* court held that a narrowly tailored subject matter could serve to bind the language completely to the commission of the actual crime. The court held that "[the book] is so narrowly focused in its subject matter and presentation as to be effectively targeted exclusively to criminals" (*Rice v Paladin Enterprises*, 1997). Furthermore, the court held that the marketing of material can affect how much protection it is afforded. As previous courts held, the *Paladin* court found that the marketing of the book was so restricted that a jury could reasonably infer that the publisher practically sought out an exclusive segment of the population that was likely to use the information provided for illegal purposes. In contrast, *Hess v Indiana* (1973) found that the First Amendment protects idle threats that by their nature lack imminence. Similarly, in *Watts v United States* (1969), the court held that the First Amendment protected an idle threat against the President in the context of a political rally, as it lacked the imminence to constitute an illegal act.

In the end, the court refused to give the book First Amendment protection and, thus, found the publisher liable for the crimes committed by readers of the book. The court held that

[t]his book constitutes the archetypal example of speech which, because it methodically and comprehensively prepares and steels its audience to specific criminal conduct through exhaustively detailed instructions on the planning, commission, and concealment of criminal conduct, finds no preserve in the First Amendment (*Rice v Paladin*, 1997).

Therefore, if the content and effect of the speech used by NAMBLA or online sex rings is similar to that used by the publisher of *Hitman*, any examination of language by the courts should be with the same sort of analysis and interpretation as used in the *Paladin* decision.

With the basic constitutional framework established, it is clear that images depicting children engaged in sexually explicit conduct are not protected by the First Amendment. Moreover, language that is used to incite listeners to illegal behavior is also unprotected. Therefore, to the extent that groups like NAMBLA and online sex rings engage in speech that is specifically directed to selected listeners, educating and directing the listeners to sexually exploit children or distribute child pornography, they are in violation of the law. This violation creates a conspiracy between the speaker and the listener. Likewise, by this speech, the speaker may become an accessory to the commission of a criminal offense by a listener. The next 2 sections will discuss how conspiracy and aiding and abetting liability is established through unprotected speech.

A Conspiracy Is Established When One Party Advocates or Provides Instruction or Opportunity to the Coconspirators

18 USCS § 2251 explicitly states that whoever conspires to sexually exploit children receives the same treatment under the law as the coconspirator who actually commits the crime. A conspiracy results when at least 2 people do 3 basic things: (1) they agree (2) to commit an act, and (3) one of the parties makes an overt act furthering that end (18 USCS § 371 [2001]). The defendant does not have to know that the act is illegal, he must merely have agreed to do it and taken a substantial step towards its completion. Therefore, the defense of mistake as to legality is no defense (*United States v Ehrlichman*, 1976). Because of the vast sea of case law interpreting and supporting this idea (*United States v Gibbs*, 1999; *United States v Ehrlichman*, 1976), charging groups like NAMBLA and online sex rings with conspiracy to commit offenses committed by their members may be a successful and effective way to combat the spread of child sexual exploitation.

Conspiracy is an effective charge because it binds all members of the conspiracy (*United States v Fusaro*, 1983), is a separate and distinct crime independent of the crime conspired to commit (*United States v Feola*, 1975; *United States v Edwards*, 1999), and survives regardless of the participation of all parties or of the possibility of the crime actually occurring (*United States v Feola*, 1975). According to *United States v Gibbs* (1999),

[t]o be found guilty of conspiracy, the government must prove that [the defendant] was aware of the object of the conspiracy and that he voluntarily associated himself with it to further its objectives. … Once a conspiracy is shown, evidence connecting a particular defendant to the conspiracy 'need only be slight.' The defendant 'need not be an active participant in every phase of the conspiracy, so long as he is party to the general conspiratorial agreement.'

Moreover, the ultimate scope and depth of potential defendants can be great because there can be multiple conspirators, each with a separate and distinct conspiracy, or with multiple conspirators in one large conspiracy. For example, *United States v Cihak* (1998) found 2 overlapping conspiracies of bank fraud and money laundering. In contrast, *United States v Peterson* (2001) found a single conspiracy with multiple defendants for crimes of mail fraud and money laundering.

Because membership in NAMBLA is restricted and limited and its goals are likewise limited to the promotion and advancement of sexual relations between adult men and minor boys, conspiracy charges can be applied to the organization as a whole for illegal acts committed by individual members (**Table 37-8**). Through the use of newsletters and exclusive, selective membership (membership applications are sent to anonymous PO boxes in San Francisco or New York with checks made out to NAMBLA; memberships are then screened and voted upon by a steering committee whose members' names and identities are kept secret), NAMBLA, and similar types of organizations, have effectively made agreements with each of their paying members to commit various and multiple acts of illegal child sexual exploitation. The information disseminated by the national organization constitutes the overt act furthering the likelihood that a NAMBLA member will exploit a child. In an article in a NAMBLA publication, the authors describe step-by-step procedures on how to evade detection by law enforcement when initiating or continuing a sexual relationship

2 parties working toward the criminal goal (*United States v Baskes*, 1981). Proof of membership in an organization like NAMBLA directly proves agreement, as the only reason to join an organization dedicated to furthering an illegal end is to aid in that task. Furthermore, as discussed earlier, membership in NAMBLA is closely protected and selective; joining NAMBLA is a difficult process. Therefore, membership implies that NAMBLA agreed to accept the individual into its group. Most obviously, the agreement between the individual and NAMBLA would manifest itself in the form of dues paid or proof of membership. Other evidence of agreement might include a newsletter from NAMBLA, letters addressed to NAMBLA by the defendant, or other publications or materials offered by NAMBLA exclusively to its members.

Once the agreement with NAMBLA is established with one defendant, the model can be repeated for every member of NAMBLA. Each member has a separate and distinct conspiracy with the national NAMBLA organization because each member is a separate individual; thus, the proof of conspiracy can be used for each individual member of NAMBLA. This is because separate conspiracies can exist as long as the central conspirator (NAMBLA) conspires with each coconspirator in a way that does not affect the success of any other conspiracy (*United States v Sertich*, 1996). Therefore, because NAMBLA sends information out to each individual member with the intention of the member using that information to exploit children sexually, separate conspiracies can exist because the success of each member is dependent upon the individual acting upon the information from NAMBLA, not on members assisting each other.

Likewise, proof of an agreement between groups like the Wonderland Club or the Orchid Club and its members would require evidence that the individual was trading with other members in a setting that was exclusively reserved for members. Fortunately, like proving membership in NAMBLA, membership in online sex rings is fairly straightforward. All of these groups require their members to post a certain number of child pornography images to join. Therefore, proof that images on the defendant's hard drive were sent by other members could suffice, as would proof that the defendant sent images from his computer to other members. Additionally, members have access to exclusive, password-protected chat rooms in which members trade images with each other. The best evidence of an agreement between members of such a group is evidence that they were in these "members only" rooms. Passwords, chat logs, or Internet site histories on the defendant's computer evidence this. Another form of evidence would be contained on a part of the suspect's hard drive known as the "F-drive" or "F-server." The "F-drive" is merely a part of the hard drive that has been partitioned from the rest of the computer. Other computers are allowed to access that area, and using a File Transfer Protocol (FTP), download or upload files, images, documents, or any other type of data.

THE ILLEGAL ACT AGREED UPON

Conspiracy law is unique in its level of proof because the underlying or target offense plays a relatively minor part in proving the larger charge of conspiracy. In a conspiracy to distribute child pornography via the mail, the target crime is the actual distribution of child pornography via the mail. Case law has held that the target act does not have to be completed (*United States v Feola*, 1975), the parties do not have to be able to complete the act (*United States v Trapilo*, 1997), and the parties need not know that the act is necessarily illegal (*United States v Trapilo*, 1997; *United States v Cangiano*, 1974). The goal of conspiracy law is to

[protect] society from the dangers of concerted criminal activity [through the identification of] an event of sufficient threat to social order to permit imposition of criminal sanctions for agreement alone, plus overt act in pursuit of it, regardless of whether the crime agreed upon actually is committed (*United States v Feola*, 1975).

Therefore, to achieve that goal, the law of conspiracy demands that the parties' specific intent to commit the crime be demonstrated, not the parties' success or even ability to complete the target crime.

A conspiracy survives even if the target act is impossible to complete or remains unfinished (*United States v Trapilo*, 1997). Most recently, the courts have applied this concept to include acts of molestation performed via the Internet. In *United States v Laney* (1999), the defendant, a member of the Orchid Club, was convicted of conspiring to exploit a minor sexually. Two members of the group decided to molest a child live via the Internet for all of the members of the club to observe. Though the defendant possessed a recording of the original Web cast but did not actively participate in the molestation or observe the live broadcast of the crime, he was convicted as a coconspirator.

In affirming his conviction, the court held that the molesters' actions were reasonably foreseeable given the interests of the group and were done to further the group's illegal purpose. Therefore, the court ruled that the defendant was a coconspirator because he was a member of the group. The court refused to consider whether the defendant participated in the molestation or whether it was impossible for him to do so, neither facts were relevant to the culpability of a conspirator. The court's conviction was that the defendant was a member in good standing of the group. In the trial of another member of the Orchid Club, the charge of conspiracy was upheld, even though the defendant did not participate in the molestation of the victim (*United States v Tank*, 2000). As the court in *Laney* (1999) found, the defendant's participation in the group was enough to bind him to the actions of his group members.

These recent rulings follow earlier lines of cases that consistently found it irrelevant whether the defendant and his conspirators could successfully, or even possibly, achieve the act to which they conspired (*United States v Giry*, 1987). The reason courts have been willing to find culpability in conspirators, despite their failure to commit the crime, is because the conspiracy itself raises danger. Thus, the agreement to commit the crime is illegal in and of itself, regardless of the plan's ultimate success (*United States v Crocker*, 1975; *United States v Giry*, 1987; *United States v Senatore*, 1981). Therefore, a conspiracy may exist because the prohibited act of conspiracy occurs at the moment 2 parties agree to commit a crime and form the specific intent to do so, regardless whether a member of NAMBLA molests a child or whether a member of a group like the Orchid Club distributes any child pornography (*United States v Hsu*, 1998).

Along these same lines of reasoning, a party may be a coconspirator even though he does not know the complete or specific plan for completing the illegal act, as long it is proven that he had knowledge of the conspiracy and was participating in it (*United States v Evans*, 1978). As the holding by the *Laney* (1999) court demonstrates in sexual exploitation cases, the participation of a defendant in an online pornography group is enough participation to consider him a coconspirator to all crimes committed by members of that group regardless of the defendant's participation in, or knowledge of, those acts. Because the defendant need not know every detail of the conspiracy, only the general scope of the agreement (*United States v Alvarez*, 1980), courts have expanded liability to include any reasonably foreseeable action taken by any member of the conspiracy (*United States v Mortinson*, 2000). This expansion of liability recognizes that among coconspirators, each conspirator may have a different task to perform independent of the other members, though, they are all working toward the same illicit goal (*United States v Branham*, 1996).

The common thread among all cases that find conspirator liability (despite impossibility, failure of completion, or lack of knowledge of the plans or participants) is that liability is attached as long as the defendant has the specific intent to commit the target crime with his coconspirators (*United States v Haldeman*, 1976). (*United States v Francis* [1999] describes the difference between general and specific intent crimes.) Thus, the conspirator must merely have the intent necessary to commit the crime, regardless of whether he commits it. To establish intent, the government must show beyond a reasonable doubt that the defendant had the intent to commit the conspired crime (*United States v Peterson*, 2001). However, the level of proof required for child pornography requires that the defendant had the intent specifically to exploit children sexually, not just commit an act of sexual exploitation. Because the lack of First Amendment protection for child pornography is dependent upon the images being of minors, the defendant must know the content of the images and that the subjects of the images are underage (*United States v X-Citement Video*, 1994).

In the instant example, there are 2 different crimes of conspiracy: groups such as NAMBLA, which conspire to sexually exploit children through the possession and consumption of child pornography or the encouragement of child exploitation by adults; and groups such as the Orchid Club, which conspire to create, distribute, and possess child pornography. NAMBLA's publications are consistently clear about its intent to promote and legitimize sexual relationships between adult males and minor boys. In one article, the authors first define what child pornography is and how different types of photos may or may not qualify as pornography. They differentiate between the source: "a photo of a naked boy from a boy-love magazine is riskier than one from *National Geographic*." They differentiate between the content: "a photo of a naked boy with legs parted is riskier than one of a naked boy simply standing" (NAMBLA, 1991). The article outlines what form government sting investigations take, how to avoid detection, where to store images, how to describe images so as not to arouse suspicion, and how and when to destroy images. Additionally, in 1986 their spokesman stated, "[w]e do not believe that sex is a bad thing; therefore, we don't believe that visual depictions of sex is a bad thing" (Hechler, 1988).

Likewise, sex rings are explicit in what type of pornography is desired by its members. Most chat rooms that host servers with child pornography have rules that must be read before trading. These rules list desired images, if the room is for traders of child pornography only, and the consequences of posting images that do not comply with the chat room's rules. Failure to follow the rules for posting specified types of pornography can lead to members losing their membership.

THE OVERT ACT TO FURTHER THE ILLEGAL ACT

The final requirement for a conspiracy is that the parties must make an overt act in furtherance of the agreed upon crime. The overt act does not have to be a crime itself; an innocent act can satisfy the overt act requirement as long as it is done in furtherance of the agreement (*United States v Dillman*, 1994). It must only be an act that makes the completion of the conspired act more likely to happen (*United States v Browning*, 1988). The overt act can be done by any of the conspirators but must be done by at least one (*United States v Messerlian*, 1987). Therefore, not all conspirators need to join in the act, and conspirators can join in after the act is done although all present and subsequent coconspirators will be held liable as coconspirators once the act is done (*United States v Bletterman*, 1960). Because only 1 party in the conspiracy needs to perform the act, federal conspiracy law allows 1 member of the conspiracy to be a law enforcement agent without fatally affecting the rest of the conspiracy (*United States v Menotas-Mejia*, 1987). Therefore, as long as the defendant was acting in concert with a person to further the conspiracy, even if that second person joined the conspiracy late or was a law enforcement agent, the defendant can be charged with a conspiracy.

In the context of a group like NAMBLA, the overt act would have to be taken in furtherance of the goal of a member sexually exploiting a child. More likely than not, an officer in NAMBLA is not going to demonstrate how to molest a child; however, the NAMBLA newsletter does provide such information through the means of essays, articles, and other writings that encourage and describe the benefits of engaging in sex with children and point out the potential pitfalls of such relationships (NAMBLA, 1991). Printed under the authority and with the guidance of the national organization, the newsletter is sent to all members of NAMBLA. To get the newsletter, a person must be a current member of NAMBLA; hence, the marketing requirements of *Direct Sales v United States* (1943) are met. Therefore, because distribution and membership is limited and protected, because a person has a newsletter, or claims membership, can serve as the agreement. Additionally, the form of the information is not as relevant as the content; just as *Hitman* and *The Turner Diaries* (MacDonald, 1978) are works of fiction that provide practical, real-world directions for how to break the law (**Table 37-9**), the content of the writings distributed by NAMBLA provide the training, direction, and encouragement to NAMBLA members to engage in sexual activity with boys under the age of majority.

Thus, the contents of the newsletter constitute the overt act. An act merely has to further the goals of the conspiracy (*United States v Bletterman*, 1960); therefore, an act of furnishing information can suffice. Information, like any other criminal tool, can further the likelihood of the commission of the crime; just as providing a crowbar to a person planning a burglary would be an overt act in a conspiracy to break into a building, NAMBLA's overt act of providing information and encouragement to child molesters on how to molest a child serves the same purpose. As will be discussed below, though the information may be offered under the auspices of lobbying to change laws or social advocacy (Hechler, 1988), the actual content of the articles, stories, and essays distributed by NAMBLA serve as a blueprint emboldening men interested in engaging in sexual relationships with children to do so. Just as one of the purposes of *Hitman* was to mentally prepare the defendant to kill a person (*Rice v Paladin Enterprises*, 1997), the materials distributed and promoted by NAMBLA help convince and support the child molester in sexually exploiting a child: "Take the risk, the consequence of the risk, and make the claim: this is something good. Paedophiles need to become more positive and make the claim that paedophilia is an acceptable expression of God's will for love and unity among human beings" (Underwager, 1993).

For example, in one NAMBLA article (1991), there are 5 topic headings: "Relationships between boys and men," "If you are a boy in a relationship with a man," "Pornography," "Dealing with police," and "Your safety as a member of NAMBLA." Within each of these subheadings are tips and pointers on how to actively participate in, and keep secret, a sexual relationship with a child. The article describes how to destroy evidence during a search, how to remain anonymous as a member of the organization, and attempts to offer legal justifications for the group's existence. Like the guidelines and advice given in *Hitman* (*Rice v Paladin*, 1997), the article in NAMBLA gives specific and detailed advice on how to exploit a child sexually and get away with it. This crosses the line from mere advocacy to teaching and instruction and establishes liability.

Table 37-9. *The Turner Diaries*

The Turner Diaries, written by William L. Pierce using the pseudonym "Andrew MacDonald" was written in 1978 and has been recognized as one of the leading sources for political thought and munitions expertise for right-wing militia groups. Timothy McVeigh was an avid reader of the book and the bomb he used in his attack on Oklahoma City was an almost exact replica of the bomb described and detonated in *The Turner Diaries*. Although Pierce was not convicted as a coconspirator, the similarities between his book and McVeigh's attack are striking.

(For more information, see also: Pankratz H. The Turner Diaries. *Denver Post.* June 14, 1997. Available at: http://63.147.65.175/bomb/bombp11.htm. Accessed June 14, 2004.)

The first section is intended for men engaged in, or preparing to engage in, a sexual relationship with a boy. The section first explains the ages of consent in various jurisdictions, as well as what physical acts may or may not be covered by those statutes. Bullet points outline what child molesters should consider when engaging in sexual activity with a boy. Notably, the language used in this part of the article assumes that the reader is, or will be, having sex with a child: "If you decide not to have sex with boys under the age of consent." The first section offers tips and instructions on how to hide an ongoing sexual relationship with a child. The tips outline what to tell the boy being molested, what the man should tell friends who ask about the boy who is around the man, how to end a sexual encounter so the boy does not tell the police, what to tell the boy to say during a police interrogation, and how to proceed legally when investigated or charged with sexual assault or molestation. This section is important in form because it provides information first on the legal considerations of beginning a relationship, how to behave during that period, and what to do at the end when police interaction is likely. This type of advice goes beyond mere advocacy and crosses the line into teaching the victim how to act and teaching the defendant how to cover up all criminal liability.

The second section is addressed to children involved in relationships with men but is clearly written to encourage and protect the illegal activity. The section is addressed to the child; however, it does little more than repeat the previous section's guidelines on what to do if a policeman asks questions about the adult male, if the boy is requested to appear at the police station, and why nobody should be told of the sexual activity. One disturbing difference with this section versus the other 4, and most of the literature reviewed written in support of these types of illegal sexual activities, is the language. The phrases and expressions used in most pro-man/boy literature is that of "relationships," "love," and "friendships" (Underwager, 1993). In contrast, in the section addressed to the child, the language used to describe these same activities is more graphic and crude; relationships are commonly described as "f***ing," bodily fluids described as "cum," and what appears to be an admonition to engage in prohibited sex safely, reduced to its most base form: "No matter who you are having sex with … don't let cum or menstrual blood get in anyone's a**, mouth … or open cuts. If you f**k, use a condom" (NAMBLA, 1991). Based on the content of the information provided, and the language used, this section does little more than reinforce the illegality of the sexual acts by emphasizing the importance of not telling anyone and illustrates the true nature of how NAMBLA views adult males engaging in sex with minors. To the outside world, it is described in terms most people would associate with healthy relationships; when addressing the victim-child, those same acts are described in cruel and demeaning slang.

The third section deals with how to safely collect and, if necessary, destroy child pornography. NAMBLA has previously supported child pornography, and this section expands upon that initial show of support (Hechler, 1988). In this section, NAMBLA defines terms such as erotica and uses them instead of pornography (NAMBLA, 1991). The article tries to differentiate pornography from erotica and offers suggestions on how to obtain child pornography without raising the suspicion of law enforcement. Police investigative techniques are then described, with tips on how to avoid becoming the subject of an undercover sting. Suggestions on how to destroy and conceal evidence is explained in detail so the defendant can decide which method is most practical if needed. This type of information that suggests that evidence of a crime can be destroyed can empower parties to the conspiracy who may have otherwise been hesitant to act out of fear of prosecution.

The fourth section is titled "Dealing with police" and details at length what to do if questioned by police, served with a search warrant, or merely approached by a law enforcement agent. Among the points made are when to ask for a lawyer, what to say to a police officer during questioning, and how to react to requests for information or consent to search. This section, while not explicitly providing ways to hinder an investigation, offers general guidelines that can be used to provide a suspect time to destroy evidence, as suggested in section 3, or discuss interview strategies with a child-victim, as discussed in section 2. Moreover, it creates a sense among NAMBLA members of a community struggling against a common foe, the police. This sense of community only strengthens the members' will to commit acts suggested and described in the NAMBLA newsletter, as well as obstructs justice during investigations.

Finally, NAMBLA's attempts to provide legal disclaimers or justifications explaining why the law protects the contents of the newsletter and why the acts encouraged are legal are an overt act in the conspiracy because they steel the will and determination of the defendant to exploit a child sexually. Throughout its literature and interviews, NAMBLA contests that it is completely legal and doing nothing wrong (NAMBLA, 1991; Hechler, 1988). Additionally, NAMBLA, through its publications and spokesmen, insists that there should be no minimum age of consent and that adult males should be free to engage in sexual relations with children of any age. These 2 arguments, first that NAMBLA, and thus its members, is not engaged in any illegal act, and second that the laws prohibiting adult males engaging in sexual activity with minors are unjust, serve to embolden child molesters to molest actively by reassuring them that they are not alone in their appetites and by appealing to other constitutional or moral sensibilities to encourage them to act.

NAMBLA's materials encourage its members to become sexually engaged with a minor by creating the illusion that many people feel the same way and it is natural and good to act on their sexual urges (Underwager, 1993). NAMBLA creates the sense of community among its members and then reinforces that community with a sense of security and protection as it reminds its members, "the NAMBLA mailing list is private and kept secured. It is never released or shared," and "since the organization was founded in 1979, no one has been prosecuted simply for participation in NAMBLA," and it provides its members with guidelines on what to say or do when questioned by police (NAMBLA, 1991). This sense of safety among members and the common cause uniting members against a society that does not approve of their choices further strengthens the resolve of members engaged in sexual relationships with minors and encourages members to do so if not already. For a person not engaged in such a relationship, but desirous to be so, such a showing of support and acceptance by its members overtly strengthens his will to find a child to exploit.

Additionally, NAMBLA encourages its members to become engaged in sexual relations with minors by appealing to other sensibilities, namely members' First Amendment freedoms to speech and choice. This type of appeal has been held unduly persuasive when used by police to encourage people to engage in sex with minors in undercover stings (*Jacobson v United States*, 1992; *United States v Gamache*, 1998), and in this setting, this type of inducement is just as overly persuasive. In 1986, then-NAMBLA spokesman Robert Rhodes appealed to what he described as political sensibilities and to cultural, historical, and logical ones as well. He asserted that sexual relations between men and boys have been part of society for centuries and the only reason they are not today is because of "an antisexual movement which seeks to arouse by fear and hatred and demagogy all sorts of primordial passions on the subjects of pornography, homosexuality, what's labeled child sexual abuse, and all of those things" (Hechler, 1988).

By couching his argument in those terms, he, and most NAMBLA material, inserted emotional, political, and social influences into the subject of the illegality of child sexual exploitation. In addition to functioning as a tangent to the larger legal argument, those statements build a sense of camaraderie and belonging to the members of NAMBLA who believe it. By imposing the specter of freely exercising freedom of choice or defining love in a new way (Underwager, 1993) on an act that is against the law and prohibited in every state in the union, NAMBLA encourages its members to commit an illegal act for social or constitutional reasons in addition to their sexual desires. Essentially, this sort of language creates further seemingly legal or moral inducements to act in addition to the sense of security, community, or other more purient desires.

Likewise, groups such as the Wonderland Club or the Orchid Club create conspiracy liability by taking the overt step of providing a forum for a select group of people to produce and trade child pornography. Once an individual becomes a member of an online sex ring, that person is given access to a private trading room. In that room, requests for specific types of pornography are entertained; from these requests, child pornography is produced and distributed among the members (*United States v Laney*, 1999). With Web cameras and video streaming technology, live acts of exploitation via the Internet are performed for members, by members, and sometimes with members requesting specific acts during the broadcast. Additionally, discussions about past or future molestations take place; serving to whet the appetite, these discussions create the need and desire for more child exploitation among the members. Although not as formulaic or precise as NAMBLA's members, the amount of knowledge provided to members by other members, as well as creating an environment that makes such behavior possible, serves as the overt act cementing the parties in a conspiracy to commit sexual exploitation.

The Possibility of Withdrawal

Withdrawal from a conspiracy is difficult and not readily accepted by the courts. To withdraw from a conspiracy completely and successfully, a person must take an affirmative step in opposition to the goals of the conspiracy to demonstrate his cessation (*United States v Gypsum Co*, 1978; *United States v Lowell*, 1980). Most commonly, and obviously, this amounts to the individual going to the police and reporting the criminal conspiracy (*United States v Juodakis*, 1987). Courts have been hesitant to recognize any less of a definitive action, holding that mere "hibernation" from criminal activity for several months (*United States v Panebianco*, 1976), frustrating coconspirators' actions without informing the authorities of withdrawal (*United States v Katz*, 1979), or cessation of associating with fellow coconspirators (*United States v DeLeon*, 1981) does not adequately mark withdrawal from a conspiracy. Therefore, failure to pay dues, post pornographic images, or trade or possess child pornography are not acts that properly vitiate a member-defendant from the criminal acts performed by the fellow coconspirators in groups such as NAMBLA or online pornography rings.

CRIMINAL LIABILITY AS AN AIDER AND ABETTOR

In addition to conspiracy liability, groups such as NAMBLA, the Wonderland Club, and the Orchid Club are exposed to liability for being aiders and abettors. The Supreme Court defined aider and abettor as "one who aids, abets, counsels, commands, induces, or procures commission of [an] act is as responsible for that act as if he committed it directly" (*Nye & Nissen v United States*, 1949). Simply stated, the aider or abettor shares the criminal intent of the person committing the crime if he purposefully participates in the activity to ensure the success of the crime (*United States v Jaramillo*, 1995). Because of distinctions between conspiracy and aiding and abetting, courts have held that the crime of aiding and abetting is different from conspiracy (*United States v Segal*, 1988; *United States v Mueller*, 1981; *United States v Phillips*, 1981), but "a conspirator is almost always an aider and abettor" (*United States v Ortega*, 1995; *United States v Corral-Ibarra*, 1994).

Aiding and abetting is distinguishable from conspiracy because the crime in a conspiracy consists of an agreement and intent to commit a crime, in addition to the overt act (*United States v Carson*, 1993). Conversely, an aider and abettor is criminally liable, regardless of whether an agreement was explicitly proven, because the illegal act was actually completed with the aid of the defendant (*Ianelli v United States*, 1975). Furthermore, unlike with a conspiracy, culpability of an aider and abettor is dependent upon the completion of the crime (*United States v Barnett*, 1982). Therefore, because the burden of proof in an aiding and abetting crime is on the completion of the criminal act, rather than on the intention of the parties as in a conspiracy, the importance of proving an agreement is minimized. Whereas in a conspiracy in which proof of an agreement and an overt act are required, in an aiding and abetting case, actions showing a desire for the successful completion of a crime, and the actual completion of the crime, must be demonstrated (*United States v Buttorff*, 1978). Aiding and abetting is a crime based on completed, not intended, criminal action.

The 2 requirements for proving aiding and abetting are completion of a criminal act by someone and the inducement or aiding in that act by another who desires its completion (*United States v Ortega*, 1995). The first requirement is easy to demonstrate: The elements of the target crime were satisfied or they were not. Thus, only the second requirement will be discussed in detail.

Courts have broadly construed the requirement of acting with the desire that the crime be completed. Generally, courts have allowed themselves the freedom to divine the desire for completion from all of the evidence presented, as well as all reasonable inferences that the aider and abettor's actions would lead to the crime's completion (*United States v Jaramillo*, 1995). In addition to judging the aider's actions by the totality of the circumstances and inferences, courts have been willing to find that the aider desired the crime from a showing that the aider knew the criminal nature of the target act and "deliberately render[ed] what he [knew] to be active aid in carrying out the act" (*United States v Ortega*, 1995; *United States v Superior Growers Supply*, 1992).

There are 3 rough divisions of cases concerning aiders and abettors. The first category covers aiders and abettors present during the crime who actively participate in everything but the actual crime. Although mere presence during a crime or mere association with the principal of the crime does not automatically create aider and abettor liability (*United States v Ortega*, 1995), if there is even the slightest form of aid provided by a person, courts are willing to hold that person liable as an aider and abettor. In one case, the court found a defendant guilty who was present at a drug deal but not directly involved in it. The defendant directed the dealer to where the drugs were kept and then stated that the quality of the narcotics were "the best." The court held that the direction to the drugs and vouching for their quality created sufficient inducement to the buyer; thus, he aided in the distribution of narcotics. Likewise, one court found that a defendant was guilty as an aider and abettor to manslaughter because, although he did not actually kill anyone, he was involved in a gunfight in which a federal agent was shot (*United States v Branch*, 1996).

The next type of aiding and abetting cases involves aiders and abettors whose participation is more passive during the commission of the crime but who take some direct action prior to the crime. In one case, the court convicted a defendant of aiding and abetting for driving a drug dealer to the scene of a deal, standing in a room with the drugs during the deal, and carrying a container large enough to carry the drugs after the deal was done (*United States v Jaramillo*, 1995). The court reasoned that although the defendant was not directly involved in the drug deal, providing the transportation and means of removal of the contraband was sufficient enough action to create culpability. These types of aiders and abettors are usually the type found in cases involving the interstate transportation of a minor for sexual activity. Generally, the person transporting the minor across state lines is liable for the actions of the person ultimately engaging in sexual activity with the minor (*United States v Johnson*, 1997; *United States v Sirois*, 1996).

Courts have recognized that defendants who enable a person to commit a crime through encouragement and support can be convicted of aiding and abetting. A defendant was convicted for aiding and abetting another defendant in defrauding the

IRS by failing to file proper currency conversion forms (*United States v Kington*, 1989). The court held that because the aider's encouragement induced the principal to commit the crime and the aider had a financial stake in the fraud, the aider was properly liable. Likewise, defendants who provide promises or conditions as a form of encouragement or inducement are criminally liable as aiders and abettors. In another narcotics case, the court held that a defendant's statements of "I can move 5 kilos [of cocaine]" and "I've got 30 000 in the car right now" (*United States v Woods*, 2000) served as sufficient inducement to a drug dealer to consummate a deal with the defendant's partner.

Finally, aiding and abetting can occur when a defendant provides the principals with information about committing the crime despite the aider and abettor being removed from the actual commission of the crime by time and geography. These cases are the ones that best resemble the facts of potential cases involving NAMBLA or online sex rings. In *Rice v Paladin Enterprises* (1997), the court held that Paladin Press was liable for the information published in the book *Hitman* because the book had no other value than as an aid in a criminal enterprise. Using similar logic, courts have found defendants guilty of aiding and abetting for providing information that counsels and creates the reasonable expectation that a crime will be committed. In *United States v Superior Growers Supply* (1992), the Sixth Circuit held that the defendants could be tried for aiding and abetting because they sold equipment and materials used in the growing of marijuana. The court reasoned that given the nature of the equipment and that they marketed the materials for their drug producing qualities, the defendants had the reasonable expectation that their customers would engage in criminal activity. Likewise, courts have convicted defendants for selling guides on how to manufacture drugs (*United States v Barnett*, 1982), reasoning that

encouraging and counseling another by providing specific information as to how to commit a complex crime does not alone constitute aiding and abetting. If, however, the person so assisted or incited, commits the crime he was encouraged to perpetrate, his counselor is guilty of aiding and abetting (*United States v Barnett*, 1982).

The type of aiding and abetting offered by a defendant removed in time or geography from the crime is directly analogous to the types of charges involving NAMBLA and online sex rings.

Because the elements of proving aiding and abetting require that the defendant act to bring about the completion of the crime, the proof of NAMBLA and online sex rings' liability is almost identical to that of their conspiracy liability. The difference is that their liability is created only when an individual sexually exploits a child. Thus, if an investigation uncovers that a member of NAMBLA has molested a child, then NAMBLA as an organization may be charged with aiding and abetting because it furnished the defendant with information intended to aid the defendant in the criminal act of molestation (*Rice v Paladin*, 1997; *United States v Superior Growers Supply*, 1992; *United States v Barnett*, 1982). Conversely, if a detective conducts a sting by posing as a child on the Internet and convinces a defendant to meet him in anticipation of sexual relations, NAMBLA might be a conspirator to the crime of traveling to exploit a child. However, since the crime did not take place, the organization did not aid in the exploitation of a child.

If an investigation reveals that a members-only chat room is engaged in creating and distributing child pornography, the members would be aiders and abettors because they created the inducement to trade and produce child pornography by creating a private forum dedicated to child pornography. They would not be considered aiders and abettors if only evidence existed of requested, but as yet nonexistent, pornographic images; rather, this type of evidence would suggest conspiracy.

When charging a pornography ring or organization with aiding and abetting, conspiracy charges are not ruled out. Conspiracy is a separate and independent crime

(*United States v Feola*, 1975) and, thus, can be charged in concert with aiding and abetting. Because the crime of conspiracy is a crime of intent, and the crime of aiding and abetting is one of completion, they can be charged together for completed crimes. Additionally, charging defendants with both crimes maximizes the effect of the evidence. Just as the defendants who completed the criminal act show that they intended to complete it, the agreement and planning necessary to prove conspiracy shows that the parties had complete knowledge of the crime committed by the principal. Therefore, when a charge of aiding and abetting is considered, the evidence should be thoroughly examined to determine whether conspiracy counts can also be added.

CONCLUSION

Groups such as NAMBLA and online sex rings such as the Wonderland Club or the Orchid Club expose themselves and their members to conspiracy and aiding and abetting liability because of the speech they engage in and the activities they encourage. The speech used by both types of groups fails to qualify for protection under the First Amendment because the content and impact of it contravenes compelling state interests denying protection to child pornography. The information and services provided by groups such as NAMBLA and online sex rings are done with the sole intention that their members use them to commit crimes of violence against children. Organizations such as NAMBLA and online sex rings incur criminal liability for the actions of their members because the information and services they provide to members serve no legitimate purpose beyond the illegal goal of sexually exploiting children. Finally, the associations created by these groups are not innocent; they exist for the sole purpose of child sexual exploitation. As the technological abilities of child molesters and exploiters evolves, so must the creativity and diligence of law enforcement.

Although standard weapons in a prosecutor's arsenal, conspiracy and aiding and abetting charges can be effective and aggressive options. Both charges can be used separately or together to cast a wide net, ensnaring any and all participants active before, during, and after the commission of the crime.

REFERENCES

Amended Complaint and Jury Demand at Docket No.00cv10956 (D Mass).

Ashcroft v Free Speech Coalition, 535 US 234 (9th Cir 2002).

Beier T, Neely S. Feature-based image metamorphosis. SIGGRAPH 1992 Proceedings. Available at: http://www.hammerhead.com/thad/morph.html. Accessed June 12, 2003.

Brandenburg v Ohio, 395 US 444,447-449 (1969).

Braun v Soldier of Fortune, 968 F2d 1110,1119 (11th Cir 1992).

Broadrick v Oklahoma, 413 US 601,615 (1973).

Central Hudson Gas and Electric v Public Service Commission of New York, 447 US 537,561-571 (1980).

Committee Reports, Senate Report 104-358, Child Pornography Protection Act of 1996, 104 S Rpt 358.

CPPA, Pub.L.No. 104-208 § 1(8), 110 Stat3009-26 to 3009-27 (1996).

Curley v NAMBLA, Docket No. 00cv10956.

Department of Justice. 1997 report on the availability of bombmaking information. Available at: http://www.cybercrime.gov/bombmakinginfo.html. Accessed July 17, 2004.

Direct Sales v United States, 319 US 703,712 (1943).

18 USC § 2251 (2001).

18 USC § 2252 (2001).

18 USC § 2256(8)(C) (2001).

18 USCS § 2251.

18 USCS § 2252 (2001).

18 USCS § 2256.

18 USCS § 371 (2001).

FCC v Pacifica Foundation, 438 US 726 (1978).

Giboney v Empire Storage & Ice, 336 US 490,498 (1949).

Ginsberg v New York, 390 US 629 (1968).

Globe Newspaper Co v Superior Court, 457 US 596 (1982).

Hechler D. *The Battle and the Backlash: The Child Sexual Abuse War*, Lexington, Mass: Lexington Books; 1988:293-299.

Herceg v Hustler Magazine, Inc, 814 F2d 1017,1023 (5th Cir 1987).

Hess v Indiana, 414 US 105,108 (1973).

Ianelli v United States, 420 US 770 (1975).

Jacobson v United States, 503 US 540 (1992).

Lanning KV. Child molesters: a behavioral analysis for law enforcement. In: Hazelwood RR, Burgess AW, eds. *Practical Aspects of Rape Investigation: A Multidisciplinary Approach*, New York, NY: Elsevier Press; 1987.

MacDonald, W. *The Turner Diaries*. 2nd ed. Fort Lee, NJ: Barricade Books Inc; 1978.

McCollum v CBS, 202 Cal. App. 3d 989 (1988).

Miller v California, 413 US 15 (1973).

Mitchell KJ, Finkelhor D, Wolak J. Risk factors for and impact of online sexual solicitation of youth. *JAMA*. 2001;285:3011-3014.

New York Times Co v Sullivan, 376 US 254,270 (1964).

New York v Ferber, 458 US 747 (1982).

North American Man /Boy Love Association. Staying safe and happy as a man/boy lover: guidelines developed by NAMBLA activists for surviving in an insane world. *NAMBLA Bulletin*. October 1991:12(8).

Nye & Nissen v United States, 336 US 613,619 (1949).

Osborne v Ohio, 495 US 103 (1990).

Pankratz H. The Turner Diaries. *Denver Post*. June 14, 1997. Available at: http://63.147.65.175/bomb/bombp11.htm. Accessed September 27, 2001.

Perry v State, 344 Md 204, 233-235 (1996).

Porn ring was real child abuse. *BBC News*. February 13, 2001. Available at: http:/ /news.bbc.co.uk/hi/english/uk/newsid_1168000/1168109.stm. Accessed December 13, 2001.

Prince v Massachusetts, 321 US 158 (1944).

R.A.V. v City of St. Paul, 505 US 377,383-384 (1992).

Rice v Paladin Enterprises, 128 F3d 233,248 (4th Cir 1997).

Shouvlin DP. Preventing the sexual exploitation of children: a model act. *Wake Forest Law Rev.* 1981;17:505-560.

Underwager R. Interview: Hollida Wakefield and Ralph Underwager. *Paidika: J Paedophilia.* 1993;3:2-12.

United States v Acheson, 195 F3d 645,649 (11th Cir 1999).

United States v Alvarez, 610 F2d 1250,1255 (5th Cir 1980).

United States v Andrale, 788 F2d 521 (8th Cir 1986).

United States v Ballard, 663 F2d 534 (5th Cir 1982).

United States v Barnett, 667 F2d 835,841 (9th Cir 1982).

United States v Baskes, 687 F2d 165,169 (7th Cir 1981).

United States v Bletterman, 279 F2d 320 (2nd Cir 1960).

United States v Branch, 91 F3d 699,732 (5th Cir 1996).

United States v Branham, 97 F3d 835,854 (6th Cir 1996).

United States v Browning, 723 F2d 1544 (11th Cir 1988).

United States v Buttorff, 572 F2d 619,623 (8th Cir 1978).

United States v Cangiano, 491 F2d 906 (2nd Cir 1974).

United States v Carson, 9 F3d 576 (7th Cir 1993).

United States v Cihak, 137 F3d 252,257-258 (5th Cir 1998).

United States v Corral-Ibarra, 25 F3d 430,435 (7th Cir 1994).

United States v Crocker, 510 F2d 1129 (10th Cir 1975).

United States v DeLeon, 641 F2d 330 (5th Cir 1981).

United States v Dillman, 15 F3d 384 (5th Cir 1994).

United States v Edelin, 128 F Supp 2d 23,32-33 (DDC 2001).

United States v Edwards, 188 F3d 230 (4th Cir 1999).

United States v Ehrlichman, 546 F2d 910,918 (DC Cir 1976), *cert denied*, 429 US 1120 (1977).

United States v Evans, 572 F2d 455,469 (5th Cir 1978).

United States v Feola, 420 US 671,692 (1975).

United States v Ferber, 966 F Supp 90 (D Mass 1997).

United States v Fleschner, 98 F3d 155,158-160 (4th Cir 1996).

United States v Francis, 164 F3d 120 (2nd Cir 1999).

United States v Freeman, 761 F2d 549 (9th Cir 1985).

United States v Frick, 588 F2d 531,535 (5th Cir 1979), *cert denied*, 441 US 913 (1979).

United States v Fuel, 583 F2d 978,981 (8th Cir 1978).

United States v Fusaro, 708 F2d 17 (1st Cir 1983), *cert denied*, 464 US 1007 (1983).

United States v Gamache, 156 F3d 1,12 (1st Cir 1998).

United States v Gibbs, 182 F3d 408 US (1999) AppLEXIS 36343 (5th Cir 1999).

United States v Giry, 818 F2d 120 (1st Cir 1987), *cert denied*, 484 US 855 (1987).

United States v Grassi, 616 F2d 1295,1301-1302 (5th Cir 1980).

United States v Gypsum Co, 438 US 422 (1978).

United States v Haldeman, 559 F2d 31,113-114 (DC Cir 1976).

United States v Hamilton, 689 F2d 1262,1270 (6th Cir 1982).

United States v Hsu, 155 F3d 189,203-204 (3rd Cir 1998).

United States v Jaramillo, 42 F3d 920,923 (5th Cir 1995).

United States v Johnson, 132 F3d 1279 (9th Cir 1997).

United States v Juodakis, 834 F2d 1099 (1st Cir 1987).

United States v Katz, 601 F2d 66 (2nd Cir 1979).

United States v Kelley, 769 F2d 215,217 (4th Cir 1985).

United States v Kington, 875 F2d 1091 (5th Cir 1989).

United States v Laney, 189 F3d 954,957 (9th Cir 1999).

United States v Lowell, 490 F Supp 897 (D NJ 1980).

United States v Mendelsohn, 896 F2d 1183, 1185 (9th Cir 1990).

United States v Menotas-Mejia, 824 F2d 360 (5th Cir 1987).

United States v Mento, 231 F3d 912 (4th Cir 2000).

United States v Messerlian, 832 F2d 778 (3rd Cir 1987).

United States v Mortinson, 2000 US AppLEXIS 31917, 6-7 (9th Cir 2000).

United States v Moss, 604 F2d 569 (8th Cir 1979).

United States v Mueller, 663 F2d 811 (8th Cir 1981).

United States v Mulherin, 710 F2d 731,738 (11th Cir 1983).

United States v Ortega, 44 F3d 505 (7th Cir 1995).

United States v Panebianco, 543 F2d 447 (2nd Cir 1976).

United States v Peterson, 244 F3d 385 (5th Cir 2001).

United States v Phillips, 664 F2d 971 (5th Cir 1981).

United States v Segal, 852 F2d 1152 (9th Cir 1988).

United States v Senatore, 509 F Supp 1108 (E.D. Pa 1981).

United States v Sertich, 95 F3d 520,525-26 (5th Cir 1996).

United States v Simmons, 679 F2d 1042,1050 (3rd Cir 1982).

United States v Sirois, 87 F3d 34 (2nd Cir 1996).

United States v Superior Growers Supply, 982 F2d 173 (6th Cir 1992).

United States v Tank, 200 F3d 627,629-630 (9th Cir 2000).

United States v Trapilo, 130 F3d 547 (2nd Cir 1997).

United States v Travis, 993 F2d 1316 (8th Cir 1993).

United States v United States Gypsum Co, 438 US 422 (1978).

United States v Woods, 210 F3d 70,78 (1st Cir 2000).

United States v X-Citement Video, 513 US 64,78 (1994).

Watts v United States, 394 US 705,707-708 (1969).

Wickedness in wonderland. *BBC News.* February 13, 2001. Available at: http://news.bbc.co.uk/hi/english/uk/newsid_1167000/1167879.stm. Accessed December 13, 2001.

Yates v United States, 354 US 298,321-322 (1956).

Young v American Mini Theatres, 427 US 50,66 (1976).

Chapter 38

THE HIDDEN TRUTH OF INVOLUNTARY SERVITUDE AND SLAVERY

Bharathi A. Venkatraman, Esq
Sp Agt Eileen R. Jacob
Sp Agt Donald B. Henley

Involuntary servitude and slavery, also known as **human trafficking**, is an often-discussed but little understood crime. Unlike trafficking in drugs or arms, human trafficking requires no movement, no selling, and no mass shipment. Unlike the slavery of a bygone era, modern-day slavery does not necessarily involve beatings, whippings, and physical torture. Human trafficking only requires breaking the will of a victim no matter what race, creed, color, age, or nationality to obtain labor or services. Human trafficking can involve the abuse of young women from Eastern Europe for commercial sex, child domestic workers from Western Africa for household labor, East Asian sweatshop workers for the manufacture of garments, and African-American agricultural workers for harvesting crops. All of these examples are drawn from real-life cases that have been investigated and prosecuted by the United States government as modern-day slavery. These facts recur in varying permutations throughout the United States and victimize Americans and foreigners, as well as the old and young. Though human trafficking is an "equal opportunity crime," all slavery involves preying on the weak and vulnerable elements of society. In human trafficking crimes, these weak and vulnerable elements are often children and women. In many cases, the victims are illiterate, unable to speak English, and the product of impoverished and desperate circumstances. Victims become enslaved precisely because their will can be broken, and their compliance can easily be achieved. Because of their helplessness and suggestibility, children are often targets of such crimes.

Human trafficking is not a small problem confined to the "gateway cities." Sadly, modern-day slavery is a persistent occurrence in the United States and worldwide. While estimates vary considerably, some indicate that up to a million people are trafficked annually within or across national borders, and thousands of potential victims are trafficked in the United States every year (deBaca & Tisi, 2002). Trafficking is not just a "big city problem" as indicated by the numerous human trafficking investigations initiated nationwide, from Idaho and Oklahoma to Alaska and New Hampshire. In fact, as of this writing, the Justice Department has not opened a trafficking investigation in only Delaware, Maine, Rhode Island, South Dakota, and Wyoming.

Despite the frequency of the crime, human trafficking operations and the individuals they victimize largely remain underground. Victims are often concealed from sight, in places such as private homes and the back rooms of seemingly legitimate businesses. Alternatively, victims are overseen by guards who monitor their movements and contacts. Such factors, coupled with a fear of law enforcement officials and/or retaliation by the trafficker, contribute to the virtual invisibility of this victimized population.

Even in the face of such obstacles, the United States government has made substantial progress in uncovering human trafficking offenses, combating the crime, and protecting victims. The United States Congress passed the Trafficking Victims Protection Act in October 2000, thereby adding a powerful set of new statutory tools to the legal arsenal. In addition to new statutes, the Act provides extensively for victim needs. According to the US Department of Justice (USDOJ), Civil Rights Division (2004a), in the 3 fiscal years since the passage of the Act, the Justice Department opened 210 new investigations, charged approximately 113 traffickers, and obtained guilty pleas from 77 defendants. These figures represent a substantial increase over the previous 3-year period, revealing a 100% increase in new investigations, a 300% increase in indicted cases, and a 50% increase in guilty pleas. With respect to sex trafficking, 79 defendants out of the 113 charged traffickers were indicted for sex trafficking crimes, and 59 defendants entered guilty pleas to sex trafficking charges over the 3 fiscal years since passage of the Act. These are the highest figures ever obtained for investigation and prosecution of sex trafficking crimes on the federal level (USDOJ, Civil Rights Division, 2004a).

Though such advances are impressive, complete eradication of modern-day slavery will occur only when first responders (police, paramedics, emergency room personnel, or good Samaritans) learn to spot the crime and get help. Through this chapter, the authors, who are all federal law enforcement personnel involved in investigating and prosecuting human trafficking offences, will introduce readers to the crime and its various manifestations by painting a realistic picture of an unfolding investigation. The example below is a fictional account but is, in many respects, typical of trafficking crimes that occur throughout the world. The story is one example of the way human trafficking can occur. Readers are encouraged to think "outside the box," given the various guises a trafficking situation can assume and the various professionals likely to encounter the crime.

THE CRIME SCENE

One summer morning many years ago, 18-year-old CS came home to her apartment in a large northeastern city and was confronted by what she described as a horrifying sight. Her 16-year-old roommate, LY, was lying unconscious in the stairwell leading to their apartment unit. Describing herself as "stunned," CS recollected that she somehow managed to stumble up to her unit for a cup of cold water to douse on the girl's face. CS knew she needed to seek help but did not know how since she was a poor, uneducated, illiterate, young woman from another country who lacked English skills. She called the only people she knew in America, her colleagues from a grocery store in the city, for assistance. Her colleagues arrived, but instead of calling emergency medical services, they took LY's body out to the alley behind the building. The workers' attempt at a stealthy exit failed when an apartment resident looked out her window and noticed the strange sight in the alley. The alarmed resident called the city police, who, along with paramedics, responded immediately. The police officers became suspicious when they learned that CS and LY spoke little or no English and lived alone and unsupervised. The explanations provided by various witnesses that the younger girl's parents lived in a different part of the apartment complex did not ring true. Likewise, 18-year-old CS's claims that she was married to a fellow grocery store employee but did not live with him struck the police officers as bizarre. Despite the heroic efforts of emergency personnel, LY died. The ensuing police investigation eventually morphed into an intensive federal investigation with participation by the Federal Bureau of Investigation (FBI), Bureau of Immigration and Customs Enforcement (ICE, formerly known as the Immigration and Naturalization Service [INS]), US Department of Labor (USDOL), Internal Revenue Service (IRS), the US Attorney's Office, and the Civil Rights Division of the USDOJ. The investigation revealed that the young girl died of a one-time asthmatic episode. Although there was no criminal cause for the child's death, the investigation of this tragedy led to a surprising and disturbing revelation—the deceased girl and her young roommate were among 25 teenaged, sexual abuse victims of a prominent and wealthy local businessman, 75-year-old John Smith.

BACKGROUND: THE STORY BEHIND A GRUESOME DISCOVERY

Smith, the businessman in question, owned a number of businesses in the city. His holdings included grocery stores, gas stations, convenience stores, parking garages, and slum real estate. He was a tycoon with an estimated net worth in the hundreds of millions of dollars. Although Smith came from humble beginnings in a foreign country, he managed to pursue higher education in the United States and discovered an aptitude for business. Smith worked for several import/export businesses after graduation, which earned him business trips to his home country and, eventually, a green card and citizenship. Smith's paychecks went toward the slow and steady acquisition of profitable grocery stores and other business investments, which led him to amass his own business empire.

Smith staffed his businesses by facilitating the illegal immigration of his native townsfolk. He initiated this scheme to obtain a cheap labor force for his businesses decades before. Few people in Smith's hometown had a college education or financial stability, so Smith's educational achievements and economic success in the United States commanded the awe and respect of his hometown neighbors. Smith capitalized on their admiration and poverty. By visiting his foreign hometown regularly, wearing fancy clothing and spending money that he often did not have in the early years, Smith created an impression that left his hometown neighbors envious and eager to replicate his success. Many townspeople sought Smith's patronage to help them start life over in the United States, and he often agreed.

Despite his apparent philanthropy, Smith had a dark side. He required his hometown beneficiaries to abide by some stringent conditions. He would help them fraudulently immigrate to the United States and meet their housing, food, and other miscellaneous needs, provided they worked for his businesses for several years. Smith's targets, many of whom were destitute people on the economic fringes, readily agreed to Smith's conditions given the distant promise of permanent residence and substantial earning potential in the United States. After their illegal entry into the United States was achieved, many of these workers were at Smith's mercy. They received little, if any, pay. They worked long hours and were on their feet all day without sufficient breaks. They lived in squalid properties owned by Smith. They usually ate dated food from Smith's supermarkets, whether they wanted to or not. In addition, they were generally required to do Smith's bidding. Many did not have health insurance or the opportunity to consult with physicians, lest their illegal status be discovered. The workers were required to answer to Smith and his higher level associates. Over time, Smith's strategy paid off. He amassed a veritable fortune that enabled him to buy more businesses, which in turn served to reinforce the power and influence he enjoyed in his homeland.

Smith's exploits were not limited to immigration fraud and unfair labor practices. Witnesses eventually revealed that Smith displayed a penchant for young, pubescent girls. In his native country and the United States, Smith engaged in sex with young girls and women. According to various victims and witnesses, Smith typically visited his native town several times a year. He often spotted girls at schools and in markets during these visits and pointed out the girls he liked to his accompanying entourage. His employees used various tactics to lure the chosen girls back to Smith's villa on the outskirts of the town. Often, Smith's power and influence drove victims and their family members to comply since they felt that they had no choice. On occasion, Smith successfully pacified protesting parents with assurances that their daughters would eventually go to the United States and have opportunities for a better life. Typically, a victim's will was broken after several unwelcome sexual encounters, and she would ultimately relent to Smith's advances. According to witnesses, many of Smith's associates and employees (eg, the groundskeeper, butler, cook, office manager) lived on the estate surrounding Smith's villa and knew of his exploits; however, on account of Smith's power, and perhaps out of a sense of loyalty, workers kept his confidences and did not, by and large, attempt to stop him.

Several of the young abuse victims lived on Smith's foreign estate and performed odd chores, such as laundry or kitchen work, even though they had family in the area. Feeling ashamed and fearful, girls often chose to remain at the estate rather than go home to their parents when opportunities arose. Parents who sought their daughters' return occasionally turned to the police for help. However, the police often turned a blind eye due, at least in part, to Smith's ability to buy police cooperation. Despite some freedom of movement, girls who were rumored to be involved with other men in relationships unsanctioned by Smith were strictly disciplined. These girls were verbally abused, occasionally subjected to rough sex or other physical discipline, and generally ostracized. This treatment resulted in suicide attempts and depression on the part of some of the young victims.

Occasionally, Smith would bring some of his young sex victims to the United States through an elaborate immigration fraud scheme. The scheme involved 1 of 2 pretexts:

1. Smith claimed native townsfolk as fake relatives or dependents.

2. Smith sponsored individuals to come to the United States under the pretext of temporary employment visas.

Smith easily obtained these employment visas because of his established and profitable businesses in the United States. He required his sponsored townsfolk to claim the young sex victims as their dependent children, thereby manipulating existing family immigration provisions with the purpose of continuing his perverse sexual activities in the United States. Smith regularly cobbled together fraudulent families and concocted false names to effectuate this scheme. In almost every case, the sponsored workers were not related to the children they claimed on paper as their own.

So it was that the young LY came to the United States. A Smith acquaintance, Matthew, who was down on his luck and studying at a vocational academy established by Smith in his native town, repeatedly asked Smith to facilitate his immigration to the United States so he could help his family get out of debt. Matthew had a wife and children, as well as an extended family of parents, in-laws, and siblings. Smith agreed to Matthew's requests and offered to sponsor Matthew as an office manager in the United States. Smith did so by falsely claiming Matthew as one of his key managers abroad, who also possessed the necessary foreign language skills and influence to manage Smith's workforce in the United States. However, Smith conditioned his offer on Matthew's willingness to claim LY as his dependent daughter even though Matthew was unrelated to the young girl. Instead of bringing Matthew's true wife into the United States to pose as LY's mother, Smith instead chose to designate an older sex victim, Rachel, to round out the "family."

Matthew was the first member of the sham family to arrive in the United States. Once in the United States, Matthew expected to work as an office manager, as was represented on the visa application; however, Smith rarely employed sponsored workers in the manner represented. Matthew was no exception to this rule. When Matthew learned that he would be bagging groceries in lieu of the promised office job, he expressed surprise and politely suggested that he work in one of Smith's offices. Smith swiftly reminded Matthew that his wife and children remained back home and that their welfare was in Matthew's hands. Interpreting Smith's response as a threat, Matthew reluctantly and resentfully accepted the bagging position.

Like many of his colleagues, Matthew worked 12-hour shifts without breaks and ate rotten food from the supermarket. All the workers, including Matthew, were transported back and forth from their shared apartments to various grocery stores. Occasionally, workers would wait hours after finishing their shifts to return home because were forbidden to leave unaccompanied. Smith exercised complete control over the lives and daily routine followed by Matthew and his colleagues. Smith or his associates dictated where the workers lived, with whom they lived, whether they could eat, what they could eat, and the people with whom they could associate. Matthew and the others rarely had social contact with individuals outside of Smith's organization. Despite their long hours and horrid working conditions, Matthew and the others were seldom, if ever, paid, and they were prevented from coming near the cash registers. Whenever Matthew and his colleagues questioned these practices, Smith and his associates reasoned that workers' salaries were adjusted for the cost of their plane tickets, visa application fees, food, and housing expenses that they incurred. Once workers began earning a positive balance after paying off such "debts," they would receive their paychecks. Often, like Matthew, other protesting workers were rebuffed with reminders that they should think of their families back home, a response the workers found threatening given Smith's power and influence.

Several months after Matthew's arrival, Matthew's fake wife, Rachel, arrived with LY, whom she did not know, but was required to claim as her daughter. LY and Rachel joined the dozens of sex trafficking and labor victims in Smith's scheme, including Matthew and CS, who worked day and night unpacking produce, bagging groceries, or cleaning stores. Within months of their arrival, the asthma attack claimed LY's life.

Smith's stores were frequented by students, physicians, lawyers, and other affluent and well-educated members of the community. Young sex victims labored in the stores, but their youthful looks did not drive patrons to ask difficult questions. Likewise, Smith's loud and threatening overseers often publicly raised their voices at the girls (albeit in a foreign language), yet no one questioned such intimidating conduct. The silence of the larger community conspired with the guarded, cautious, and secretive attitude adopted by Smith's tightly knit, ethnic community to create a seemingly unsolvable puzzle for investigators.

INVESTIGATING THE CRIME
THE WISDOM OF A TEAM APPROACH

Uncovering the extent of Smith's criminal activities was a work-intensive and personnel-intensive endeavor lasting years. The investigation into Smith's actions was staffed by a multitude of agencies, including, but not limited to, the city police department, INS (now ICE), the US Attorney's Office, USDOJ Civil Rights Division, FBI, IRS, USDOL, and the local prosecuting authority. Nongovernmental organizations (NGOs) and private attorneys including immigrants' rights activists, ethnic organizations, and womens' groups, also played a role.

Each agency made a unique contribution to the investigation. INS, the only agency with jurisdiction to handle immigration matters, investigated the extent of Smith's immigration fraud. Agents of the INS single-handedly unraveled the complex web of false relationships and identities that beset the investigation by combing ethnic enclaves in the United States to find ex-Smith employees who came into the United States fraudulently. Similarly, agents traveled to Smith's homeland to conduct a vital overseas investigation and provide witnesses safe passage to the United States. The INS investigators determined that Smith had filed a number of false visa petitions himself by conducting handwriting exemplars on critical documents, such as visa applications.

The FBI assisted in 3 major ways. One FBI agent assigned to the investigation was an expert in interviewing minor victims of sexual abuse and managed to elicit key incriminating information from several young and traumatized victims. A second FBI agent collected and condensed reams of documents, reports of investigations, and boxes of evidence into a coherent and user-friendly guide. A third agent, working out of the US Embassy in Smith's home country, found several sex abuse victims who were smuggled out of the United States and back to their native country when the charges against Smith first broke; he personally escorted these victims back to the United States.

The city police department was instrumental in acquiring intelligence from key players on the street. Two city officers gained the trust of knowledgeable witnesses and cultivated confidential informants. These officers remained in constant communication with informants, as well as other members of the community who eventually trusted the police officers and provided them with critical information. Some of the most crucial witnesses developed in the case were procured through the efforts of the local police officers.

The 2 prosecutors on the case brought different, but equally important, strengths to the effort. The US Attorney's Office proved to be the staging ground for this massive effort with an Assistant US Attorney (AUSA) assigned to the case. Working with him was a trial attorney from the Civil Rights Division in Washington, DC. While the AUSA served as the programmatic overseer, the Civil Rights Division attorney was the prosecutor most involved with the "nuts and bolts" of evidence collection and the daily operations of the team.

The Civil Rights Division specifically worked with the prosecution of involuntary servitude, slavery, and trafficking. As a result, its prosecutor focused on developing evidence of these crimes. In an effort to fulfill his mission, the prosecutor relocated for several years to the northeastern city where the investigation was underway. This Civil Rights prosecutor provided strategic counsel and insights that informed the team's approach in questioning witnesses and determining what evidence could be realistically retrieved from abroad. He participated with the agents in almost every victim interview and many other witness interviews, stayed up late at night to contact and interview witnesses abroad, and made an investigative visit overseas to track down critical government documents filed by Smith and his associates.

Other team members included agents of the IRS and the USDOL. The IRS agents confirmed that Smith failed to issue paychecks or withhold taxes for claimed employees. The USDOL agents investigated Smith's wage and hour abuses.

NGOs played a pivotal role in attending to the victims' extensive needs. From completing the victims' lawful immigration applications and maintaining contact with the victims' family members in their native country, to helping the victims learn English, find employment, and navigate their way through the city, these NGOs proved to be the victims' lifeline by taking over the victims' care and sustenance from the Smith family. Beyond the ethnic and women's groups caring for the victims, volunteer attorneys protected victims' rights and interests, including their immigration and financial status. They protected the victims from incurring criminal liability and played an important role in preparing victims to cooperate with the federal investigation.

The different members of the team used their individual expertise to strengthen the group effort. For example, in the wake of Smith's arrest, a city police officer determined through street intelligence that Smith arranged for several of the sex victims to leave the United States so that these girls could evade investigative questioning. Upon learning this information from the police officer, INS officials examined passenger manifests and other travel data to pinpoint the approximate dates of travel and the destination cities. The lead FBI agent coordinated interviews with the cooperating victims and witnesses in the United States to locate the whereabouts of those victims who had fled. After questioning cooperating witnesses regarding telephone numbers (whenever available) and other contact information to locate the absconders, the lead INS and FBI agents telephoned the absconded witnesses to secure their cooperation. Then the team worked to establish a plan for those who had fled to meet an American agent in their country so they could be safely escorted back to the United States.

THE FIRST BREAKS

The first obstacle confronting the team was determining what crimes were committed. Clearly, the apartment dweller who looked out her window to see grocery workers carrying LY's body in the alley was justified in suspecting that something was wrong. But what exactly was it? How were investigators to determine whether this was a murder investigation, an immigration fraud case, a case of child abuse and neglect, or something else?

The fact that the 2 young girls were living alone and without supervision or a lifeline to the English-speaking world seemed suspicious. Although the girls lived in a lower-income neighborhood, their rent would have been unaffordable if solely financed by their grocery store jobs. As a result, the police officers pursued evidence relating to the girls' living arrangements. These officers attempted to interview witnesses on the scene and at the hospital regarding the young roommates' living situation and the whereabouts of their parents. However, their efforts were frustrated by Smith's associates who insisted on answering the officers' questions on behalf of the workers and giving the excuse that the workers did not speak English. Tipped off by this odd behavior, the police officers called INS to run some checks.

The INS investigators began to participate with the city police officers in questioning CS, Matthew, and Rachel. These 2 sets of investigators worked together to determine that the fake couple knew little about their purported (and now deceased) daughter, LY. Uncharacteristic of grieving parents, they displayed little emotion in connection with LY's death.

In the midst of these witness interviews, the agents received an anonymous telephone call captured on tape, which was presumably from a disgruntled Smith associate. This telephone call, which was in broken English, exposed the complex network of false relationships that Smith used to staff his businesses. Investigators eventually began to focus their questions around the specific information provided in the telephone call, which proved to contain accurate and important facts regarding the identities, whereabouts, and true names of individuals fraudulently smuggled into the United States over the years. The anonymous caller's information included details about the sex victims.

Matthew was the first to "break." He confessed that Smith had masterminded a vast immigration fraud scheme. Matthew advised that he, Rachel, and CS had been coached by Smith and Smith's associates to provide evasive or false answers to investigators' questions. During this interview with Matthew, investigators discovered that Smith had completed Matthew's fraudulent visa paperwork by hand himself. As such, Smith's carefully constructed, decades-long immigration fraud was exposed in part by his own carelessness: Matthew's information enabled agents to obtain handwriting samples from Smith, which confirmed that Smith had personally completed numerous, false applications by hand. Smith had thus been caught red-handed.

This evidence resulted in forced labor, immigration fraud, and obstruction of justice charges being filed against Smith, and several obstruction and tampering charges against Smith's associates. After Smith was arrested on these charges, the evidence began to mount. No longer were community members convinced that Smith was untouchable. They began to worry that they would be implicated for lack of cooperation with the government or that they would be arrested for immigrating to the United States illegally under Smith's scheme.

CS and Rachel, who had been arrested by the INS for their attempts to cover up the immigration fraud (per Smith's instructions), began to follow Matthew's example and cooperate with authorities, resulting in their release from detention. CS and Rachel implicated Smith in illicit sexual activity, which countered their initial denials. CS confirmed that she did not want to be sexually involved with Smith and that Smith had raped her during her childhood, which taught her to comply or face physical punishment for failure to cooperate. CS now "tolerated" sex with Smith out of habit and fear, as well as out of the hope that her liaison with Smith would one day result in a good job through which she could support and help her family back home. Once she arrived in the United States and realized that she would not be paid, CS tried to leave Smith's organization by surreptitiously speaking with townspeople who had successfully left Smith's businesses in favor of other work, but Smith learned of CS's efforts and threatened her with deportation for disobeying him. CS feared deportation because she knew that the police and Smith's associates in her native country would sexually abuse her and generally ostracize her and her family if she were sent back. She also feared that her parents would be evicted from their small, thatched-roof home on Smith's estate.

Rachel provided significant, circumstantial corroboration of CS's account since Rachel had seen Smith inappropriately touch CS, LY, and other young girls in his company. Rachel reported several instances, primarily at the grocery stores, in which she saw Smith lightly brushing girls' thighs, breasts, and buttocks during his oversight visits. She presumed that some of these instances led to sexual encounters between Smith and the girls since she noticed that the girls he touched would follow him into his store office and return from the office shortly thereafter looking disheveled. Rachel did not know what went on inside the office since 2 or 3 men would typically stand outside the office in an effort to discourage others from eavesdropping. Rachel could provide little insight into LY's dealings with Smith, and though she represented herself to be LY's mother, they were not close. Rachel recounted her own sexual victimization at Smith's hands when she was a child in their native town; however, she noted that Smith lost interest in her when she grew up. She claimed that she and Smith had not been sexually involved since she had arrived in the United States with LY.

The investigative team moved the 3 cooperating witnesses (Matthew, CS, and Rachel) to a nearby, undisclosed location outside of the city where they could live, work, and meet with investigators without attracting too much attention from their tightly knit ethnic community. A number of social service groups came forward to represent the interests of these 3 witnesses, which helped to ease the transition to their new environment. Eventually, word spread among other victims and witnesses within the city that Matthew, CS, and Rachel were cooperating with the investigation without negative repercussions. This resulted in a domino effect.

Thus, an investigation that initially focused on murder charges grew into an immigration fraud, rape, and obstruction of justice investigation. As witnesses began to come forward with facts supporting an unholy picture of Smith and his associations with young girls and women, word of Smith's exploits began to leak to the press.

Hiccups

Despite the momentum gained by Smith's arrest and the cooperation of numerous victims and witnesses, the complications for the investigation and prosecution team were just beginning. Interviews with cooperating victims and witnesses in the United States revealed that a number of young victims had returned to their native country and then scattered. The team felt the need to make contact with these victims given the possibility that these victims could be influenced, further intimidated, or in danger.

Complicating the agents' efforts to make contact with these victims was that the local police in Smith's native town were hardly cooperative. In fact, certain officers seemed determined to protect Smith and tip off his local associates to the arrival of the US agents. As a result, the agents were thwarted by their local "partners" in the investigative effort.

The local police officers in Smith's native town began harassing the victims' family members by raiding their homes in the middle of the night, seizing their passports, threatening them, and generally intimidating witnesses who were otherwise pre-disposed to cooperate with the US investigative effort. Perhaps because of the heavy-handed approach used by the town's police officers to ensure that victims in their township did not attempt to contact or cooperate with US investigators, the victims who had left the United States eventually came forward of their own accord. In addition, a close Smith associate, who did not cooperate with the US investigative efforts though he was reportedly critical of Smith's behavior, had his house set on fire by unidentified arsonists. All of these events conspired to cause deep-seated fear among the people of the town that refusing to cooperate with US agents was no insurance policy against harm. The tide began to turn, and witnesses began seeking US patronage and protection when their local authorities failed to protect them.

THE END RESULT: SHEER DETERMINATION AND A LOT OF LUCK

With the domino effect of victims and witnesses coming forward in the United States and abroad, the team eventually crafted a multi-count indictment, which implicated Smith and his associates. Among the statutes charged were forced labor (18 USC § 1589), immigration fraud conspiracy (18 USC § 371), harboring illegal aliens (8 USC § 1324(a)(1)(A)(iii)), transportation of minors for illegal sexual activity (18 USC § 2423(a)),* child sex tourism (18 USC § 2423(b)),* illegal importation for immoral purposes (8 USC § 1328), false statements to federal law enforcement (18 USC § 1001), and tampering with witnesses and obstruction of justice (18 USC § 1512(b)(3)). These charges were supplemented by various tax violations.

Ultimately, Smith pled guilty to various offenses when he realized that multiple witnesses were prepared to come forward and expose his exploits. In considering the proper disposition of this case, the prosecution team weighed factors such as the possibility that the vulnerable victims would be retraumatized during a trial. Smith's convictions on multiple felony counts after his guilty plea involved immigration, transportation for illicit sex, obstruction of justice, and other charges. Smith's associates pled guilty to lesser immigration charges. Smith is expected to spend the rest of his life in prison.

HOW TO DETERMINE WHETHER YOUR CASE IS A TRAFFICKING CASE

THE IMPORTANCE OF IDENTIFYING THE CRIME

Trafficking offenses masquerade as other crimes. Vice, domestic violence, immigration offenses, and other types of criminal activity provide the context for unearthing trafficking crimes. Investigators and prosecutors occasionally encounter situations in which a victim's neighbor calls the police after hearing screams and violent noises coming from the victim's home. Once law enforcement officials respond, the crime is investigated as a domestic violence offense, when, in fact, the situation involved a human trafficking violation (eg, a pimp who is beating an unwilling victim to force her to engage in prostitution).

In a case recently prosecuted by the USDOJ Civil Rights Division, a local sheriff who was looking for a missing child in a wooded area happened upon a beaten and bloody yet alive African-American trafficking victim instead. This victim, a fruit-picker, was beaten by his employer for seeking new employment after he had complained about the employer's practices of paying him in crack rather than in cash.

Trafficking is a crime wherein a victim's will is overborne by force, fraud, coercion, or some other threatened harm such that the victim believes that he or she has no choice but to perform the labor or services demanded by the trafficker. Though many trafficking victims are foreign-born, trafficking does not necessarily involve move-

---

* *Both offenses listed under 18 USC § 2423 are known as* Mann Act *offenses.*

ment or transportation of a victim from one point to another. A victim can be born, bred, and enslaved in a single location.

It is important to identify a trafficking or servitude crime for what it is, rather than allow this crime to be classified otherwise. One reason for ensuring the proper identification of trafficking crimes relates to the specialized assistance that victims of trafficking receive. The Trafficking Victims' Protection Act (TVPA) of 2000 considers trafficking victims to be victims of a violent crime; therefore, these victims are a breed apart from victims and witnesses in immigration and other cases. In trafficking cases, victims are often brainwashed by the trafficker into believing that US law enforcement officials will behave in a punitive manner. Some past investigations and cases unfortunately reveal that traffickers may have been justified in warning their victims about the danger of detection by US authorities. Before the passage of the TVPA, victims were occasionally placed in immigration detention while the authorities attempted to find suitable housing and financial assistance to meet the victims' needs. Alternatively, in situations where victims simply lied or attempted to mislead investigators, they risked exposure to criminal liability and/or administrative action by the immigration courts. With the "special victim status" conferred by the TVPA, qualified individuals are streamlined through government channels to receive immigration benefits, psychological counseling, employment authorization and training, housing and food assistance, medical care, and other benefits. These benefits can be crucial to establishing rapport and trust with the victim and to countering negative propaganda about the insensitivity of US law enforcement officials. Such benefits are not tied to the successful prosecution of a case; victims can access temporary immigration, healthcare, employment, and other benefits even while the investigation is pending. Information about such benefits is available through the Victim Witness Specialist at the USDOJ Civil Rights Division, Criminal Section in Washington, DC, and through Victim-Witness Coordinators at FBI, ICE, and US Attorneys' offices nationwide.

Besides specialized relief provisions for trafficking victims, other compelling reasons call for the proper identification of trafficking crimes. One such reason is that trafficking offenders are punished more stringently than immigration violators or domestic batterers. For example, in January 2004, the lead defendant in the unreported case *United States v Soto* (a sex trafficking case prosecuted by the USDOJ Civil Rights Division and the US Attorney's Office for the Southern District of Texas) was sentenced to 23 years in federal prison. The defendant was the leader of a sex-slave ring near the United States/Mexico border that held women against their will, raped them, and forced them to work without pay. Similarly, in August 2003, 2 female defendants in the unreported case *United States v Jimenez-Calderon* (a sex trafficking in juveniles case prosecuted by the Civil Rights Division and the US Attorney's Office in New Jersey) were sentenced to more than 17 years in prison after their convictions on federal conspiracy and sex trafficking charges. These female defendants supervised young Mexican trafficking victims who were lured into the United States under false pretenses and then forced into prostitution through threats of physical violence. Both cases could have easily been prosecuted as other crimes—the former as an immigrant-smuggling case and the latter as a prostitution case; however, since both cases were prosecuted as trafficking crimes, the defendants received swift and severe punishments. Subject to the application of the Federal Sentencing Guidelines, most trafficking offenses carry a maximum statutory penalty of 20 years imprisonment and, in the case of certain juvenile sex trafficking victims, the maximum term of imprisonment is life.

Finally, the TVPA requires defendants who are convicted of trafficking crimes to pay mandatory restitution to their victims. Such restitution can provide victims with the necessary support they need to piece their lives together. The Smith case illustrates the poverty that drives many trafficking victims into unsavory situations, and financial restitution may enable victims to attain some degree of self-sufficiency. Victims who receive restitution through successful trafficking prosecutions have gone on to college, secured stable and rewarding jobs, and learned English and other life skills, such as driving. Most importantly, many victims whose cases were resolved have options they never had before, making them less vulnerable to revictimization.

LEGAL PARAMETERS: VICTIMHOOD DEFINED

Different forms of relief, which involve separate and distinct requirements, are available to trafficking victims. Generally, however, the TVPA requires that a victim must be defined as a "victim of a severe form of trafficking" who is a potential witness in a case (to qualify for temporary immigration benefits under the "continued presence" immigration provision) and/or one who demonstrates a willingness to assist law enforcement officials in their investigation and prosecution efforts (to qualify for longer-term and potentially permanent T-visa benefits). (For more on the T-visa and the range of assistance and relocation options available to trafficking victims, see **Table 38-1**.) Thus, any law enforcement official encountering a potential trafficking situation must first determine whether the situation involves a "victim of a severe form of trafficking." The term "severe form of trafficking" encompasses certain trafficking offenses to which a victim must have been subjected to receive appropriate classification. 22 USC § 7102 (2004) recognizes the following offenses as sufficient to trigger the benefits provisions of the TVPA:

— A commercial sex act induced by force, fraud, or coercion, or one in which the person induced to perform such an act is younger than 18 years old

— The recruitment, harboring, transportation, provision, or obtaining of a person for labor or services, through the use of force, fraud, or coercion for the purpose of subjection to involuntary servitude, peonage, debt bondage, or slavery

Once classified as a victim, the law enforcement agency works in conjunction with the US Department of Health and Human Services to "certify" the victim to receive state refugee benefits in the locality in which he or she resides.

A number of different violations qualify for classification as trafficking crimes, entitling victims to receive the enumerated benefits. These violations include the following:

— *Involuntary servitude.* A victim is required to work or perform services through force, threats of force, or threats of legal coercion (18 USC § 1584).

— *Forced labor.* A victim is required to work under threats of "serious harm," including psychologically coercive ploys aimed at a victim's family members, and/or schemes, plans, or patterns intended to lead a victim to believe that the victim or another person would suffer serious harm or physical restraint for failing to perform the requested services (18 USC § 1589).

— *Sex trafficking of children or by force, fraud, or coercion.* A victim is required to perform a commercial sex act through force, fraud, or coercion, or a minor victim is required to perform a commercial sex act (18 USC § 1591).

These statutes are not mutually exclusive. All 3 statutes (and others) may be charged in the appropriate case. Though these are the primary statutes qualifying victims for enumerated benefits, other trafficking violations may provide similar scope. The bottom line is that the trafficker must have used some compelling behavior, such as force, fraud, or coercion (physical, legal, or psychological) to overpower the victim's free will for purposes of extracting work or commercial sexual services. However, where a minor is required to perform a commercial sex act, no force, fraud, or coercion need be shown.

In the case of juvenile victims of trafficking, separate benefits apply. Minor victims are eligible to participate in the Unaccompanied Refugee Minor (URM) Program run

Table 38-1. Other Assistance Available to Trafficking Victims

T-visa benefits impose the additional requirement of establishing extreme hardship upon removal to the victim's home country. Not all victims have chosen to remain in the United States; some have requested repatriation to their home countries during the investigation or after its conclusion. In one case, a group of juvenile victims requested to be reunited with their families in their native country though the victims expressed a willingness to return to the United States to testify against the traffickers. In another investigation, a victim of Indo-Nepalese origin requested repatriation to India so she could be reunited with her daughter. In such instances, federal personnel have assisted in securing victim benefits pending repatriation.

Despite the requirements for continued presence and T-visa status, victims can access immediate services upon liberation even before receiving official "certification" as a victim of a severe form of trafficking. The USDOJ has funded grants for emergency medical attention, food, shelter, vocational and language training, mental health counseling, and legal support available during the precertification stage. The Office of Victims of Crime provides grants to nongovernmental agencies for the specific purpose of assisting victims "between the period of time they are encountered by law enforcement, and when they are 'certified' to receive other benefits through the Department of Health and Human Services" (Trafficking in persons, 2004).

by the US Department of Health and Human Services. Though minor victims must qualify for continued presence or other immigration relief, their sustenance needs may be more easily met through the URM Program, and, unlike adults, they do not require certification to receive such benefits. Hence, the process is even more streamlined for children so they can access the necessary benefits quickly. In addition, victims who are between the ages of 16 and 24 and have work permits may be eligible for Job Corps, a program run by the US Department of Labor.

Spotting a Victim

Trafficking victims come in all packages: They may be US citizens, foreigners, female, male, young, or old. They may work in a wide range of industries or be forced to perform various services. As previously discussed, federal trafficking offenses have been noted in all but 5 US states and territories. Since trafficking crimes are becoming so ubiquitous, first responders (whether they be medical personnel, social workers, law enforcement officials, ministers, or good Samaritans) must be prepared to identify victims (**Table 38-2**).

Federal law enforcement authorities have noticed a pattern of recurrence in certain industries or services such as massage parlors, strip clubs, brothels, garment manufacturing plants (also known as *sweatshops*), farms and other agri-businesses that employ migrant labor, restaurants that employ busboys and dishwashers, and homes that employ domestic help. (See the USDOJ, Trafficking in persons information Web page at http://www.usdoj.gov/trafficking.htm) Some apparently "benign" businesses (eg, manicure salons, massage parlors) may offer commercial sexual services (deBaca & Tisi, 2002). Law enforcement officers involved in vice operations or other professionals who work on vice-related issues should note particularly young looking prostitutes even if such individuals claim to be adults.

Sexual abuse of trafficking victims, even in cases not involving sex trafficking and/or commercial sex, has been noted by USDOJ attorneys in several recent matters,

---

Table 38-2. Contexts in Which Child Victims of Trafficking Are Encountered

In a study aimed at identifying juvenile trafficking victims, the United States Conference of Catholic Bishops and the Institute for the Study of International Migration (ISIM) at Georgetown University identified 16 contexts in which law enforcement and social service agencies could encounter child victims of trafficking. The identified locations and groups include the following:

1. Hospital emergency rooms

2. Child protective services agencies

3. State and local juvenile justice departments

4. Domestic violence centers

5. Covenant House type shelters

6. Ethnic community-based organizations

7. Churches and religious centers

8. Healthcare providers

9. School counselor offices

10. Refugee service providers

11. Labor unions/garment industry workers

12. Legal aid agencies

13. Street outreach programs

14. Soup kitchens/homeless shelters

15. Domestic servants

16. Adult prostitutes

Data from Bump M, Duncan J. Conference on identifying and serving child victims of trafficking. Int Migr *[serial online]. December 2003;41:201-218. Available at: http://www.blackwell-synergy.com/ links/doi/10.1111/j.0020-7985.2003.00266.x/enhancedabs/. Accessed August 9, 2004.

---

particularly in cases involving juvenile domestic servants. Such workers are arguably the most cloistered and isolated of all victimized groups since they normally work in private homes. However, even these isolated victims may be visible when working in the yard, walking a dog, taking children to school, or tending children in public areas (eg, malls, parks). Be aware of domestic workers, especially juveniles, who may be introduced to visitors or other inquiring parties as "relatives." In fact, traffickers often procure their kin for trafficking into domestic servitude, other labor, or commercial sex (see Dhakal, 2004). A claim of kinship can be a ruse to mislead inquiring individuals or the reason a victim was targeted to work for the trafficker in the first place. Thus, a claim of blood ties or other relationship does not undercut a trafficking investigation.

Some common characteristics shared by trafficking victims, regardless of the type of work or services they perform, include long work hours, little or no salary, fear of employers, restrictions in movement, and/or being watched or guarded by other employees or family members of the defendant. Victims of trafficking may appear haggard or fatigued, or display bruising or other evidence of injury. Trafficking victims can be withdrawn and afraid of contact with "unsanctioned" outsiders. In addition, victims may find their statements and attempts at communication stifled or censored by others (deBaca & Tisi, 2002; Venkatraman, 2003). Such was the case in the Smith example, when Smith's associates arrived to speak for all the workers and victims on the scene soon after emergency personnel responded. Medical professionals, in particular, should be wary of "employers" or other individuals who silence the patient or insist on acting as the "interpreter."

Seemingly unhelpful facts (eg, a significant salary, failure to flee the trafficking situation despite multiple opportunities, initial consent to substandard working conditions or commercial sex) do not necessarily undercut the viability of a trafficking prosecution. In instances in which the defendant used unlawful means to overcome the victim's will and force his or her performance, statutory requirements for slavery and trafficking offenses can potentially be met.

Generally, formal questioning of a suspected trafficking victim is best left to investigators; however, threshold questions may occasionally be warranted. Such questions may include the following (deBaca & Tisi, 2002; Venkatraman, 2003):

— How did you come to work for [the defendant]?

— Describe your work.

— Were you paid?

— Could you come and go at will?

— Could you talk to anyone you wanted to talk to?

— How did you arrive in the United States?

— Did anyone take your passport or papers?

If the victim resists answering, appears to be withholding information, or is not being truthful, reassure the victim that he or she is not in trouble. Do not persist in questioning recalcitrant victims. All cases warrant immediate contact with law enforcement officials, and any basic questions should be asked through a trust-worthy interpreter.

HOW TO OBTAIN HELP

Once a trafficking situation is identified, numerous ways exist to alert law enforcement officials. Usually, when the case is of an emergency nature and a victim must be liberated immediately, the complainant should call emergency services. An overwhelming number of human trafficking cases are initiated through the USDOJ Trafficking in Persons and Worker Exploitation Complaint Line (888-428-7581). The complaint line is operational 24 hours a day and is staffed during business hours (Eastern Standard Time) by the Civil Rights Division. The complaint line uses TTY services for hearing-impaired callers, and a telephonic interpretation service capable of facilitating communication in 150 languages for callers who are not fluent in English. A number of resources are accessible through the complaint line, including specialized prosecutors at the Civil Rights Division who work exclusively on human trafficking prosecutions, as well as a full-time Victim Witness Specialist who assists trafficking victims and their representatives in obtaining benefits, accessing representation, finding helpful social service groups near the victim's residence, and arranging for competent and neutral interpretation services. Complaints are considered confidential. Callers include good Samaritans, members of nongovernmental groups, members of ethnic organizations, federal and state law enforcement officers, and the victims themselves. Besides contacting the complaint line, complainants can initiate federal investigations by notifying field offices of various federal law enforcement agencies. Local branches of the FBI, ICE, and the US Attorneys' offices have Victim-Witness Coordinators on staff to help arrange for victim safety and security. Complainants, therefore, have a number of investigative and prosecutorial agencies available to assist them. By federal mandate, all trafficking investigations and prosecutions are monitored by the USDOJ Civil Rights Division, even in those instances in which the Division is not the primary prosecutorial agency (USDOJ, Civil Rights Division, Criminal Section, 2004b).

LESSONS LEARNED: INVESTIGATIVE "BEST PRACTICES"

At this time, few states have anti-trafficking laws; Washington, Texas, Missouri, and Florida are the notable exceptions (Washington Revised Code, 2004; Texas Penal Code, 2004; Missouri Statutes, 2004; Florida Statutes, 2004). Despite the relatively small number of state laws on the books, local law enforcement officers are full partners in the anti-trafficking effort, as demonstrated in the Smith case example. Ideally, investigations involve a joint team of local and federal investigative agents working in tandem with prosecutors. Investigative tools often used in trafficking cases include extensive victim interviews with sensitive and preferably specialized interviewers; surveillance of the subject's home and/or business; undercover investigation (especially in sex trafficking cases); use of polygraphs; use of mechanisms such as "pen registers" and "trap and trace orders" to track phone calls and e-mails; immigration paperwork (ie, "A-files" that include visa and naturalization applications); document and handwriting analysis on immigration paperwork; bone-density tests for age determination; use of confidential informants; use of travel records and flight manifests; and foreign investigation and/or interviews of witnesses in the victim's and/or subject's home country. As in most criminal investigations, a key requirement in trafficking investigations is the existence of corroborative evidence. Such corroboration can include live witnesses or additional victims, medical evidence, bruising, scarring, documentary evidence showing false information on visa paperwork, logs of deductions taken for debts incurred by trafficking victims who are unwittingly made to reimburse their traffickers for various expenses, and so on.

As demonstrated in the Smith example, investigators, prosecutors, and other professionals involved in trafficking cases can expect to face complications. However, key lessons have emerged from the real-life challenges faced by numerous anti-trafficking professionals (**Table 38-3**). Though some of the tips are geared toward healthcare providers and others toward law enforcement investigators, many are best executed by a multidisciplinary team.

Table 38-3. Key Lessons and Tips for Investigating Trafficking Cases

1. *Get victims stabilized before debriefing them.* Such measures build trust. Victim-Witness Coordinators should be brought on board early in an investigation to ensure that the proper services are in place when victims come into law enforcement custody. Refrain from arresting the victim and find alternatives through the Victim-Witness Coordinator or Specialist. Such a professional (from the USDOJ Civil Rights Division, US Attorney's Office, FBI, or ICE) can ascertain a potential victim's rights and benefits options. Coordinators can work with NGOs, attorneys or other advocates, immigration authorities, and US Department of Health and Human Services officials to expedite a victim's lawful presence in the United States, work authorization, and other public benefits.

2. *Pay attention to the companions of the suspected victim.* Do they fit the profile of a "guard" or overseer who is monitoring the victim? Do they permit the victim to speak for himself or herself? Does the companion insist on interpreting for the victim or being present during questioning? Does the companion appear angry?

(continued)

Table 38-3. Key Lessons and Tips for Investigating Trafficking Cases *(continued)*

3. *Be aware of people who "clam up" or refuse to answer questions about their employment, injury, medical condition, living conditions, and/or other salient facts.* Be particularly suspicious when such people are minors presenting sexually transmitted diseases (STDs), pregnancy, signs of trauma, extreme fear, evidence of abortion, and/or signs of depression. Take special notice of non-English speakers who are fearful of your questions. Such people may be accompanied by a "guard" or overseer who seeks to monitor their communications. Some victims may be excessively protective of their captors. For example, some victims trafficked into prostitution consider their pimps/traffickers husbands, while other victims are scared of the power their traffickers wield.

4. *Strongly resist any attempts by a companion to speak or interpret for a suspected trafficking victim.* Instead, ascertain the potential victim's language and seek a neutral interpreter. Insist on speaking with the potential victim in private.

5. *Do not expect the victim to open up immediately.* Victims have often been conditioned to hide their victimization out of fear of the trafficker, mistrust of Americans or US law enforcement officers, or out of shame. If appropriate, question a possible victim on what he or she has heard about US law enforcement and from whom.

6. *Be suspicious of a discrepancy between a victim's stated age and appearance, particularly in patients showing signs of STDs, pregnancy, trauma, fear, abortion, and/or depression.* Reliable evidence of a victim's age may be ascertained through dental examinations, bone-density tests, seizure of school records, ration cards, or other official documents from the victim's home country, if births are not routinely recorded. Gather evidence from abroad quickly to avoid the possibility that evidence may be altered or tampered with.

7. *Conduct a comprehensive medical work-up when treating a potential trafficking victim.* Consider pregnancy, STDs, and psychiatric evaluations whenever isolation or trauma is suspected. When dealing with non-English speakers from developing nations, test for tuberculosis (TB), intestinal parasites, and other diseases that may occur with greater frequency in such countries.

8. *Be sure to ask potential victims whether they are scared or suspect they are in immediate danger.* Ask about the possibility of the victim being harmed in the future. Has the victim ever seen or heard of a weapon (firearm, knife, or another instrument) being used to threaten/harm him, her, or another person? Ask the victim whether anyone else in the household or organization is being mistreated.

9. *Be sure to ask potential victims whether they have children, and if so, where the children are and why they are there.* Trafficking victims may have children in their country (or state) of origin who are being held by the trafficker's associates or family members.

10. *Use specialized interviewers such as child sex experts and cultural specialists.* Federal investigative agencies often have specialized interviewers on staff. Cultural specialists can provide insight into the victim's and/or trafficker's social status in their native culture. Differences in social status can be significant in trafficking cases, which recognize psychological coercion as a means of exercising control over a victim. In many cases, psychological control may start with cultural status or power differences (**Table 38-4**). When using a cultural specialist from the victim's native country, ensure the victim and specialist do not know each other and the victim is comfortable with the specialist. Consider the possibility that the cultural specialist may have his or her own biases regarding certain communities in the culture. Test for impartiality, and check the specialist's background.

11. *Use an independent interpreter.* Contact federal agencies for assistance. The USDOJ Civil Rights Division, Criminal Section, maintains a nationwide list of independent interpreters for most languages. Test for interpreter bias, victim comfort level, and possible familiarity between the victim and interpreter (especially with respect to more obscurely spoken languages in the United States). If possible, conduct a background check for the interpreter. Do not assume a victim from a particular country speaks the prevalent language of that country. For example, a Guatemalan

(continued)

Table 38-3. *(continued)*

victim may speak Mixtec and not Spanish. Use separate law enforcement and social services interpreters to avoid claims of bias in any legal proceedings. Each interpreter's role should be specific and limited.

12. *Do not assume that the victim can read and write in his or her native language.* The victim may be illiterate.

13. *Ensure the team members interviewing the victim do not "trigger" him or her.* For example, consider the appropriateness of using a bearded interpreter if the child-victim was abused by a bearded individual.

14. *Do not attempt to tackle a trafficking case without interagency help.* Interagency partnerships are crucial to the anti-trafficking effort. Different investigative agencies have unique and specialized expertise: ICE in immigration, USDOL in employment-based visa applications, FBI in child sexual exploitation, Civil Rights Division in human trafficking prosecutions and victim support, local law enforcement agencies in key street intelligence, and NGOs in managing daily victim needs. Each agency is indispensable to the effort and can develop evidence on alternative charges in case the primary trafficking charges are insufficiently supported. Identify the nongovernmental groups, attorneys, medical personnel, law enforcement officials, and the Victim-Witness Coordinators who will be part of your "team." Establish a task force.

15. *Consider obtaining legal representation for the victim.* The trafficker may attempt to send in an attorney who claims to represent the victim. Be wary of this. NGOs are a good resource for legitimate attorneys. Bear in mind, however, that the interests of the victim and those of the investigative team can diverge. Expect that the victim's counsel will zealously protect the interests of the victim should the investigation reach such a juncture.

16. *Form links with ethnic, community-based organizations to develop trust.* Such organizations, which include "social hubs" where members of the community congregate, can assist the team's efforts in proactive and reactive ways. Proactively, such groups can provide community members with vital information about victim services since trafficking victims and the good Samaritans who help these victims may surface in temples, mosques, churches, ethnic shopping centers, and so on. Specific measures may include posting culturally appropriate, victim-assistance information at these social hubs or conducting workshops to familiarize community members with your services in tandem with a reliable interpreter. Reactively, ethnic community groups can provide key assistance when the team encounters a trafficking victim. Ensure the community members who assist the team are not connected to the suspected trafficker.

17. *Take anonymous tips seriously.* Even when the tipster has a hidden agenda or motive, certain information gleaned from the tip can help investigators. In the Smith example, an anonymous phone call helped unravel the complex web of false relationships that Smith had constructed. Such information accurately identified fictitious claims and sham relationships, thereby distinguishing such situations from lawful claims and beneficiaries.

18. *Do not record statements from victims and witnesses in the first person.* In court proceedings, victims may be considered to have "adopted" such statements, thereby subjecting themselves to potential cross-examination regarding the content of those statements. The Jencks Act (18 USC § 3500) requires the prosecutor to disclose, in certain situations, statements in the government's possession that were made by the witness, where such statements relate to the subject matter of the witness's testimony. Victims on the witness stand who give answers that are inconsistent with their statements may be challenged by defense attorneys, thereby resulting in trauma and compromised credibility.

19. *Document all benefits and gifts that the victims receive including work permits, psychological and medical care, and other assistance.* In the event of a prosecution, such information must be provided to the defense as part of the laws governing disclosure of benefits, promises, or other

(continued)

Table 38-3. Key Lessons and Tips for Investigating Trafficking Cases *(continued)*

special consideration that a witness may have received in exchange for testimony. For more information on the potential relevance of such benefits on a case, see *Giglio v United States* (1972).

20. *Remain in touch with possible witnesses in the victim's home country.* If safety concerns dictate, arrange for possible witnesses to come to the United States. Consult federal law enforcement officials regarding such issues. Ensure that the victims and witnesses who remain abroad are not subject to witness tampering, obstruction, or intimidation.

21. *Do not assume that law enforcement officials abroad will cooperate with the investigation and/or protect witnesses abroad.* Though most law enforcement officers worldwide are ethical and responsible, occasional exceptions are possible.

22. *Photograph victims and witnesses.* Law enforcement officers should use such photographs when interviewing victims and witnesses about various players in the trafficking scheme. In many trafficking cases, witnesses and victims will have aliases. The witnesses may not know each other by their true names, so photographs may prove helpful during interviews.

23. *Ensure that all travel documents, whether they are those of victims, witnesses, or potential defendants, are within law enforcement's custody and control.* No officer wants to be surprised by the revelation that the defendant was abroad when the victim alleges being raped in the United States. However, avoid relying on the passport as an accurate indicator of age. Victims who were trafficked into the United States under an alias may actually be younger than the passport indicates. Age is an important factor to ascertain for charging decisions in the event of a prosecution.

24. *Expect that defendants are possibly coaching and contacting witnesses and victims, even if the witnesses and victims have been relocated.* Use reliable methods of monitoring telephone calls and other modes of communication.

25. *Investigators, social service providers, and other team members are especially subject to stress when dealing with child slavery and trafficking.* Be aware of irritability, short tempers, and depression. Support each other through the process.

Table 38-4. The Significance of Power and Status in a Trafficking Case

The first conviction under the new forced labor statute added by the Trafficking Victims' Protection Act at 18 USC § 1589, was in the unreported case *United States v Blackwell*, a case prosecuted by the USDOJ Civil Rights Division and the US Attorney's Office for the District of Maryland. In that case, the victim, a domestic servant from Ghana, had been tricked and trafficked by politically powerful Ghanaian traffickers, one of whom was a high-level Ghanaian government official. The defendants' status partially served to maintain the victim in a condition of compelled service.

CONCLUSION

Though slavery and trafficking cases, especially those involving children, are among the most difficult and heart-wrenching injustices of the modern day, they can also be highly rewarding. Successfully identifying a trafficking victim is a challenge. With appropriate rehabilitation assistance for liberated victims, their lives can be transformed. Many victims who began their ordeal in a destitute and defenseless state go on to lead productive lives after liberation and appropriate rehabilitation. Trafficking success stories abound with examples of poor, illiterate, violently brutalized, and sexually abused victims learning to read, write, speak English, and earn a college degree, and generally becoming confident, law-abiding members of society. The gratitude and respect that victims feel for the professionals who liberated and cared for them, the lifetime bond that can develop as a result, and the anti-trafficking work that some former victims have themselves undertaken, provide those who are involved in combating such crimes with deep and meaningful validation. As anyone who has worked a successful trafficking investigation will attest, the true reward of such work is in witnessing liberated victims regain control of their lives, regardless of the outcome of any prosecution effort.

REFERENCES

Bump MN, Duncan J. Conference on identifying and serving child victims of trafficking. *Int Migr* [serial online]. December 2003;41:201-218. Available at http://www.blackwell-synergy.com/links/doi/10.1111/j.0020-7985.2003.00266.x/enhancedabs/. Accessed August 9, 2004.

deBaca L, Tisi A. Working together to stop modern-day slavery. *Police Chief Magazine*. August 2002;69(8):79-80.

Dhakal S. Nepal's victims of trafficking shy away from justice. *One World South Asia.* January 8, 2004. Available at: http://southasia.oneworld.net/article/view/76359/1/. Accessed August 9, 2004.

18 USC § 1584 (2000).

18 USC § 1589 (2004).

18 USC § 1591 (2004).

18 USC § 3500 (2004).

Fla St § 787.06 (2004).

Giglio v United States, 405 US 150 (1972).

Mo St 566.203, 566.206, 566.209, 566.212, 566.215, 566.218, 566.223 (2004).

Tex Penal Code §§ 20A.01, 20A.02 (2004).

Trafficking Victims Protection Act of 2000, Pub L No 106-386, 114 Stat 1464.

Trafficking in persons. Office of Victims of Crime Web site. Available at: http://www.ojp.usdoj.gov/ovc/help/tip.htm#4. Accessed August 9, 2004.

22 USC § 7102 (2004).

US Department of Justice (USDOJ), Civil Rights Division. *Anti-Trafficking Newsletter.* February 2004a;1(2):2-3.

US Department of Justice, Civil Rights Division, Criminal Section. Trafficking in persons: a guide for non-governmental organizations [brochure]. Washington, DC: USDOJ; 2002. Available at: http://www.usdoj.gov/crt/crim/wetf/trafficbrochure.pdf. Accessed March 19, 2004b.

US Department of Justice. Trafficking in persons information. Available at: http://www.usdoj.gov/trafficking.htm. Accessed March 19, 2004.

Venkatraman BA. Human trafficking: a guide to detecting, investigating and punishing modern-day slavery. *Police Chief Magazine*. December 2003;70(12):41.

Wash Rev Code §§ 9A 40.100, 9A 20.021(1)(a), 7.68.350 (2004).

Keeping the Faith: A Call for Collaboration Between the Faith and Child Protection Communities

Victor I. Vieth, JD

"If I am my brother's keeper, it's not enough for me to learn about or even pray about his troubles. I'm called upon to act on his behalf, even when that requires fighting injustice and tyranny" (President Jimmy Carter, 1997).

The child protection and faith-based communities are often at odds with one another. Although both professions are charged with the protection of children, members of the faith community often see themselves as keeping families together and believe that the child protection community breaks families apart. The child protection community, having had a negative experience with some members of the faith community, assumes that all members of the faith community are problematic. At the core of the dilemma is that both groups know far too little about the work of the other. The sad consequence of this distrust is that children are more likely to fall through the cracks in our faith and child protection communities. The sources of this conflict, the consequences of the conflict, and suggestions for crossing the bridge that now divides these communities are fully explored in the following text.

THE CONFLICT

There are numerous factors contributing to conflict between faith communities and child protection professionals. No factor is necessarily more important than another, and many of these factors overlap.

First, members of the faith-based community often show up as character witnesses for the accused. In speaking at a child abuse conference, I asked the prosecutors in the room to raise their hands if they had cross-examined a clergyperson appearing as a character witness for the accused. All hands went in the air. When I asked how many had ever used a clergyperson as a witness for the victim, all hands dropped. To illustrate the frustration some prosecutors have with members of the faith community, consider the following scenario. In a case where the defendant was found guilty of raping a minor, a minister testified that the defendant had a good reputation in the community and that he was a truthful person (*Tennessee v Stewart*, 1993). In making this claim, the minister was compelled to admit that the defendant's previous guilty plea to 2 counts of sexual battery "did not in any way affect [his] opinion of the defendant" (*Tennessee v Stewart*, 1993). Such testimony leaves prosecutors and jurors alike skeptical about the ability of clergy to empathize with, much less protect, child victims of abuse.

To the extent this inability exists, it may simply reflect the lack of understanding many clergypersons have about sexual abuse and how easily manipulated they are. A member of the clergy once told my colleague that he knew the defendant was innocent because he "had looked him in the eye and he told me he didn't do it." Perhaps this is not surprising. Many clergy receive little or no training about the dynamics of child physical or sexual abuse. For example, the following seminary catalogs listed no courses covering the subject of child sexual abuse or pedophilia: Asbury Theology Seminary, Bethel Seminary, Christian Theological Seminary, Colorado Theological Seminary, Eastern Mennonite Seminary, Fuller Theological Seminary, The King's Seminary, St. Patrick's Seminary, Trinity Theological Seminary, Valley International Christian Seminary, Wisconsin Lutheran Seminary, and Woolston-Steen Theological Seminary. Even with training, clergy may be ill-equipped to deal with child abusers who are extremely manipulative. As described by Leberg (1997), sex offenders "cannot deal openly and honestly with who they are or what they have done. This is not surprising. With something to hide, they have become practiced at hiding it, often (in part) from themselves as well as others."

The allegiance of some clergy to perpetrators may not result from being outwitted by the offender. Instead, this allegiance to sex offenders may be mandated by church rules and statutory law. This results when penitent privilege statutes gag the clergyperson from testifying regarding inculpatory statements made by criminals, such as confessions to child abuse or domestic violence. These statutes require the consent of the penitent in order for the clergyperson to testify on matters disclosed to him in the course of his religious duties. The following is an example of this type of state privilege statute (Conn Gen Stat Ann § 52-146b [West 2001]):

A clergyman, priest, minister, rabbi, or practitioner of any religious denomination accredited by the religious body to which he belongs who is settled in the work of the ministry shall not disclose confidential communications made to him in his professional capacity in any civil or criminal case or proceedings preliminary thereto, or in any legislative or administrative proceeding, unless the person making the confidential communication waives such privilege herein provided.

See also Ariz Rev Stat § 13-4062(3) (2001); DC Code Ann § 14-309 (2001); Iowa Code § 622.10 (2002); Mass Gen Laws Ann ch 233 § 20A (2001); Minn Stat § 595.02 (2000); Mont Code Ann § 26-1-804 (2001); Nev Rev Stat § 49.255 (2000); NH Rev Stat Ann § 516:35 (2000); Ore Rev Stat § 40.260 (1999); 42 Pa Cons Stat § 5943 (2001); RI Gen Laws § 9-17-23 (2001); Tenn Code Ann § 24-1-206 (2001); Wash Rev Code Ann § 5.60.060(3) (2001); and W Va Code § 57-3-9 (2001).

Second, members of the clergy fail to understand, much less report, abuse. The pastoral care department of the Children's Hospital Medical Center of Akron, Ohio, surveyed 143 clergy of numerous faiths and found that 29% believed that actual evidence of abuse, as opposed to suspicion, was necessary before a report could be made. The same study found that only 22% of the respondents were required by their denomination/faith group to receive child abuse training. This study also documented an underreporting of suspected abuse cases, with the most prevalent reason being a lack of trust in children's services bureaus (Grossoehme, 1998). The 143 clergy responding to this survey have an impact on, at some level, the lives of 23 841 children (Grossoehme, 1998).

Third, some churches are perceived as "hiding" clergy accused of abusing children. Catholic Cardinal Bernard F. Law said he was "profoundly sorry" for sending a pedophile priest to a new assignment rather than turning him over to the authorities (Robinson & Paulson, 2002). In 2002, the Vatican issued "new rules for Roman Catholic churches around the world to deal with pedophile priests, saying they should stand trial in secret ecclesiastical courts" (Reuters News Service, 2002). The notion of secret courts compounds a long-standing criticism that the Catholic Church is protecting child abusers. In 1992, Catholic priest and novelist Andrew M.

Greeley wrote, "bishops have in what seems like programmed consistency tried to hide, cover up, bribe, stonewall; often they have sent back into parishes men whom they knew to be a danger to the faithful" (1992). Dealing secretly with church child molesters is not a recent phenomenon, nor is it limited to Roman Catholicism. For example, Horatio Alger was a Unitarian minister who, when accused of molesting children, was not turned over to the police but was quietly dismissed from his pastoral duties (Pollenberg, 1997).

Fourth, many congregations rally around the perpetrator and, in some cases, even blame the victim or the victim's parents. In one case, in Minnesota, the pastor concluded that half the congregation believed "the girl seduced the perpetrator" (Delaplane, 1988). A Lutheran minister once confided to me that he was shocked when an older boy in his congregation sexually abused his daughter. The minister was even more alarmed that the church council was critical of the pastor's decision to report the incident to the police. In the mind of many, the juvenile's sexual conduct was simply a case of misplaced hormones that could be handled exclusively within the church. (The problem of taking juvenile sex offenses seriously is a significant problem in assisting young offenders. See Vieth, 2001.)

Even when guilt is unequivocal, some prominent members of the faith community blame the victims rather than the offenders. In response to a $119 million verdict against the Dallas diocese for the serial molestation of altar boys by a priest, the former vicar general, Msgr. Robert Rehkemper, stated, "no one ever says anything about what the role of the parents was in all this." Msgr. Rehkemper also insisted that the child victims "knew what was right and what was wrong. Anybody who reaches the age of reason shares responsibility for what they do" (Dreher, 2002).

The phenomenon of supporting perpetrators over victims may reflect a long-standing, deeply ingrained belief that God has placed children under the province of parents or other caretakers and that no one, certainly not the government, should interfere. In reference to his rural boyhood in Georgia during the depression era, former President Jimmy Carter writes, "[t]he role of our three churches was gently but carefully circumscribed. Whether Baptist, Methodist, or Lutheran, our families did not expect the pastor, deacons, stewards, or other congregation leaders to interfere in private or personal affairs" (2001).

The aversion to government may reflect a view that lawyers and courts are people and places the faithful should avoid. John Calvin believed a Christian could never go to court out of anger or vengeance but only out of love. Specifically, Calvin said of lawsuits "however just, can never be rightly prosecuted by any man, unless he treats his adversary with the same love and good will as if the business under controversy were already amicably settled and composed" (Allegretti, 1996). Martin Luther echoed these sentiments, claiming "that all those who go to law and wrangle in the courts over their property and honor are nothing but heathen masquerading under the name of Christians" (1962). Even today, Christians openly question whether they can serve as lawyers or otherwise participate in the legal system. (For further discussion of this issue, see Schutt, 1999.)

Fifth, in cases of child and domestic abuse, some members of the faith community counsel victims to forgive their abusers without accountability under the criminal law and suggest that the doctrine of submission requires endurance of the abuse. In permitting ongoing sexual abuse by clergy, one author comments that "the concepts of mercy, redemption, and humility come into play" (Dreher, 2002). The concept of "he who is without sin, cast the first stone" works to forgive a surface repentant without requiring true reform in behavior (Dreher, 2002). One survey of Protestant clergy found that 71% of them would not advise a battered woman to leave a spouse immediately because of abuse, and 92% would not advise divorce as an option (Alsdurf & Alsdurf, 1988). The need to forgive and to preserve the marriage was so pronounced that 45%

of the surveyed pastors said the violence of the husband should not be "overemphasized and used as 'a justification' for breaking the marriage commitment" (Alsdurf & Alsdurf, 1988).

Sometimes, a member of the faith community may not actively counsel or condone abuse but may nonetheless fail to speak out. Silence in the face of evil is tantamount to harboring the sin. Even so, the pressure to be quiet is great and deeply ingrained in our culture. Jewish Rabbi Julie Spitzer writes of the silence surrounding family violence in the Jewish community and laments that she grew "tired of being one voice among so many who refused to listen" (1999).

Sixth, members of the faith-based community often claim scriptural authorization for corporal punishment. When this happens, a clash between church and state may occur if the latter deems the discipline to be excessive. Case law is replete with examples of the government prosecuting church members who use the Bible for justification of their violence. In a North Carolina case, 5 Christian daycare providers used hands and paddles to hit children "pursuant to the policy of the church." A North Carolina Baptist Church administered corporal punishment to an infant less than 1 year old. (For references to these cases and a fuller discussion of religion and corporal punishment, see Vieth, 1994.) Christian psychologist Dr. James Dobson advocates hitting children and, as scriptural support, cites the following verse: "Withhold not correction from the child; for if thou beatest him with the rod, he shall not die" (Proverbs 23:13, 14). (Modern translations do not use the word "beat" but do acknowledge using the rod to "punish" the child. See New International Version of the same verse.) Commenting on this verse, Dobson opines, "Certainly if the 'rod' is a measuring stick, you now know what to do with it!" (1970).

Many theologians, however, disagree with this interpretation of the verse in Proverbs. According to this view, "rod" is a shepherd's staff used to guide and not strike sheep. To these theologians, the proverb "seems to imply that parents who love their children are careful to discipline them, and those parents that don't provide guidance aren't adequately caring for their children" (Carey, 1994).

It is not, however, the place of a front-line social worker or other child protection professional to debate scripture with a parent who may have used excessive force. Indeed, nearly every state permits parents to use "reasonable" force on their children. Even if such debate were permissible, it is unlikely that one group or the other would be converted to adopt a different interpretation of scripture. The social worker can, of course, argue that corporal punishment is not an effective means of discipline and can support this argument with research. (See Carey, 1994.) An intellectual argument such as this, however, is also unlikely to be effective with a parent who believes God is commanding him or her to use physical discipline.

Seventh, many remedial measures taken by the church, such as treatment centers and policies, have proven to be relatively ineffective and may actually result in sending offenders back to their victims. For the most part, the Catholic Church uses 2 treatment centers for pedophile priests: St. Luke Institute in Maryland, and the facility operated by the Servants of the Paraclete in Jemez Springs, New Mexico. An interview with officials at St. Luke reveals that the center is openly used to help priests avoid prosecution for sexual abuse of children and that the staff promotes keeping pedophiliac priests in the ministry, albeit closely monitored (Niebuhr, 1993; Steinfels, 1992). St. Luke staff members agreed that offending priests should not be put in settings placing future children at risk but rejected the proposal that molesting priests be automatically barred from the priesthood or church posts (Niebuhr, 1993; Steinfels, 1992). Likewise, the New Mexico facility has been referred to as a "dumping ground for pedophile priests." "The church had them say prayers and rosaries, then they released them for sexual sabbaticals with young boys," commented victims' attorney, Bruce Pasternack (Kurkjian, 1992, 1993). Furthermore, although

130 people have accused former priest Father John Geoghan of molesting and raping them as children throughout the course of his 36-year career, he has been described as a "veteran of institutions that treat sexually abusive priests." (NOTE: On February 21, 2002, Father Geoghan was sentenced the maximum sentence of 9 to 10 years in prison for fondling a 10-year-old in a swimming pool in 1999. In addition, the Catholic Church has paid $10 million to settle 50 civil suits, while 84 civil suits and 2 criminal trials are still pending against Father Geoghan. See Belluck, 2002.) Finally, Rudy Kos, a former priest who faces a life sentence for serial molestation of altar boys, regularly telephoned one of his victims while under treatment at the Servants of the Paraclete (The Kos Files, 2002).

Certain churches and dioceses have instituted their own "child safety policies" that address child sexual abuse (**Table 39-1**). Cardinal Law announced a "zero tolerance" policy against child sexual abuse and agreed to hand over the church's records to the authorities in response to findings of child sexual abuse within the Dallas diocese (Engel, 2002). Nevertheless, enforcement of such policies has been met with cynicism, and cases against clergymen continue to emerge. A leading victims' attorney said of Law's new policies and the Catholic Church's decade-old "quiet" policy of excluding homosexuals from the seminary, "I don't want to hear about another new policy until someone says to me that someone other than the fox guarding the henhouse has examined the files" (Dreher, 2002).

Cleric sex offenders pose every bit the danger to children and society as do noncleric offenders. Cleric sex offenders share many characteristics with noncleric offenders (Haywood et al, 1996; Langevin et al, 2000) although cleric offending may be related more to psychosexual adjustment and development issues and less to severe mental disorder (Haywood et al, 1996).

It can even be argued that cleric sex offenders are more skilled than their less-educated counterparts and, thus, may be particularly adept at selecting their victims and avoiding detection. In one study, researchers found that a "substantial number of complainants were children and adolescents, and therefore did not complain to authorities until years later. Thus, there may be some selection of susceptible victims who were confused and less likely to report the clerics' inappropriate behavior" (Langevin et al, 2000). The same study found that "significantly more" clerics used force than noncleric offenders. In terms of treating cleric sex offenders, researchers

---

Table 39-1. Policies That Outline Child Sexual Abuse as Prohibited Conduct

— West Olive Christian Reformed Church, Abuse Prevention and Child Protection Policy (West Olive, Michigan, May 1997)

— Greater Tulsa Christian Church, Policy and Guidelines of Greater Tulsa Christian Church to Ensure the Safety and Well-Being of Our Children (Tulsa, Oklahoma)

— North Shore Congregational Church, Child Safety (Fox Point, Wisconsin)

— Epworth United Methodist Church, Personal Safety Policy (Gaithersburg, Maryland, August 29, 2001)

— Child Abuse Policy of the Diocese of Tuscon (Available at: http://www.diocesetucson.org/restore2.html. Accessed February 25, 2002)

— Episcopal Diocese of Albany, New York, Sexual Misconduct Manual, Policy Statements (Available at: http://www.albanyepiscopaldiocese.org/ documents/sxmisconduct/policy.html. Accessed February 25, 2002)

have found that "they appear to suffer from the same problems as sex offenders in general and they should be assessed in the same fashion" (Langevin et al, 2000). To do this, however, the church must report abuse and the child protection and criminal justice systems must respond with equal vigor to a case of sexual abuse at the hands of a cleric as at the hands of any other molester.

Eighth, the child protection community often assumes the hostility of the faith-based community and fails to involve it. Child protection professionals often fail to solicit clergy for membership on our multidisciplinary teams (MDTs). We also fail in keeping clergy informed of services such as Parents Anonymous that could be accessed to help parents on edge. We fail to attempt education of the faith-based community on issues surrounding cases of child abuse. When we fail to reach out and educate the clergy, we perpetuate myths that may be harmful to children. Once, while I was teaching a class to clergy, an older pastor commented to me, "I suppose you're going to tell me that if I give a child a hug, that's sexual abuse." Obviously, this pastor bought into the idea that child protection professionals are zealots looking to fill the prisons by misinterpreting innocent behavior. I was able to correct this perception by commenting to the effect, "No, an abused child who wants or needs a hug should not be denied that comfort. It is not a crime to hug a child. It is a crime to touch a child's genitals for your own sexual gratification or to cause a child to manipulate your genitals. That's what we're going to talk about."

THE COST

When faith-based and child protection professionals clash, there are at least 4 consequences. *First, children are lost in the church.* I had a case in which the pastor and church elders showed up at the trial as a show of support for the member of their congregation accused of sexually abusing his cognitively impaired daughter. The pastor even testified as a character witness for the accused. All of this was no doubt troubling to the victim, herself a member of the congregation, who may well have wondered if this meant God did not believe her. She certainly understood that her church did not believe her.

Second, victims of domestic violence are lost in the church. One study of victims of spouse abuse found that 71% of the victims reported a "dissatisfactory" contact with clergy or a "very unsatisfactory" relationship with a religious leader. Those victims who had a positive experience received "validation" and "approval" from their religious leader (Horton et al, 1988).

Third, perpetrators are lost in the church. A perpetrator receiving quick or cheap forgiveness may assume the sin was not great and may reoffend. After all, if forgiveness is this easy, the offender can get it any time. Over 60 years ago, German theologian Dietrich Bonhoeffer called this phenomenon "cheap grace," which means "grace sold on the market like cheapjacks' wares. The sacraments, the forgiveness of sin, and the consolations of religion are thrown away at cut prices" (1959).

Cheap grace often, if not always, poisons a perpetrator's chance to shed the sin of sexual abuse. According to Horton & Williams' (1988) study of incest perpetrators:

The perpetrators stated that "Hail Marys" and "kneel therapy" are not enough. Most offenders want clergy to be informed, sensitive, and understanding, but they agree that sexual abuse treatment is best left to the experts. They emphasize the need to coordinate and cooperate. Many services are required for the incestuous family. Law enforcement, treatment, and spiritual recovery need to be combined as a joint effort to ensure total care for all family members.

Fourth, the faith needs of children are lost in the system. Faith issues often come up in cases of child abuse. I have had cases, for example, in which a victim asked if she was still a virgin in God's eyes. I had one case in which a victim told me she could not report her abuse because she knew that sex outside of marriage was a sin and did not want to be condemned by the church or her parents. These are faith and mental health issues that are often ignored by MDTs.

CROSSING THE BRIDGE THAT DIVIDES

The cost of continued conflict between the faith and child protection communities is simply too high a price to pay. Crossing the bridge dividing these important disciplines may include the following steps.

First, prosecutors and other child abuse professionals should recognize the key role that clergy play in communities. Often, the most respected leaders in communities do not occupy a position on the school or township board. Instead, they preach from a pulpit. Moreover, families in crisis typically do not call social services; these families may call their pastor, priest, rabbi, or iman. Accordingly, prosecutors and other members of the child protection community need to reach out to local ministerial associations. The outreach can be as simple as offering to give a presentation on local efforts to combat child abuse.

Second, conduct a mandated reporter training for clergy. It is appropriate to conduct separate mandated reporter training for members of the clergy. In part, a separate training is warranted because mandated reporting laws for clergy may differ from those for other professionals. In Minnesota, for example, a member of the clergy is not required to report the possibility of abuse or neglect if the information is obtained while receiving a confession or from a person seeking "religious or spiritual advice" (Minn Stat § 626.556, Subd 3(2)). (For an overview of the mandated reporting statutes for all 50 states, see US Department of Health & Human Services, 2002.)

Third, develop and use other training materials for the faith-based community. There are myriad resources available for such training. For example, the video *Hear Their Cries,* produced by the Center for Prevention of Sexual and Domestic Violence, is an excellent training resource. (For information, contact the center at 1914 North 34th Street, Suite 105, Seattle, WA 98103, (206) 634-1903.) A book containing great suggestions and helpful resources for Catholic parish and school staff is entitled *Creating Safe and Sacred Places,* by Gerard McGlone and Mary Shrader.

It will be particularly helpful to train members of the faith community about the games pedophiles use in obtaining access to children in churches and other faith centers. As noted by one imprisoned pedophile:

I considered church people easy to fool ... they have a trust that comes from being Christians. ... They tend to be better folks all around. And they seem to want to believe in the good that exists in all people ... I think they want to believe in people. And because of that, you can easily convince, with or without convincing words (Salter, 2003).

Upon his release from prison, one pedophile asked an unsuspecting minister if he believed in forgiveness. When the minister said his church forgave all the truly penitent, the pedophile falsely told the minister that he had just been released from prison for passing bad checks. In reality, the offender had been in prison for sexually abusing children. The pedophile gave this sob story to the minister:

While I was there (in prison), I found the Lord, and there was this hymn I dearly loved. And I knew it would be a sign from God, whatever church was playing that hymn, that was the church for me. And Father, when I walked by your church this morning, you were playing that hymn (Salter, 2003).

Moved by this lie, and without determining the pedophile's true criminal history, the minister permitted the offender to be in charge of the church's children's choir. When the authorities caught up with this offender, they found he was actually operating in 2 churches (Salter, 2003).

In educating the faith community about these types of manipulations by offenders, it may be possible to limit the access pedophiles presently have to a number of children in the faith community.

Fourth, receive training from members of the leading faiths in your community. It is difficult, if not impossible, for child protection professionals to work effectively with or respect the culture of the victims unless these workers have as full an understanding as possible of the victims' belief systems. This may be as simple as attending various worship services and asking families about religious practices or beliefs.

Fifth, invite members of the faith-based community to be part of MDTs. Once clergy see the inner workings of a local child protection system, they will be in a position to rebut myths by their fellow clergy regarding the system. For example, clergy on an MDT can educate their brethren that rigid legal standards are in place to prevent the taking of a child into protective custody on a mere whim and that even if a given social worker or police officer went too far, a judge must review and approve the decision within a matter of hours. More importantly, a faith-based member of the MDT can help other members of the team recognize and respond to faith issues raised by various victims.

Sixth, involve members of the faith-based community in your prevention programs. In the county where I prosecuted, we had a committee established to address child abuse at the front end through various prevention efforts. One year, for example, we identified a need for and then developed a Parents Anonymous program. By involving clergy in such efforts, the members of the faith-based community will be aware of and hopefully refer parishioners to these local resources. Because clergy work with so many families in crisis, these professionals can also help identify programs most needed in a given community.

Think of creative ways to involve the faith community in your child protection efforts. When, for example, local training of child protection professionals is conducted, consider asking local churches, temples, and synagogues to donate space for the training or otherwise involve members of the faith community in the training. Using the church for such training sends a subtle message to all members of that congregation that the church is opposed to child abuse and is supporting local efforts to combat this sin.

Seventh, teach parishioners how to respond to cases of child abuse and how to protect their children. Topics can include child personal safety as well as Internet safety. **Appendix 39-1** contains several simple but concrete steps parents and others can take to protect children in their homes and congregations.

Eighth, when dealing with an aspect of child abuse involving a family of faith, take the time to learn about the family's religion and culture and, if possible, work within it. For example, I had a child protection case of excessive corporal punishment. The mother/offender, with the support of her pastor, insisted that corporal punishment is necessary and is sanctioned by God. There is a recurring strain in some segments of Christianity that children must be disciplined sternly in order to avoid a path that may lead to condemnation. Martin Luther once said there "is no greater tragedy in Christendom than spoiling children" (Owen, 1993).

In the case mentioned above, the mother's source for her belief was the book *Dare to Discipline* by Dr. James Dobson. Our child protection workers read the book and found references to avoiding excessive discipline, not disciplining a child for involuntary acts such as bed-wetting, and an acknowledgment that not all children need to be hit. Indeed, Dobson writes that one of his greatest fears is that his recommendations of corporal punishment will lead some parents to "apply the thrashings too frequently or too severely" (1970). We asked the mother if she agreed with these parts of the book as well and if we could teach her to use less aversive forms of discipline. The mother agreed and learned to use other forms of discipline effectively.

Ninth, realize that, at times, a clash is unavoidable. The policy of the National District Attorneys Association (NDAA), for example (**Table 39-2**), is to oppose religious exemptions from child abuse laws and, if possible, to prosecute those who withhold medical care from children based on religious grounds. In instances such as these, there will be a conflict. When these occur, the best a prosecutor can do is be respectful of someone's faith but be unflinching in the protection of the child.

Table 39-2. National District Attorneys Association Position

"WHEREAS, all children are entitled to equal access to all available health care, and WHEREAS, all parents shall be held to the same standard of care in providing for their children, and that all parents shall enjoy both equal protection and equal responsibilities under law, regardless of their religious beliefs, BE IT RESOLVED that the National District Attorneys Association shall join with other child advocacy organizations to support legislation to repeal exemptions from prosecution for child abuse and neglect."

Reprinted from NDAA Position Paper on Religious Exemption. National Center for Prosecution of Child Abuse Update. American Prosecutors Research Institute. Alexandria, Va; September, 1991. (For a more complete discussion of this issue, see Asser & Swan, 1998.)

Tenth, help the faith-based community establish a system that responds appropriately to the needs of child abuse victims. **Appendix 39-2** describes a 5-step plan for use by congregations desiring to do all they can to protect the children in their midst.

Eleventh, help the faith-based community establish a system that responds appropriately to the needs of domestic violence victims. When teaching congregations about protecting victims of domestic terror, I offer 7 suggestions. These suggestions are contained in **Appendix 39-3**.

Twelfth, consider religion throughout the case. If a child asks, "Am I still a virgin in God's eyes?" the MDT must deal with this issue as part of therapy and should involve a religious leader who shares the child's faith to ease his or her anguish about God's reaction to the victimization. Hopefully, a caring clergy member can explain the difference between sinning and being the victim of someone else's sin.

Thirteenth, include religion as part of victim assistance services. Ask a nonoffending parent, for example, if the child has religious questions about the abuse such as, "Why didn't God protect me?" If so, perhaps the MDT can help the family access religious services that will help the child cope with this crisis of faith.

CONCLUSION

The National Cemetery Administration authorizes 32 different religious symbols to be used on headstones in the 120 national cemeteries it oversees (Youso, 2002). Tour any of these cemeteries and you will find the Latin cross, the Star of David, the Muslim Crescent and Star, and the Angel Moroni (Youso, 2002). The members of these divergent faiths shared in life and death a common purpose in defending their nation. In the same vein, the members of our country's divergent faiths must band together not for the purpose of intermingling or in any way altering our faith traditions but to protect from abuse the children God has placed in our care. To this end, it becomes necessary to cooperate not only with other faiths but also with a secular government whose assistance is essential if we are to protect children. By the same token, child protection authorities can not minimize and must never ignore the role of the faith community in detecting abuse and assisting families to heal. In crossing the bridge that divides, the faith and child protection communities offer the victims of abuse the best hope for a better life.

REFERENCES

Abel GG, Becker JV, Mittelman MS, Cunningham-Rathner J, Rouleau JL, Murphy WD. Self-reported sex crimes of nonincarcerated paraphiliacs. *J Interpers Violence.* 1987;2:3-25.

Allegretti JG. *The Lawyer's Calling: Christian Faith and Legal Practice.* New York, NY: Paulist Press; 1996.

Alsdurf JM, Alsdurf P. A pastoral response. In: Horton AL, Williamson JA, eds. *Abuse and Religion: When Praying Isn't Enough.* Lexington, Mass: Lexington Books; 1988:165-172.

Ariz Rev Stat § 13-4062(3) (2001).

Asser SM, Swan R. Deaths from religion-motivated medical neglect. *Pediatrics.* 1998;101(4 pt 1):625-629.

Belluck P. Ex-priest in child abuse case sentenced to 9 to 10 years. *New York Times.* February 22, 2002;A16.

Bonhoeffer D. *The Cost of Discipleship.* Fuller RH, trans. New York, NY: Macmillian; 1959.

Carey TA. Spare the rod and spoil the child. Is this a sensible justification for the use of punishment in child rearing? *Child Abuse Negl.* 1994;18:1005-1010.

Carter J. *Sources of Strength: Meditations on Scripture for a Living Faith.* New York, NY: Times Books; 1997.

Carter J. *Christmas in Plains: Memories.* New York, NY: Simon & Schuster; 2001.

Conn Gen Stat Ann § 52-146b (West 2001).

DC Code Ann § 14-309 (2001).

Delaplane DW. Stand by me: the role of the clergy and congregation in assisting the family once it is involved in the legal and treatment process. In: Horton AL, Williamson JA, eds. *Abuse and Religion: When Praying Isn't Enough.* Lexington, Mass: Lexington Books; 1988:173-180.

Dobson J. *Dare to Discipline.* Glendale, Calif: Regal Books; 1970.

Dreher R. Sins of the fathers, pedophile priests and the challenge to the American church. *National Review.* February 11, 2002:27-29.

Engel M. Sex abuse cover-up rocks Boston's Catholic Church. *The Guardian.* February 23, 2002.

Greeley AM. Foreword. In: Berry J, ed. *Lead Us Not Into Temptation: Catholic Priests and the Sexual Abuse of Children.* New York, NY: Doubleday; 1992:xiii-xiv.

Grossoehme DH. Child abuse reporting: clergy perceptions. *Child Abuse Negl.* 1998; 7:743-747.

Haywood TW, Kravitz HM, Wasyliw OE, Goldberg J, Cavanaugh JL Jr. Cycle of abuse and psychopathology in cleric and noncleric molesters of children and adolescents. *Child Abuse Negl.* 1996;20:1233-1243.

Horton AL, Wilkins MM, Wright W. Women who ended abuse: what religious leaders and religion did for these victims. In: Horton AL, Williamson JA, eds. *Abuse and Religion: When Praying Isn't Enough.* Lexington, Mass: Lexington Books; 1988:235-246.

Horton AL, Williams D. What incest perpetrators need (but are not getting) from the clergy and treatment community. In: Horton AL, Williamson JA, eds. *Abuse and Religion: When Praying Isn't Enough.* Lexington, Mass: Lexington Books; 1988: 259-266.

Iowa Code § 622.10 (2002).

The Kos Files. Showdown in Dallas. Available at http://www.thelinkup.org/kos.html. Accessed February 25, 2002.

Kurkjian S. Priest accused of abuse while at parish in mass. Sexual misconduct allegations widen. *Boston Globe.* December 21, 1992. Cited by: Christian Sex Crimes. "Massachusetts-to-New Mexico Pervert Pipeline." 1992. Available at: http://www.belial.org/enbib/libxabu2.htm. Accessed July 17, 2003.

Kurkjian S. Two accuse ex-Worcester priest of molesting them, lawyer says. *Boston Globe.* January 8, 1993. Cited by: Christian Sex Crimes. "Massachusetts-to-New Mexico Pervert Pipeline." 1992. Available at: http://www.belial.org/enbib/libxabu2.htm. Accessed July 17, 2003.

Langevin R, Curnoe S, Bain J. A study of clerics who commit sexual offenses: are they different from other sex offenders? *Child Abuse Negl.* 2000;24:535-545.

Leberg E. *Understanding Child Molesters: Taking Charge.* Thousand Oaks, Calif: Sage Publications; 1997.

Luther M. *Martin Luther, Selections From His Writings.* Dillenberger J, ed. Chicago, Ill: Chicago Quadrangle Books; 1962.

Mass Gen Laws Ann ch 233 § 20A (2001).

Minn Stat § 595.02 (2000).

Minn Stat § 626.556, Subd 3(2).

Mont Code Ann § 26-1-804 (2001).

NDAA Position Paper on Religious Exemption. National Center for Prosecution of Child Abuse Update. American Prosecutors Research Institute. Alexandria, Va; September, 1991.

Nev Rev Stat § 49.255 (2000).

NH Rev Stat Ann § 516:35 (2000).

Niebuhr G A place of 'conversion' for priests who abused children *Washington Post.* January 2, 1993. Cited by: Christian Sex Crimes. "St. Luke's Helps Priests Evade Prosecution?" 1992. Available at: http://www.belial.org/enbib/libxabu2.htm. Accessed July 17, 2003.

Ore Rev Stat § 40.260 (1999); 42.

Owen B, ed. *Daily Readings From Luther's Writings.* Minneapolis, Minn: Augsburg; 1993.

Pa Cons Stat § 5943 (2001).

Pollenberg R. *The World of Benjamin Cardozo: Personal Values and the Judicial Process.* Cambridge, Mass: Harvard University Press; 1997.

Reuters News Service. Vatican issues new rules on podophile priests. January 8, 2002.

RI Gen Laws § 9-17-23 (2001).

Robinson WV, Paulson M. A 'grieving' law apologizes for assignment of Geoghan. *Boston Globe.* January 10, 2002.

Salter, AC. *Predators: Pedophiles, Rapists, and Other Sex Offenders: Who They Are, How They Operate, and How We Can Protect Ourselves and Our Children.* New York, NY: Basic Books; 2003.

Schutt MP. What's a nice Christian like you doing in a place like this? *Regent U Law Rev.* 1998-1999;11:137.

Spitzer JR. Without justice, there can be no healing. *Relig Abuse.* 1999;1:7-8.

Steinfels P. Giving healing and hope to priests who molested. *New York Times.* October 12, 1992;A11 Cited by: Christian Sex Crimes. "St. Luke's Helps Priests Evade Prosecution?" 1992. Available at: http://www.belial.org/enbib/libxabu2.htm. Accessed July 17, 2003.

Tenn Code Ann § 24-1-206 (2001).

Tennessee v Stewart, No. 01-C-01-9301-CR-00007, 1993 Crim App LEXIS 845, at 9-10 (Tenn Crim App Dec 16, 1993).

US Department of Health and Human Services (USDHHS). Statutes-at-a-glance: 2002. Available at: http://www.calib.com/nccanch/statutes/manda.cfm. Accessed August 7, 2003.

Vieth VI. Corporal punishment in the United States: a call for a new approach to the prosecution of disciplinarians. *Juv Law.* 1994;22:27-30.

Vieth VI. Drying their tears: making your congregation safe for child abuse victims. *Northwest Lutheran.* October 1, 1994;81:10.

Vieth VI. In my neighbor's house: a proposal to address child abuse in rural America. *Hamline Law Rev.* 1998;22:143.

Vieth VI. When dad hits mom: seven suggestions to make your congregation safe for victims of domestic violence. *Northwest Lutheran.* October 1, 1996;83:10.

Vieth VI. When the child abuser is a child: investigating, prosecuting and treating juvenile sex offenders in the new millennium. *Hamline Law Rev.* 2001;48:54-56.

W Va Code § 57-3-9 (2001).

Wash Rev Code Ann § 5.60.060(3) (2001).

Youso K. Religious symbols intermingle in nation's cemeteries. Available at: http://www.startribune.com/stories/389/28555937.html. Accessed May 27, 2002.

APPENDIX 39-1: TEACHING THE FAITH-BASED COMMUNITY TO TEACH THEMSELVES AND THEIR CHILDREN PERSONAL SAFETY

I have been blessed on several occasions to teach pastors and parishioners alike to, in turn, teach children in their homes and congregations about personal safety. Unless and until we empower children to report abuse, we can expect widespread silence to remain the norm. Many congregations have misgivings about personal safety that is based on a misunderstanding of what it is we need to teach our children. In teaching the 7 points below, though, I have found practitioners of conservative and liberal faiths accepting of these simple truths and expressing a willingness to follow this advice.

1. *Create an atmosphere in which children feel comfortable talking to you about difficult subjects.* Many children suffer silently, afraid to tell a parent of the evil taking place in their own home or the home of a neighbor, relative, or friend.

   Teach your children the difference between a good touch and an uncomfortable touch. Let them know that if the unthinkable occurs, you will not be angry but will support and protect your child as best you can. Teachers and parents routinely speak to children about fire safety. While it is appropriate to teach a young-ster to stop, drop, and roll, children are far more likely to encounter child abuse than they are a fire. Therefore, it is equally and perhaps more important to teach a child personal safety. Though a parent may feel uncomfortable speaking to a child about abuse, failure to do so lessens the chance your child will approach you in the event abuse occurs.

Many parents confuse a good touch/bad touch curriculum with sex education. The instruction is not the same. When speaking to a child about touches, simply instruct that while hugs and kisses are generally good, private parts of the body are off limits. If the child is unsure of the location, tell him or her a private part of the body is that covered by a bathing suit. Tell your child that while a doctor may have occasional need to examine genitalia, and a parent may need to clean intimate parts, these body parts should not otherwise be touched by others. Most importantly, give your child a game plan of what to do if inappropriate touching occurs. The game plan can be as simple as reporting any such touching to you.

If your school has a good touch/bad touch curriculum, do not assume that this guarantees your child will talk to you if abused. Tell your child you are aware of the curriculum, that you approve of it, and that you would like your son or daughter to tell you if anyone makes him or her feel uncomfortable.

Some parents mistakenly assume it is enough to teach a child to avoid strangers. This assumption is mistaken because the child may be harmed by someone who is not a stranger. Moreover, children often violate the rule against speaking to or going somewhere with a stranger. Tell your child you understand mistakes happen and that if he or she forgets and has contact with a stranger he or she can tell you about the contact without fear of reprisal.

2. *Listen to your children.* A child revealing abuse may begin with a tentative, ambiguous disclosure. The child may be testing the water in an effort to de-termine whether it is safe to reveal more. A child may say, "I don't like it when Uncle Bobby hugs me." Not understanding the significance of the comment, a parent may smile and say something like, "Do his whiskers tickle?" Even worse, a parent may admonish the child, telling the child that he or she sees the uncle only sporadically and the least he or she can do is share a hug. A parent respond-ing along these lines may close off communication with the child and fail to learn why Uncle Bobby's hugs are disturbing.

Rather than dismiss the child's statement, explore with him or her why the uncle's hugs are viewed unfavorably. Praise the child for sharing his or her feelings and ask the child if there is anything else the uncle does that makes him or her feel uncomfortable.

3. *Assure a child who reveals abuse that he or she did nothing wrong and that your love for him or her is unending.* Many parents are understandably shocked at the revelation and ask the child why the abuse was not revealed sooner. Parents pos-ing such a question unwittingly place blame on the child.

4. *Speak to a pediatrician and a child psychologist about the specifics of the abuse so that you can be sure that your child's physical and mental health needs are being addressed.* Your child may or may not need counseling, medical care, or other services. By consulting with trustworthy professionals experienced in handling cases of child abuse, you are better equipped to address your child's needs.

5. *Be prepared to respond to the spiritual damage inflicted on your child.* Many child abusers twist and pervert scripture as a means of keeping the child quiet. The perpetrator may tell a young girl that her "seductive" behavior caused the abuse. Pointing to the biblical condemnation of sex outside of marriage, the perpetrator

may tell a child that if she speaks of abuse, the church will condemn her. In response, a parent may tell a child victim that God condemns child abusers, not victims. Point out the difference between sinning and being the victim of someone else's sin. Tell your child he or she does not need God's forgiveness as a result of the abuse, the perpetrator does.

At some point, your child may ask you difficult, heartbreaking questions. Why didn't God answer my prayers when I asked him to stop Uncle Bobby from hurting me? If God loves me, why didn't he help me sooner? There is no simple answer to questions such as these. Perhaps the best parents can do is to acknowledge that we do not have all the answers. If I am teaching in a Christian congregation, I may suggest the parents can point to Christ's unjust suffering and express the belief that God has a sympathetic ear.

6. *Make sure that, in addition to yourself, your church is also prepared to address the needs of a child abuse victim.* In assessing your church's readiness, ask the following questions:

— Have the pastors and teachers in your church received any training on child abuse issues?

— Do your pastors and teachers know the police officers, social workers, and prosecutors who handle child abuse cases in your community?

— Are your pastors and teachers familiar with mandated reporting laws and the procedures to be followed if abuse must be reported?

— Does your church library have materials to assist a child or family victimized by abuse?

— Does your church school have a good touch/bad touch curriculum?

— Do your church workers know where to refer a child abuse victim in need of professional help?

By answering these questions now, your congregation will not only be better prepared to help a child abuse victim but you will also create an environment in which children can reveal abuse.

7. *Report the abuse to the police.* Well-meaning parents often choose not to report the abuse out of a sincere desire to protect their child from having to relive the ordeal in court. This decision all but guarantees that the perpetrator will reoffend.

Few, if any, perpetrators offend only once or offend against only one child. According to one study, men who molest girls average 19.8 victims, and men who molest boys average 150.2 victims. In a study of 561 sex offenders, these offenders accounted for the abuse of an astonishing 195 407 victims (Abel et al, 1987). Confidently relying on the silence of their victims, most child abusers escape justice. Indeed, a child molester's chance of getting caught is calculated to be as low as 3%.

Reporting abuse to the police does not necessarily mean your child will have to testify at trial. Not all cases result in the filing of charges. Most cases that do result in charges end in a plea of guilty. If your child does have to testify, the process is often more stressful for the parent than the child. More than one study finds that most abused children view the court process positively. Many children feel empowered by having confronted their abuser in court.

Obviously, no one can guarantee that your child will have a positive experience with the legal system. By coming forward, though, you send the unmistakable message that it was wrong for the perpetrator to violate your child's body and injure his or her spirit. Evil flourishes when good people remain silent.

Indeed, it is not parents alone who are responsible for protecting our children. Anyone with knowledge of abuse has a moral responsibility to speak for those too frail to help themselves. It always amazes me that when a child is dead, there is so often a flood of relatives and neighbors proclaiming a lack of surprise at the child's fate. These bystanders then relate scenes when the child was struck, cursed, and otherwise mistreated. Unfortunately for the deceased, the moral outrage of neighbors seldom translates into a phone call to social services.

Child abuse is appropriately described as a footprint on the heart. May we never lose our resolve to spare children from this sin. In the event abuse finds them, let us support our children with all the love they deserve.

APPENDIX 39-2: MAKING CONGREGATIONS SAFE FOR CHILD ABUSE VICTIMS*

As a prosecutor, my most difficult cases are those involving allegations of child abuse. I do not recall the name of each child victim I have worked with, but I remember each face. I recall the courage of more than one child forced to confront his abuser, a jury filled with strangers, and a legal system that is not childproof. With every case, my heart breaks.

The abuse of children is intolerable in our faith communities. Unfortunately, the faith community is not immune from this sin, and we often unwittingly permit this sin to flourish in God's houses. I have seen it happen.

In my experience, children are safe in congregations that adopt the following approach to an allegation of child abuse.

1. *Abused children are safe in congregations that understand child abuse can happen anywhere.* We can not live under the false assumption that child abuse can not happen in conservative congregations filled with respected members of our faith. The sin of child abuse does not check itself at the door of our churches, synagogues, and temples.

   Child abusers are rich and poor, male and female, college professors and high school dropouts, and they are found in every racial and religious class. Even social workers, police officers, and prosecutors assigned to the protection of children have been convicted of abuse.

   Studies indicate that as many as 38% of women and 16% of men have been sexually abused as children. Each year, our nation subjects 7 million children to caretaker violence, and as many as 2000 of these children die as a result. Moreover, some studies conclude that child abuse is more prevalent in rural than in urban communities (Vieth, 1998). (See also Salter, 2003 for citation and discussion of a number of studies on the prevalence of child sexual abuse. This includes some studies suggesting that the sexual abuse of girls may be as high as 37% and the abuse of boys as high as 30%.)

   If these studies are accurate, on any given Sunday, the pews of your congregation will likely hold at least one child abuser and one victim. Realizing this, we will not blind ourselves when the signs of abuse become obvious.

2. *Children are safe in congregations where child abuse is not covered up.* On more than one occasion, child abuse victims have been told to forgive their abusers and to remain silent about the abuse. Similarly, congregations have told abusers to ask God's forgiveness and to "sin no more." This is not enough.

---

* ***Appendix 39-2*** *reprinted with permission from Vieth VI. Drying their tears: making your congregation safe for child abuse victims. Northwest Lutheran. Octorber 1, 1994;81:10*

Abused children need to be able to speak about abuse as a means of healing. Abused children told to keep the secret pay a terrible price. I have known several who chose suicide rather than silence.

Abusers need forgiveness, but they also need to deal with their sin and its consequences. Typically, this includes professional counseling and some level of punishment. A congregation would never tell a parishioner with a heart disease to say a prayer but ignore the need to see a doctor. In the same vein, a parishioner confessing the sin of child abuse, particularly the sin of child sexual abuse, needs professional psychiatric or psychological care to address his or her abnormal behavior. Moreover, the parishioner should recognize his or her criminal behavior and turn himself or herself over to the authorities. If you would urge a confessed burglar to turn himself in to the police, why would you not urge a confessed child abuser to also reconcile himself or herself with the law?

3. *Abused children are safe in congregations that recognize them as victims and not as sinners.* A child abuse victim once told me she could not tell a pastor, teacher, or church elder about a sexual relationship with a parent because she knew that sex outside of marriage is a sin, and she was afraid of being condemned. Children need to know the difference between sinning and being the victim of someone else's sin. Children need to know that adults also understand this difference.

4. *Children are safe when congregations do not ostracize children who reveal abuse.* A child who reveals abuse is often isolated. The nonoffending parent and other siblings may rally around the perpetrator and, for all practical purposes, disown the victim. Typically, the victim—not the perpetrator—is removed from the home. The child's friends may tease and abandon him or her. A boy revealing a sexual relationship with his father may be labeled homosexual. The combined effect of this treatment is to compel the child to minimize the abuse and, in some cases, to recant the allegation altogether.

The victim's isolation is compounded when a congregation stands behind the perpetrators and implicitly condemns the child making the accusation. Tragically, this is often without full knowledge of the accusation or the evidence.

In one case, a pastor testified to the good character of an accused molester. Months later, the pastor confided to me that if he had known additional facts, his testimony would have been different.

In another case, a pastor and other community members wrote a letter professing the innocence of an accused molester and condemning the children for bringing their accusation years after the fact. Presumably, these parishioners did not realize that the accused molester had testified under oath that he had in fact molested 6 children. Apparently, the molester had not been forthright with the members of his church.

This is not to say that while an investigation is pending, a congregation must assume the guilt of an accused. Although children rarely lie about abuse, some adults have been falsely accused. When the veracity of an allegation is unclear, the congregation can support the accused and the accuser by praying that the truth be known.

5. *Children are safer in congregations where abusers receive tough love.* Forgiveness is an important aspect of most faiths. Certainly, Christians will claim that Christ died for the sins of child abusers as much as anyone else. Although our faith traditions can and should offer God's forgiveness, we must also insist on true repentance and changed behavior. We must recognize that child abuse rarely happens only once and that most abusers wrap themselves in a blanket of denial. We can support child abusers by letting them know we will not abandon them for telling

the truth and that we will not support them in continued lying or minimizing of their conduct.

In the words of Erik Erikson, "Someday, maybe, there will exist a well informed, well considered, and yet fervent public conviction that the most deadly of all possible sins is the mutilation of a child's spirit." May we pray that the faith community never contributes to this mutilation.

APPENDIX 39-3: SEVEN SUGGESTIONS TO MAKE CONGREGATIONS SAFE FOR VICTIMS OF DOMESTIC VIOLENCE*

In my career as a prosecutor, I have worked with hundreds of victims of domestic violence. I have seen the toll that domestic violence takes on the bodies, spirits, and children of these women. Sadly, more than one mother has removed herself from the faith community when she perceived the community's indifference to her need to survive.

Domestic violence is nothing less than a direct attack by the devil on our families and our faith. As members of the faith community, we must dedicate ourselves to understanding the dynamics of violence and ensure that we do not take any action that contributes to the cycle of abuse.

In my experience, congregations adhering to the following guidelines are the best prepared and the most effective in combating the sin of domestic violence.

1. *Our clergy and our congregations need to ensure the safety of domestic violence victims.* The goal of family preservation can not be achieved by returning a victim home to endure additional poundings. All too often, such advice leads to serious injury or death to our mothers, the imprisonment of our fathers, and the foster care placement of our children.

    Each year, 4000 women in the United States are killed by their spouses. The United States Surgeon General cites domestic violence as the leading cause of bodily injury to American women. Much of this violence could have been avoided, and many families saved, if we had not insisted on continuing a dangerous living arrangement.

    In many cases, family preservation is possible only after the victim and perpetrator are living apart, and the perpetrator accesses spiritual and professional help. Domestic abusers are so dedicated to the use of power to maintain their relationships that these complex dynamics can not be addressed until there is a separation.

    In conservative Christian congregations, the scriptural belief that the couple must stay together no matter what is often expressed. When, however, an abusive husband fails to love his wife as Christ loved the church, he has abandoned her, and this abandonment is a scriptural basis for divorce (1 Corinthians 7:15).

2. *We need to care for the spiritual needs of women victimized by violence.* Some victims of violence are confused by the abuse and believe that if God chose their husband, God wills the violence. The faith community must in no uncertain terms remind these women that violence is inconsistent with God's will for their marriages.

3. *Our congregations need to tend to the spiritual and physical needs of children growing up in violent homes.* Children raised in such homes have higher rates of truancy, drug and alcohol problems, and suicide. Many of these children choose a life of

---

* **Appendix 39-3** *reprinted with permission from Vieth VI. When dad hits mom: seven suggestions to make your congregation safe for victims of domestic violence.* Northwest Lutheran. *Octorber 1, 1996;83:10*

crime. Ninety percent of the men in Minnesota prisons grew up in homes where violence was the norm.

When children turn to crime, drugs, and suicide, it is a clarion call to recognize and address their spiritual needs. When church-going dad beats church-going mom, and congregation looks the other way, it is understandable why many children abandon their faith and look elsewhere for comfort. Reaching out to children of violent homes is not always easy but, if the faith community does not act, the devil and his agents are eager to fill the void.

4. *We must insist that domestic abusers be accountable for their sin.* In the book of Genesis we are told that Adam was the first man to blame his wife for his sin (Genesis 3:12). Domestic abusers are adept at continuing this tradition.

As a prosecutor, it is disheartening to view the photographs of bruised and blood-ied women and then to read the statements of abusers who blame the beating on the victim. I know domestic abusers who blame their violence on the alleged nagging, obesity, cooking deficits, and sexual shortcomings of their wives. Abusers use such excuses as blatant attempts to whitewash their sin.

In the Genesis account, God did not allow Adam to blame his sin on Eve. In the same vein, the faith community today must be vigilant in reminding domestic abusers that they alone are responsible for their sin, and they alone must answer to God.

5. *We should encourage domestic abusers to make themselves right with the law.* After decades of avoidance, police and prosecutors at long last have begun to take seriously the crime of domestic violence.

Unfortunately, many abusers blame the victim when a police officer makes an arrest or a prosecutor seeks jail or other sanctions against an abuser. Some abusers hire unscrupulous defense attorneys or otherw.ise seek to use the legal system to further intimidate or manipulate the victim. Such conduct may be legal, but it is sinful and should be condemned by the faith community.

6. *The faith community must resist the temptation to be silent about the sin of domestic violence.* Preachers must preach and teachers must teach that husbands who love their wives do not beat them. The faith community must call to repentance those who do abuse and forgive those who heed this call by taking the steps necessary to forever reform their behavior. Abusers who do not heed this call should be disciplined pursuant to the tenets of our nation's various faiths.

7. *The faith community must pray that God will guide our efforts to end the assault of our spouses and the emotional torture of our children.* May God speed the day when our families are safe in heaven, and the violence we knew on earth is only a memory.

Exiting Route: A Peer Support Model for Exiting and Healing Programs

Fadi Barakat Fadel

"I don't want somebody coming up to me saying, 'You're wrong, you're doing it because you're stupid.' You need somebody out there who actually has had experience, somebody to tell you their story: 'This is what I did to get out of it; this worked for me, it might work for you; it might not; and if it does, great, and if it doesn't, we'll find some other way."

This chapter discusses the issue of commercial sexual exploitation of children (CSEC) from the point of view of the children and explores the process of exiting and healing. The ideas presented here go beyond the personal experience of the author to reflect the voices of hundreds of other *experiential children and youth* (ie, those who have been involved in commercial sexual exploitation by working in the sex trade) throughout the Americas. These voices were in the transcripts of consultations held prior to "Out From the Shadows: International Summit of Sexually Exploited Youth of the Americas," a summit held in Victoria, British Columbia, in 1998, and in the focus groups that resulted in the report *Sacred Lives: Canadian Aboriginal Children and Youth Speak Out About Sexual Exploitation.* They were also recorded at a number of youth forums and community meetings throughout Canada as well as during one-on-one interviews (Mark & Kingsley, 2001). The transcripts present the experiences and insights of sexually exploited children and youth in their own words as they describe their life experiences and make recommendations for addressing the critical issues they face on a daily basis.

The model introduced in this document was developed as a result of engaging child survivors of the sex trade as key intervenors and actors in efforts to address CSEC. It is a model for healing using group interaction combined with teachings derived from the Aboriginal Medicine Wheel (introduced later in this chapter) as a means to engage survivors of commercial sexual exploitation on the road to successful recovery. The image of a spinning top symbolizing the precariousness of the process, the powerful forces in play, and the need for balance within the young person completes the picture.

The need for such a model was revealed at the Victoria Youth Summit as youth began to emerge from the shadows and participate in projects aimed at combating CSEC. With the United Nations Convention on the Rights of the Child as its ground, a youth-driven model has been designed whose main purpose is to enhance the campaign to stop the use of children as sexual commodities and to enable them to exit the sex trade and heal. It is based on the premise that exploited children and youth have the right to participate in their own protection. The Exiting Route model offers opportunities and skill development mechanisms to enable children who have exited the sex trade to resist returning to it, to listen to others who are still trapped in it, and to be the public voice educating the larger community about the complex nature of the sex trade.

The model presented here should not be considered a stand-alone solution for exiting and healing but rather a way of binding services and youth in a safe and welcoming environment. Children and youth exploited in the sex trade have unique issues, such as addictions and traumas, and they need a wide range of services to help them deal with these issues. But they also need to be able to explore and come to terms with their devastating experiences and renew a balanced sense of self in the presence of others who have also "been there." This model allows groups of exploited children and youth to experience camaraderie and closeness so they can share, struggle, and inspire one another to exit and heal.

UNDERSTANDING COMMERCIAL SEXUAL EXPLOITATION OF CHILDREN

Experiential children share common social conditions and histories, and they undergo similar psychosocial effects despite personal differences. By analyzing the contents of their stories, common points were identified that helped to understand the "process" of being commercially sexually exploited. It became clear that permanent exiting for children in the sex trade depends on their ability to define their reality, shape their personal identity, find inner balance, and take their place in the wider community. In other words, exiting means acquiring equality and the ability to enjoy human rights.

Based on transcripts and interviews as well as anecdotal evidence, the following characteristics appear to be true for children and youth who are commercially sexually exploited:

— The average age of entry is 14 to 15 years.

— They are coerced, lured, and forced (it is not about choice).

— They come from varied ethnic and social backgrounds, especially in major urban areas.

— Aboriginal (indigenous) children and youth are overrepresented.

— Low wages and youth unemployment make it hard for youth to live independently.

— They have inadequate family and community support, as well as involvement in the state care system and/or institutionalization.

— The average stay in the sex trade is 5 years.

— Drugs and alcohol are used as entrapment tools; addictions keep children and youth in the sex trade.

BARRIERS AND CHALLENGES TO EXITING

For children and youth who have been isolated from the community, with little formal education, and with health and/or substance abuse problems, the barriers to exiting the sex trade are considerable. They have learned to distrust adults, and their self-esteem has usually been seriously eroded. For many, the support they need in order to stay off the streets has to come from someone who has experienced what they have experienced.

"I think we need more places for kids to go. They say there is no funding, no place to put them. There are lots of side-by-side apartment blocks boarded up in this city, lots of places kids on the street could go for shelter if these buildings were fixed up and there were enough resources."

"I need someone to love me. I was hungry for love and attention. Not sexual love, but someone to hold me and love me, to say encouraging things. I didn't have that."

"[I need] people like me to help me. There are agencies out there, but they couldn't help me get clean. They needed experience to feel my pain, my scars; the centers just continued to fail."

"At least one person to support you, not to be judgmental, to be there for you if you screw up; someone to talk to, to sort out feelings; one person to say, 'I believe you'; someone to encourage you and say you are a good person."

Some young people are constantly looking for ways out, while others seem to stumble upon an opportunity to exit. Both, however, have reported that the decision to exit was made due to a variety of reasons from "I have had it" to "I want to take care of myself and my friends."

"I realized I had to love myself more. I had to be away from the streets, from my friends, from my mother. But I still feel a need to be out there because my friends are still suffering. I need to get myself out first."

"I got donations of clothing and make-up, furniture, and money. Talking to people, support from my family, and having people tell me they believed in me."

Unforeseen circumstances, such as a drug overdose, pregnancy, violence, and sometimes rape are also triggers that motivate youth to seek a path of exiting.

"I got pregnant. I was working all the time, but my relationship with my baby's dad, he did not give me any money, not even for stuff like tampons. To get away from this guy, I needed my own money."

"Seeing the people around me. I was scared all the time. I was tired of being raped and seeing my friends die. I wanted a better life for my child."

Even after making the decision to exit the sex trade, young people struggle and often fall back into the trade due to the gaps in existing crisis intervention services. The complexity of social security systems, long waiting lists, and lack of resources at the front line dramatically reduce the chances of successful and permanent exiting. According to the May 1999 Jurisdictional Scan Report prepared for the British Columbia Ministry of Health and the Inter-Ministry Steering Committee on Prostitution, the main gaps include the following:

— Insufficient outreach personnel

— Insufficient detoxification and treatment beds for youth

— Lack of residential mental health facilities

— Lack of safe, supportive, residential environments specifically designed for commercially exploited youth

For many youth, the suffering experienced while in the trade poses the biggest barrier to overcome. The damage caused by the sexual, physical, and emotional abuse they encountered stays with them when they leave the trade. Healing begins by accepting the fact that children are victims of abuse and exploitation and that they did not choose the sex trade but were instead forced into it physically or financially.

Although it may be impossible to forget the experiences of trauma and abuse from the sex trade, experiential young people have identified the need to forgive themselves for what happened to them.

"In my mind, I'll never forget; I'll always have nightmares. I'll always cry about it."

"Forgiveness; you have to learn to forgive yourself for what you have done to yourself."

One major part of healing is to resolve the confusion between love and sex. Exploited sexual relations are detached from any understanding of love. Love is an emotional connection, while exploited sex is an activity void of any meaning. The sexual abuse experienced by the young people has taught them not to love or trust and not to let their guard down.

"It damaged my self-image, my self-worth, and my self-esteem. I needed counseling for child abuse. I had to learn how to have healthy relationships with my family, friends, and boyfriends."

"The sexual abuse. There wasn't a day that would go by that I wouldn't think about it, about the people that hurt me. I am full of shame and regret."

Sexually exploited youth are more vulnerable to physical health problems such as human immunodeficiency virus/acquired immunodeficiency syndrome (HIV/AIDS) and sexually transmitted diseases (STDs). Drug use also increases the chances of contracting hepatitis. Children and youth are often powerless to insist on condoms, and many have little information about sexual health and reproduction. Pregnancies are problematic because exploited youth are unlikely to receive adequate prenatal care and early childbirth can be dangerous. Children and youth, by virtue of their age, have more delicate inner tissues and are more vulnerable to internal tears, infections, inflammatory disease, and infertility. Sexually abused children have also been found to suffer from malnutrition, untreated wounds, and tuberculosis.

"Risks: pregnancy, standing on the street and getting kidnapped and getting the shit beaten out of you, being taken away to another city … AIDS, STDs, all forms of violence and abuse."

On the mental health side, researchers have noted that survivors of prolonged sexual abuse suffer from complex posttraumatic stress disorder (PTSD). Their self-esteem is extremely low and, overall, they feel a sense of helplessness, shame, and guilt (Robinson, 1997).

The inability to access affordable housing and low or inaccessible welfare assistance are other obstacles preventing children and youth from exiting the sex trade. Experiential youth rarely have the resources or support to change their environment and attain stable and sustainable living arrangements, a crucial first step toward exiting. Available assistance programs often require the youth to commit to an intervention plan that is unrealistic given the severity of the issues and trauma they have experienced. Meeting basic needs for survival is vital for successful exiting and healing as well as their participation in any programs that support the process. Children and youth have the right to protection, survival, participation, promotion, and development.

Children must also be able to participate in the conception, design, and implementation of their exiting plans. We believe that any other way is bound to fail. For children and youth, services that utilize reprimands and punitive actions simply mirror the exploitation and abuse they have already experienced. Safety, food, and housing must be offered as the first step of intervention without enforcing any conditions in order to provide an environment that encourages and maintains the exiting process.

"Positive people around me, people who had been there, who have done it, and who knew about it. I don't want to listen to people who just read books."

Even after overcoming the barriers to exiting the sex trade, youth face multitudes of obstacles and hurdles while staying out. Being out is not enough. Young people must be able to stay out. To do so, experiential youth need a support system that meets the needs of their new lifestyle. Existing community outreach programs do offer some of the help needed to exit and stay out. But youth report that commonly used harm-reduction models do not address the complex variety of issues they deal with. Services that only sustain the survival of young people on the street make them dependent on these services, thus maintaining their involvement in street lifestyles. Most (if not all) programs to help sexually exploited children get off the streets have been developed and managed by professional social workers and therapists. Without experiential involvement in designing and carrying out such programs, many issues experienced by exploited children may not be addressed or resolved. Experiential young people have often stated that they do not feel any connection with outreach workers. They do not want to talk to people who have "just read the book," as one experiential female stated. They feel that professionally trained workers can not possibly understand what they have suffered. These workers have not experienced the sex trade themselves; they need to "feel (the) pain, (and) scars," said another experiential female.

Opportunities for involvement in advocacy or community activities often enable young people to connect with peers and other youth and to feel good. Experience has proven that in most cases, participation activities are the triggers needed for youth to make a decision and begin the process of exiting and healing (Rabinovitch, 2001).

SUCCESSFUL EXITING AND HEALING

Successful exiting means that young people have developed the capacity to cope with and heal from the effects of CSEC. Issues of trauma and abuse will be revisited until they are resolved. Exploited children and youth have learned a set of survival skills more suited to the sex trade and the street than to "mainstream" culture. They lack interpersonal skills as well as the ability to resolve conflict and manage money. Exiting is the process of providing healing activities as well as education and capacity-building that empower the youth.

"Experiential young people need options to off-street incomes."

Successful exiting and healing requires support mechanisms that can provide a place to live, a job, and an education. Experiential children and youth identified the need for shelters and safe houses to help them stay on their feet until they are financially secure to provide for themselves the basic necessities of life.

Exploited children and youth have identified a number of prerequisites for successful exiting:

1. *Housing.* Without a stable address, the exploited young person can not acquire identification documents or access social programs and services.

2. *Access to quality services and peer support.* Peer support programs should be run by people who have had the same experiences as those seeking help. Peer counselors, incorporated in drug and alcohol treatment programs, counseling, and other services, keep the young person focused on his or her goals and reduce the negative effects of relapse.

   "We need a healing center for anybody exiting that is run by survivors."

   "It empowered me to speak out, to have a voice, to feel like I wasn't just a hooker, but that I actually was somebody."

   "I was able to be honest and not judged for not exiting. At a spiritual level, it has an impact. It got me away from the trade more."

   "… empowered myself to give hope to other people, to myself; I grew from it. Helped me to believe in myself and can change people's opinions."

3. *Economic opportunities and skills development.* Employment opportunities and human resource services provide exploited youth not only with work experience but also with positive role models for exiting and healing.

"Bridging program, things to teach how to write resumes and how to conduct yourself in a different environment."

4. *Strong and meaningful support from individuals and community services.* The Victoria Declaration and Agenda for Action states that exploited children and youth are not prostitutes but victims of abuse and exploitation. Communities need to reach out to these youth and let them know that they are part of the community. Being marginalized by the community is often the entry point into the sex trade and a real barrier to exiting.

5. *Ability to adopt healthy behaviors.* Exploited youth need to learn to cope with the history and effects of sexual, physical, and emotional abuse.

EXITING ROUTE MODEL

Exiting the sex trade begins with a wish for an imagined new self; staying out, however, can be achieved only when the young person is able to protect and maintain his or her physical, mental, emotional, and spiritual health. The ancient North American Aboriginal teaching of the Medicine Wheel (**Figure 40-1**) offers great insight and understanding on how to protect and maintain these aspects of self.

The Medicine Wheel includes spiritual, emotional, mental, and physical components; its study promotes personal accountability and healthy lifestyles. Over the years, it has been taught as a community service leadership model to Native youth as a way of sharing teachings on Aboriginal values, culture, and traditions. Young people are encouraged to develop a stronger self-concept and healthy goals as well as to embrace the values of respect, reverence, and reciprocity that help them become effective leaders in their communities. In the past, the Medicine Wheel was a reflection of an individual's strengths and weaknesses that gave one guidelines to follow for personal growth on what the individual needed to learn and what he or she needed to teach.

The Medicine Wheel is a circle divided by a cross to create 4 directions and 4 realms. A person in both Aboriginal and non-Aboriginal cultures is thought to comprise 4 realms: the physical, mental, spiritual, and emotional. The North is the place of beginning, the place of rebirth; the East represents the new light of day, the place for new thoughts; the South, as the highest point of the sun, represents the opportunity to make connections with powers greater than the self; and the West is the place for letting go, of introspection. The 4 directions line up with the 4 realms: North = physical realm; East = mental realm; South = spiritual realm; and West = emotional realm.

Unlike western models for psychology that begin personal work with looking into incidents of the past to explain the present, the Medicine Wheel begins in the South, the realm of spirituality. The personal work of the South means healing the past in order to shed it. Healing is attained when the past no longer owns the person. It is in the southern direction that people become free; this is where the choice for a new self is born and the mastery of one's skill and performance is achieved. Moving to the western direction, personal work consists of facing death and personal fears, investigating the center of violence and transforming the self; this is where change occurs. The North works to connect with ancestors; this is where wisdom develops and new beginnings take root. The work of the East is abstract and deals with seeing new ways. It serves to connect and bond the self with wisdom and experience. Therefore, the Medicine Wheel is a valuable tool for understanding exiting and healing from commercial sexual exploitation.

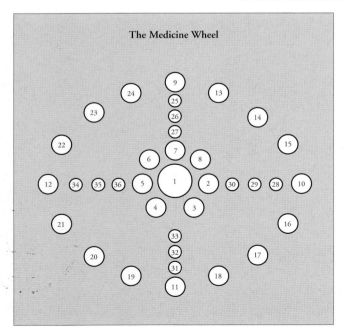

Figure 40-1. *The North American Aboriginal Medicine Wheel.*

The Medicine Wheel

The teachings of the Medicine Wheel are the principles of the Exiting Route. This model creates a third dimension for the Medicine Wheel that further explains the complexity of exiting and healing. The Medicine Wheel is transposed into a rotating top (**Figure 40-2**). When released with sufficient energy and sent in a certain direction, the top will rotate on its principal axis and move in a chosen direction for a long period of time even if there are disturbances. The faster the spin, the more it will withstand disturbances. This motion explains the beginning of an exiting path (**Figure 40-3**). An event, negative or positive (eg, overdose, pregnancy, assault), triggers the top to spin and the exiting process to begin.

However, without a constant input of energy, the spinning top is unstable. There will come a time when the spin diminishes. When this happens, the top will wobble, move off its axis, and eventually fall to one side. To spin again, it must be picked up, given energy, and rereleased. Once directed, it will rotate its weight, shape, and contact point in a perfect balance.

Getting the top to spin on its axis (signifying a perfect balance of physical, emotional, mental, and spiritual realms) is started by the decision to exit and is sustained and energized through experiential peer participation, expert facilitation, and collaboration of systems.

When the top (representing the youth's energies and balance) stops and falls, the young person is alerted that his or her self is not in balance (**Figure 40-4**). To spin again and move forward, he or she has to heal all aspects of his or her being and understand that these aspects are always interconnected. The road to exiting and healing is dependent on how interconnectedness is sustained among all 4 realms of the person. Practice is the only way to flag what is throwing the top off balance and to correct the problem before a fall or a relapse occurs. If a relapse occurs, the person has to start spinning again until a new consciousness is formed. The best way to do

Figure 40-2. Components of the Medicine Wheel transposed into a top.

Figure 40-3. The motion of a spinning top can be used to represent the exiting process.

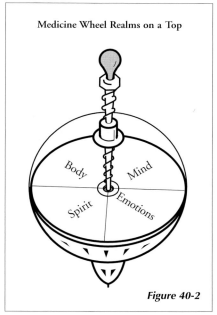

Medicine Wheel Realms on a Top

Body · Mind · Spirit · Emotions

Figure 40-2

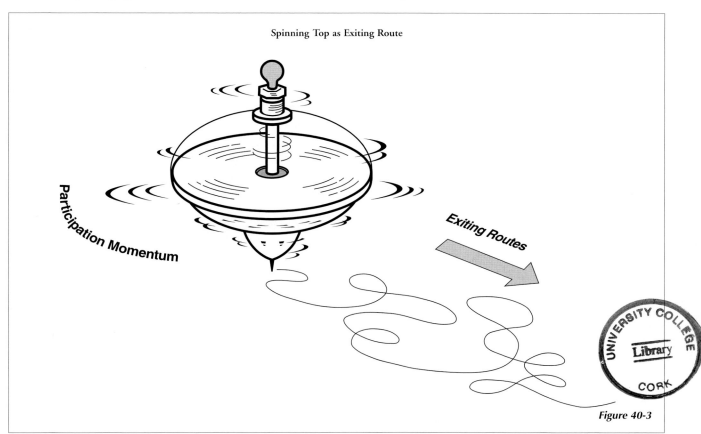

Spinning Top as Exiting Route

Participation Momentum

Exiting Routes

Figure 40-3

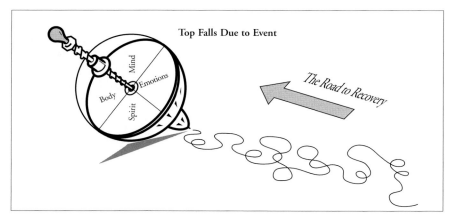

Figure 40-4. *The falling top suggests that the dimensions of the self are out of balance.*

this is through an experience of group dynamics carefully designed and facilitated by a helping organization.

Experience shows that the process of exiting and healing has a higher chance of success when it is in a safe and community-like environment. This can be realized by bringing together groups of 4 to 6 sexually exploited children and youth and providing them with stable and secure access to housing, food, and adequate social care and healthcare.

In the field of applied social sciences, many theories explain group dynamics in terms of reference points for participants' behavior. A well understood group dynamics theory, Lacoursiere's theory of the Life Cycle of Groups, underlies the Exit Route model we propose for this process. According to this theory, any group has a progressive 5-stage life cycle: inclusion, conflict, resolution, production, and termination (**Table 40-1**). These stages occur in a regular sequence; though they may overlap and blend one into another, they are separate and distinct. This does not mean that once a stage is passed, issues central to that stage do not reappear. On the contrary, traces of earlier stages can be seen in later ones and vice versa. For example, aspects of inclusion are dealt with throughout the life of the group and feelings of dissatisfaction are not isolated to just one stage. In other words, participants will revisit issues of trust, relapse, and addiction until those issues are resolved. The length of the stay at each stage varies with the size of the group and the resources available to sustain an exiting group of young people (Kass, 1996).

Lacoursiere's theory combines therapy and skill training. It provides a safe environment for participants to learn how to heal and cope with issues of trauma and abuse while working on a task. A task-training component is essential. It means that members of the group, the young people, participate in a community development project that enables them to acquire work skills and experience toward independence. Task behaviors are related to defining and testing the feasibility of suggestions and ideas, learning and applying skills related to the task, assessing what needs to be achieved, and determining how to achieve it.

Socioemotional behaviors are related to reactions, feelings, and interactions of group members toward the task, the group facilitator, and other members. Having to accomplish a task provides a safe and protective environment for the young person to engage in a certain activity but at the same time be able to explore personal issues

Table 40-1. Stages of the Life Cycle of Groups

1. Inclusion
2. Conflict
3. Resolution
4. Production
5. Termination

Adapted from Kass R. Theories in Group Development. *Montreal, Canada: Concordia University; 1996.*

without fear or prejudice. It also provides young people with a chance to be a part of the community without having to be put under the spotlight and labeled as sex trade workers. Eliminating the shame factor is key to getting young people involved. It is also a way to deal with community prejudice and eventually change people's attitudes.

One example of a group task was Street Fest 2001, a 1-day street festival held in March 2001 in Vancouver, British Columbia, Canada, designed and implemented by a group of 15 experiential youth who formed a steering committee. The committee met weekly to organize, fundraise, advertise, and carry out the festival. The task was the catalyst to motivate young people to get involved in their community, begin to trust adults, and explore exiting possibilities. Facilitating the participation of the youth was not an easy task. Much preparation and thought was put into the process. Overall, Street Fest 2001 aimed to bring public awareness to the true worth of street youth as integral members of the community in Vancouver. It was devised to promote a culture of peace where all members of the downtown community would come together and showcase the talents of youth through art, music, film, and the spoken word. Approximately 200 youth and 25 service providers attended the 9-hour event.

Group dynamics rely on experienced facilitators who understand members and are capable of acquiring the members' trust. The facilitator, ideally a survivor of sexual exploitation who has successfully exited and acquired intervention and training skills, will use the Life Cycle theory to help sexually exploited children and youth exit, heal, and do the following:

— Achieve stable living patterns

— Become trained citizens able to participate in the well-being of the community

— Become employable and skilled persons ready to enter the job market

— Become individuals with strong and meaningful support from an alternative family (can include biological family but should involve friends and peers) and community

— Become healthy individuals with strong and sustained experience to deal with drug and alcohol addictions and other socioemotional effects of commercial sexual exploitation

In classic groups, where the focus is less personal, task and socioemotional behaviors are quite separate and easily distinguishable. In exiting and healing groups, the focus is personal and interactive so that tasks and socioemotional behaviors are inseparable and often difficult to isolate.

The Exiting Route model aims to help children and youth overcome fear and trust issues, relate their stories and accounts of violence, validate their experiences, provide them with exiting opportunities, and link them to local support and services. It combines goals, tasks, skills, and knowledge and sets practice standards sensitive to the special needs of exploited youth. For the model to work, expectations must be clarified and communicated to staff, partners, and beneficiaries. A baseline for work must be set and a mechanism provided for the monitoring, review, and further development of work.

STAGES OF AN EXITING AND HEALING GROUP LIFE CYCLE FOR SEXUALLY EXPLOITED YOUTH

INCLUSION

This is the initial stage of group development. Participants first get informed and oriented to the group, its members, and the facilitator. This is probably the first time these young people are meeting peers in a safe and understanding environment. Young people get acquainted and accept membership to a group that will "stick together" for the period of the project. The experiential facilitator has a major role to play; he or she acts as a translator and mediator between the youth and the organization sponsoring the project or the community in which the group exists. It is also a time for defining the task and what needs to be achieved. Lacoursiere suggests that most people (other than those forced to participate) enter the new group experience with enthusiasm, positive expectations, and optimism. While there may be some preoccupation and anxiety about this new situation, hope far outweighs anticipatory fears that participants may have concerning the task, the new job, the new environment, or other issues for exiting and healing (Kass, 1996).

During this initial period, there is heavy reliance on the group leader for guidance, content, and structure. Maintaining a healthy dependence is vital because it propels participants to ask for ground rules and gives rise to group norms. At this stage, information and opinions are given and sought and tasks are specified. Powerhouses and rank are also established as is the nature of all street-related relationships. Roles of leadership are defined. Members of the group become leaders, followers, and stoppers. The facilitator's role is crucial because he or she is responsible for ensuring that everyone participates actively, each within one's own capacity. Members are looking to the facilitator for leadership, reassurance, and orientation and to test feasibility.

CONFLICT

As the most difficult but important stage of exiting, the conflict stage is characterized by frustration, ambiguity, and anxiety (Kass, 1996). Reality sets in, and youth participants begin to realize the enormous task ahead. Chances of relapse are high. The facilitator's role is to ensure that each member understands the Medicine Wheel model for achieving balance. The Aboriginal "talking circle" is used to arrive at decisions and work collaboratively. This involves each person speaking freely and without interruption, yet treating all other speakers with respect even when he or she disagrees with them, thereby creating a shared consensus (Talking Circle, 2003). The facilitator works with members to build the foundation that will bring the topsy-turvy self into balance. At this time, members who have experienced extreme trauma may need referrals to a qualified counselor or specialist.

The reality of the group encounter during this stage may not only be unpleasant but also is often experienced as a shock. It usually brings into sharp focus discrepancies among the expectations and the experiences of the various members, constituting a major obstacle for the group to overcome.

As the group examines what needs to be done, the possible (the real world) comes into conflict with the ideal (unrealistic expectations). Frustration and anger set in as members begin to realize that they may not be able to accomplish what they had hoped to do as easily as they had expected. They may also see that the initial reason they joined the group was not what it seemed to be. The anger they feel is a direct reaction to the frustration they experience. The "top" begins to wobble. However, there is new energy as children and youth survivors of the sex trade begin to deal with issues of anger and abuse. This stage is critical in the exiting process. Members start to learn how to deal with feelings generated by disappointment, resentment, discouragement, sadness, doubt, resistance, anxiety, anger, confusion, disequilibrium, fear, crisis of confidence, and more. These feelings are explosive, and working with them is difficult. The morale of the group may sink. Some members may drop out for varied reasons, such as separation from familiar relationships, disconnectedness, and relapse. If negative feelings prevail, they may outweigh the more positive ones experienced. At this early point of exiting, running away, relapsing, and returning to earlier negative patterns are quick and easy solutions for participants, because they are not too far "out."

Relapse, dropout, and "group arrest" are inevitable and present a danger to the exiting process. Group arrest occurs when the exiting group becomes trapped in the conflict stage. At this point, an outside intervention must be introduced to stop the arrest.

Losing members along the way can be a threat to the rest of the life cycle of the group. Outside help is needed so that members can understand what is happening to their personal selves and be linked to appropriate services and programs. Kass (1996) believes that this stage, so full of intensity, can take well over 40% or more of total group time. Sadly, this large portion can be quite unpleasant.

Before individual tops spin out of control, the facilitator has to move the group into the resolution stage by resolving the conflict. Progress into this stage depends largely on how the conflict stage has been handled. These 2 stages are closely connected. Peer and professional support will be needed to address issues and help members move on.

One must keep in mind that survivors of sexual abuse and exploitation are remarkably resilient and eager to exit the sex trade. However, if the commitment to exit and heal is solid, the group may take less time. No matter how well inclusion has been handled, the realities of their situations are never clearer or more obvious to the group than now.

RESOLUTION

This stage is characterized by reconciliation between reality and the expectations of members, organization, and outside players. The group begins to examine goals in the light of time available, the task it has to accomplish, the restrictions of the situation, and the skills accessible within the group. The resolution stage falls between conflict and production, and what happens at this time (Kass, 1996) will influence the depth, quality, and success of the exiting and healing process. The facilitator must evaluate whether there should be redefinition or clarification of what still needs to be done, reassessing priorities and needs. Essentially, it means contracting to continue to work as a group.

The resolution process allows for open discussion, ownership of dissatisfaction, and willingness to compromise on the part of the group. It sets the tone for building cohesion and creates a climate for change. Children and youth survivors of sexual exploitation can begin to establish an equilibrium that will allow them to move on. As structures and procedures are sorted through and decided on, resources will begin to be used and pooled, and skills will be learned. The facilitator is obligated to promote the skills of the members by linking them with community players and involving them in leisure and creative activities. Seeing small successes and community support helps to lower the tension, decrease dissatisfaction, increase self-esteem, accept differences, and lessen anxiety. If the process used by the group matches the needs of the individuals, the norms that emerge will usually be constructive and useful.

If the conflict stage has not been completely resolved or if there is relapse that reverts the group back into conflict, the resolution stage can take a long time. Successful exiting means that needs are met and issues resolved. This is a hard and long process. Exiting is not an overnight treatment.

PRODUCTION

This is the most productive stage in the group's life cycle. Attention is focused on the task with renewed anticipation, hope, and positive feelings of eagerness to participate.

Members begin to acquire new learning as well as to apply and practice new skills and opportunities. Acquiring new skills raises positive feelings that influence self-esteem, feelings of adequacy, and a renewed sense of excitement (Kass, 1996).

TERMINATION

Termination for the group means that the process has reached the end; the task has been completed or the time allotted has run out (Kass, 1996). If termination comes after the task has been completed or after the group has worked though issues of interdependence and cohesion, members will benefit enormously. If, however, the group terminates before this stage has been reached, outcomes can be quite negative.

In exiting and healing groups, this process is complex because termination is part of the task the group needs to grapple with. On a personal level, the group has been privy to painful, critical, and demanding encounters among members. Bonding has taken place at a deep level that can make closure particularly difficult. With sexually exploited children and youth, disclosure of profoundly traumatic experiences and feelings has often been a first-time experience and involves real risks. Members may choose to keep meeting after the group is terminated and should be supported to do so.

MORE INSIGHT

Exiting and healing from sexual exploitation presents many unique issues and dilemmas for those who work with such a group. Mechanisms, structures, and values of hosting organizations need to be adapted in order to ensure that members of the group are not ghettoized and that efforts to work with them are lasting. This requires ongoing attention and awareness-raising on the part of the host organization; the staff must have a clear understanding of the issues of sexually exploited youth and the challenges they face in exiting. Also, host organizations should promote the groups they are facilitating and ensure that members are not just passive service recipients.

It is important to provide appropriate services that cater to the specific needs expressed by the group regardless of gender, race, culture, sexuality, disability, or other differences. Group members need to acquire a balanced self-identity in the face of their past experiences to secure long-lasting exiting and healing.

The role of experiential youth and their democratic participation and collaboration can not be underestimated in determining the success or failure of exiting and healing. Many young people who have been sexually exploited have developed extremely resilient but highly individualistic survival strategies. Carrying out a project of group work and reaching out to the community can become a rite of passage for experiential children and youth, enabling them to enter the community and take their place as citizens. Nevertheless, adequate resources and outside support must be in place to meet their needs.

PRINCIPLES OF GOOD PRACTICE

Over the years, the young people who have helped develop the Exiting Route model described above have identified 12 principles to help guide good practice work with commercially sexually exploited children and youth. Over the years, they have proven to be useful in carrying out youth-driven projects and exiting activities.

1. *The principle of meaningful and visible decision-making of experiential children and youth.* Experiential children and youth must play a meaningful and visible decision-making role in the development of any efforts. Wherever possible, they should play a role in the development of the participation process itself.

2. *The principle of realistic participation.* Opportunities, support, and resources for participation must be realistic and address the circumstances under which experiential youth live. Some ways to facilitate this include the following: paying for youth expertise; using nonintimidating processes; interpreting the culture of government and law in plain language; showing a willingness to listen and learn from the youth's experiences; engaging in open dialogue and providing room to speak openly; and creating trust that supports meaningful and pragmatic outcomes, such as covering the costs of transportation and daycare.

3. *The principle of capacity-building.* Commitment to a capacity-building approach to addressing the commercial sexual exploitation of children and youth means that those who have personally experienced exploitation will be supported through the creation and delivery of services. Youth have repeatedly asked for the opportunity to connect with those who have successfully exited the sex trade.

Those who have successfully exited the sex trade have repeatedly asked for the opportunity to play a meaningful role in providing outreach, support, public education, and advocacy and in mentoring young people in the sex trade.

4. *The principle of recognition of expertise.* The only real experts on the commercial sexual exploitation of children and youth are those who have experienced sexual exploitation. They must be considered an integral part of all local, regional, national, and international dialogue and be respected and supported by cultures, communities, and families. They should be paid for their expertise and be seriously considered for any employment opportunities created in the development of strategies designed to address the commercial sexual exploitation of children and youth.

5. *The principle of meaningful exchange.* All efforts to address the commercial sexual exploitation of children and youth must include the capacity or opportunity for meaningful exchange among the partners. System professionals can learn from those who have experienced living on the streets, and the young people can acquire marketable skills so they can move beyond the limitations of the sex trade. Processes that use the experiences and expertise of commercially sexually exploited youth must create a better life opportunity for those youth; if they do not, they serve to perpetuate exploitation.

6. *The principle of safe, voluntary, and confidential participation.* The safety of youth who participate in the development and implementation of solutions and strategies must be a primary concern. Their anonymity must be respected if they so choose, confidentiality must be explicitly acknowledged, and all involvement must be voluntary. If any disclosure laws apply to their participation, they must be told before any disclosure takes place.

7. *The principle of self-help.* It is important to acknowledge the value of the ability of youth to help themselves and each other. Recognizing that considerable time, effort, and resources of state, culture, community, and family will be required to help heal from the traumatic effects of commercial sexual exploitation, opportunities must be created for these youth to gather together and to talk to each other without fear of repercussion.

8. *The principle of accountability.* Young people must be able to play a role in monitoring and evaluating the actions taken by government and the community in addressing the commercial sexual exploitation of children and youth.

9. *The principle of flexibility.* Meeting times, styles and locations must reflect the needs of the youth and not those of the facilitators or the community organizations. For example, it may not always be necessary that the same youth participate at each step of the process. It must be recognized that the need for continuity can have more to do with institutional culture than the needs of the project. Everyone must be willing and able to change the approach when needed.

10. *The principle of commitment to outcomes.* Experiential youth are engaging in this process because they believe it will make a difference. Everyone involved must be committed to change. It is important to recognize that everyone involved is challenging the status quo by engaging in this process.

11. *The principle of long-term vision.* This process takes time, therefore, deeply rooted change can be slow. It requires focusing on underlying factors and not merely surface symptoms.

12. *The principle of meeting people where they are.* This means physically going to locations where youth feel safe and comfortable or imaginatively finding ways to accommodate the needs of experiential youth so that the process belongs to them.

CONCLUSION

This framework is the product of extensive work with survivors of sexual exploitation over the years. Its design began in the form of a wish that was transformed into the Victoria Declaration and Agenda for Action, which was written by the 54 youth delegates in 1998. Its effectiveness has been tested by countless children and youth survivors of sexual exploitation who have become leaders and social activists.

An approach grounded in Aboriginal healing has proven to work with Aborginal and non-Aboriginal children and youth exploited in the sex trade. This approach uses the teachings of the Medicine Wheel coupled with the non-Aboriginal model of the spinning top and applies it to group dynamics. The true path of healing and exiting is not a linear and solitary one. Relapses are inevitable. When young people relapse to substance abuse or to the sex trade, the focus must shift to understanding and addressing the factors that have led to relapse.

Legacy projects of the Victoria Youth Summit have proven that participation brings about positive change. Participation, however, can be problematic at best because meaningful participation requires a framework that defines and monitors the level and validity of child participation within an organization or project. The framework presented here empowers young people who are survivors of sexual exploitation to exit and heal by means of helping others. It provides ways to engage young people in the design, implementation, and evaluation of programs that are "for youth, by youth."

REFERENCES

Kass R. *Theories in Group Development.* Montreal, Canada: Concordia University; 1996.

Mark M, Kingsley C. *Sacred Lives: Canadian Aboriginal Children and Youth Speak Out About Sexual Exploitation.* Vancouver: Save the Children Canada; 2001.

Out From the Shadows: International Summit of Sexually Exploited Youth Final Report. Victoria, Canada: University Press; 1998.

Rabinovitch J. *Impossible, Eh?* Vancouver: Save the Children Canada; 2001.

Robinson LN. The globalization of female child prostitution: a call for reintegration and recovery measures via article 39 of the United Nations Convention on the Rights of the Child. *Indiana J Global Leg Stud.* 1997;5(1):239-255.

Talking Circle. Turning point: native peoples and newcomers on-line. Available at: http://www.turning-point.ca/forum/list.php?f=1. Accessed July 24, 2003.

Chapter 41

The AMBER Alert Program: Missing Children Before and After

Sharon W. Cooper, MD, FAAP

Although a missing child is a parent's worst nightmare, national attention to the plight of these parents and children was delayed for several decades. According to the US Department of Justice (USDOJ), 74% of the children who are kidnapped and later found murdered were killed within the first 3 hours of their abduction (National Conference on AMBER Alert, 2003). For this reason, a missing child who has been abducted under certain circumstances may constitute an emergency and, therefore, mandates an immediate, competent law enforcement response. Though there have been thousands of missing and sexually exploited children, there are a few whose legacies continue in the form of foundations and victim support services. **Table 41-1** provides contact information for these foundations and victim support services.

Table 41-1. Currently Active Foundations and Victim Support Services
National Center for Missing & Exploited Children (NCMEC)
— 1-800-THE-LOST
— http://www.missingkids.com
Jacob Wetterling Foundation
— http://www.jwf.org
The Polly Klaas Foundation
— http://www.pollyklaas.org
KlaasKids Foundation
— http://www.klaaskids.org
Megan Nicole Kanka Foundation
— http://www.megannicolekankafoundation.org
The Jimmy Ryce Center for Victims of Predatory Abduction
— http://www.jimmy-ryce.org

CHILDREN WHOSE LIVES BEGGED FOR A BETTER RESPONSE

Many children's stories led to the development of a concerted effort to search for children effectively. The following are a few of these stories and the resulting strategies developed to help in the search for such children. **Table 41-2** provides a synopsis of these tragic situations.

Table 41-2. Select Missing and Abducted Children in American History			
YEAR	CHILD'S NAME	OCCURRENCE	STATE
1979	Etan Patz	Disappeared, never recovered	New York
1979-1981	29 African-American Children	Abducted, murdered	Georgia
1981	Adam Walsh	Abducted, murdered	Florida
1989	Jacob Wetterling	Abducted, never recovered	Minnesota
1993	Polly Klaas	Abducted, murdered	California
1994	Megan Nicole Kanka	Abducted, raped, murdered	New Jersey
1995	Jimmy Ryce	Abducted, raped, murdered	Florida
1996	Amber Hagerman	Abducted, murdered	Texas

ETAN PATZ

In May 1979, Etan Patz (**Figure 41-1**), a 6-year-old boy living in New York City, asked his mother to let him walk to the school bus alone. His subsequent, mysterious disappearance led to the work of numerous volunteers and police officers to find him. His father's photos of Etan were posted everywhere in the neighborhood. Eventually, in the effort to locate him, his picture was the first to be placed on milk cartons. Sadly, he was never located. In his honor, May 25 was named as National Missing Children's Day by President Ronald Reagan.

THE ATLANTA MURDERS

In the history of the United States, few child murders obtained as much attention as that of the Atlanta child murder victims (**Figure 41-2**). From July 1979 through May of 1981, 29 victims were killed or are still missing from the Fulton County jurisdiction surrounding Atlanta, Georgia. Serial murders are undoubtedly the most frightening of crimes, since community hysteria and paranoia can readily result from the media reports of victims. The Atlanta murders were no different, and the additional concern of the possibility of a crime spree based upon race brought many political leaders forward to appeal to the community to help stop the killings and increase public safety.

The child murders began in July of 1979. The cases of the first 2 victims, Edward Smith and Alfred Evans, were immediately connected by investigators because they

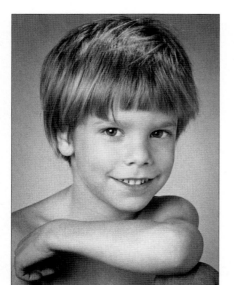

Figure 41-1. *Etan Patz, 1979.* Permission from and photo by Stanley K. Patz.

were friends, they were both 14 years old, and although they disappeared at different times, their bodies were discovered together though they were killed by different means. Less than 6 weeks later, Milton Harvey, another 14-year-old, disappeared from a middle-class neighborhood in Atlanta and was found 2 months later. Nine-year-old Yusuf Bell was the last child to be abducted in October of 1979 and his remains were discovered a month later in a deserted elementary school. The Federal Bureau of Investigation (FBI) eventually placed these children's names on a list (**Table 41-3**) as it became more evident that there might be a pattern to the victimization based upon the location of their disappearances in Atlanta and that all of the victims were African Americans.

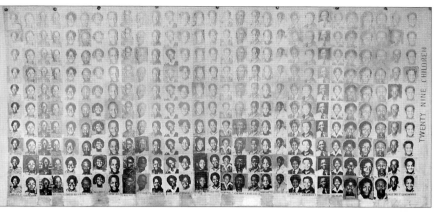

Figure 41-2. Commemorative artwork of the 29 victims of the Atlanta murders by artist John P. Weber. Permission from and on display at the National Center for Missing & Exploited Children.

In 1980, 13 children were abducted and killed from March through November. In July, when Earl Terrell was abducted and possibly transported across the state line into Alabama, the FBI was finally able to be officially involved in the investigation, though in fact, it had been involved from behind the scenes earlier (Dettlinger & Prugh, 1983). During the subsequent months, 12 other children were killed by various means.

By early 1981, 17 African-American children had been slain in 20 months. There arose an immense community outcry and response to include a benefit organized by Frank Sinatra and Sammy Davis, Jr, which raised more than a quarter of a million dollars to assist in the investigation. The Reagan administration provided $1.5 million in federal funds and local citizens raised more than $100 000. Tragically, there were 12 more victims killed in 1981 whose names were included on the FBI list.

Though there were 29 names on the original list, 24 were minors by federal guidelines. Eventually, a suspect was captured on June 21, 1981 who was later prosecuted and convicted primarily on circumstantial evidence for the deaths of Nathaniel Cater and Jimmy Payne. Tremendous concern remained in the case, as 63 other victims

Table 41-3. Victims of the Atlanta Murders

1979	1980	1981
— Edward Hope Smith, age 14	— Jefferey Mathis, age 10	— Lubie Geter, age 14
— Alfred Evans, age 14	— Angel Lanair, age 12	— Terry Pue, age 15
— Milton Harvey, age 14	— Eric Middlebrooks, age 14	— Patrick Baltazar, age 11
— Yusuf Bell, age 9	— Christopher Richardson, age 11	— Curtis Walker, age 13
	— LaTonya Wilson, age 7	— Joseph Bell, age 15
	— Aaron Wyche, age 10	— Timothy Hill, age 13
	— Anthony Carter, age 9	— Eddie Duncan, age 21
	— Earl Terrell, age 11	— Larry Rogers, age 20
	— Clifford Jones, age 13	— Michael McIntosh, age 23
	— Darron Glass, age 10	— Jimmy Ray Payne, age 21
	— Charles Stephens, age 12	— William Barrett, age 17
	— Aaron Jackson, age 9	— Nathaniel Cater, age 27
	— Patrick Rogers, age 16	

were killed over the period of time from 1979 through 1983 whose names were never included on the FBI list. In addition, 25 of the victims whose names were not included on the list were killed after the arrest of Wayne Williams, who was convicted and is presently serving 2 consecutive life sentences.

ADAM WALSH

In 1981, Adam Walsh (**Figure 41-3**) was abducted while with his mother in a store at a mall in Florida. Despite his mother's efforts to convince the store personnel that Adam's disappearance was not a benign occurrence, Revé Walsh was unsuccessful in locating her son and was instructed to leave the store by employees. The local law enforcement agency was not trained to initiate an immediate search for a child. Two weeks after his abduction, Adam's body was discovered more than 100 miles from the site of his abduction. These delays and lack of experience are believed to have contributed to the tragic outcome in Adam's brutal death. As a result of their experience, Adam's parents, John and Revé Walsh, have devoted their lives to improving and coordinating a team response to situations involving missing and abducted children.

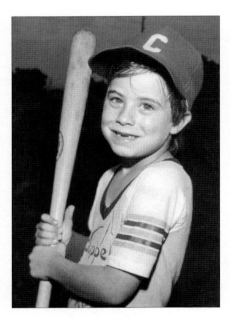

Figure 41-3. Adam Walsh, 1981. Permission from John and Revé Walsh.

The Walsh family especially wanted to ensure that employees in local stores and businesses take the disappearance of a child as a serious event and have a coordinated, careful response. Since 1994, more than 45 000 major retail stores have implemented one of the country's largest child safety programs, aptly named "Code Adam." This initiative allows the store to "lock down" all store exits whenever a child is reported as missing within the store. In addition to making an announcement that a child is missing, a verbal description of the child is relayed to the employees and customers. The store employees are allowed to stop their work and help search the store for the missing child. If the child is not found within a certain amount of time, law enforcement officials are notified.

Cunning on the part of predators warrants education of families and the public about the real and certain danger that might exist if a child is missing, even in a public place of commerce. In one such incidence that occurred in 2004, an 11-year-old girl named Carlie Brucia was abducted while walking near a commercial carwash; she was subsequently murdered even though her abduction was captured on a video surveillance camera.

In addition to helping initiate "Code Adam," Adam's death contributed to the inception and continuation of a popular American television program that airs on the FOX network, called *America's Most Wanted*. This program, hosted by Adam's father, has been lauded by numerous law enforcement agencies for its help in solving crimes, some of which are missing persons crimes. Typically, the people featured on the program are fugitives, have existing warrants for capture, and often present a continued threat to society by the nature of the crimes they have committed. Often, when the public viewers recognize a picture of a known felon, they call the toll-free number posted on the television show and, as a result, assist in the capture of people who have committed various crimes.

John and Revé Walsh became the cofounders of the National Center for Missing & Exploited Children (NCMEC) in 1984. Since its creation, the NCMEC has worked closely with officers and investigators from the nation's 18 000 law enforcement agencies to learn to provide the most professional and comprehensive work in searching for missing, abducted, and exploited children. The resources of the NCMEC include the following:

— Technical assistance given in cases of missing and exploited children

— A 24-hour, toll-free hotline to receive reports of missing children or sightings of missing children, with the appropriate dispositions made immediately to the specified law enforcement agency

— Nationwide distribution of photographs and descriptions of missing children

— Preparation of age-enhanced photographs for long-term missing children and analysis of case information and leads

All of these services and more are provided free of charge to victims and their families.

Jacob Wetterling

Jacob Wetterling was an 11-year-old boy from Minnesota who was bicycling home from a convenience store one evening with his 9-year-old brother and an 11-year-old friend. A gunman appeared from a driveway and forced the 3 boys to throw their bicycles in a ditch and lay on the ground. He allowed 2 of the boys to run toward the surrounding woods, but when they turned back to look for Jacob, he was gone. Jacob has never been seen since that time. His family has established the Jacob Wetterling Foundation for families of children who have been abducted, are missing, or have never been recovered. This active foundation provides a great deal of information to families. In addition, its Web site offers important links to missing children services.

Polly Klaas

Polly Klaas (**Figure 41-4**), a 12-year-old girl, was having a slumber party at her home on October 1, 1993, in Petaluma, California. During the night, she was abducted at knifepoint and was missing for the next 65 days. Hundreds of community volunteers searched for her, but her remains were not discovered until December 4, 1993. During the search for Polly, the Polly Klaas Foundation was established to help find missing children and prevent children from going missing in the first place. This organization has been instrumental in achieving nationwide acceptance of the AMBER Alert initiative. When only 14 states had statewide programs based upon the AMBER Alert concept, the Polly Klaas Foundation actively lobbied with numerous governors, helping to bring the number of states into compliance to 49 in only 2 years. It is anticipated that the state of Hawaii will bring this program into a fully effective initiative on all national levels. A second organization that memorializes Polly is the KlaasKids Foundation. Although research has shown that fewer than 100 children are actually abducted on an annual basis by the stereotypical stranger, the sober reminder of this second organization that works in the field of missing children is its motto: "a mile a minute … that is how fast your child can disappear."

Megan Nicole Kanka

In July 1994, 7-year-old Megan Nicole Kanka was raped and murdered by a previously convicted sex offender who had recently moved into a house across the street from her home in Hamilton Township, New Jersey. This tragic occurrence led the New Jersey State Legislature to pass the now famous "Megan's Law," which requires that if a convicted sex offender assumes residence, neighbors have the right to be notified. "Megan's Law" also became the basis for the sex offender registry system required in more than half of the states in the United States.

Jimmy Ryce

In 1995, 9-year-old Jimmy Ryce (**Figure 41-5**) was kidnapped at gunpoint, raped, and murdered. Donald and Claudine Ryce, Jimmy's parents, have worked tirelessly since their son's death to help in victim recovery as well as the education of parents regarding predatory abductors. In coordination with 4 other families of abducted children, his parents helped establish the Jimmy Ryce Law Enforcement Training Center located in Alexandria, Virginia. Working in concert with the Office of Juvenile Justice and Delinquency Prevention of the USDOJ, the NCMEC, and the FBI, this agency offers numerous training opportunities for law enforcement officers to learn ways to respond to a missing child report and ways to assess the degree of danger that might exist for that victim. The major emphasis of the Jimmy Ryce Center is to educate communities and municipalities about the risk for victims of

Figure 41-4. *Polly Klaas, 1993.* Permission from the Polly Klaas Foundation.

Figure 41-5. *Jimmy Ryce, 1995.* Permission from Donald Ryce.

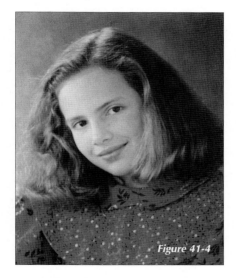

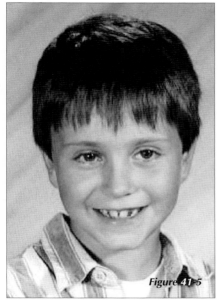

predatory abductors. **Table 41-4** lists the primary goals of the Jimmy Ryce Law Enforcement Training Center.

The efforts of the Jimmy Ryce Center for Victims of Predatory Abduction have led to a Web site that offers learning opportunities for children of various ages about ways to escape an abduction scenario. These scenarios are all taken from true situations and are referred to as the Great Escape Maneuvers (GEMS) Program. As an interactive training tool, children and teenagers have the chance to learn about strategies, such as yelling when someone who picks up a child is not that child's parent or knowing that it is better to run away even if a predator threatens the child with a weapon. Parents are advised to interact with their children as they read through the various scenarios, so the family can discuss this serious subject.

Table 41-4. Primary Goals of the Jimmy Ryce Law Enforcement Training Center
— Distribute pictures of children who have been abducted by predators and advocate for adequate media coverage of the missing child's case.
— Increase public awareness of the dynamics of sexual predators and abductions through the development and dissemination of brochures and newsletters and through the use of public forums, radio and television broadcasts, and other means.
— Educate teachers and parents about ways they can help their students and/or children know what to do if they are ever abducted in addition to strategies to avoid an abduction scenario.
— Identify model legislation and programs designed to better protect children from sexual predators.
— Provide well-bred search dogs (eg, bloodhounds) as a donation to law enforcement agencies.
— Assist various law enforcement agencies to develop more effective strategies and procedures in handling sexual predators.
— Provide empathetic support to parents of children who have been abducted by sexual predators.
— Work to improve coordination and cooperation among state missing children clearinghouses, missing child nonprofit organizations, and law enforcement agencies.

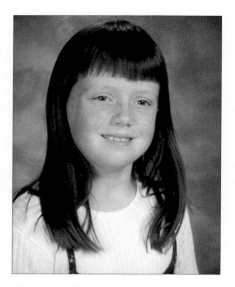

***Figure 41-6.** Amber Hagerman, 1996.*
Permission from Donna Norris.

AMBER HAGERMAN

While riding her bicycle in Arlington, Texas in 1996, 9-year-old Amber Hagerman (**Figure 41-6**) was kidnapped and brutally murdered. Efforts to search for her and a resident's suggestion to broadcast special "alerts" over the airwaves led to the first team response by the Dallas-Fort Worth police officers and the local broadcasters who devised an early warning system to notify the public that a child had been abducted. The outcome of these efforts came in 2001 when the National Center for Missing & Exploited Children launched the AMBER Alert, which is an acronym for America's Missing: Broadcast Emergency Response.

Shortly after this notification system was placed into effect in Texas, other states began to use the technology. For example, in 2001, Utah had implemented the Rachael Alert system. This was activated on June 5, 2002, within hours of the kidnapping of Elizabeth Smart, a 14-year-old child who was abducted from her own home by a vagrant worker. The case of Elizabeth Smart received national attention for several weeks, and television stations and various cable networks frequently flashed updates on the investigation of her case. Although Elizabeth remained missing for 9 months, a cooperative effort involving the NCMEC, as well as the Utah law enforcement forces and the FBI, eventually assisted in her recovery. It was with immense relief that her family was able to be present with Elizabeth when the AMBER Alert became a national law in the United States (Smart & Morton, 2003).

THE AMBER ALERT

AN OVERVIEW

The AMBER Alert process is initiated whenever a child is missing and considered to be in imminent danger. A coalition involving the emergency broadcast system, law enforcement agencies, and the department of transportation provide an essential response capability to enhance the recovery of abducted children.

In various parts of the United States, concerns exist regarding the appropriate initiation of an alert. For example, an observation has been made that a longer delay in the initiation of an alert is occurring with missing African-American and Hispanic children. Consequently, there continues to be a need to enforce a uniform policy regarding the appropriate execution of the process regardless of the region of the country or the victim's ethnic origin.

In September 2003, the 100th child was saved through the AMBER Alert system by using all major components of the program (ie, law enforcement officials, broadcasters, transportation departments, and the people within the community). The system works by having law enforcement officials verify that an authentic need exists for an alert to be initiated. This verification results in broadcasting a message via radio and/or television as well as being displayed on highway signs. Often this leads to assistance by private citizens, who search for the described vehicle and license plate number so law enforcement officials can be notified as soon as possible after a sighting. The ensuing search-and-rescue mission has frequently ended in a safe outcome for the child victim. Although more than 100 children have been saved through this program, more than half of these children were recovered after 2002, when President George W. Bush announced a call to action at the White House's Conference on Missing, Exploited, and Runaway Children.

THE NOTIFICATION PROCESS

The backbone of the AMBER Alert process is the immediate notification to the public that a child is missing and may be in imminent danger. Each of the team's agencies plays a specific role in the process of alerting the public to become vigilant to the plight of a missing child.

Law enforcement officials help validate the degree of threat of harm for a child who has just been reported. Several circumstances increase the risk for harm such as whether the abductor is known, has a history of substance abuse and/or violence, has a prior criminal record, or whether a witness reports the presence or possession of a weapon. The investigators must then notify a designated local broadcast system and confirm the appropriate range of dissemination of the information.

The message may be broadcast via television and/or radio as well as by transportation signs on the highway system. The local department of transportation facilitates this latter type of notification and is especially necessary if the initial law enforcement report includes a vehicle's description and/or license plate information. Citizen reports become the key element that assists in the recovery of children who are abducted in this manner. As a result of using the emergency broadcast system for this reason, many abductors relinquish custody of their victims and turn themselves in to investigators after realizing the futility of attempting to escape such a coordinated community search.

ROLE OF THE NATIONAL AMBER ALERT COORDINATOR

The AMBER Alert process achieved a national focus in 2002 when the Department of Justice appointed the Assistant Attorney General for the Office of Justice Programs as the National AMBER Alert Coordinator. To ensure a seamless system of notification, this coordinator is responsible for assisting state and local officials as they develop and enhance AMBER plans and promote statewide and regional coordination among the plans. In April 2003, President George W. Bush signed into law the Prosecutorial Remedies and Other Tools to end the Exploitation of Children Today (PROTECT) Act of 2003, making the National AMBER Alert Network into law and more thoroughly outlining the coordinator's tasks, which include the following:

— Facilitate the AMBER network development.

— Provide support for the development of state AMBER plans and efforts.

— Increase efforts to eliminate geographic gaps in AMBER networks.

— Provide regional AMBER network coordination.

— Establish guidance criteria to ensure an AMBER Alert.

The establishment of guidance criteria became necessary as a result of the irregular patterns of issuing alerts in different parts of the country. For example, some regions feared that too frequent alerts would desensitize the public to the importance of the process, which caused these regions to delay alerts until the use was marginalized. Conversely, some regions required too much information before beginning notification, thereby potentially thwarting the success of the alert process.

ABDUCTION OF INFANTS AND THE AMBER ALERT

The AMBER Alert process has assisted in the tragedy of infant abduction scenarios. Although infant abductions are a particular concern for hospitals that have birthing units or newborn nurseries, an additional risk exists during the neonatal period of 4 weeks postpartum, when infants may have been discharged to their homes and home health care agencies are providing services. Announcements may be posted in newspapers or attractive gender specific signs may be placed in the front yards of homes to announce a baby's birth, thereby unintentionally putting the newborn at risk for possible abduction attempts.

In June 2003, such an attempt prompted an AMBER Alert. While still in the hospital, a young mother of a newborn son was visited by a woman who claimed to be a church employee whose job was to visit new mothers who may need baby supplies and services. Two weeks later, this woman visited the mother and her newborn baby in their home and offered to provide the transportation for them to agency assistance. After a brief walk in a park, the woman placed the infant in her van and asked the mother to run into a nearby store for some snacks. When the mother returned to the park, the woman and her son were gone. She notified authorities immediately, and an AMBER Alert was issued. After receiving more than 500 tips because of the alert, the authorities discovered that one tip was from the suspect's daughter, who reported that her mother had brought the infant to her and asked her to babysit. When she recognized the newborn from the information provided in the AMBER Alert, she called the police. Police officers safely recovered the newborn and returned him to his mother.

ABDUCTION OF TEENAGERS AND THE AMBER ALERT

Teenager abductions may result in trafficking across state lines for the purpose of sexual exploitation through prostitution, extortion, forced child labor, or sexual slavery. Although sexual slavery is thought to be rare, the highly publicized case of John Jamelske is a sober reminder of the serious nature of this type of sexual offense.

Jamelske, a 68-year-old man from Syracuse, New York, abducted 5 women and girls during a 15-year period. His victims ranged in age from 13 to 53 years old. He kept them in a concrete dungeon that was constructed beneath his home and used his victims as sexual slaves for as long as 2 years. He used frequent doses of a sexual performance drug and repeatedly sexually assaulted these women and girls. Since the nature of the abuse was so bizarre, and since these victims did not know where they had been held captive and were unable to identify their captor, they were often unable to convince law enforcement officers of the validity of their experience once they were released from their prison. Although his criminal activity began before the AMBER Alert initiative was enacted, had there been more publicity of the missing people, such as the alert process, the subsequent results may not have occurred so repetitively over such a long period of time.

An AMBER Alert was initiated by teenager abductions in August 2002. Sixteen-year-old Tamara Brooks and 17-year-old Jacqueline Marris were parked at a local "lover's lane" with their boyfriends in Orange County, California. Even though they were in 2 separate cars, an abductor approached the vehicles and forced all 4 people at gunpoint to leave their vehicles. After tying up the young men, the abductor took Tamara and Jacqueline in one of the vehicles. An AMBER Alert was issued, and the case immediately became a huge media story. A description of the girls, the vehicle, and the license plates was broadcast over local stations and displayed on electronic highway signs. A short while later, an animal control officer spotted the vehicle, which had left the highway and headed into the desert. Law enforcement officials were notified, and both girls were successfully recovered.

AN AMBER ALERT SUCCESS STORY

In March 1999, 9-year-old Fleisha Moore was walking home from school with a friend in Saginaw, Texas. A man drove up and enticed the girls with stories about kittens in a nearby field, then grabbed Fleisha and threw her into a truck. Her friend was able to give the Dallas-Fort Worth law enforcement officers enough information about the vehicle and the abductor that an AMBER Alert was issued. About 5 hours later, Fleisha was seen walking along the highway alone. The abductor had ordered her out of his vehicle when he heard the information about the kidnapping and a description of his truck on the radio. Not only was Fleisha rescued, but her abductor was later apprehended.

STRATEGY FOR AMBER COORDINATION

In an effort to assist the National AMBER Alert Coordinator, a national advisory group has been established. This group includes the USDOJ, US Department of Transportation, the NCMEC, television and radio broadcasters, and law enforcement officers. Together, they work to develop a strategy for support in states and communities in which the system is beginning to be used.

To assure the program's success, many factors must be taken into consideration. One major consideration is the nature of a community. Urban communities have considerably different dynamics than rural communities with respect to the nature of the crime of abduction, the skill of the local law enforcement officers, and even the caliber of the transportation department support capability. In many rural communities, for example, electronic road signs that would provide motorist information are not used. Additionally, local law enforcement manpower in rural areas may be significantly limited, making it difficult to ensure that the appropriate contingency of responders is available at short notice, which may be necessary in the event of a child abduction.

The following are 3 important aspects of the national strategy for AMBER coordination:

1. The assessment of current AMBER activity.

2. The creation of a coordinated AMBER network.

3. The communication of "lessons learned."

ASSESSMENT OF CURRENT AMBER ACTIVITY

In assessing the status of current AMBER activity, an initial determination of the number of existing local, state, and regional plans must be made. Currently, 49 state AMBER plans exist in the United States, and 9 international plans exist (the majority of which are located in the Canadian provinces).

The AMBER Alert is managed by different organizations from state to state, including law enforcement agencies, the state broadcasters' association, or the state Attorney General's Office. Several states use their local missing children's clearinghouses as the primary cite for the AMBER plan.

As a result of such diverse management agencies, the national strategy plans to include a comparison of these plan operations and establish clear community notification criteria for each local AMBER Alert group. In addition, the national strategy plan includes an assessment strategy to evaluate each community's available technology.

CREATION OF A COORDINATED AMBER NETWORK

The second component of the national strategy for AMBER Alert coordination is the creation of a cohesive network of providers. In collaboration with the national advisory group, the national coordinator will seek to develop guidelines regarding the appropriate criteria used to issue an AMBER Alert. Such guidelines are necessary to train local agencies regarding the risk factors that elevate the degree of urgency in a case necessitating an alert. The AMBER network plans to establish federal, state, and local partnerships so communities share the success of the AMBER Alert process.

In addition, this national strategy plans to promote the technological compatibility among the different communications systems. This aspect of the strategy will require expert technology consultation coordination so that a universal cyberspace language will exist when one emergency notification agency communicates with another. Funding for this aspect of the strategy will require assistance both from the federal government and the previously cited local partnerships.

COMMUNICATION OF "LESSONS LEARNED"

The final component of the national AMBER strategy is the communication of "lessons learned." The goals of this component are to do the following:

— Provide experiential learning for all participants as they establish working relationships between law enforcement agencies and local broadcasters who are seeking to address the various issues surrounding missing children and the proper issuance of AMBER Alerts.

— Assist state and community officials as they develop their AMBER Alert plans so the errors of older, more established programs are not repeated.

— Raise public awareness regarding ways to protect children and prevent abduction.

CHILD LURES PREVENTION

Probably the most well-recognized and original child abduction and sexual abuse prevention program in the United States is Child Lures Prevention designed by Ken Wooden. This educational program is geared to parents and children as well as educators and has been endorsed by numerous organizations, including the American Medical Association, American Academy of Pediatrics, and American Osteopathic Association. Since many schools throughout the United States implement the carefully structured curriculum especially designed for children of varying age groups, the National Association of Elementary School Principals and National Association of Secondary School Principals have partnered with Child Lures Prevention. As of 2004, the Child Lures Prevention Safe Environment Program has been developed and is being implemented in the Catholic dioceses in the United States.

Before developing the Child Lures Prevention program, Wooden canvassed thousands of incarcerated child-sex offenders and catalogued and collated their numerous self-reported techniques. He placed specific techniques into victim age groups and then devised educational programs for each age group (ie, early childhood children, school-aged children, and adolescents). For a number of years, Wooden's program has been used nationally and internationally to train law enforcement officers, multi-disciplinary child abuse investigation teams, school personnel, and public officials.

In addition to the Child Lures Prevention program, *Child Lures: What Every Parent and Child Should Know About Preventing Sexual Abuse and Abduction* (1995) presents reported abduction and sexual offense situations as well as suggestions for alternative actions that a child might use to escape or avoid being victimized in this manner.

An example of a child lure technique discussed in Wooden's (1995) book involves the risks associated with children wearing clothing imprinted with their names. Serial killer Ted Bundy tragically abducted Kimberly Leach, a 12-year-old girl who was on her Florida school grounds wearing a sweatshirt with the name "Kim" on the back. He was able to call out her name, immediately making him seem familiar and trustworthy. Bundy, wearing a name tag reading, "Richard Burton, Fire Department," told her of a family emergency, after which she became distraught and left with Bundy in a van. Ted Bundy was eventually executed for the murder of Kimberly Leach.

The Child Lures Prevention program recognizes that child abductions are often well thought out and may include a careful ruse. An example of one such abduction, which was an ultimate AMBER Alert success story, occurred in Houston, Texas in April 2001. Five-year-old Maria Cuellar was lured with 5 other children (all between the ages of 4 and 8) from their apartment complex into a stolen ambulance under the guise that the vehicle was a playroom. The other children were able to escape from the abductor, but Maria was unable to get out before the abductor drove away. Shortly thereafter, an AMBER Alert was issued with a description of Maria, her abductor, and the ambulance. After the alert was broadcast along the airwaves, a citizen reported seeing a child with a man in his neighborhood who matched the kidnapper's description. Within 3 hours of the AMBER Alert, Maria was successfully recovered and returned to her family.

ATTEMPTED NONFAMILY ABDUCTIONS
NATIONAL INCIDENCE STUDY OF MISSING, ABDUCTED, RUNAWAY, AND THROWNAWAY CHILDREN

A discussion of abducted and missing children must include further information regarding the complex nature of the definition of the term "missing." Many decisions in the AMBER Alert process require a careful understanding of how a child may have come to be missing. At times, children are missing because they are lost or because they have run away from home. At other times, children are thrown out of their homes and often no report is made at all of their missing status.

In an effort to assess the actual incidence of missing, abducted, runaway, and thrownaway children in the United States, the USDOJ commissioned the *National Incidence Study of Missing, Abducted, Runaway, and Thrownaway Children* (NISMART) (Finkelhor et al, 1990). This study polled law enforcement agencies and households.

The law enforcement component of the study concluded that between 200 and 300 ***stereotypical kidnappings*** (nonfamily abduction in which a child is kept one night, transported 50 miles, held for ransom, or killed [Sedlak et al, 2002]) occur each year. However, within the legal definition of abduction, 3200 to 4600 cases were documented during that same time frame. The study also assessed household data based upon a national telephone survey of 10 367 households. The reliable estimate was that 114 600 children (ie, between 79 900 and 149 400) had experienced an attempted nonfamily abduction in 1988; most of these experiences occurred with strangers in passing cars (Finkelhor et al, 1990).

Attempted nonfamily abductions are defined as "any incident in which a nonfamily member tried to take, detain, or lure a child, and if the action had been successful, the situation would have probably met the criteria for a completed nonfamily abduction" (Finkelhor et al, 1990). In the study, the screener questions included whether a time occured when someone tried to sexually molest, rape, attack, or beat the specific child. Families were also asked whether anyone other than a family member had tried to take the child away against the family's wishes. Of the families who responded "yes," in 19%, the child was either 4 or 5 years old, 26% were either 8 or 9 years old, and 20% were either 10 or 11 years old. Of the children who had experienced an attempted nonfamily abduction, 56% were female and 44% were male. The police were notified in 42% of the episodes.

Conclusions of the NISMART analysis of attempted nonfamily abductions revealed that most of the attempts were lures wherein strangers tried to get the child to accompany them in their cars. It was also found that when children had experienced a near abduction, a statistically significantly increased incidence of preexisting parental anxiety was associated with their own childhood traumas and abuse. Finkelhor et al (1990) explained that a degree of subjectivity existed in the household survey with respect to whether force was used in the attempted abduction. However, the conclusion remained that the description of such episodes suggested that most events were not cases in which the child had misconstrued the intent of a completely innocent encounter with a stranger who may simply have been asking for directions. Indeed, there seemed to be a threatening component to the encounter, enough so that the parent perceived a real threat. A final and provocative conclusion of the first report of this kind was that the single most powerful predictor of an attempted, nonfamily abduction event was whether the victim's parent had a history of being abducted, sexually or physically abused, or had been a runaway or had been missing from the home long enough for the police to be called.

NATIONAL INCIDENCE STUDY OF MISSING, ABDUCTED, RUNAWAY, AND THROWNAWAY CHILDREN-2

In 2002, a NISMART-2 was published (Sedlak et al, 2002). This second study used 4 studies (household surveys of youth and adult caretakers and studies of law enforcement and juvenile facilities) to derive a unified estimate of the number of missing children in the United States. In-depth surveys of adults and youths, more than 400 county sheriff departments and 3700 municipal law enforcement agencies, and facility staff members from a nationally representative sample of juvenile detention centers, group homes, residential treatment centers, and runaway and homeless youth shelters helped make this study more comprehensive than the first NISMART.

In this second study, the researchers advised that the results should not be compared to the first study because the definition of "missing" had changed. The criteria for "missing" in the NISMART-2 study included that a victim was younger than 18 years of age and fell into one of the following 5 categories (Sedlak et al, 2002):

1. The victim experienced a nonfamily abduction, which included the subcategory of a stereotypical kidnapping, during which a child was taken by the use of physical force or was threatened with bodily harm and then was detained for at least 1 hour in an isolated place. In the case of a stereotypical kidnapping, the child was taken and detained at least overnight, transported at least 50 miles from his or her home, held for ransom, and risked permanent abduction or death.

2. The victim experienced a family abduction, which was in violation of a custody order, decree, or other legitimate custodial rights, during which the child was concealed or transported outside of the state with the intent to prevent the child from returning to his or her rightful caregiver.

3. The victim experienced a runaway or thrownaway episode. A *runaway* is considered to be a child who voluntarily leaves his or her home at least overnight and is younger than 14 years old, or is 15 years old or older and stays away for 2 nights. A *thrownaway* child refers to a child who has been asked or told to leave his or

her home by a parent or other household adult without an adequate alternative-care option arranged by that caregiver, and in addition, the child remains out of the house at least overnight.

4. The victim experienced an involuntarily missing, lost, or injured episode during which the child's whereabouts are unknown to the caregiver for at least 1 hour and with a responding alarm of that caregiver. In this circumstance, the child was unable to contact the caregiver because the child was lost, stranded, or injured, or the child could not contact the caregiver because the child was too young to know how to do so.

5. The victim was *caretaker missing*, or was missing with a benign explanation in which a child's whereabouts were unknown to the caregiver, causing that caregiver to become alarmed and try to locate the child. The victim is considered *reported missing* once the local authorities are contacted for purposes of locating the child. This experience is considered benign as long as the child was not actually lost, injured, abducted, victimized, or classified as a runaway or thrownaway child.

NISMART-2 recorded demographics such as age, gender, and race of missing children. Eighty-four percent became missing when they ran away or because of benign misunderstandings. This is consistent with the fact that approximately 75% of children who went missing were 12 years old and older, an age range in which children become more independent and more conflicts occur with caretakers. The NISMART-2 study found no significant gender differences in missing children but did find that White children had a significantly lower risk. This study found that, contrary to popular belief, children became missing very rarely because of abduction, and most of these occurrences were family abductions. A summary of the estimated number of children missing calculated from this study can be found in **Table 41-5**.

Table 41-5. Estimated Total Number of Children With Episodes and the Percent Who Were Counted as Caretaker Missing and Reported Missing

EPISODE TYPE	TOTAL NUMBER OF CHILDREN WITH EPISODES (MISSING AND NONMISSING)	PERCENT COUNTED AS CARETAKER MISSING	PERCENT COUNTED AS REPORTED MISSING
Nonfamily abduction	58 200	57	21
Family Abduction	203 900	57	28
Runaway/Thrownaway	1 682 900	37	21
Missing involuntary, lost, or injured	198 300	100*	31
Missing benign explanation	374 700	100*	91

* By definition, all children with episodes in this category are caretaker missing.

Note: These estimates can not be added or combined. All estimates are rounded to the nearest 100.

Reprinted from Sedlak AJ, Finkelhor D, Hammer H, Schultz DJ. Second National Incidence Studies of Missing, Abducted, Runaway, and Thrownaway Children in America (NISMART-2). Washington, DC: US Dept of Justice, Office of Justice Programs, Office of Juvenile Justice and Delinquency Prevention; 2002.

CONCLUSION

The data presented in this chapter reveal that missing children come from a diverse, complex mix of circumstances. As a result, this affects the methods of locating a missing child as well as the need for appropriate public policy. The most common type of missing child is the child who has run away, or who was thrown away, followed by the child who has been abducted by a family member. Recognizing the risks of sexual exploitation and harm will continue to be paramount in public policy decisions.

The AMBER Alert initiative remains an important means of recovery for missing children who meet the correct criteria. The adoption of the AMBER Alert in the United States constitutes an important means of continuing to keep children safe.

REFERENCES

Dettlinger C, Prugh J. *The List*. Atlanta, Ga: Philmay Enterprises; 1983.

Finkelhor D, Hotaling G, Sedlak A. *National Incidence Studies of Missing, Abducted, Runaway, and Thrownaway Children in America* (NISMART). Washington, DC: US Dept of Justice, Office of Justice Programs, Office of Juvenile Justice and Delinquency Prevention; 1990.

National Conference on AMBER Alert, conference proceedings report [press release]. August 3-5, 2003; Dallas, Texas. Available at: http://www.ojp.usdoj.gov/amberalert/docs/AMBER-r1.pdf. Accessed October 11, 2004.

Sedlak AJ, Finkelhor D, Hammer H, Schultz DJ. *Second National Incidence Studies of Missing, Abducted, Runaway, and Thrownaway Children in America* (NISMART-2). Washington, DC: US Dept of Justice, Office of Justice Programs, Office of Juvenile Justice and Delinquency Prevention; 2002.

Smart E, Morton L. *Bringing Elizabeth Home*. New York, NY: Doubleday; 2003.

Wooden K. *Child Lures What Every Parent and Child Should Know about Preventing Sexual Abuse and Abduction*. Arlington, Tex: Summit Publishing; 1995.

Chapter 42

The Impact of News Coverage: How the Media Can Help

Migael Scherer

When children are kidnapped by strangers or killed in a school shooting, the violence is explosive. Police and emergency medical technicians rush in, and with them comes the news media. Through their reports, the impact is felt by the wider community and at times by the nation and the world. The public rallies, empathizing with the victims and their families: "That could have been my child!" Many are moved to help, and try to prevent the crime from happening again.

But when violence takes the form of child abuse or child sexual exploitation, the explosion is muffled, as though it were taking place far underground. The public as a whole is unaware. If they know about it at all, most people keep their distance. They fabricate excuses or explanations that allow them to turn away and continue on without altering their view of the world.

Where is the public outrage, the demands that policies or laws be changed so that children are safer?

In the recommendations that follow their 2001 study, The Commercial Sexual Exploitation of Children in the U.S., Canada and Mexico, Richard Estes & Neil Weiner list "protect the children" as number 1. "Public media," they state, "… share a heavy responsibility for disseminating age-appropriate and accurate messages concerning the nature, extent, and seriousness of child sexual exploitation (CSE) in contemporary American society." Estes and Weiner point especially to television, movies, and music, which are primarily entertainment industries.

Equally important is the news media. How can journalists rally readers and viewers around this issue? Have they ever done so, and what will encourage them to continue?

This chapter provides a brief view into the world of news coverage—primarily print journalism—and its impact on the community's response to the sexual exploitation of children. The aim here is not to bash journalism but to encourage effective reporting on this issue. Promoting changes in news coverage, as in legal or medical procedures, requires an understanding of the process as it exists. The first part of this chapter explains some of the basics of journalism, as well as the pressures under which journalists work and what they value. A look at research on the coverage of domestic violence homicides illustrates how news gathering and writing can influence the outcome of a story, from the readers' and journalists' perspectives. Because much can be learned by examining what works rather than what does not, this chapter provides examples of news coverage that have had a positive effect on the community's understanding of CSE, with a look behind the scenes at how those stories came about and the obstacles faced by the reporters writing them. The chapter concludes with ideas about how to influence the news in ways that respect journalists' work and at the same time protect victims.

The words and perspectives here are, for the most part, those of journalists. Along with journalism and mass communications educators (and the researchers among them), they are the "experts" whose work is cited and discussed.

UNDERSTANDING JOURNALISTS

"Good journalism is collecting a lot of facts in a very short time, figuring out what you don't know and organizing what you do know in some coherent way, and telling people about it accurately and in language they can understand. With the names spelled right" (A. R. Isaacs, former reporter for *The Baltimore Sun*, e-mail communication, April 28, 2000).

It is impossible to condense the entire field of journalism into a single chapter. News writing for a metropolitan daily differs from writing for a community weekly, or a monthly news magazine, to say nothing of radio and TV broadcasts. The focus here is on print journalism, yet there are commonalities in how all reporters do their work, as well as in their values and pressures.

News writing starkly contrasts academic and legal writing. Reporters use short paragraphs (a common length is 60 to 90 words) and relatively simple sentences, avoiding complex and even compound sentence structures. Often, paragraphs consist of no more than a sentence. The assumption is that readers (and, even more so, listeners and viewers) are on the run and that there are many other stories competing for attention. Thus, headlines, lead paragraphs, and nut paragraphs (those which contain the main news item) distill the story into its main elements: who, what, where, when, and (whenever possible) why and how. And since so many people skim the news and rarely have time to follow the story to its end, these elements are covered early in the article.

The practice of putting everything important at the beginning has an added advantage: with space always at a premium, the story can be cut to fit, from the bottom up. Indeed, stories are often assigned by the inch, with 1 inch containing about 30 words of print. In broadcast, the measure is in seconds of airtime.

Photojournalists work under similar pressures, only visually, and with more equipment: through the lens of a camera, they must capture the subject in the right angle and lighting to tell the story in a single frame.

The brevity and clarity of news at its best is all the more remarkable for being done on time, day after day. From assignment to production, everything happens on deadline: conferring with editors, researching, getting to the scene, interviewing, organizing the information, writing, fact-checking, copy editing, layout—everything. For a morning paper, a story that breaks in late afternoon generally needs to be filed by 11:00 PM. A reporter for an evening paper has at most a few hours. Television ratchets this up further: from assignment to air can be as little as half an hour. And bear in mind that most reporters work on several stories at once, under multiple deadlines. Some must also produce online versions for their paper's Web site. With high-profile breaking news, the competition can be intense. Editors and producers put pressure on their news staff to "get it first," and in the rush, "get it right" may suffer.

But making deadlines and reducing language and images to fit in limited space are just entry-level skills. Good journalists have a "nose for news" that can sniff out a compelling story. They are skilled at getting people to talk, at observing and recording details, at *showing* rather than *telling* so that readers are drawn in. The best reporters make complex issues clear without over-simplification. They know that people remember and are moved by stories, not statistics, and that a news account about one individual has more impact than generalizations about a group. Most editors would agree with Tracy Grant, managing editor of the online afternoon edition of the *Washington Post*, when she describes a good reporter as "someone who has an intellectual curiosity, who always asks the next question, who is not satisfied with the pat answer—somebody who writes lyrically, who can really take you some-place as a writer, as well as be a good reporter" (Gorney, 2000).

JOURNALISM VALUES

Journalism values are no less daunting. Accuracy is one. This means accurate descriptions, numbers, quotes, and correctly spelled names. Credibility and accountability are equally important and demand the use of multiple sources for information and confirmation. And though it may be the most difficult to achieve, context is critical; it drives the story beyond what happened and shows readers where an event fits into the larger world and why they should care.

Journalists may differ in their belief in "objectivity," but they try to keep themselves and their opinions out of the news, and they put a high value on fairness. To achieve fairness, they try to cover all sides of an issue, or at least 2 sides, balancing a quote from one, for example, with a quote from the other. This practice of setting one side "against" the other may also expose (critics would say *create*) conflict that attracts reader and viewer interest. But the primary goal is fairness and balance.

The news value about which journalists are most defensive is press freedom. News organizations will go to court over freedom from censorship and freedom of access to information. Reporters are suspicious of secrecy, especially when the information is, or in their opinion should be, available to the public. The reason is deeper than the needs of a particular story. Beneath the focused rush to deadline and between assignments, when they come up for air, journalists have no trouble explaining what motivates them: a desire to inform, a need to explain events so the public can understand and take action, and the hope for a safer community. They really mean it, some with the fervor of a vocation, as when Max Frankel, former executive editor of *The New York Times*, described news as "the oxygen of our liberty" in the introduction to a collection of September 11 front pages (2001). Added Jim Naughton, president of the Poynter Institute, a school dedicated to teaching and inspiring journalists and media leaders, "News is what breaks, not soothes … Real news, hard news, matters again. People want to know what governments—theirs and others'—are doing" (2001). The rewards for individual reporters are not monetary. The average salary for a newspaper reporter in a mid-size city is about the same as a public school teacher's or less. In their résumés, print journalists list the newspapers they have worked for, fellowships they have earned, and the prizes they have won, especially those judged by other journalists. Pulitzer prizes, which are well-known outside the profession, are not the only awards included; other awards given by peer organizations such as the Society of Professional Journalists (SPJ), the American Society of Newspaper Editors (ASNE), Investigative Reporters & Editors, and the National Press Photographers Association, to name a few, are also highly regarded (**Table 42-1**).

Table 42-1. Examples of Prizes Awarded to Journalists

CASEY MEDALS FOR MERITORIOUS JOURNALISM

Honors distinguished coverage of disadvantaged children and families and the institutions charged with serving them; $1000 is awarded in various categories. Funded by the Casey Journalism Center for Children and Families (http://www.casey.umd.edu).

THE DART AWARD FOR EXCELLENCE IN REPORTING ON VICTIMS OF VIOLENCE

A $10 000 prize for newspaper story or series that best illustrates the effects of violence on its victims and the ways individuals cope with emotional trauma. Funded by the Dart Center (http://www.dartcenter.org).

When others back away, run, or stand and gawk, reporters move closer in order to explain what happened and why—toward the fire, the bomb blast, the car crash, the shooting. They do this as the event is unfolding with all of its energy, chaos, and danger. Caught up in the demands of their work and untrained for the most part about issues of trauma, they expose themselves to stressful and sometimes horrific incidents day after day. Do the pressures of covering violence have an impact on journalists? Since a 1996 survey of reporters, editors, and photographers found "a level of symptoms one might find among public safety workers" such as police and firefighters, the research continues to show that journalists are affected (Simpson & Boggs, 1999). How trauma affects journalists is beyond the scope of this chapter, but many journalists are beginning to pay attention to the emotional impact that their work has on their own lives.

THE IMPACT OF NEWS

"We are neither therapists nor advocates. We are not trained or equipped to treat mental illness. And we are bound by standards of impartiality and truth, as well as competitive pressures that sometimes clash with our best intentions toward the suffering. With this in mind, and though we sometimes misstep, we are trying to do right by other human beings and not inflict further pain" (Silvestrini, 2001).

All the strengths, skills, talents, and good intentions of journalists can backfire of course. Everyone in law enforcement and social services has at least one story to tell about "bad" news coverage. Complaints range from the emphasis on perpetrators over victims, the focus on grisly details, the repetition of traumatizing images, and simple yet upsetting errors. Advocates know that the media spotlight often makes it harder for victims who face the already confusing maze of the criminal justice system. Victims of sex crimes especially expect to be blamed—they have seen it happen to others in the news and, fearing media attention, may refuse to testify or report in the first place.

Yet these complaints do not erase the fact that news coverage has a positive impact, if only because news makes an event "real." Far more people read newspapers and watch television than review court cases or police reports, to the extent that, except perhaps in the smallest communities, it can be said that only when a news story about CSE is printed or broadcast can it be truly made public. The act of news reporting alone gives a sense of worthiness to a case and those involved in it. In "Setting the news story agenda," Frederick Fico and Eric Freedman of Michigan State University confirm what observant readers and viewers already know intuitively: "Agenda-setting research has established that news media attention to issues subsequently influences the public's assessment of the importance of those issues" (2001). To be newsworthy is to be worthwhile.

But worthwhile in what sense? In its 2002 study, Coverage in Context, the Casey Journalism Center on Children and Families found that in news stories focusing on youth crime and violence or abuse and neglect, fewer than 1 in 20 gave the public information to help connect events to broader patterns and trends (Kunkel et al, 2002). It is not enough for an issue like CSE to be viewed as newsworthy; the coverage must promote constructive action as well as alarm. For this to occur, change must occur on many fronts, journalism among them.

It does little good to criticize with a broad brush. What is it about coverage as it stands that may keep readers from taking action? And what, precisely, does "right" look like?

A brief look at research on news coverage of a related, so-called private crime, domestic violence, may help answer these questions, shedding some light on the subtle and often complex ways that media coverage can influence public opinion. In contrast to CSE, domestic violence has been the topic of clinical research for 4 decades and of journalism research for about 10 years. The Estes & Weiner study (2001) identifies domestic violence as contributing to CSE, and there are other parallels as well. Like the battered spouse, the CSE victim is often blamed for the abuse, especially when the child is older than 12. Staying in "the life," like staying in a violent relationship, is perceived by many people as a choice.

In a recent study at the University of Washington School of Communications, researchers Bullock & Cubert (2002) examined newspaper coverage of domestic violence homicides in Washington State during 1998. Using content analysis and frame analysis, they explored how newspapers portrayed these fatalities, and how accurately the portrayal reflected what past research has revealed about victim experience and the broader social problems. They followed up with a 2001 survey of newspaper journalists (also in Washington State). Together, the study and survey illuminate the readers' and the journalists' perspectives and help pinpoint specific areas where—and, of most importance to readers here, may suggest *how*—news coverage can improve.

Bullock & Cubert (2002) looked at 44 cases from arrest through arraignment—a total of 230 articles. They broke each article into headlines, subheads, leads, and paragraphs, noting the terms and phrases used to describe the violence, the victim, and the perpetrator, as well as the sources that the reporter referred to or quoted. What they found in this content analysis was an overall absence of the *context* in which domestic violence occurs. The coverage they examined "seldom labeled a killing as domestic violence" (fewer than one third), "tended to omit the idea of a pattern of abuse" (90% portrayed the homicide as an isolated incident), and described the violence "overwhelmingly in terms of physical harm, while the psychological component was largely ignored" (2.2% showed psychological abuse). Articles drew heavily on such "official" sources as police, court documents, and legal personnel and much less on those "who could put a human face on domestic violence." Domestic violence experts were rarely cited.

In their frame analysis of these same articles, Bullock & Cubert (2002) identified themes or patterns in the coverage. News framing refers to words, images, and sources journalists choose to use and not use and the organization of stories that suggest attitudes and opinions for the public. Bullock and Cubert looked at the choice of topics, sources, facts, and words, as well as the placement and repetition of information. The frames that emerged also misrepresented the problem of domestic violence. One, the police ("just the facts") frame, offered no information that the killing was part of a larger situation. Another frame portrayed those involved as "different" or as a crime that happens only to certain people, in certain places. Another blamed the victim and/or excused the perpetrator. Overall, these frames tended to provide unrealistic, simple solutions to complex problems.

For readers of these articles, the picture of domestic violence as portrayed in the news was a distorted one—no surprise for anyone who works with victims or perpetrators. The relevance of this study here is that it identifies where and how the distortions occur. Bullock & Cubert speculate that "the coverage has the potential to insulate readers from the idea of domestic violence, allowing them to conclude that it couldn't happen to them and that there is no need to discuss it or take action" (2001).

Their study also uncovered some positive surprises. One of these was that the news coverage, on the whole, did *not* exonerate the perpetrator, though almost half the articles suggested a motive or excuse that could be interpreted as such. Also surprising was that victims were blamed in fewer than 20% of the articles. Twenty percent is still too often for victim advocates, but it is important to note that 80% of the time, the press did *not* blame the victims.

Just as important, Bullock & Cubert noted the "handful" that showed more accurate portrayals (2001):

Some articles illustrate domestic violence as a social problem by tying in other domestic violence cases, quoting domestic violence experts, discussing the work of domestic violence-related agencies, or including domestic violence hotline numbers. Some carefully describe the victim and perpetrator's history of physical and psychological abuse. Some put a human face on the crime through family members, friends, and others who know the victim and perpetrator.

What is especially heartening is that these approaches are also "within the boundaries of current journalistic norms and practices" (Bullock & Cubert, 2002). Tying in other cases, quoting experts, and acknowledging agencies that help, as well as putting a human face on the crime and describing victim and perpetrator history—all of these approaches give a story context, credibility, and balance; make it more accurate; and involve readers.

In a follow-up survey, Bullock & Cubert (2001) asked questions of journalists to determine reporters' knowledge, assumptions, and approaches to domestic violence, as well as the factors they feel affect their reporting. It would seem that journalists possess the same knowledge as the rest of society. Most acknowledged that the violence was psychological as well as physical, though few gave a sense that it worsened over time. Their impressions of victims and perpetrators were realistic and distorted.

Perhaps the most interesting insights, for the purposes of this chapter, were the journalists' answers to questions about their work. When asked how they *decide* to cover domestic violence, they mentioned impact, proximity, novelty, audience interest—criteria used with any news story. Several mentioned the benefit to the community and concern for victims.

When asked how they *approach* their coverage, they found "[i]t appears that some journalists favor an approach that places domestic violence incidents in a broader context, while others focus on the facts of the incident—depending on the type of story" (Bullock & Cubert, 2001). Two thirds of the respondents said that context was important, although space was a constraint in police beat summaries and first.0day incident stories.

What hinders collecting information about domestic violence? Journalists in this survey mentioned ethical concerns such as victim safety and privacy, rules of the court, uncooperative or unresponsive sources, and overprotective advocates. "Factors such as these can certainly help explain, at least in part, why articles often fail to place domestic violence in a broader context" (Bullock & Cubert, 2001).

Bullock and Cubert describe their survey as a "first step." And though they do not state it specifically, their study and survey together point to some good news that can help reverse the discouraging lack of context found in the Casey study on news coverage of children: Journalists are concerned about the issues, and they want to get them right.

COVERAGE THAT WORKS

In January 2001 readers of *The Atlanta Journal-Constitution* opened their Sunday papers to the front-page story, "Selling Atlanta's children" (**Figure 42-1**). The enlarged text next to the headline bluntly explained, "Runaway girls lured into the sex trade are being jailed for crimes while their adult pimps go free." The photo, placed prominently above the fold, was stunning and unforgettable: the shackled ankles of a 10-year-old girl (**Figure 42-1**).

"Selling Atlanta's children" continued through Monday and Tuesday. The response was immediate. "Thank you for the incredible articles on child prostitution," wrote one reader. "It is an outrage and needs to be exposed." Another wrote, "It is shocking … that I could have been oblivious to its existence." Many were moved to action: "I will be writing my representatives to plead with them to change this situation."

The Atlanta Journal-Constitution

January 7, 2001

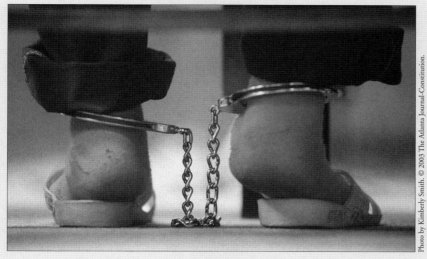

Shackles bind the legs of a 10-year-old girl, an alleged prostitute, at a Fulton County Juvenile Court hearing. *Reprinted with permission from* The Atlanta Journal-Constitution.

SPECIAL REPORT: PROSTITUTING OUR YOUNG

Selling Atlanta's Children

Runaway girls lured into the sex trade are being jailed for crimes while their adult pimps go free

BY JANE O. HANSEN, Staff Writer

The courtroom door opened, and a guard led the defendant inside. She was dressed in standard jailhouse garb—navy jumpsuit, orange T-shirt, orange socks and orange plastic flip-flops. Metal shackles around her ankles forced her to shuffle.

"All rise," the bailiff said. The judge entered and took her seat on the birchwood bench while the defendant sat down at a table and chewed her finger.

At issue was what to do with her.

She had been in and out of an Atlanta jail since August. It was now November. Her sister was in another jail. As lawyers and officials debated whether she should remain behind bars, probation officer Gail Johnson asked whether the defendant could address the court.

A little girl, her hair pulled into a tiny pigtail and her head bowed, rose from the defendant's table. She was 10 years old, a runaway and an alleged prostitute.

"I think I have been locked up long enough," the girl said in a small, high-pitched voice. She began to cry and rubbed

her eyes with balled-up fists. "If you would just let me go home ..."

But for children like her and her 11-year-old sister, also an alleged prostitute, it's not that simple.

In Atlanta, prostituted children often go to jail while the adults who exploit them go free, a review of court records shows. Attitudes toward prostitution are partly to blame, say Juvenile Court judges and others. But a lack of children's programs in Georgia, particularly for girls, has left some judges no choice but to place exploited children, such as these, in detention for their own safety.

"The last thing I want to do is detain her, because it comes across as punitive," said Fulton County Juvenile Court Judge Nina Hickson. "But I've got to make sure that she's safe."

In Georgia, pimps are rarely arrested, even when the prostitute is a child. When pimps are charged, their cases often are dismissed or result in a small fine, court records show.

No reliable statistics are available to

gauge the number of prostituted children, although Atlanta judges say they are seeing an alarming growth in their courtrooms. But statistics for adults show a clear disparity in the system's treatment of pimps and prostitutes. Since 1972, 401 adults—nearly all women—went to prison in Georgia for prostitution. No one went to prison for just pimping.

"I think there was an unwitting bias that the woman was the perpetrator," said Mike Light, Department of Corrections spokesman and a former parole officer. "She was the one out having sex. ... The pimp was just collecting the money."

Atlanta police say it's harder to arrest pimps than prostitutes. And prosecutors say it's difficult to build a case against pimps because prostitutes often are reluctant or scared to testify against them.

"We need evidence," said Carmen Smith, solicitor general for Fulton County State Court. "We need witnesses."

But critics say too often, police and prosecutors fail to distinguish between prostitutes who are adults and those who are children, such as the 10- and 11-year-old sisters. Many child prostitutes are runaways who are often escaping physical or sexual abuse at home and then are exploited on the streets.

Yet in the eyes of law enforcement, said Judge Hickson, "These girls aren't seen as victims. They're seen as consenting participants."

Juvenile Court judges and others have begun pressing for change in Georgia to bring harsher penalties against those who exploit children. They want the Georgia Legislature to make the pimping of children a felony punishable by up to 20 years in prison. They want authorities to become more aggressive in arresting and prosecuting men who pay to have sex with underage prostitutes, as well as the adults who sell them. And they want some alternative for helping these girls other than putting them behind bars.

In recent months, local and federal prosecutors have begun to respond. The Fulton district attorney's office has brought felony charges against about a dozen alleged pimps believed to have prostituted children. The U.S. attorney's office hopes to bring federal charges against pimps under the nation's racketeering laws.

Still, says DeKalb County Juvenile Court Judge Nikki Marr, not enough is being done for children whose lives may already have been destroyed.

"It's not a priority," she said. "That's what it comes down to."

By March, the Georgia legislature had passed 2 laws, one making it a felony to pimp any child 18 or younger (until then it had been a misdemeanor "no more serious than a parking ticket"), and another giving courts the authority to seize assets used in the business of pimping children. By the end of the year, 14 pimps had been indicted on federal racketeering charges that resulted in prison terms (8 pled guilty; the rest were convicted). An Atlanta Women's Foundation donor purchased a home for the young victims, and a special fund was created to treat and protect them.

What was it about this story that moved the community to take such swift action? Like the "handful" of domestic violence homicide articles discussed earlier, much of the effectiveness of "Selling Atlanta's children" was due to its accuracy, credibility, and balance. From the first paragraph, the series put a human face on CSE. By the eighth paragraph (still on the front page), the crime was tied to other cases. Experts in juvenile court and juvenile detention, as well as police, were quoted throughout, but the story never let the reader forget that 10-year-old girl or stop caring about her and her 11-year-old sister. A companion article ("Prostitution's middle men usually slide by") described the perpetrators and their history, even including the rap sheets on 3 of them, and explained some of the problems with law enforcement. A third article ("Promise of the easy life pulls the young to streets") explored how and why the girls became prostitutes, in part through the experts but primarily through the voices of the girls themselves.

That Sunday, readers learned a great deal. Writing, layout, and photos worked together to expose the problem of CSE, with all its complexity, heartbreak, and viciousness. And though none of the girls were named, nor were their faces shown, the reality of their stories made people sit up and take notice.

The next day, the series focused more on the experts ("Prostitutes getting younger as sex trade grows, judges say") and described how other states have handled the problem ("Feds, police elsewhere finding solutions"), underscoring the need for action. Statistics were presented in simple bar and pie charts. On Tuesday, the series ended with a story of mothers whose daughters had been lured into prostitution through chat lines ("When danger is as close as a phone"). The article included advice for parents, as well as specific ways for readers to help through volunteering, contributing, and lobbying.

The power of the series was also due to the talent and tenacity of reporter Jane Hansen. Hansen, who has been with the *Journal-Constitution* since 1982, began writing about kids by covering education issues. In 1990, she was a Pulitzer finalist and won several journalism awards for "Suffer the children." This 7-part series uncovered the suffering of abused and neglected children and showed how the abuse occurred in foster homes as well as in natural homes. The *Journal-Constitution* sued to get the records she needed of children killed while under the "protection" of Georgia's child welfare system, challenging that "confidentiality" should not apply to protect the privacy of children who were already dead.

"The harder they fought, the harder I fought," Hansen says, reflecting on that experience. "I was convinced it was a total cover-up" (J. Hansen, interview, January 2002). The court agreed. Ten years later, when she was working on "Georgia's forgotten children," the *Journal-Constitution* sued again for access to documents that a state law (which was enacted after "Suffer the children" was published) had already made available. Hansen is emphatic about the importance of her newspaper's support through these "two expensive lawsuits" and of her editor, Hyde Post.

By the time Hansen began the work that would become "Selling Atlanta's children," she was a veteran at scaling obstacles put in her way by state agencies and the court, and at questioning policies. In her experience, "Confidentiality laws have done more to protect tormenters and harm children." She also was clear about her motives. "As a journalist, I am often driven by the public's need to know about people who lack a voice," she wrote in a guest article for Georgia's forensic science newsletter, "Children, for instance" (Hansen, 2001b).

The idea of covering CSE in Atlanta came to her indirectly, through a column she had written in 1991 about a private Christian school that would not hire Jews. The mother of one of the students Hansen had interviewed called to compliment her. Nine years later, the same mother became familiar with the problem of child prostitution in Atlanta through her volunteer work in the courts and called Hansen again. Would she be interested in hearing more? Hansen was, but she was working on other projects and could not get to it at the time.

When she later spoke with the mother, Hansen knew the story was important. She also knew there would be resistance, within the newspaper and among readers. The problem of CSE had been explored before, usually dealing with immigrant children or kids in other countries, making it, from the perspective of editors, an "old story." The fact that these were local girls in Atlanta made it "new" enough, but even judges had trouble getting the district attorney to prosecute because prostitution was considered a "victimless" crime. The public generally assumed that teenage prostitutes were not victims because they chose to sell their bodies.

To overcome reader bias, Hansen needed a very young girl. Reporting about a child prostitute would frame the story more powerfully than the testimony of agencies and experts alone. "When talking about child sexual abuse, we have many statistics and research, but numbers make people *numb*," she explains. "If I can write about one child behind those numbers, and if the story is compelling enough, then it will have impact. Then it will move people" (J. Hansen, interview, January 2002).

Learning about a 10-year-old girl's case (and that of her 11-year-old sister) was only the beginning. Juvenile hearings are closed by law, and it took months of reassurance on Hansen's part before Judge Hickson would let her inside the courtroom or, for that matter, be introduced to the girl. Hansen talked to other judges who knew her reporting on previous cases and could recommend her to Hickson. She offered past news stories that showed she was protective of confidentiality and provided photos that showed they could be taken without identifying the girl, agreeing to let the judge see photos before they ran. At the same time, Hansen worked to win the confidence of the child advocate and probation officer in the case.

The resistance did not end with Judge Hickson's approval. When Hansen showed up with photographer Kimberly Smith, the bailiff stopped them; after Hickson upheld the permission in chambers, the Department of Child and Family Services objected. It took another hearing that day before the photographer was allowed to take the picture that was so riveting to readers. "You have to really believe a story needs to be told," says Hansen, looking back on the effort behind that front page and what kept her going.

Across the country in Wyoming at the *Casper Star-Tribune,* city editor Deirdre Stoelzle voices similar frustrations. Vast as it is, Wyoming is sparsely populated, making the state essentially "a small town," and making privacy—let alone confidentiality—an especially sensitive issue (D. Stoelzle, interview, February 2002). Stoelzle's reporting is also shaped by her own experience: as a child she was molested by her grandfather. "I've got some perspective on interviewing victims," she admits. She works to engender trust, and she does not ask questions that she would "be terrified to answer" herself. Afterward, her practice is to read back quotes after interviews and encourage survivors to call her later.

Like Hansen, Stoelzle is accustomed to being kept away from child victims by prosecutors and psychologists. She understands their distrust and protectiveness. "But *we* think we're being helpful: to the investigation because we can tell others about it, to families because we can reassure them that child abuse happens a lot and pass along what and who can help them" (D. Stoelzle, interview, February 2002). An article that she wrote about a soccer coach who was charged with manufacturing child pornography illustrates the kind of help she describes and is a good example of the impact that news writing can have. In "Facing fears of molestation" (**Figure 42-2**), she tackles a complex issue that is frightening for parents and explains it with authority and clarity, using 2 local experts—all in less than 400 words.

Sometimes she gets lucky, as when her subsequent coverage of the soccer coach case featured one of the coach's victims. In "Back in control" (Stoelzle, 1999), John Warnick, now 20, described how the coach had molested him when he was 10 years old, the painful journey afterward, and his courageous participation in a sting operation that led to the coach's arrest. Warnick had approached Stoelzle, and what made his story newsworthy beyond its timeliness was Warnick himself. "He looked healthy, strong, commanding, and so nice," explained Stoelzle. "Not who we might stereotype as a victim. Yet he had lived with his secret for so long." Stoelzle is adamant about getting beyond the reflexive disgust people feel when they read about child sexual abuse and exploitation. "We need to take that initial horror and tell stories in ways that don't harm victims." By "harm" she includes the implication that what they've gone through is insurmountable. "They've survived. They deserve to be praised in some way" (D. Stoelzle, interview, February 2002).

Stoelzle's loudest complaint is, interestingly enough, lack of timely access to child abuse experts. When a story breaks late in the afternoon, she can always reach someone at the local nonprofit agency. But articles about CSE need resources who are "higher up the food chain." For readers, the psychiatrists and psychologists who are the leaders in the therapeutic community are more believable and credible. "If a doctor says it," Stoelzle acknowledges, "it means more." In her experience, these experts are also less likely to return her urgent phone calls. "They don't have to care

Figure 42-2. "Facing fears of molestation." Reprinted with permission from Deirdre Stoelzle, City Editor, Casper Star-Tribune; *Casper, Wyo.*

Casper Star-Tribune
October 8, 1999

Facing Fears of Molestation

By Deirdre Stoelzle, City Editor

CASPER – Parents who are worried their children might have been subject to sexual molestation should be delicate in their initial questioning, says a prominent local child psychiatrist.

Dr. Stephen Brown suggests parents familiar with a local soccer coach now accused of distributing child pornography approach the situation tangentially.

A parent might begin by saying, for example, that they understand this soccer coach may be in trouble or that there's some talk that he may have been doing things with kids that he shouldn't have, said Brown.

Parents then could ask their children how they feel about this talk that the coach may be in trouble. Parents should gauge their child's reaction to determine whether to pursue the matter, Brown said.

"But you also don't want to put things in kids' heads," he said.

It's best to let police handle the questioning after that, says Cari Rothenhoefer of the Self Help Center. She acknowledges that reporting sexual assault incidents is tremendously difficult for both male and female victims because of stigmas attached to the crime.

Boys may be even more hesitant to do so, she said.

"Sometimes boys will worry, 'Does this mean that I'll be a homosexual?'"

"I think they worry about what people will think of them if they find out. In some circumstances, there's probably reason to worry if a perpetrator will ever retaliate against them—for example, 'What if he gets out of jail and comes looking for me because it would be my fault that he's in jail?'"

But stepping forward is crucial to stopping perpetrators from repeating their crimes, she said. And while reporting a case certainly changes an incident from a family secret to a law-enforcement matter, she said, victims' names are kept secret outside court documents.

"I would like to think that if they do report, that it would then be brought to the parents' and families' attention—and that maybe other boys would realize, 'I wasn't the only one,'" said Rothenhoefer, who counsels children.

"Sometimes kids can feel like they were the only one, and so it's their private secret," she said. "But they might feel better knowing that it wasn't only them, that (such an incident) happened to other boys, and now that a person's caught, no other boys will hopefully be affected by that person."

about my deadline," she says. "But if they care about the issue, we need a response" (D. Stoelzle, interview, February 2002).

WORKING WITH THE NEWS FOR THE SAKE OF EXPLOITED KIDS

"Citizens in a democracy must know about violence if they are to make responsible decisions about how to protect themselves, their families, and their communities. The job of the media is to tell them accurately, fairly, and comprehensively" (Cote & Simpson, 2000).

By now it should be clear that, while news coverage has an impact on public opinion, what is also true is that "the public" has an impact on journalism. The two are necessarily interrelated, with the beliefs, knowledge, and opinions of one affecting the other. But while journalists accept that their job is to search out, confirm, and present timely information to the public, "the public" generally assumes a passive role, taking whatever news comes. It does not have to be this way. In her study that examines how prochoice and prolife groups competed for media coverage and favorable public opinion, Andsager summarized past research showing that "interest groups that must compete to gain media coverage are most successful when they ... understand how news is constructed, positioning their communications in terms of traditional newsworthiness values such as timeliness, conflict, prominence, proximity, and impact" (2000).

IMPROVING ATTITUDES ABOUT JOURNALISTS

So far, this chapter has focused on understanding the news, particularly print journalism. The next section will discuss specific ways to promote news coverage that moves the community to protect exploited children.

It will help first to stop thinking of journalists as the enemy. *Atlanta Journal-Constitution* reporter Jane Hansen, who worked on the White House staff under then-president Carter, knows what it feels like to be unfairly written about in the news. "My experience there taught me to fear reporters, but it also inspired me to become one," she wrote in a guest editorial (2001b). She urges readers to keep an open mind. "As in any profession, some of us are insensitive, arrogant, and rude. And yes, some of us are dumb, biased, liberal, and evil. But most of us are committed to high standards of journalism" (Hansen, 2001b).

Casper Star-Tribune editor Deirdre Stoelzle wishes prosecutors and psychotherapists would see reporters as allies. "What counselors want more than anything is for victims to talk," she explains. "We're professional communicators. We know how to help people express themselves. Use us as a resource!" (D. Stoelzle, interview, February 2002).

One of the best ways to find the good reporters Hansen refers to is by looking for articles related to an area of expertise. Legal or clinical experts are in a better position than most readers to recognize when a news story on CSE is written with accuracy, context, and balance. When there is an article like this, note the byline (some newspapers include the reporter's direct phone number and e-mail address). The idea is to catch reporters doing a good job and to tell them so—by phone, fax, or e-mail. This does not have to be a thought-out letter to the editor, just a quick note; but be specific about what was "right" in terms of the reality of CSE and community safety. The reporter will appreciate the praise, and will have been introduced to a resource for future stories.

Learn more about the news business, too, by reading trade publications now and then and checking the Web sites of professional organizations (**Table 42-2**). There are always articles and postings about journalism ethics and practices, many of them examining the decisions behind going with a story (or not), questioning trends, and challenging the way things have "always" been done. A sample from the December

---

Table 42-2. A Sample of Journalism Publications and Web sites

— American Journalism Review (http://www.ajr.org)

— Columbia Journalism Review (http://www.cjr.org)

— Society of Professional Journalists (http://www.spj.org)

— Casey Journalism Center for Children and Families (http://www.casey.umd.edu)

— Dart Center for Journalism & Trauma (http://www.dartcenter.org)

— Poynter Institute for Media Studies (http://www.poynter.org)

— Associated Press Managing Editors (http://www.apme.com)

— National Press Photographers Association (http://www.nppa.org)

2001 editions of *Quill* and the *American Journalism Review (AJR)* reveals some of the newsroom struggles after the September 11 terrorist attacks:

— "Ethics and war: critics claim journalists go too far—and, sometimes, not far enough" (*Quill*)

— "Asleep at the switch: nonths ago, journalists failed to alert the public about terrorist threats" (*Quill*)

— "The anthrax enigma: did news outlets keep their audiences informed without unduly heightening the fear?" (*AJR*)

More routine concerns of falling revenues, attracting readers, information access, and the credibility of online news are also discussed in these publications. In addition, ethics issues are covered in ombudsman columns of local newspapers.

GETTING NEWS ATTENTION

Journalists are always looking for stories. They welcome tips, particularly a local angle on a national story, or a new angle on a chronic problem. Such tips are "the lifeblood of a reporter," says Janet Grimley, assistant managing editor for the *Seattle Post-Intelligencer* (J. Grimley, interview, February 2002). She urges people to "get on that phone" when they know of a local tie-in. Stoelzle agrees wholeheartedly: "After 9/11, tons of calls came in, telling us about a friend who worked near the Trade Center, or a kid stranded in an airport that day. If there's just been an arrest for Internet porn and someone's got a link or information we can use, call us right away" (D. Stoelzle, interview, February 2002). Do not be discouraged, however, if your tip does not get covered. It is not personal. "I give reporters tips all the time that go nowhere," Grimley admits.

An effective way to work with media is through contact lists within your professional organization (eg, the American Psychological Association has a media referral service). But do not overlook the power of a direct contribution, such as a letter to the editor or broadcast call-in. Better yet, try for a guest editorial. You can send in a finished piece or call, e-mail, or write to pitch your idea to the editorial department, which operates separately from the newsroom. Timeliness and the credibility of the person submitting the piece increase the chances of getting published. A 2001 opinion piece in the *Seattle Post-Intelligencer* by child advocate Laurence Gray on trafficked children was published as the Second World Congress Against Commercial Exploitation of Children was getting under way in Yokohama; in addition, the humanitarian organization Gray works for has its US office in Federal Way, a Seattle suburb. Psychologist Robert Baugher's essay, "How long (according to the media) should grief last?" was published in the *Columbia Journalism Review* in March/April 2001, coinciding with anniversary coverage of the Oklahoma City bombing and the Columbine school shootings.

When an organization or agency has new information to announce to all media at once, a press release is the standard method of getting attention. News agencies receive many press releases every day, and the competition for coverage is keen. A good press release grabs attention and keeps it with short sentences and paragraphs. It is a skill worth learning and why many in public relations were trained as reporters. The Estes & Weiner (2001) study provides a good example of the contrasting styles between press releases and executive summaries, as shown in **Table 42-3**.

Again, timeliness is important; unfortunately, despite the most careful plans, this can not be controlled. As alarming and newsworthy as the Estes and Weiner study was, it was virtually buried by events the day after it was released—September 11, 2001.

WHEN A REPORTER CALLS

At 5:30 in the afternoon, a high school teacher has been arrested after asking one of his students if he could take pornographic photos of her to post on the Internet. Police found computer disks in his car and home that contained images of girls engaged in explicit sexual conduct. All that reporters have is the police report and hundreds of questions. Among these questions are: how common is this kind of exploitation? Why does it happen? What can schools and parents do to stop it? The answers will put the news in context, help the community respond with outrage at the crime and with empathy for the victims, and possibly encourage more victims to come forward to help police and prosecutors make a better case.

But again, at 5:30, child abuse experts have already left the office, or are on their way home, or are busy with clients.

"I would love to have an expert's direct or home phone number for times like that," says *Seattle Post-Intelligencer* managing editor Janet Grimley (interview, February 2002). "But the reality is that we'll run the story with only the cop report, if that's all we've got." Other news outlets have the story, too, and people who hear about it on TV and radio expect it in their newspaper the next day. The story is hot now, and "we can't wait for all the information."

Given that a scenario like this rarely occurs at a convenient time, legal and clinical experts should consider how they or their office would react to a reporter's call. This is where the "heavy responsibility ... for accurate messages concerning the nature,

---

Table 42-3. Examples of Contrasting Writing Styles

EXECUTIVE SUMMARY	PRESS RELEASE
"The benefits of economic globalization, internationalization, and free trade have brought with them an unanticipated set of social problems. Among them is what appears to be a dramatic rise worldwide in the incidence of child exploitation" (Estes & Weiner, 2001).	"Tens of thousands of U.S., Mexican and Canadian children and youths become victims of juvenile pornography, prostitution and trafficking each year. So significant is the problem that even most law-enforcement and child-welfare officials do not realize its scope" (Commercial child sexual exploitation, 2001).

extent and seriousness of CSE" that the Estes & Weiner (2001) study places on media rests for a while on your shoulders. The timing will never be better: you have the information, and the reporter wants it.

This does not mean you have to respond instantly. Ask the reporter a few questions first. What is the deadline? Is this interview for background or attribution? What kind of information is needed? "We can tell you exactly what questions we want to ask," *Casper Star-Tribune* editor Deirdre Stoelzle says (interview, February 2002).

Sometimes the reporter may be trying to reach you for advice before interviewing a victim or family member who has already agreed to talk to them. Stoelzle, who as a Dart Fellow received specialized training from Dart Center faculty and the International Society of Traumatic Stress Studies, still appreciates a reality check. The insight of child abuse experts helps her understand more about the victim's experience. "Without their help, I may ask a lot of dumb questions."

During the interview, explain any medical or legal terms you use, as well as words or acronyms that mislead journalists and readers. It may be appropriate within your profession to speak of prostitutes exiting from street life, but the term *exiting* connotes a casual walking away that is hardly the reality for girls. In the short time you have with the reporter, be as clear as you can, and meticulous with your facts. If the interview turns its focus on medical or legal practices, expect to feel defensive, but try not to give in to that feeling; in attempting to avoid responsibility, it is easy to inadvertently shift the blame to the victims.

An unexpected call from a reporter is less of a surprise if you are prepared for quick media response. Before you need it, put together a press packet, a sort of media first aid kit that will provide the kind of information journalists need when covering CSE. In it, include fact sheets *with attribution*, related short articles, and a list of local and national resources and their Web sites. Anticipate when news interest in a specific case may peak—at sentencing hearings, for example, or anniversaries. Also consider the visual needs of newspapers as well as television, and think about whether and where you could accommodate a photographer. For yourself, identify resources to call on for backup, including other professionals and victims' advocates who are comfortable with reporters, can speak in sound bites, and are prepared to answer questions without too much warning.

HELPING VICTIMS WHO GO PUBLIC

Since reporters often have no way to connect to victims other than through prosecutors, advocates, or therapists, expect to be asked if you know of one who would be willing to be interviewed. It may feel as if you are being treated as a broker, but try not to be offended by the question. Real victims make for compelling, credible news stories that convince readers and viewers that the problem is important.

Victims who are ready and willing to tell their story to the media can still benefit from a little coaching. **Table 42-4**, For Survivors Who Go Public, is included here to help you to help them. Many of the tips can apply to you as well.

CONCLUSION

The causes and effects of CSE are complex, as are the solutions. As professional communicators who influence public opinion, news media play an important role. Their breaking stories, features, and reports on the latest research can help create empathy for victims, pressure police and prosecutors to investigate and prove cases, convince agencies to revise policies and procedures, and persuade elected officials to improve the laws. This kind of reporting requires the understanding and cooperation of medical and legal professionals who are experts in the field.

Reporters and experts do not have the same goals or responsibilities, nor should they. There will always be tensions between them. But the values of solid reporting—

accuracy, context, credibility, and balance, and the overriding concern for the community—are something they share and are argument enough for the 2 groups to find ways to work together.

Table 42-4. For Survivors Who Go Public

1. **Set limits.** What do you not want to talk about? What won't you do (eg, filming in your home, appearing with partner or children, appearing with an offender)? How much time are you willing to spend? Do not be afraid to communicate these limits before the interview or appearance.

2. **Ask about format.** Is the article a lengthy feature or a short news piece? A 2-minute spot or a half-hour interview? Live or taped? Call-in? If a panel, when do you come on, how are you introduced, who else is on the panel, and who is in the audience?

3. **Ask about the focus.** What point is being made? How does your participation help make this point?

4. **Don't overlook the commercial aspect.** Is a product being promoted? If so, what is it?

5. **Be extra careful if a case is in progress.** Anything you say to media can be used against you in a trial. A good idea is to check with an advocate, prosecutor, or detective first.

6. **Guard against "off the record" statements.** Assume that reporters are always listening and taking notes and that microphones and video recorders are always turned on.

7. **Have an advocate or buddy present.** The stress of going public is considerably reduced when you can share observations. In addition, your "media escort" can take care of transportation details and—if necessary—terminate the interview for you.

8. **Always debrief within the week.** Plan for this. Debriefing can take many forms: a phone call, a walk, talking over coffee or a drink.

9. **Beware of talk shows and town meetings.** These are considered entertainment, not journalism. The host is a "star" whose livelihood is closely tied to ratings. Viewers are accustomed to tuning in to see conflict, not to be educated. The adversarial tone and dizzying pace can be overwhelming.

10. **Be ready for disclosures.** Journalists and photographers are people. They have their own histories; some have stories that will be triggered by yours. You may be the first person they have ever told.

Reprinted with permission from Scherer M. Why I turned down Oprah Winfrey. Nieman Reports. Fall 1996;50(3):35-37.

REFERENCES

Andsager JL. How interest groups attempt to shape public opinion with competing news frames. *Journalism & Mass Communications Quarterly.* Autumn 2000;77(3): 577-592.

Baugher R. How long (according to the media) should grief last? *Columbia J Rev.* March/April 2001. Available at: http://www.cjr.org/year/01/2/baugher.asp. Accessed July 28, 2003.

Bullock CF, Cubert J. Inside the newsroom: journalists' views of domestic violence and what shapes coverage. Lecture presented at: 2001 International Society for Traumatic Stress Studies Annual Meeting. December 8, 2001; New Orleans, La.

Bullock CF, Cubert J. Coverage of domestic violence fatalities by newspapers in Washington State. *J Interpers Violence.* 2002;17(5):475-499.

Commercial child sexual exploitation: "the most hidden form of child abuse," says Penn professor [press release]. University of Pennsylvania News Bureau. September 10, 2001. Available at: http://caster.ssw.upenn.edu/~restes/CSEC_Files/CSE_Final_Press_Release_010910.pdf. Accessed August 27, 2003.

Cote W, Simpson R. *Covering Violence: A Guide to Ethical Reporting About Victims and Trauma.* New York, NY: Columbia University Press; 2000.

Estes RJ, Weiner NA. The commercial sexual exploitation of children in the US, Canada and Mexico: executive summary. September 2001. Available at: http://www.ageofconsent.com/comments/Exec_Sum_010910.pdf. Accessed August 14, 2003.

Fico R, Freedman E. Setting the news story agenda: candidates and commentators in news coverage of a governor's race. *J Mass Commun Q.* 2001;78(3, Autumn): 437-449.

Frankel M. The oxygen of our liberty. *Poynter Report.* November 12, 2001. Available at: http://www.poynter.org/dg.lts/id.6401/content.content_view.htm. Accessed August 27, 2003.

Gorney C. Superhire 2000. *Am J Rev.* December 2000. Available at: http://www.ajr.org/article.asp?id=386. Accessed August 27, 2003.

Gray L. High cost of sexually abused children. *Seattle Post-Intelligencer.* December 19, 2001:B6.

Hansen JO. Selling Atlanta's children. *Atlanta Journal-Constitution.* January 7-9, 2001a:A1, A10.

Hansen JO. From investigation to print. *The Final Analysis.* Georgia Bureau of Investigation Division of Forensic Science Newsletter; April 2001b.

Kunkel D, Smith S, Suding P, Biely E. Coverage in context: how thoroughly the news media report five key children's issues. Commissioned by the Casey Journalism Center on Children and Families; February 2002.

Naughton J. The oxygen of our liberty. *Poynter Report.* Fall 2001.

Scherer M. Why I turned down Oprah Winfrey. *Nieman Reports.* Fall 1996;50(3): 35-37.

Silvestrini E. Survivors and the media. Gift From Within Web site. October 2004. Available at: http://www.giftfromwithin.org/html/survive.html. Accessed February 7, 2001.

Simpson R, Boggs J. An exploratory study of traumatic stress among newspaper journalists. *J Commun Monogr.* 1999;1(1):1-26.

Stoelzle D. Facing fears of molestation. *Casper Star-Tribune.* October 8, 1999.

Stoelzle D. Back in control. *Casper Star-Tribune.* October 17, 1999.

Working With the Tourism Industry to Prevent Child Sexual Exploitation: An Individual Perspective

Bernadette McMenamin, AO

Child prostitution and the sexual abuse of children by foreigners have existed since ancient times. Historically, soldiers, sailors, and traders have been known to sexually abuse children in the countries to which they traveled. Recorded examples of individuals traveling to exotic, tropical, and primitive locations to have sex with children dates back as far as the last century. While the sexual abuse of children by foreign travelers is not new, it has dramatically increased during the last 3 decades, coinciding with the explosive growth of international travel and tourism, particularly to third world countries. Tourism-related child prostitution has become such a significant problem globally that a term exists to describe this practice—***child sex tourism***.

Since the 1970s, child prostitution has become a lucrative industry in many third-world, tourist-receiving countries. This demand for children has come from locals and foreigners, including tourists, military, travelers, businessmen, and expatriates. The causal factors leading to this growth are multiple, interrelated, and complex. Poverty is undoubtedly the catalyst rendering children, their families, and their communities vulnerable to exploitation. However, child prostitution and child sex tourism could not exist if not for the exploiters—pimps, traffickers, corrupt authorities, lax law enforcement officers, and, most importantly, child sex abusers.

Although historical, cultural, social, and political factors contribute to the existence of child prostitution, globalization is considered the major force behind the rapid international increase and expansion of the child sex trade. The increasing interconnectedness of economies, technologies, and communities that characterize globalization has opened access to vulnerable children everywhere. In particular, the massive increase of international travel, growth of tourism to poor countries, and promotion of child sex tourism through media such as the Internet all contribute to the growth of the global child sex trade. Another contributor to the growth in child sex tourism is that many Western countries have recently begun to crack down against child sex offenders. These countries have done this by enacting stronger laws, increasing law enforcement efforts, tightening employment screening measures, conducting police checks, and compiling and maintaining sex offender databases to track offenders. This tighter scrutiny in some countries has "encouraged" many sex offenders to travel outside of their own country to destinations where they are unknown.

The exact number of children who become victims of child sex tourism is impossible to know. In the early 1990s, it was estimated that in Asia hundreds of thousands of children were exploited in prostitution, and a significant proportion of this demand was coming from sex tourism. During the last decade, child sex tourism has grown into a significant global problem that involves millions of children across Asia, Latin America, Eastern Europe, Africa, and the Pacific Rim Countries.

CONCERN RAISED FOR EXPLOITATION OF CHILDREN THROUGH SEX TOURISM

Although campaigns against sex tourism began in the 1970s when women's groups vocally opposed the sexual exploitation of women by military personnel and tourists in Southeast Asian countries, it was not until the mid-1980s that the exploitation of children in sex tourism was raised as a concern. This acknowledgment resulted from the following factors:

— A visible increase in the numbers of children engaging in prostitution in Southeast Asia

— Global minimization and even denial of the reality of the existence of child prostitution

— The historical formation of the End Child Prostitution in Asian Tourism (ECPAT) organization; in 1996, this organization changed its name to End Child Prostitution, Child Pornography and Trafficking of Children for Sexual Purposes

INCREASE IN NUMBERS OF CHILDREN INVOLVED IN PROSTITUTION IN SOUTHEAST ASIA

One factor that contributed to the concern about child exploitation was the visible increase in the number of children engaging in prostitution on the streets, in bars, on beaches, in brothels, and in tourist areas of Southeast Asia. Various forms of media were instrumental in exposing the growth of child prostitution and child sex tourism by working closely with child rights advocates to investigate the cases. In the late 1980s, several horrific incidents received international attention. In one case, 5 children were found dead and chained to beds after a brothel burned down in Thailand. In the Philippines, an 11-year-old girl was left to die in the street in plain view after an Austrian tourist sexually abused her and left a broken vibrator inside of her body. Also in Thailand, 3 Americans were discovered to be running a shelter for homeless children as a cover for sexual exploitation to visiting pedophiles. Despite this shocking media exposure, Southeast Asian government officials did not react immediately.

MINIMIZATION OR ACTUAL DENIAL OF THE EXISTENCE OF CHILD PROSTITUTION

Another contributing factor that increased the concern about child exploitation was the worldwide minimization or actual denial of the existence of child prostitution. As stories about child prostitution became more publicized, some Asian government officials initially minimized or denied the existence in their countries. This was particularly true for those countries which feared the loss of tourism money. Minimal real data existed to validate that sex crimes, particularly against children, occurred in many countries. Therefore, western government officials denied the involvement of their nationals in child sex tourism because they had no reference database to prove its existence. As a result of the dramatic, worldwide exposure to the problem, combined with the persistent and strategic lobbying of nongovernmental organizations (NGOs) (especially ECPAT), governments and communities in rich and poor countries were forced to admit that child prostitution did exist, that local and foreign nationals were involved, and that governments everywhere had a responsibility to act locally and globally to protect the most vulnerable children in the world from sexual exploitation.

FORMATION OF THE END CHILD PROSTITUTION IN ASIAN TOURISM
CAMPAIGN

The creation of the ECPAT campaign in 1990 at the Bangkok-based Ecumenical Coalition on Third World Tourism (ECTWT) was an important contributing factor that increased the worldwide recognition of child exploitation. In the late 1980s, the ECTWT commissioned research into the existence of tourism-related, child prostitution in 4 Southeast Asian countries.

This research found that child prostitution was evident in these countries and reaching alarming levels in Thailand, the Philippines, and Sri Lanka. In addition, the research found that although historical practices and local abusers contributed to the sexual demand for children, the demand for child prostitutes from foreign tourists, military personnel, and businessmen had increased significantly. As a result of these findings, a number of Asian-based, NGOs formed a network that grew into the international campaign to end child prostitution in Asian tourism, ie, ECPAT.

Originally, ECPAT's message and slogan were simply "End Child Prostitution in Asian Tourism"; in 1996, this changed to "End Child Prostitution, Child Pornography and Trafficking of Children for Sexual Purposes." This designation change was made in an effort to be more internationally applicable and to reflect all of the various forms of sexual exploitation of children. The ECPAT campaign aimed to raise international awareness of the problem, build active grassroots advocacy groups, effect a global network, and encourage governmental organizations (GOs) and communities to implement laws and policies to stop child sexual exploitation. The organization's vision was to build a lateral, democratic, global network of organizations and individuals working together with a common vision.

Although the Convention on the Rights of the Child (CRC) provided the impetus for the birth of ECPAT, its mission was specifically based upon Articles 34 and 35 of the CRC, which called for the eradication of the sexual exploitation of children in prostitution, pornography, and sex trafficking. The ECPAT campaign wants to expose these problems, and it aims to promote solutions by advocating practical strategies with achievable outcomes.

CREATING A GLOBAL NETWORK

ECPAT has a view of child sex tourism as a transnational problem and the result of global trends. To counter this force, ECPAT believed it necessary to create global opposition in the form of an active, international network of individuals and organizations. Acting as a catalyst, ECPAT facilitated the formation of national, grassroots ECPAT campaigns throughout the world (**Figures 43-1-a** and **b**). Although all the ECPAT groups were shaped (and constrained) by social, cultural, and political contexts, all groups share a vision and apply similar campaign strategies. The global network's overall goal is for ECPAT campaigns to educate and lobby locally within their own countries and to support international actions to pressure world leaders and GOs to eradicate child sex tourism. Such actions would include but not be limited to legislation, proactive law enforcement deterrents, and the establishment of good victim services. The term *governmental organization*, or GO, is an internationally accepted and frequently used designation of an agency. This is in contrast to a *nongovernmental organization*, or NGO, such as a private business, church, or other type of non-profit organization.

As previously discussed, ECPAT initially consisted of only Asian-based campaigns, but once the problem of child sex tourism was exposed outside of Asia, individuals and groups around the world eagerly joined the campaign and formed local groups. Groups in Thailand, Sri Lanka, the Philippines, and Taiwan developed and initiated the first ECPAT campaigns. Australia, France, Germany, the Netherlands, Austria, Belgium, New Zealand, and the United States later joined in support. Within 3

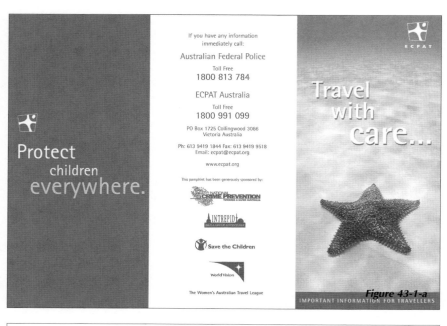

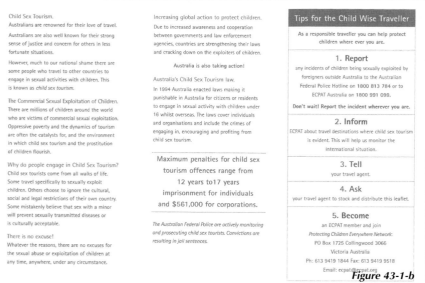

Figures 43-1-a and b. Brochure from the ECPAT campaign group in Australia. Reprinted with permission from Child Wise.

years, more than 20 ECPAT groups had formed. The ECPAT network grew rapidly and extended into Latin America, Africa, and Eastern Europe as these regions became concerned as the commercial sexual exploitation of children (CSEC) increased in their countries. As of 2004, more than 70 ECPAT groups exist worldwide.

A MULTIDISCIPLINARY APPROACH

ECPAT adopted a multidisciplinary and multilayered approach to combat child sex tourism and child prostitution because these problems were seen as the result of numerous complex forces that required understanding to develop preventive strategies. Although the campaign remained focused, members of ECPAT worked with community groups, government officials, individuals within the private sector, and people within the media industry. The ECPAT groups encouraged these people to take action and do all they could to prevent child sexual exploitation. In addition, the ECPAT groups launched educational campaigns around the world in an effort to expose the hidden problem of child prostitution and child sex tourism.

Members of ECPAT successfully lobbied the governments of 40 countries to enact extraterritorial child sex tourism laws that prosecute their nationals for child sexual abuse committed in other countries. In the absence of child protection laws in child sex tourism destinations within Asia, ECPAT encouraged GOs in those specific countries to introduce laws that would protect children from all forms of sexual exploitation.

Recognizing that laws alone would be ineffective without active enforcement, government authorities were encouraged to enforce their laws and prosecute the child sex tourists and traders. Members of ECPAT worked closely with the International Criminal Police Organization, or Interpol, and local police forces in exchange for information about offenders and their destinations. In addition, they facilitated the establishment of specialist police units within Interpol as well as many other countries.

Although ECPAT began as a small network with limited resources, these groups effectively used mass media channels and partnered with world media organizations to expose the involvement of their country's nationals in child sex tourism and convince their GOs to take proactive investigative and prosecution measures. This media exposure eventually forced government officials to take action and address the CSEC.

TRAVEL AND TOURISM INDUSTRY EDUCATION AND ACTIONS

One of ECPAT's most successful collaborations has been with the international travel and tourism industry. In the early days of the campaign, ECPAT members approached groups within the travel and tourism industry to form a working partnership and address the sexual exploitation of children within the tourism industry. Although the tourism industry was not to blame for child prostitution, the industry did have an opportunity to play a vital role in its prevention.

At that time, a responsible tourism movement was growing within the tourism sector, which was concerned with the negative impact of tourism on vulnerable communities. Although attention was primarily given to the impact of tourism on the culture and environment, child prostitution began to be discussed. Within the tourism industry, a belief emerged that child sex tourism was a growing concern and detrimental to sustainable tourism.

The ECPAT's approach was well received by key international travel and tourism industry groups, such as the World Tourism Organizations (WTO) and the United Federation of Travel Agents' Association (UFTAA). Both organizations agreed to support ECPAT by educating individuals within the industry about and taking action to prevent the sexual abuse of children in tourism. In 1993, the WTO adopted a statement against organized sex tourism and formed the Tourism and Child Prostitution Watch Task Force to monitor child sex tourism and promote good practices. In November 1993, the UFTAA launched the Child and Travel Agents' Charter, which was signed by national associations worldwide. Article 3 of this charter states that UFTAA will give every assistance to the various organizations, campaigns, and charitable associations concerned with the welfare of child victims of sex tourism. Article 6 states that UFTAA members and affiliates will inform their customers about the consequences to tourists who sexually exploit children. Other international associations followed this example and adopted similar resolutions against child sex tourism.

TOURISM CAMPAIGNS IN SENDING COUNTRIES

Many ECPAT groups in "sending countries" (ie, those countries which are residences to frequent offenders) formed local partnerships with the travel and tourism industry to raise awareness and encourage action within the travel industry and among travelers. These awareness campaigns have occurred in Australia, New Zealand, the United States, and the European Union (Austria, Belgium, Cyprus, Czech Republic, Denmark, Estonia, Germany, Greece, Finland, France, Hungary, Ireland, Italy, Latvia, Lithuania, Luxembourg, Malta, Poland, Portugal, Slovakia, Slovenia, Spain, Sweden, the Netherlands, and the United Kingdom).

Such campaigns have primarily involved the distribution of printed materials by travel agents, in airports, through visa and passport offices, and at other travel-exit points. Most of these campaigns have received government financial support. The message was spread in some countries, such as Australia and New Zealand, through television and radio advertisements as well as poster, postcard, and luggage-sticker campaigns (**Figures 43-2-a** and **b**).

Although all of these awareness campaigns against child sex tourism are quite different in style, their messages remain universal:

— Children should not be sexually exploited anywhere.

— Laws exist that protect children from being sexually exploited in tourism.

— Any concerns should be reported to the authorities.

In Italy, the tourism industry is required by law to notify travelers of the child sex tourism law. Some European airlines have joined the campaign and are screening an in-flight video on flights to child sex tourism destinations that informs passengers of

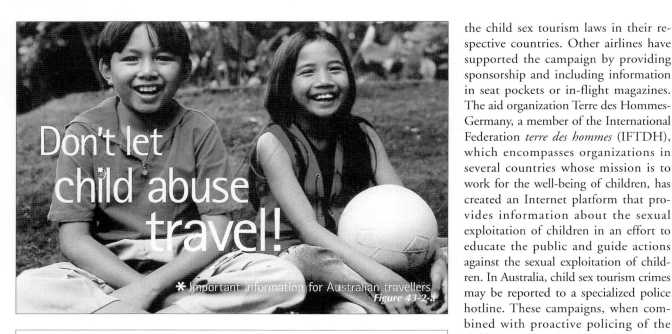

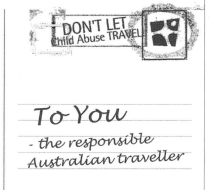

Dear Traveller

Australians are renowned for their love of travel. Sadly there are some Australians who travel overseas to sexually exploit children.

To protect children overseas, Australia has enacted The Crimes (Child Sex Tourism) Amendment Act 1994. It is a crime for Australians to engage in or benefit from sexual activity with children (under 16 years of age) whilst overseas. This law carries penalties of up to 17 years imprisonment, and up to $561,000 in fines for companies. The Australian Federal Police are actively monitoring and prosecuting child sex tourists. Convictions are resulting in significant gaol sentences.

Report concerns of any Australian/s sexually exploiting children overseas to the Australian Federal Police **1800 813 784** www.afp.gov.au

Join the global campaign against child abuse. For more information or donations contact **Child Wise™ (ECPAT in Australia) - 1800 991 099 or www.childwise.net**
This project has been funded by the National Crime Prevention Program, Australian Government Attorney-General's Department

To You
- the responsible
Australian traveller

Figure 43-2-b

Figures 43-2-a and b. *Postcard campaign from Child Wise geared toward Australian travelers. Reprinted with permission from Child Wise.*

the child sex tourism laws in their respective countries. Other airlines have supported the campaign by providing sponsorship and including information in seat pockets or in-flight magazines. The aid organization Terre des Hommes-Germany, a member of the International Federation *terre des hommes* (IFTDH), which encompasses organizations in several countries whose mission is to work for the well-being of children, has created an Internet platform that provides information about the sexual exploitation of children in an effort to educate the public and guide actions against the sexual exploitation of children. In Australia, child sex tourism crimes may be reported to a specialized police hotline. These campaigns, when combined with proactive policing of the child sex tourism legislation, have led to a significant number of prosecutions under the child sex tourism law in sending countries.

TOURISM CAMPAIGNS IN DESTINATION COUNTRIES

Tourism destinations in which child sex tourism has become a problem have been running campaigns to deter and identify child sex tourists. This is becoming an increasing trend as government officials and the local tourism industry organizations have begun to recognize the problem or acknowledge that they are potentially at risk of becoming a child sex tourist destination.

In addition to the enactment and enforcement of child protection legislation, GOs have been sending out strong messages to child sex tourists. For example, the National Tourism Administration in Brazil (ie, Embratur) ran a highly visible poster campaign with the slogan: "Beware, Brazil is watching you." This poster campaign included a police hotline telephone number, which was printed on hotels' "do not disturb" signs. In another example, the Cambodian Ministry of Tourism produced a small travelers guide book that promotes Cambodia's child protection laws. Sri Lanka, Vietnam, Mexico, the Philippines, Kenya, and the Dominican Republic have run similar awareness campaigns targeting tourists. A number of locations around the globe have taken further action, such as those listed in **Table 43-1**.

OTHER TOURISM INCENTIVES

CHILD WISE TOURISM

Since the late 1990s, Child Wise (the Australian representative of ECPAT International) has delivered the innovative Child Wise Tourism program across Southeast Asia (**Figures 43-3-a** and **b**). Child Wise Tourism is a training and net-

Table 43-1. Global Actions Against Child Sex Tourism
— In Thailand, any minor who enters a first-class hotel must now register.
— In Taiwan, hotels provide intensive education programs about child sex tourism to their employees and prohibit children who are younger than 18 years old to visit hotel rooms.
— In the Philippines, notices are provided in hotel rooms informing guests that child prostitution is illegal.
— In Brazil, by-laws have been enacted prohibiting minors in hotels and taxis without parental consent.
— In the Dominican Republic, a code of conduct has been developed for tourism workers.
— In Samoa, the Police Minister sent out a global press release after the successful prosecution of an Australian child sex tourist who had visited Samoa; this press release warned pedophiles not to visit Samoa and that if they did, they would be treated harshly.
— In Asia, the Accor Hotel Group partnered with the region's ECPAT groups to begin training their staff members to protect children and respond to child abuse and sexual exploitation situations.

work development program that seeks to build partnerships among government agencies, nongovernment agencies, and the tourism industry in order to protect children from sexual abuse. In an effort to help prevent child abuse, this program especially focused on training people in Southeast Asian countries (Brunei, Cambodia, Indonesia, Laos, Malaysia, Burma, the Philippines, Singapore, Thailand, and Vietnam) who work on tourism's front line (hotel staff members, tourism managers, tourist police officers, tourism trainers, trainers in tourism institutions, and others in the tourism industry). Child Wise Tourism also hosts the Association of Southeast Asian Nations (ASEAN) Regional Think Tank. This Think Tank provides organized venues for communication among government national tourism authorities, travel industry representatives, and child protection agency officials for the purpose of developing and strengthening working relationships and stressing the reality of a need to prevent child sex tourism. In addition, the ASEAN Think Tank has recommended future regional actions such as an ASEAN regional, educational campaign against child sex tourism and the promotion of an ASEAN Travellers Code. This Travellers Code would encourage travelers to do the following:

— Help prevent the abuse and exploitation of people, since everyone has the right to be protected from exploitation and abuse

— Consider people's human rights, especially those of women and children

— Consider the activities they undertake and the businesses they support while traveling

THE CODE OF CONDUCT FOR THE PROTECTION OF CHILDREN FROM SEXUAL EXPLOITATION IN TRAVEL AND TOURISM

The Code of Conduct was developed by ECPAT Sweden along with Nordic tour operators and was written for the activities provided by these tour operators with respect to combating commercial sexual exploitation of children. This Code of Conduct project has been adopted by ECPAT groups in Germany, Italy, the United Kingdom, the Netherlands, and Austria. Presently, the Code of Conduct is designed

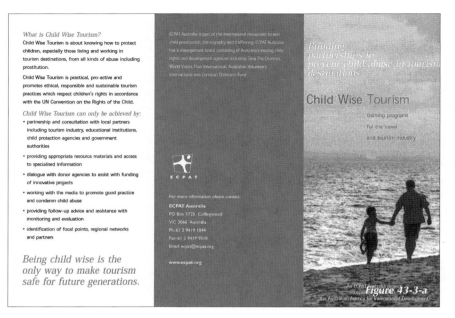

What is Child Wise Tourism?
Child Wise Tourism is about knowing how to protect children, especially those living and working in tourism destinations, from all kinds of abuse including prostitution.

Child Wise Tourism is practical, pro-active and promotes ethical, responsible and sustainable tourism practices which respect children's rights in accordance with the UN Convention on the Rights of the Child.

Child Wise Tourism can only be achieved by:
• partnership and consultation with local partners including tourism industry, educational institutions, child protection agencies and government authorities
• providing appropriate resource materials and access to specialised information
• dialogue with donor agencies to assist with funding of innovative projects
• working with the media to promote good practice and condemn child abuse
• providing follow-up advice and assistance with monitoring and evaluation
• identification of focal points, regional networks and partners

Being child wise is the only way to make tourism safe for future generations.

ECPAT Australia is part of the international movement to end child prostitution, pornography and trafficking. ECPAT Australia has a management board consisting of Australia's leading child rights and development agencies including Save The Children, World Vision, Plan International, Australian Volunteers International and Christian Children's Fund.

Building partnerships to prevent child abuse in tourism destinations

Child Wise Tourism

training programs
for the travel
and tourism industry

For more information please contact:
ECPAT Australia
PO Box 1725 Collingwood
VIC 3066 Australia
Ph 61 3 9419 1844
Fax 61 3 9419 9518
Email: ecpat@ecpat.org

www.ecpat.org

An ECPAT Australia project supported by the Australian Agency for International Development

Figure 43-3-a

Child prostitution and child sex tourism
The prostitution of children in tourism destinations, commonly called child sex tourism, is definitely a tourism industry issue. We know that tourism is not the cause of child exploitation but it does provide potential abusers the anonymity and the environment to seek out vulnerable children. The abusers are not always tourists, they can be business travellers or expatriates. Local people are often involved.

Child sex tourism is a phenomenon that affects children all over the world. The prostitution and exploitation of children is internationally condemned and should not be tolerated under any circumstance.

Can the travel and tourism industry help?
The problem for most hotels, tour guides, travel agencies and airlines is that they do not have the specialist knowledge to deal appropriately with child sex tourism. They think it wont involve their clients or staff and they become reluctant to interfere.

ECPAT believes that all travel and hospitality businesses should know about child sex tourism and what to do about it. The tourism industry can help to put an end to child sex tourism.

Child Wise Tourism Training is a training program that provides information and teacher training on the prevention of child sex tourism. It provides information on policy development and practical guidelines.
It connects the tourism industry to community based organisations to promote corporate-community partnerships in combating child sex tourism.
It recognises that information materials alone are not sufficient to develop sustainable training programs. The issue of child sex tourism is so sensitive in some communities that it requires a process of consultation and the nurturing of support from key industry bodies and government authorities.

The Child Wise Tourism concept recognises the importance of :
• a 'working together' approach
• promotion of good practice models
• the development of specialist knowledge

In 1999 ECPAT Australia worked together with the travel industry and travel educators in Thailand and Vietnam to pilot the Child Wise Tourism training concept in Asia. This pilot was supported and endorsed by PATA (the Pacific Asia Travel Association)

Background
ECPAT Australia has worked closely with the tourism industry forging successful links with local and regional partners. ECPAT Australia has produced resources which have been used extensively by the tourism industry and for tourism training.

Great progress has also been made at an international level with ECPAT developing close working relationships with the world tourism bodies. These developments include declarations by:
• the World Tourism Organisation
• The Universal Federation of Travel Agents Associations (UFTAA)
• The International Air Transport Association (IATA)
• The International Hotels & Restaurant Association (IHRA)
• The International Federation of Womens Travel Organisations (IFWTO)

In 1995 ECPAT Australia was awarded the Australian Federation of Travel Agents award for the most significant contribution to the travel industry.

In 1996 ECPAT Australia was successful in encouraging the Australian Federation of Travel Agents (AFTA) to include condemnation of child sex tourism in their industry code of ethics.

In 1996 ECPAT Australia won the Australian Human Rights Commission - Human Rights Award

In 1999 ECPAT Australia won the Australian Council for Overseas Aid - Human Rights Award

Figure 43-3-b

Child Wise Tourism

Figures 42-3-a and b. *Brochure from the Child Wise Tourism program.* Reprinted with permission from Child Wise.

to raise awareness of child sex tourism among European tour operators, their local partners in tourist destinations, and travelers. Based on the United Nation's (UN's) Declaration of Human Rights and the UN Convention on the Rights of the Child and with an emphasis on Article 34, the Code of Conduct is included in the follow-up work of the World Congress' Agenda for Action, which was held in Stockholm in August 1996.

Socially responsible travel and tourism companies that sign onto the Code of Conduct agree to incorporate the following 6 practices into their operations:

1. Establish an ethical corporate policy against the sexual exploitation of children.

2. Provide information to travelers by means of catalogues, brochures, Web sites, posters, in-flight films, ticket slips, home pages, and so on, as appropriate.

3. Educate and train personnel in the country of origin and travel destinations.

4. Introduce a clause in contracts with suppliers that makes a common repudiation of sexual exploitation of children.

5. Provide information to local official "key persons" at the destination.

6. Report annually on the implementation of these criteria.

That a tour operator adopts the Code of Conduct against commercial sexual exploitation of children does not mean the tour operator guarantees that sexual exploitation does not occur at the operator's travel destination. Rather, this Code of Conduct states the tour operator's awareness of the problem and indicates that the tour operator will take active measures to prevent the child sex trade. Coordination with similar measures on an ethical level is also important.

THE YOUTH CAREER INITIATIVE
The Youth Career Initiative was launched by Pan Pacific Hotels and supported by the International Hotel & Restaurant Association (IH&RA) and the United Nations Children's Fund (UNICEF). Thailand became one of the first countries to provide opportunities in tourism for young people between the ages of 17 and 19 years of age from the poorer and rural provinces. The project includes a basic introductory course to the hospitality industry that is aimed at empowering young people who are considered at risk specifically for sexual abuse to make choices about their future and the opportunity to enter the workforce in the tourism industry. A large percentage of class time is spent teaching these young people life skills.

CONCLUSION

The sexual exploitation of children in prostitution and sex tourism was almost a hidden phenomenon in 1990. While the world remained blissfully ignorant, hundreds of thousands of young girls and boys, mainly from poor communities, were being traded, trafficked, and sold into sexual slavery. For most of these children, prostitution was a death sentence because of the high rate of human immuno-deficiency virus (HIV) and/or acquired immunodeficiency syndrome (AIDS) among prostitutes. This age-old but rapidly growing form of child abuse through sexual exploitation went largely ignored and denied by members of the government and communities. At that time, few third world countries had laws prohibiting the sale and sexual exploitation of children, and most law enforcement agencies profited from the trade and turned a blind eye to child traffickers and abusers. Preventive programs and services did not largely exist to help rescue the child victims of sexual exploitation. Throughout the 1980s, the child sex trade reached epidemic proportions in many parts of the world.

Since 1990, significant efforts have been made to protect children from sexual exploitation at every level of society and everywhere. The international ECPAT campaign has been instrumental in bringing about these social and political changes by building a global movement dedicated to combating the commercial sexual exploitation of children.

ECPAT has raised international awareness of the problem and motivated hundreds of thousands of people in every region of the world to join its campaign to protect children from sexual exploitation. Government organizations in rich and poor countries alike have listened to the ECPAT message and been encouraged to implement laws, policies, and practices that have led to the better protection of children. Now law enforcement officials actively enforce international child sexual statutes, and traffickers and offenders are being successfully prosecuted in increasing numbers; both of these actions send a strong message that children have a right to be protected from sexual exploitation. The international travel and tourism sector continues to educate and encourage its members and travelers to take action. The travel industry's partnership with ECPAT has been one of the most innovative and effective programs in the campaign against child sex tourism.

Despite these great efforts, the child sex trade continues to flourish, expand into new areas, and develop into new forms. The resilience of the child sex trade clearly demonstrates its deep and ancient roots as well as its interconnectedness to inequality and poverty. Emerging trends, such as the promotion of child sexual exploitation via the Internet, have facilitated a further growth in demand for child sexual abuse. No easy solution exists to such a complex problem. Multiple factors contribute to the existence of the child sex trade. These factors require wide-ranging and sustainable interventions to tackle the root causes that render children and their communities vulnerable to exploitation. Although ECPAT paved the way, government organizations, members of the tourism industry, and community groups everywhere must intensify their efforts and give far more attention to the prevention of child sexual exploitation and the promotion of children's rights.

Internet Hotlines and the History of INHOPE: The Association of Internet Hotline Providers

Cormac Callanan, BA, MSc
Thomas Rickert

Worldwide, the Association of Internet Hotline Providers in Europe (INHOPE) (http://www.inhope.org) coordinates Internet-related hotlines that are an essential element of a coordinated response to the illegal and harmful use of the Internet. Its mission is to eliminate child pornography from the Internet and protect young people from harmful and illegal uses of the Internet. INHOPE advocates shared responsibility for this protection by government, educators, parents, and the Internet industry. INHOPE is partly funded by the European Union (EU) Safer Internet Action Plan, which supports the following 3 programs: hotlines, filtering and rating, and awareness. The Safer Internet Action Plan is a funding program established by the EU to encourage initiatives which improve online safety for adults and children. INHOPE was established by this program and continues to be partly funded under this program.

What is an INHOPE Hotline?

INHOPE hotlines receive complaints from the public about alleged illegal Internet content, use of the Internet, or both, and have effective, straightforward procedures for dealing with the reports. Individual INHOPE hotlines have the support of their national governments, the Internet industry, law enforcement officials, and Internet users in their countries. In addition, members of INHOPE cooperate with other members by exchanging information about illegal content, sharing their expertise, maintaining confidentiality, and respecting the procedures of other members.

Historical Background

The members of INHOPE know the Internet has had a positive effect on the lives of many people and, when used properly, is a wonderful tool. It is educational, informative, and an efficient and inexpensive method for communicating with friends and family worldwide. However, the Internet has negative aspects and can create harmful situations for children. Though some filtering software can prevent children and young people from viewing illegal and harmful material, it does not affect the accessibility of the information on the Internet. Measures need to be taken to stop the distribution of illegal material and identify the distributors. Identifying the distributors of child abuse material on the Internet is important because many of the victims featured in the pictures or movies are still being abused and could be removed from their dangerous situations if they were found.

By 1995, Internet users, the Internet industry, governments, and law enforcement agencies were aware that the Internet was being used by pedophiles to publish and exchange child pornography. Internet users who accidentally encountered this material often did not know whom to contact. INHOPE hotlines can be used as a single resource for a swift investigation by law enforcement officials of illegal Internet material and for quick, efficient removal of the material. Hotlines promote international collaboration among the various members of INHOPE.

Between 1995 and 1999, various national initiatives were launched to prevent illegal Internet activities, especially the abuse of children on the Internet. In Germany, numerous separate initiatives were first discussed in 1995 and 1996 during the proceedings of several high-profile court cases and parliamentary debates. With the support of the police, in 1996, the first Internet child pornography hotline was established in the Netherlands by concerned Internet users and individuals in the Internet industry. Hotline initiatives were developed in Norway, Belgium, and the United Kingdom before the end of 1996.

Other countries began to become involved, and plans for hotlines were finalized in Austria, Ireland, Finland, Spain, and France. The issue was extensively debated in other European countries as well. In 1998, the National Center for Missing & Exploited Children launched its CyberTipline, which quickly became established as one of the busiest hotlines for illegal Internet material.

The INHOPE Forum was created in 1998, allowing hotlines from various nations to meet and discuss common issues of concern. Following this, 8 hotlines joined forces to create the INHOPE Association. The organization meets regularly to share knowledge and discuss best practices in the operation of Internet hotlines. In 2004, INHOPE had 20 hotlines in 18 countries, and other countries were in the process of becoming members (**Table 44-1**).

From the beginning, INHOPE has managed to bring together different individuals at national and international levels and has forged trust and respect among those with whom it interacts. The professionalism and dedication demonstrated by the members of INHOPE will continue to make INHOPE even more successful in the future.

HOW DO INHOPE HOTLINES OPERATE?

When an INHOPE hotline receives a report, the information is logged into the hotline database system. Reports are usually received from users who complete a form on the hotline Web site. Sometimes people send reports by e-mail, fax, letter, or telephone. If the report has not been submitted anonymously, a confirmation of receipt is sent to the reporter. Hotline staff members, who are specially trained in assessing Internet content, determine whether the reported material is illegal according to local legislation (though the material may not have originated in that country). If the material is legal, the report process is complete. However, even if deemed legal, the hotline staff members may forward the report to a partner hotline.

If the reported material could be illegal according to the local legislation of the hotline, the hotline staff members begin an investigation to identify the origin of the material. This is a time-consuming process that requires technical expertise. Web site addresses can provide important information but can be misleading. Addresses are composed of ***domain names***, single words or initials that are combined to create a unique name. For example, Web addresses with ".de" are allocated by the German domain name registry and in the past might have suggested a Web site located in Germany. However, regardless of the domain name, such a Web site can be located anywhere in the world. Indeed, often these registrations contain false information as is the case with most ".com" addresses since checking of registrations is performed only in a small number of domain name registries.

Table 44-1. INHOPE Members

Country	Membership Status	Organization Name	Web Site Address	Membership Date
Australia	Full	Australian Broadcasting Authority (ABA)	http://www.au.inhope.org	1999
Austria	Full	Stopline	http://www.at.inhope.org	1999
Belgium	Full	Child Focus	http://www.be.inhope.org	2001
Denmark	Full	Red Barnet	http://www.dk.inhope.org	2002
Finland	Full	Save the Children (STC) Finland	http://www.fi.inhope.org	2002
France	Full	Association des Fournisseurs d'Accès et de Services Internet (AFA), or Internet Service Providers Association	http://www.fr.inhope.org	1999
Germany	Full	ECO	http://www.de.inhope.org	1999
Germany	Full	Freiwillige Selbstkontrolle Multimedia-Dienstanbieter (FSM), or Voluntary Self-Control for Multimedia Service Providers	http://www.de.inhope.org	1999
Germany	Full	jugendschutz.net	http://www.de.inhope.org	1999
Greece	Provisional	Safeline	http://www.gr.inhope.org	2004
Iceland	Full	Barnaheill	http://www.is.inhope.org	2001
Ireland	Full	Internet Service Providers Association of Ireland (ISPAI)	http://www.ie.inhope.org	1999
Italy	Full	STC Italy	http://www.it.inhope.org	2003
Netherlands	Full	Meldpunt	http://www.nl.inhope.org	1999
South Korea	Associate	Information Communication Ethics Committee (ICEC)	http://www.kr.inhope.org	2003
Spain	Full	Protegeles	http://www.es.inhope.org	2002
Sweden	Full	STC Sweden	http://www.se.inhope.org	2002
Taiwan	Provisional	End Child Prostitution, Child Pornography and Trafficking of Children for Sexual Purposes (ECPAT) Taiwan	http://www.tw.inhope.org	2004
United Kingdom	Full	Internet Watch Foundation	http://www.uk.inhope.org	1999
United States	Full	CyberTipline	http://www.us.inhope.org	1999

Available at: http://www.inhope.org/en/about/members.html. Accessed October 21, 2004.

A domain name can be used to refer to any Web server anywhere in the world. The domain name is converted into an ***Internet protocol (IP) address***. This address is used by a computer to establish an Internet connection with a ***Web server***, which has an actual physical location. However, a Web Server can have content that is hosted from many parts of the world and all the IP numbers must be traced by the hotline to determine where the Web server and content are located.

If hotline staff members find that the reported material is being hosted on a local server, they involve local law enforcement officials, the relevant Internet Service Provider (ISP), or both. If the material is located on a server in a foreign country, matters become more complicated. In most cases, the individual hotlines do not cooperate directly with foreign organizations, except those that are hotlines and direct members of INHOPE. When a global medium such as the Internet is involved, the hotline activity should not stop at national borders; therefore, the INHOPE hotline forwards the report to the hotline in the country with the originating Web server. If the country does not have an INHOPE hotline, INHOPE responds to the material by cooperating with a range of supranational organizations such as the United Nations, the Council of Europe, Interpol, Europol, the Organisation for Economic Co-operation and Development (OECD), the Organization for Security and Co-operation in Europe (OSCE), the G8, and a range of nongovernmental organizations (NGOs).

The decision to initiate a criminal investigation is made by law enforcement officials. The ISP is responsible for timely removal of the content from their servers to ensure that other Internet users can not access the material. After the hotline has notified law enforcement and the ISP, the case can be closed.

INHOPE ACTIVITIES

WORKING GROUPS
In January 2002, INHOPE established working groups that addressed Internet content, the INHOPE Code of Practice, statistics, awareness and visibility, and membership fees. Each group has a chairperson and rapporteur. Some hotlines also exchange information on a one-on-one basis with other hotlines about methods of sharing technology, processes, procedures, and results of hotline reports.

BEST PRACTICE PAPERS
The INHOPE Code of Practice was adopted in May 2003 and is available on the INHOPE Web site (http://www.inhope.org/doc/inhope_cop.pdf). However, guidelines for INHOPE can be found in the Best Practice Papers, which cover specific areas of hotline activity in-depth. The following Best Practice Papers have been developed:

— Staff Welfare

— Exchange of Reports

— Membership Application Form/Completion Form

— ART-1 and ART-2 Principles for the Operation of a Hotline (ART-1 stands for "Availability, Reliability, Transparency" and ART-2 stands for "Accountable, Responsible, Trustworthy")

— Common Statistics Format

Continually improving its practices, INHOPE has ongoing discussions on raising awareness and improving hotline visibility, self-assessment of hotlines, and handling reports about peer-to-peer activities on the Internet.

INTERACTIONS WITH LAW ENFORCEMENT OFFICIALS
INHOPE uses the acronym REACT to describe the benefits of its network of hotlines: **R**eport-receiving mechanisms, **E**xpertise, **A**ccleration, **C**ontacts, and **T**rends. INHOPE reacts to reports that are received about alleged illegal content on the

Internet, whereas law enforcement agencies are entitled to take a proactive approach investigating content and pursuing perpetrators, so the roles of hotlines and law enforcement agencies are complementary.

Report-Receiving Mechanisms

Some may wonder why hotlines are needed when Internet users can notify law enforcement agencies directly about any illegal material they encounter. INHOPE members know that law enforcement agencies operate their own hotlines in many countries, and INHOPE hopes to serve as an alternative resource. In addition, some citizens in Germany (and other countries) who reported illegal content to non-INHOPE official hotlines—especially child pornography—became the subject of police investigations or prosecution. Individuals are not at risk when they report to INHOPE, which could be one reason that the hotlines are so successful. However, INHOPE does not encourage individuals to act as "cyber vigilantes." INHOPE members warn individuals who submit reports frequently that they should not actively search for illegal material.

Because hotline staff members examine the material reported and do not forward to the police the reports about obviously legal material or general questions (eg, regarding filtering software), they save valuable time for law enforcement agencies. The time-consuming and difficult procedure of tracking and tracing of illegal material is carried out by INHOPE and may not have to be pursued by the police.

Expertise

INHOPE members have at their disposal the knowledge of experts on technological, legal, child protection, and psychological issues. Therefore, hotline representatives are frequently asked to participate in training seminars or deliver national and international lectures. Numerous people in the INHOPE network train law enforcement agencies how to track and trace illegal material on the Internet. Though a growing number of specially trained and equipped police units are being developed, if requested, INHOPE members educate law enforcement officials about their experiences and approaches.

Acceleration

INHOPE hotline staff members examine whether reported material is illegal, and they trace its apparent origin. The term *apparent origin* is used because the geographical origin can not be unambiguously determined in every case. If an INHOPE hotline exists in the country of origin, the report is forwarded to the country's hotline, which makes the process progress more quickly than it would otherwise. For example, reports that were received in Germany were forwarded to the US Cyber-Tipline, and the child pornographic material was removed from the Internet in fewer than 48 hours. In cases such as this, criminal investigations are performed and evidence is preserved before the material is removed.

Contacts

INHOPE members have excellent contacts, including Internet users and individuals in the government, law enforcement agencies, and the Internet industry. Formal and informal arrangements of cooperation are in place to tackle the encountered issues. Therefore, reports being made to people in a foreign country are handled by people in that country, which is more effective in many cases.

Trends

INHOPE hotlines serve as indicators of criminal trends. Underground criminal activity is a major problem for law enforcement all over the world since it is difficult to identify such activities and trends so appropriate resources can be available when required. Therefore, when forwarding reports and identifying trends, INHOPE can help police forces organize their resources.

Workload of the Member Hotlines

The members of INHOPE are receiving an increasing number of reports as the exposure of the hotlines increases. Hotline staff members are often asked questions by government members, Internet users, and journalists regarding their workload, the numbers of reports received and investigations completed, the type and source of illegal material being reported, and the number of convictions resulting from hotline activity. Such questions can not easily be answered.

INHOPE detailed statistics are confidential and only available to members of INHOPE. Currently, it would be inappropriate to release the INHOPE collated statistics because the information that has been collected does not reflect accurately the breadth and depth of activity of the membership hotlines and because reporting on trends about criminal activity on the Internet particularly in such an important area as child abuse requires extra caution and sensitivity. However, summary trends and statistics are published regularly on the INHOPE Web site and detailed hotline activities are often available from the individual hotline Web sites. A template to provide a reasonable summary of the workload and results of the association has been developed, and the version is now in regular use. The statistics are primarily being assessed to meet the needs of INHOPE. However, INHOPE does know that its work has generated substantial interest among a wide range of groups, including among governmental organizations and NGOs.

Statistics can be helpful, but aggregated statistics do not necessarily reflect the true picture of each individual hotline. INHOPE's experience is that the majority of child pornography content is not hosted in Europe. However, because one INHOPE hotline is receiving numerous reports of alleged illegal material in newsgroups that are relayed by German providers, that hotline considers those reports as being hosted in Germany.

Statistics Reference Period

The statistical results include information from March 2003 to February 2004. During this period, more than 272 000 reports were received by the INHOPE network, with more than 35% involving child pornography and more than 50% of the total reports referring to Web sites. Statistics from all members are included. Because INHOPE is growing, the number of statistics is increasing.

Analysis of Trends

An analysis of trends can be done on a purely empirical basis because figures do not permit a strict statistical approach. Discussions during INHOPE meetings have revealed that hotline staff members have noticed the following:

— A growing number of reports about child pornography *spam*, or e-mails received by consumers without their consent

— Many reports of Web sites *apparently* hosted in Russia

— A growing number of reports about child pornography hosted in a specific European country on the server of a specific hosting provider; the INHOPE network helped this hotline encourage the hosting provider to take appropriate measures which reduced the amount of child pornography being distributed through that server

— A growing number of reports about rape-related material

— Closer cooperation of INHOPE members with their local police forces

Numerous reports are sent to police because much of the reported material is hosted in countries with no INHOPE hotline. The material is normally reported to the local police in the country of the receiving hotline. Reporting would be more efficient if the INHOPE network were extended.

The total number of reports is higher than the total number of actions taken because no action is taken on reports of material that hotline staff members assess to be legal. Some hotlines can not yet count reports for which no action has been taken. In addition, this statistic is complicated because one report can lead to numerous actions (eg, transmission to police, transmission to the ISP).

SUCCESS STORIES

OPERATION MARCY

In September 2003, the German police in the eastern state of Saxony-Anhalt and prosecutors in the city of Halle exposed one of the largest child pornography networks in the world—one that involved 26 500 Internet users in 166 countries. The Operation Marcy investigation, which took more than a year, was launched after a tip was received at the INHOPE member hotline in Spain. The tip was sent to the German hotline, FSM, which transferred it to another German hotline member—ECO's Internet Content Task Force hotline. The tip was finally sent to the German federal police (BKA), which in Spring 2002 was able to launch an investigation.

The suspects were traced using computer files seized from a man in Magdeburg, Germany. The files contained a huge e-mail distribution list used by suspected pedophiles to exchange pornographic images of children, some as young as 4 months of age. In Germany alone, Operation Marcy involved some 1500 police officers, hundreds of raids, and the seizure of 745 computers and more than 35 500 CDs, 8300 floppy disks, and 5800 videos.

OPERATION HAMLET

In 2002, a member of the public made a child pornography report to the Swedish INHOPE hotline. When the report was processed and the images were reviewed, the hotline staff members recognized a logo on a t-shirt worn by the possible perpetrator. The logo led them to believe the perpetrator was in Denmark, so the report was forwarded to the Danish INHOPE hotline and Danish police for additional investigation.

As a result of a swift investigation, Operation Hamlet, the pedophile was arrested and the victim was rescued and taken out of the abusive situation. A follow-up joint investigation by the US Customs Service and the Danish police further identified a ring of pedophiles who molested their own children and distributed the images on the Internet; the perpetrator was a member.

By March 2003, Operation Hamlet had resulted in the issuance of 16 US search warrants, 19 arrests in the United States, 12 arrests in other countries, and more than 100 children being rescued and removed from abusive situations.

SPAIN

As a result of trend analyses by the INHOPE network, INHOPE found that a large volume of child pornography was being distributed from servers located in Spain. The trend was discussed and debated at the INHOPE meeting in Cambridge, England, in September 2002. After the meeting, staff members from Spain's hotline, Protegeles, held several meetings with the director of security from the relevant ISP. The director was grateful for the feedback from INHOPE and held several internal meetings to develop an action plan. (The majority of the Web sites hosted by the ISP consisted of completely legal material.)

Later, the ISP's director of security informed Protegeles of the steps being taken by the company to combat the problems. The ISP had immediately blocked its 300 000 personal pages, making it immediately and temporarily impossible to place any additional material online. The ISP manually reviewed the contents of all its publicly accessible personal pages and identified and reported those with illegal content.

The ISP has instituted procedures that require users to transfer a symbolic amount of money to the ISP (approximately 10 Euros each year) to acquire a personal Web site.

Following the suggestions of the Spanish hotline, all users who want to create a personal page must provide a valid e-mail address to receive the password that allows them to create the page. The ISP began measuring the bandwidth of personal pages to detect those with significant amounts of photographic content. In addition, the ISP no longer permits entrance from foreign *proxies* (ie, intermediaries between a user and the Internet). An internal hotline has been created at the ISP which is directly linked to Protegeles. Protegeles has access to all of the reports received, processes all of them, and sends them to the police when appropriate. New personnel have been hired to work on these issues, and they have weekly meetings with the company's directors. As predicted by INHOPE, the number of reports about material located on this particular Spanish ISP's servers decreased by over 90%.

SHADOW CHILDREN: ADDRESSING THE COMMERCIAL EXPLOITATION OF CHILDREN IN RURAL AMERICA

Victor I. Vieth, JD
Erika Rivera Ragland, JD

INTRODUCTION

A number of scholars suggest there may be between 100 000 to 300 000 children "at risk" of or who are in fact being commercially exploited in cities and towns across the United States (Clayton, 1996; Estes & Weiner, 2001; Robinson, 1997). The US Department of Justice Office of Juvenile Justice and Delinquency Prevention (OJJDP) estimated that in 1999, 1 190 000 (or 71%) of the runaway and/or thrown-away youth could have been endangered during their runaway and/or thrownaway episode because of factors including physical and sexual abuse (Hammer et al, 2002). The General Accounting Office of the United States estimates that these numbers may even be higher and reach into the 600 000s (Children of the Night, 2004). On average, each child can be expected to "service" between 4 and 10 customers a day (University of Pennsylvania, 2001). These numbers roughly translate into approximately 1460 and 3650 sexual victimizations each year per child victim. Yet, even in the face of these alarming statistics, the commercial exploitation of children continues to exist largely unnoticed by policy makers, law enforcement officials, and ordinary citizens alike, despite its persistent presence in cities and towns across the nation. This is particularly true in rural communities in the United States, which supply a significant percentage of this nation's commercially exploited children.

The language used to discuss the problem likely contributes to its lingering presence. For instance, the word "prostitute" dilutes the brutality of the victimization experienced by these child victims and serves only to criminalize the desperation that leads children to sell their bodies on the street. Further, the word "prostitute" distracts from the reality that is the prostitution of children by calling forth popular media images from the film *Pretty Woman* or the character of the "good-natured whore." In 1976, James wrote that "[t]he desire for a higher income and an independent, exciting lifestyle are the major motivating factors for most prostitutes" and "[p]rostitution is a victimless crime—a crime without a complaint, in which, typically, all those involved are willing participants." Though these sentiments date back to the 1970s, the belief persists among the public that prostitution is a "chosen" profession, a fact that is evidenced by the way law enforcement officials continue to criminalize prostitutes instead of treating the problem via social means, that is, by providing access to services for prostitutes to escape the streets and/or by focusing on more aggressively prosecuting the customers, called *johns*.

In reality, child prostitution, like all prostitution, is the commodification of the body of a human being; it is a type of sexual exploitation. Estes & Weiner (2001) defined sexual exploitation as "[a] practice by which a person achieves sexual gratification, financial gain or advancement through the abuse or exploitation of a person's sexuality by abrogating that person's human right to dignity, equality, autonomy, and physical and mental well-being." In addition, because of children's inherent vulnerability—in terms of their physical stature, development, and emotional immaturity—the commercial exploitation of children is particularly violent, cruel, and ugly.

Estes finds that "child sexual exploitation is the most hidden form of child abuse in the United States and North America today" (University of Pennsylvania, 2001). Thus, in light of a thoughtful definition of the problem and the staggering figures, commercial exploitation of boys and girls is an issue of child abuse and protection rather than a victimless crime as some people believe.

This chapter provides an overview of this crime as well as some specific examples illustrating the grave difficulties that the commercial exploitation of children present. This chapter especially focuses on the recruitment of children from small towns and rural communities and discusses recommendations for addressing this aspect of the problem.

A Harsh Existence: Who Are the Commercially Exploited Children?

Commercially exploited children are not who people might expect them to be. In fact, there is no typical profile of a prostituted child. What is known from research and studies of these populations is that these minors are usually teenagers (Clayton, 1996; Flowers, 1998); they originate from cities, towns, and rural communities; and they come in all races, sizes, shapes, and socioeconomic classes (Flowers, 1998). Surprisingly, a large number of them come from middle-class homes and backgrounds (Estes & Weiner, 2001; Seng, 1989).

Regarding the gender breakdown, it is generally believed by experts that there are more female prostituted children than male prostituted children (Flowers, 1998). However, records from 1995 show roughly equal numbers of male and female prostitution arrests (Flowers, 1998).

Unlike their foreign counterparts in third-world countries who are forced into prostitution via kidnapping, sold into the illegal sex trade (Todres, 1999), or turn to prostitution out of poverty-stricken desperation (Reaves, 1993), American children are often fleeing seemingly normal lives in middle-class homes in an effort to escape their abusive home environments (Flowers, 1998; Whitcomb et al, 1998). Children run away for various reasons, including drug addiction, loneliness, and delinquency. These abusive environments include mental, physical, sexual, and/or domestic abuse (Flowers, 1998).

According to the US Department of Justice, there are more than 1 million runaway and thrownaway youth on the nation's streets at any given time, with more than one third leaving home because of sexual abuse (Paul & Lisa Program, 2004). The implication from these findings indicates that these children are so desperate to make a break from their terrible home situations that living on the street begins to emerge as a viable option.

Survival Sex

A national study determined that living on the streets for longer than 30 days is the single greatest predictor of whether a teenager will turn to prostitution (Hofstede Committee Report, 1999). Once on the street, runaways quickly find themselves without money, food, or shelter; they hang out in bus depots, arcades, or malls; and they possibly panhandle to gain enough money to buy dinner and a place to stay for the night. These typical hangouts turn out to be prime locations for would-be pimps waiting to spot a new target who will make them money. Without a home, these children find themselves immersed in a world of opportunistic predators, thrownaway children, and drug addicts.

Thrownaway children are those who are forced out of their homes. According to Flowers (1998), they are "typically suburban youths who involuntarily leave home due to family financial problems, incorrigibility, sexual identity issues, promiscuity, drug abuse, and/or parent-child disagreements," including abuse. Thus, because these children are essentially abandoned by their families, they are often not reported missing.

Another group of maltreated children that often escapes detection by the authorities is the relatively small percentage of children who are abducted or forced into prostitution by their own parents. On January 16, 2003, a *New York Times* article reported that the Detroit police broke up a Midwestern sex ring that abducted "girls from the streets, kept them captive, and coerced them to peddle jewelry and sex" (Teenage prostitution ring).

For newly homeless girls, including runaways and thrownaways, a typical initiation into prostitution via the pimp presents itself like this: the pimp approaches the teenager and seduces her with promises of love, friendship, care and/or food, shelter, or drugs (Flowers, 1998). The pimps might impress the girls with stylish clothing, cars, or other material goods. Sadly, for many of these vulnerable teenagers from dysfunctional homes, it is the attention and affection that makes them feel special (Flowers, 1998) and ultimately draws them toward a would-be pimp. Sensing this, the pimp exploits this weakness once trust has been established and ultimately uses the "companionship" shown to the child against her, demanding services and/or repayment for the "kindness" and care. Other times, the exploiter skips these steps altogether and shows brutality from the outset. Yet, regardless of the particular methods employed, the miserable initiation into prostitution has begun.

"[T]here is an orientation where they are told, essentially, that your life as you know it is over, you are essentially owned by me. I'm your daddy," said Avery Friedman, a lawyer representing a 17-year-old victim (Teenage prostitution ring, 2003). This *New York Times* article also explained the process by which the pimp, in this case 32-year-old Henry Charles Davis, treated his victims. His house looked like a

classic pimp's lair, where girls were treated alternately with lavish generosity and raw violence. 'He would buy them clothes, he would give them money to get their hair done and nails done, they were fed very well, and as long as everyone complied, everything was OK,' but [Investigator Kimberly Kovacs of the Detroit police] added: '[e]verybody's scared. If they don't do what they have to do, they get violated, (Teenage prostitution ring, 2003).

Young prostituted males, on the other hand, are much less likely to have any involvement with a pimp (Whitcomb et al, 1998). This differing response to exploitation of males and females raises questions regarding gender socialization and male and/or female responses to victimization. Boys may have difficulty admitting their victimization and/or discussing it because of their perceived role in society as strong and invulnerable. In turn, prostituted males may have difficulties with psychologically processing the trauma they have experienced. Females, some believe, are usually more able to admit being victimized.

Although the research is unclear, some of the literature proposes that high numbers of young prostituted males—as opposed to young prostituted females, who are likely heterosexual—leave home because of conflicts in their families regarding sexual identity. According to Stronski Huwiler & Remafedi (1988), "[a]n estimated 70% of male prostitutes identify as homosexual," and

[a]fter disclosing their sexual orientation to parents, many homosexual adolescents experience rejection. Some parents are unable to adopt a supportive attitude, and a substantial number of gay adolescents run away or are evicted. Half of gay adolescents in a convenience sample had run away from home at least once, citing reasons of family and sexuality-related conflicts.

Some studies allege that these young men engage in prostitution for the sake of the sex, not the money. Seemingly specious at best, this claim instead likely reflects homophobia and gender socialization differences between males and females in terms of comfort level acknowledging and discussing victimization rather than a nuanced understanding of these male victim populations and their motivations for entering into prostitution.

Although some young, gay, male prostitutes claim to be selling their bodies for the sex itself, a close look at the statistics and reality of prostitution—the poverty, homelessness, drug use, and exposure to violence—undermines any credibility of this claim. Even if the prostitute is a drug addict who turns to prostitution to support that drug habit, it is likely that a review of the family history will yield evidence of family dysfunction and/or childhood victimization. According to Whitcomb et al (1998), approximately 50% to 80% of prostituted juveniles were victimized sexually or physically as children.

Thus, the situation is best described in Seng's (1989) words: "[A]dolescent prostitution can be viewed as behavior that results from the necessities of street life—it is survival behavior more than it is sexual behavior." Further, while

[m]ost teenage prostitutes enter the business as part-time prostitutes, usually hoping to earn a few quick bucks for food, cigarettes, drugs, shelter, or pocket money, for many, this part-time work quickly becomes a full-time profession. Studies indicate that the typical female teen prostitute will be turning tricks on a full-time basis within eight months to a year after her initial prostitution experience (Flowers, 1998).

THE HORRORS OF CHILD PROSTITUTION: BROKEN LIVES

So what exactly does a life of sexual exploitation hold in store for the average prostituted teenager? According to the Children of the Night (2004) organization, prostituted children can expect to become well acquainted with the physical dangers of living and working on the streets. This includes becoming familiar with all forms of violence, particularly sexual violence, with each child prostitute enduring an average of 1300 rapes per year. Many of these children are robbed, and some are murdered. Moreover, child and/or teenage prostitutes are not likely to be in a position to demand condom use, which means they risk exposure to and transmission of sexually transmitted diseases (STDs), such as chlamydia, syphilis, and human immunodeficiency virus (HIV) and/or acquired immunodeficiency syndrome (AIDS).

In addition to the risks imposed upon their bodies, their minds suffer psychological devastation from being forced to lay aside their personhood day after day so that their bodies can be used at will for someone else's sexual gratification. Keep in mind that the typical commercially exploited child has sexual contact with an average of 4 to 10 men per day (University of Pennsylvania, 2001). Given this data, it comes as no surprise that the psychological devastation manifests itself in the form of low self-esteem, self-destruction, mutilation, and/or suicidal tendencies, feelings that may behaviorally express themselves through drug use or addiction.

Finally, in terms of the sociological impact, prostituted children will likely experience an "inability to enter mainstream society, and ostracism" (Revaz, 2002). Thus, in calculating just some of the more apparent risks, which include the physical dangers, psychological trauma and devastation, and ostracism and criminalization that follow child prostitution, clearly all the ingredients of a vicious cycle are sewn into the lives of these teenage victims. Consequently, for too many of these still-developing children, it is nearly impossible to escape from these traps.

HISTORIES OF COMMERCIALLY EXPLOITED CHILDREN: FACES BEHIND THE LABEL

Sadly, death was the escape from prostitution for Christal Jean Jones of Burlington, Vermont. She was just 16 years old when she was murdered by asphyxiation on January 3, 2001 (Stone, 2003), and later found dead and half-clothed in a New York apartment. What makes her case different from many others frequently discovered across the country is that Jones was in the custody of the Social and Rehabilitation Services Department, a branch of Vermont's Human Services Agency. As a result, the state of Vermont launched an investigation into the policies and practices of its agencies that are charged with caring for troubled and endangered youth.

Aside from this difference in home life, some parts of Jones' background appear strikingly similar to histories of the many child prostitutes working streets throughout the United States. Records reveal that Jones was born in 1984, and her parents divorced around the time she was 4 years old. A few years later, her mother became involved with an abusive partner, a man whom her mother eventually fled to escape the abuse when Jones was between the ages of 5 and 8 years old. When Jones was about 12 years old, she entered the child protection system via a report of suspected abuse, an incident claimed by her mother to have been a skirmish between Jones and her sister. From this time until her death at 16 years old, Jones began chronically running away and eventually became involved with a child prostitution ring.

Not surprising in the least, Jones' history reveals a troubled childhood. As occurs in most pimp-seduction scenarios, a pimp (allegedly Jose Rodriguez) (Hemingway, 2001) capitalized on her vulnerability and then lured Jones from Vermont to New York with promises and lies. According to various accounts, "the girls were lured from the foster homes and state-run shelters where they lived around Burlington by expressions of love and promises of $2000" (Robinson, 1997). Next, like a predictable and badly written script, upon arriving in the Bronx, 2 girls reported being threatened against leaving and forced to pay back the money "owed" to the pimp—it is unclear whether Jones was one of these girls. Sadly, Jones believed Rodriguez loved her, and she wanted to be his girlfriend, according to a 19-year-old woman familiar with Rodriguez. Her murder remains unsolved.

Jill Leighton, on the other hand, lived to tell about her nightmarish experience as a commercially exploited teenager. Like many others, Leighton appeared to have no difficulties other than the average problems afflicting teenagers in her small town of 9000 people. However, outward appearances can be deceiving. In Leighton's case, although she appeared to come from a "good" family, behind closed doors she was suffering physical and sexual abuse at the hands of her mother's boyfriends. Unable to stand it any longer, she ran away from home at the age of 14 with only $100 and hopes of escaping the abuse.

Not surprisingly, she traded in one set of problems for another. Life on the streets became a desperate exercise in survival. With no place to stay and little to no money for meals, restaurant trash bins became a fruitful source of food until "[i]nto [the] hunger, loneliness and desperation came a man named Bruce" (DePasquale, 1997). As one might expect, Bruce had the physical trappings of success, good looks, and charm; he quickly promised her work, food, shelter, and clothing. Thinking this opportunity might end the days of cleaning up in public restrooms and sleeping in cemeteries, Leighton eagerly accepted his suggestion that they go to his "office."

Once inside, the humiliation immediately began. She was blindfolded and bound with leather straps, hung from a stage half nude and subsequently raped. This degradation of the human psyche introduced Leighton to her fate for the next 3 years. Against her will, and out of fear of being subjected to increased beatings and sexual torture, Leighton endured the "work" she was offered by Bruce, which included subjecting herself to acting as a slave for clients who wanted to act out their various bondage and/or torture fantasies. These "fantasies" included gang rape, torture, starvation, and other atrocities.

Leighton avoided being killed several different times, and in 1984 her ordeal ended when Bruce was arrested on unrelated charges. When the police entered the apartment where she was staying, they found her malnourished and locked in a closet (DePasquale, 1997). Physically and emotionally scarred, she is alive and continues to reconstruct her life out of the shame, humiliation, and devastation wreaked upon her human spirit. She speaks out against prostitution as a community outreach educator, advocate, and counselor with Project Prosper, a national educational organization with locations in Pennsylvania, North Carolina, and Minnesota (STORM, 2004).

CURRENT APPROACH BY LAW ENFORCEMENT AGENCIES AND THE NEED FOR SOCIAL SERVICE RESOURCES

What emerges from the facts is clear—the prostitution of children is child abuse and exploitation. It is not a chosen occupation in any real sense, considering the emotional, physical, and developmental immaturities and vulnerabilities of the children whose bodies are being sexually exploited, nor is it a glamorous profession or a victimless crime. Consequently, those who solicit or sell children for sexual purposes must be treated as they are—child abusers and/or sex offenders who should serve prison time and register as sex offenders.

In addition, there needs to be greater emphasis upon programs that serve the needs of sexually exploited children. For instance, a national survey conducted by the OJJDP, an arm of the Office of Justice Programs of the US Department of Justice, concluded in its final report, *Program to Increase Understanding of Child Sexual Exploitation*, that while child sexual exploitation is considered important by law enforcement agencies and youth-service providers in the large cities that were studied, the lack of resources and focus left these crimes unattended. Moreover, "in only a handful of communities were there youth-serving programs with a special emphasis on the specific needs of sexually exploited youth" (Whitcomb et al, 1998). Although little research exists about child sexual exploitation in rural communities, it is assumed that if major cities provide in-adequate training and resources to address this issue, then it is also true of small or rural communities. Indeed, the danger of an inadequate response is greater in small communities that do not believe their children are at risk of commercial exploitation.

Thus, despite society's current inability and perhaps unwillingness to acknowledge and address the prostitution of children, the fact remains that these victims are children. As a "civilized" society, everyone must take responsibility for the well-being of these children.

THE SUPPLY OF COMMERCIALLY EXPLOITED CHILDREN IN SMALL TOWNS AND COMMUNITIES

Small rural communities in the United States may not have the spectacle of children selling their bodies on local street corners, but these communities do supply a significant percentage of this nation's commercially exploited children. Poor inner-city children are often aware of the dangers of the street and are better equipped to ward off entreaties to enter the world of commercial exploitation. In contrast, the naïveté of rural children makes them easier targets (Frank, 2003).

The primarily rural state of Minnesota is the nation's number one supplier of commercially exploited children. In the year 2000, the Federal Bureau of Investigation reported there were more children from Minnesota arrested as prostitutes than in the states of Michigan, Massachusetts, and Maryland combined (Critchell, 2003). Las Vegas pimps call Minnesota "the factory"; a Minneapolis judge likens his state to an "assembly line" of commercially exploited children (Critchell, 2003).

As an example of the vulnerability of small town children, consider the case of Sara, a girl who hung out at the local roller rink in Coon Rapids, Minnesota. Sara was subsequently introduced to an older girl who was compassionate when Sara spoke of her father's drinking and her difficulties in school. Sara was a prime candidate to run away, and when offered a chance to escape to Texas, she took the opportunity. With no money to get back home, she became a commercially exploited child (Critchell, 2003).

CUTTING OFF THE SUPPLY OF COMMERCIALLY EXPLOITED CHILDREN FROM SMALL OR RURAL COMMUNITIES

Once rural communities recognize they are not immune from the social ill of commercially exploited children, a number of concrete steps can be taken to protect children from living and dying on the streets (**Table 44-1**).

USE OF COMMUNITY POLICING PRACTICES

Rural communities must develop good working relationships with the managers of local roller rinks, movie theatres, pool halls, and any other places where teenagers hang out. These managers should be asked to alert the authorities if older persons, particularly persons new to the community, start spending time at the facility and speaking to local teenagers.

In addition, local newspapers and shoppers should be asked to immediately contact the authorities if individuals outside the community place an advertisement for teenage models or other seemingly glamorous jobs outside of the town. If the newspapers are uncooperative, explore the possibility of using an administrative subpoena or other police power to investigate the reasonable possibility that such advertisements are a front for the commercial exploitation of children.

USE OF A COMMUNITY NETWORK TO IDENTIFY CHILDREN AT RISK

The children most likely to be lured into commercial exploitation are those having difficulties at home. Although many of these children are abused, the abuse may be more benign. Children whose parents are divorced, alcoholic, or are otherwise creating an unhealthy environment are also at risk for being lured to the street. Many chil-

Table 44-1. Steps Rural Communities Should Take to Protect Children from Exploitation

1. Use community policing practices
2. Use the community network to identify children at risk
3. Educate children about the dangers of the street
4. Educate parents to keep their children safe
5. Closely monitor local strip clubs
6. Develop a network of state and national contacts
7. Work at addressing child abuse at the earliest ages
8. Develop forensic interviewing skills for children of all ages
9. Develop investigative abilities for child sexual exploitation
10. Work closely with social services
11. Publicly advocate for commercially exploited children in an effort to acquire the necessary resources to address child exploitation issues

dren who themselves become involved with drugs or alcohol or who are displaying promiscuous or other dangerous behaviors are good candidates to escape their current lives for another they believe can not be worse.

All of the area schools need to be members of the local child protection team. At least once a month, these schools should present to the team a list of children with whom they have concerns. Next, a prevention program should be tailored for each of these families in order to create a healthier life for the child, thereby reducing the child's risk of running away from home.

If a child fitting within one of these categories has several unexplained absences from school, the authorities should be notified immediately. A police officer should visit the child's house to determine his or her whereabouts. This officer should not be satisfied with parents who claim the child is visiting relatives or have another seemingly plausible explanation and should follow up with the "relatives" until the child is located. Many parents do not report their children as runaways, because they know the child has fled since he or she is escaping sexual abuse or other maltreatment at home.

One reporter says that "wounded children are like a neon light" to recruiters of commercially exploited children (Frank, 2003). Wounded children must also be a neon light to members of small communities seeking to protect their children.

EDUCATION OF CHILDREN ABOUT THE DANGERS OF THE STREET

Just as educators and other professionals teach young children personal safety in hopes that they will report people who prey on them, the same must be done with adolescents and teenagers. Teenagers should understand the dangers of strangers who appear "too good to be true" with offers of glamorous or exciting adventures in metropolitan communities. Sometimes this education must be blunt. One police officer told a teenager from the small town of Mille Lacs, Minnesota, of a girl who told her pimp she was proud of her washboard stomach only to have the pimp scar the stomach with a hot curling iron (Frank, 2003). Blunt education such as this takes away any glamorous thoughts about life on the street.

EDUCATION OF PARENTS TO KEEP THEIR CHILDREN SAFE

Most parents would not allow a stranger to enter the bedroom of their adolescent or teenage children but freely allow their children to access the Internet in their bedrooms and visit chat rooms while online. One study concluded that 20% of all children between the ages of 10 and 17 had been solicited online (Medaris & Girouard, 2002). Inform parents of the risks and teach common-sense practices of having Internet-accessible computers in family rooms as well as prohibiting children from entering chat rooms.

CLOSE MONITORING OF LOCAL STRIP CLUBS

Strip clubs are notorious breeding grounds for the commercial exploitation of children (Frank, 2003). Even many small communities have a strip club, typically outside of town, to which the men of several small communities flock. Police officers should regularly visit these clubs and routinely check the identification of the dancers as well as the waitresses and others who may work in the establishment. Keep in mind that many victims may have obtained fake identification. Accordingly, check the identification with driver's license records or other information networks. Investigators and prosecutors should work with city councils and county boards to require strip clubs to conduct a thorough screening of workers to ensure they are of age. One such regulation would be to enact an ordinance requiring workers to produce a birth certificate and for employers to keep a copy on file at the club.

Investigators and prosecutors may want to work with city councils and county boards to prohibit lap dancing and other activities that make it easier to solicit sexual activity. Indeed, lap dancing is a form of sexual contact and, if done with a minor, may constitute a felony crime. Even if the dancer is of age, in some states the act may constitute an act of prostitution because the dancer is hired to perform in someone's lap. For example, Minnesota defines prostitution as engaging in sexual penetration or sexual contact for hire (Minnesota Statute, Section 609.321, Subdivision 9, 2002). Sexual contact is defined as including the "intentional touching by a prostitute of another individual's intimate parts" (Minnesota Statute, Section 609.321, Subdivision 10ii, 2002). Under this definition, a man hiring a woman to grind her legs or buttocks into his genitals until he ejaculates has arguably made himself a john and should be prosecuted accordingly; however, the defense could argue that the woman did not touch the man's intimate parts but rather the clothing covering the intimate parts. As a result, under a strict interpretation of the statue, a crime has not occurred. This distinction, however, is absurd, because an act of fellatio remains an act of fellatio whether or not the penis is covered by a condom. Even so, the Minnesota legislature specifically defines sexual contact in other parts of the code as including the touching of clothing covering intimate parts (Minnesota Statute, Section 609.341, subdivisions, 2002) but curiously does not make this clear in the code prohibiting prostitution.

DEVELOPMENT OF A NETWORK OF STATE AND NATIONAL CONTACTS

If a child does run away and is in danger of being commercially exploited, law enforcement officials should know whom to call. They should identify the closest metropolitan communities to which the child may have gone, as well as who works the juvenile prostitution cases within these metropolitan communities. In addition, they need to make these connections ahead of time to help locate a child quickly before he or she is trafficked to several cities.

ADDRESSING CHILD ABUSE AT THE EARLIEST AGES

If as many as 90% of the commercially exploited children in the United States are running away from homes in which they were physically and sexually abused (Flowers, 1998; Paul & Lisa Program, 2004; Whitcomb et al, 1998), then the underlying cause of much of the commercial exploitation of children is family abuse. Accordingly, it is imperative that all communities work to end child abuse. A number of papers exist to assist rural practitioners in developing a community response to reduce the incidence of child abuse (Vieth, 1998); in addition, a number of organizations exist to assist in implementing these reforms. The American Prosecutors Research Institute (APRI) trains thousands of front-line professionals each year, with most of these trainings conducted at the state and local level tailored to local needs (Vieth, 2004). For more information, contact APRI's National Center for Prosecution of Child Abuse or the National Child Protection Training Center at Winona State University.

Every child spared from familial abuse lessens the pool of children commercial exploiters recruit for further harm.

DEVELOPMENT OF FORENSIC INTERVIEWING SKILLS FOR CHILDREN OF ALL AGES

An essential component of detecting child abuse at its earliest ages is the art and science of forensic interviewing. Accordingly, every community must have investigators thoroughly trained in the skill of interviewing children. With an increasing number of states developing these programs, this skill is becoming easier to acquire. (For further information about state forensic interview training programs, see Holmes & Vieth, 2003.)

Forensic interviewing strategies applicable to young children are often inappropriate with older children who are susceptible to being enticed into a life on the street or who may, in fact, be living on the street. These children are wary of speaking to the authorities and are sometimes just as afraid of returning home as they are of continuing life in the sex industry. These children may seek to shock the interviewer with their language and/or behavior. Some of these children may have been aggressive in pursuing a street life in their attempt to escape other negative aspects of their existence and may not view themselves as victims. (For futher discussion of this dilemma, see Lanning, 2002.) Accordingly, if those in authority hope to connect with at-risk adolescents and teenagers, then police officers, social workers, and prosecutors must be skilled in conversing with this population. Training on this topic is available; for example, APRI offers such training as a part of its *Beyond Finding Words* course.

DEVELOPMENT OF INVESTIGATIVE ABILITIES FOR CHILD SEXUAL EXPLOITATION

In addition to educating parents about the dangers of the Internet, small town investigators and prosecutors must develop the skills to investigate and prosecute those who solicit children online. In addition to pimps who may solicit children for a life of exploitation, small towns have traveling salespersons and others who may go online seeking a child for a shorter, but equally exploitive, sexual encounter. In addition to acquiring the forensic interviewing skills needed to work with these victims, the authorities must develop the skills to handle other aspects of this crime, including the ability to conduct a legally defensible sting operation. APRI is one organization that conducts such training. Indeed, APRI is the only organization that conducts multidisciplinary training on child sexual exploitation issues through a course titled *Safety Net*. (For further information, contact APRI.) If it is true that 20% of all children between the ages of 10 and 17 have been solicited online, then law enforcement officials are clearly catching very few of those who prey on children over the Internet. During a 2-year period, America's Internet Crimes Against Children (ICAC) task forces claim to have arrested more than 550 individuals for child sexual exploitation offenses. Although this is encouraging, it means that only a small percentage of online solicitors are being apprehended. This figure is not likely to improve until all communities have at least some investigators capable of addressing this crime (Medaris & Girouard, 2002). This fact will not change unless a larger percentage of this nation's investigators are trained, including those in rural communities and small towns.

One part of the problem is that training regarding child sexual exploitation must be hands-on and can typically only be done with small groups of professionals. For example, in training investigators to conduct legally defensible, online sting operations, the students need their own laptops and the class size will need to be small. One idea to overcome this is to help states set up their own child sexual exploitation training programs consistent with national standards. This is what has happened in the field of forensic interviewing; APRI has assisted states in setting up their own courses through the *Half a Nation* project. If a similar model was employed in the area of child sexual exploitation, thousands of additional professionals could be trained, thereby impacting the lives of hundreds of thousands of children.

CLOSELY WORKING WITH SOCIAL SERVICES

The commercial exploitation of children is as much of a concern for social workers and child protection attorneys as it is for professionals handling the criminal aspects of this social ill. The job of social services is to work with troubled youth and transition them to a healthier life. Unfortunately, few resources have been committed to training social workers and child protection attorneys in order to address this problem. Moreover, since most of these children are runaways who flee the local jurisdiction, there is a significant financial incentive to ignore the cases. To do otherwise would mean incurring thousands of dollars in costs for rehabilitative services. All communities must commit to protecting children who flee their home jurisdiction to the same extent as those who remain at home. Training opportunities equal to those who handle the criminal aspects of child exploitation must be provided for those who handle the civil aspects. Congress made one step in this direction by appropriating a little less than a million dollars to create the National Child Protection Training Center (NCPTC). This program is a joint effort between the APRI and Winona State University. One of the training center's goals is to provide training, technical assistance, and publications to child protection attorneys and other professionals who handle civil child protection cases. (For more information, contact the NCPTC.)

PUBLIC ADVOCATION FOR COMMERCIALLY EXPLOITED CHILDREN IN AN EFFORT TO ACQUIRE THE NECESSARY RESOURCES TO ADDRESS THIS SOCIAL ILL

Few investigative and much less preventive programs are being funded at the state or national levels to address the commercial exploitation of children. For example, Minnesota has only one officer in the state exclusively assigned to responding to these cases (Critchell, 2003).

In a paper discussing the modern political history of child abuse and neglect, Krugman (1999), Dean of the University of Colorado School of Medicine, offers this analysis of the problem:

Effective policy making requires an "iron triangle": an effective lobbying organization, several congressional "champions," and inside help from a supportive bureaucracy. In contrast to the many instances of effective political efforts in health and defense, for example, the child protection system is ineffective. There are few notable congressional advocates, a weak lobby, and an even weaker bureaucracy.

The situation described by Krugman will not change until front-line child advocates learn ways to communicate the needs of exploited children to local, state, and federal governments, as well as to private organizations. Those working with these children and those toiling on the front lines must address the needs of children, not only during the course of an investigation or prosecution but also when the needs of children are being considered by governments and private organizations.

CONCLUSION

Erik Erickson said "(s)omeday, maybe, there will exist a well-reasoned, well-informed, and yet fervent public conviction that the most deadly of all possible sins is the mutilation of a child's spirit" (Vieth, 1994). If the day Erickson dreamed of is to arrive for the commercially exploited children of the United States, all segments of society must firmly commit to the goal of significantly reducing the numbers of children abused in this way. This means that the supply line of these children from many of the small towns and suburbs of this country must also be addressed. If this does not occur, then this problem will continue to be addressed only at its margins.

REFERENCES

Children of the Night: Rescuing America's Children From Prostitution. Frequently asked questions. 2004. Available at: http://childrenofthenight.org/site/faq.html. Accessed September 13, 2004.

Clayton M. In United States, Canada, new laws fail to curb demand for child sex. *Christian Science Monitor.* September 5, 1996:11.

Critchell D. Inside the teen-hooker factory. *Rolling Stone.* October 16, 2003:78-80.

DePasquale KM. The Effects of Prostitution. 1997. Available at: http://www.feminista.com/archives/v1n5/depasquale.html. Accessed September 13, 2004.

Estes RJ, Weiner NA. The commercial sexual exploitation of children in the US, Canada and Mexico. September 2001. Available at: http://caster.ssw.upenn.edu/~restes/CSEC.htm. Accessed June 11, 2004.

Flowers RB. *The Prostitution of Women and Girls.* Jefferson, NC: McFarland & Co; 1998:69.

Frank P. Lives destroyed: recruitment of youth for massive American sex trade happening here. January 23, 2003. Available at: http://www.pineandlakes.com/main.asp?Search=1&ArticleID=726&SectionID=23&SubSectionID=27&S=1. Accessed September 13, 2004.

Hammer H, Finkelhor D, Sedlak AJ. *Runaway/Thrownaway Children: National Estimates and Characteristics.* Washington, DC: US Dept of Justice, Office of Justice Programs, Office of Juvenile Justice and Delinquency Prevention; October 2002. NCJ 196469.

Hemingway S. Locking up Rodriguez will not solve Vermont's problem. May 9, 2001. Available in archives at: http://www.burlingtonfreepress.com. Accessed June 11, 2004.

Hofstede committee report: juvenile prostitution in Minnesota. 1999:6. Cited by: Nandon SM, Koverola C, Schledermann EH. Antecedents to prostitution: childhood victimization. *J Interpers Violence.* 1998;13:206-207.

Holmes LS, Vieth VI. Finding words/half a nation: the forensic interview training program of CornerHouse and APRI's National Center for Prosecution of Child Abuse. *The APSAC Advisor.* Winter 2003;15(1):4-8.

James J. Motivations for entrance into prostitution. In: Crites L, ed. *The Female Offender.* Lanham, Md: Lexington Books; 1976:177-198.

Krugman R. Convening a national call to action: working toward the elimination of child maltreatment: the politics. *Child Abuse Negl.* 1999;23:963-967.

Lanning KV. Law enforcement perspective on the compliant child victim. *The APSAC Advisor.* Spring 2002;14(2):4-9.

Medaris M, Girouard C. *Protecting Children in Cyberspace: The ICAC Task Force Program.* Washington, DC: Office of Juvenile Justice and Delinquency Prevention; January 2002. NCJ 191213.

Minnesota Statute, Section 609.321, Subdivisions 9 and 10ii, 2002.

Minnesota Statute, Section 609.341, Subdivisions 5, 2001.

Paul & Lisa Program, Inc. Who we are: facts & stats & definitions. Available at: http://www.paulandlisa.org. Accessed February 13, 2004.

Reaves G. Trading away youth: impoverished Thai parents sell girls into prostitution. Dallas Morning News. March 21, 1993:1A. Cited by: Levesque RJR. Sexual use, abuse and exploitation of children: challenges in implementing children's human rights. *Brooklyn L Rev.* 1994;60:959, 980.

Revaz CR. Hearing on optional protocols. Presented at: the United Nations Convention on the Rights of the Child Before the Congressional Human Rights Caucus, 107th Congress; June 6, 2002; Washington, DC. Available at: http://www.house.gov/lantos/caucus/TestimonyRevaz060602.htm. Accessed February 12, 2004.

Robinson LN. The globalization of female child prostitution: a call for reintegration and recovery measures via article 39 of the United Nations Convention on the Rights of the Child. *Indiana J Global Leg Stud.* 1997;5:239-255. Citing: Beyer D. Child prostitution in Latin America, in forced labor: the prostitution of children. *US Dept of Lab Ed.* 1996;32:32. Also citing: Schabner D. Fatal attraction: 16-year-old Vermont girl lured into prostitution, death in NYC. Available at: http://abcnews.go.com/sections/us/dailynews/prostitution_vt010206.html. Accessed June 11, 2004.

Seng MJ. Child sexual abuse and adolescent prostitution: a comparative analysis. *Adolescence*. 1989;24:665-675.

Stone E. Who killed Christal Jones? December 30, 2001. Available in archives at: http://www.burlingtonfreepress.com/. Accessed June 11, 2003.

STORM. July 1, 2004. Available at: http://www.thestormproject.com. Accessed September 13, 2004.

Stronski Huwiler SM, Remafedi G. Adolescent homosexuality. *Adv Pediatr*. 1988;45: 107-144.

Teenage prostitution ring broken in Detroit. *New York Times*. January 16, 2003;sect A:22.

Todres J. Prosecuting sex tour operators in US courts in an effort to reduce the sexual exploitation of children globally. *Boston Univ Public Interest Law J.* 1999;9:1,7.

University of Pennsylvania News Bureau [news release]. Discussion of: Estes RJ. *The Commercial Sexual Exploitation of Children in the US, Canada and Mexico*. Philadelphia: University of Pennsylvania, School of Social Work, Center for the Study of Youth Policy. September 10, 2001.

Vieth VI. In my neighbor's house: a proposal to address child abuse in rural America. *Hamline Law Rev*. 1998;22:143.

Vieth VI. The mutilation of a child's spirit: a call for new approach to termination of parental rights in cases of child abuse. *William Mitchell Law Rev*. 1994;20:727.

Vieth VI. The national child protection training center: a partnership between APRI and Winona State University. *Prosecutor*. January/February 2004;38:33.

Whitcomb D, DeVos E, Smith B. *US Dept of Justice, Program to Increase Understanding of Child Sexual Exploitation*. 1998:3.

Chapter 46

RECOMMENDATIONS FOR ACTION FOR DEALING EFFECTIVELY WITH CHILD SEXUAL EXPLOITATION*

Richard J. Estes, DSW, ACSW
Angelo P. Giardino, MD, PhD, FAAP
Sharon W. Cooper, MD, FAAP

RECOMMENDATIONS

Only a comprehensive approach to the elimination of child sexual exploitation (CSE) can succeed. Realization of the 14 recommendations that follow requires a higher level of public policy focus, commitment, and coherence as well as new human and fiscal resources to support the activities of federal, state, and local governments, service providers, human service planners, child advocacy organizations, researchers, and others seeking to protect children from sexual exploitation. Additionally, a higher level of public-private cooperation in combating CSE is necessary. In every case, these recommendations are mutually reinforcing; considered together, they form an integrated plan of attack on CSE. They reflect our view concerning what is needed nationally and internationally to combat all forms of CSE effectively: child pornography, the prostitution of children, Internet cyber enticement, child sex tourism, and the human trafficking of children.

PROTECT THE CHILDREN

Child victims of sexual exploitation can rarely protect themselves from the abuse and assaults inflicted on them by adults. The situation is especially serious for those children who fail to recognize or are unable to prevent the coercion that typically accompanies CSE. Thus, efforts to protect children from sexual exploitation must emphasize prevention as the first priority as well as early case finding, early and effective intervention once CSE has occurred, and limiting the impact of sexual exploitation on those children who have been repeatedly victimized.

PROTECT THE CHILDREN: THE ROLE OF THE FAMILY

Families are in a unique position to identify and intervene early in situations involving CSE. At a minimum, we recommend:

— Families receive accurate and timely information concerning the nature, extent, and seriousness of CSE in contemporary society.

— Families receive accurate and timely information concerning ways to protect children from CSE, including monitoring children's access to the Internet, helping children avoid adults and other juveniles who seek out children for sexual exploi-

* Neil A. Weiner, PhD of the Center for Research on Youth and Social Policy of the University of Pennsylvania is acknowledged for his contribution to the earlier formulation of some of the recommendations contained in this chapter (Estes & Weiner, 2001).

tation, and maintaining close contact with children after school if they do not have parental supervision.

— All victims of violence, including CSE victims, be empowered to report incidents of illicit sexual contact to law enforcement and human service authorities, consistent with the recommendations of the World Health Organization's (WHO's) World Report on Violence and Health (WHO, 2002).

— Children be protected from the fear of reprisal by the alleged perpetrator when making reports of CSE.

PROTECT THE CHILDREN: THE CONTRIBUTION OF TEACHERS, CLINICIANS, AND OTHER ADULTS WHO COME IN DIRECT CONTACT WITH CHILDREN

Teachers, clinicians, sports coaches, religious leaders, counselors, and other adults regularly come in contact with children and can serve as potential resources for protecting children from CSE and, when necessary, helping children receive timely and effective help to halt CSE. Teachers, clinicians, and other adults can be particularly helpful to children in reducing CSE situations that occur in the child's own home. Thus, we recommend that those who interact with children on a regular basis receive accurate and timely information concerning:

— The nature, extent, and seriousness of CSE in contemporary society.

— Ways in which children can be protected from CSE, including monitoring children's access to the Internet and helping children avoid adults and other juveniles who seek out children for sexual exploitation.

— The type of evidence required to refer a suspected case of CSE for investigation and, simultaneously, the service networks and other resources that exist for receiving such referrals for investigation.

Given the critical roles that schools perform in the lives of children and communities we recommend that educators:

— Develop and implement campaigns in their schools concerning the dangers of cyberspace in facilitating CSE.

— Monitor "special needs" students who, because of their increased vulnerability, are at high risk of being victims of CSE.

— Monitor all staff closely because abusers often position themselves where children are easily accessible.

— Keep parents appraised of measures to prevent exploitation through take-home correspondence and in-school meetings.

— Work with law enforcement to bring additional training for children into the classroom.

PROTECT THE CHILDREN: PROMOTE COMMUNITY INVOLVEMENT IN EDUCATION AND ADVOCACY

Communities that take an active role in protecting children from CSE are successful because they create a "family" of people who are strongly invested in the future of children. Organizations, law enforcement, and the media provide outlets for effective protection from and prevention of CSE. Thus, we recommend:

— Members of community law enforcement agencies take an active role when CSE is suspected, including investigating a suspected abuser and serving as caring authority figures for children to look up to.

— Communities develop and support culturally sensitive programs that educate and aid minority groups.

— The highest possible level of support be given to community organizations that provide services in court, case management, and community education to CSE-affected children and their families.

— Communities provide safe living options and a full spectrum of "wraparound" services to CSE victims (eg, medical diagnosis and evaluation services, health-care, emotional counseling, drug detoxification services, remedial schooling, job training).

— The public media, particularly television networks and the movie industry, share a heavy responsibility for disseminating age-appropriate and accurate messages concerning the nature, extent, and seriousness of CSE in contemporary American society.

PROTECT THE CHILDREN: THE ROLE OF THE GOVERNMENT

Given the cross-jurisdictional nature of many sex crimes involving children, we recommend a lead federal agency be given primary responsibility for protecting children from sexual exploitation. In identifying such an agency, we further recommend:

— Local and state human service and law enforcement agencies be given access to sufficient resources to fully investigate all suspected cases of child sexual abuse, child sexual assault, and other manifestations of CSE.*

— Local and state human service and law enforcement agencies be given access to sufficient resources to adequately supervise adults convicted of sex crimes against children.

— Safety nets created to protect children from CSE have access to sufficient resources to respond adequately to the service needs of local and transient children who take up temporary residence in local communities (including child protection agencies, victim assistance agencies, mental health centers, medical facilities, runaway shelters, drop-in centers, outreach projects, independent or transitional living programs for youth, and youth service programs).

TARGET ADULT SEXUAL EXPLOITERS OF CHILDREN, NOT THE CHILDREN, FOR PUNISHMENT

Tragically, sexually exploited children are often revictimized by the law enforcement and human services agencies created to serve them. Revictimization may take several forms: (1) blaming child victims for their own exploitation; (2) treating child victims as criminals; (3) an unwarranted emphasis on the part of law enforcement and other CSE first responders on the arrest of child victims of sexual exploitation rather than the adults who benefit from CSE, especially pimps, traffickers, and others; and (4) neglect on the part of many service providers of expensive, long-term care needs for sexually exploited children and youth due to fiscal constraints. Rather than focusing on the criminalization of child victims of sexual exploitation, we recommend:

— Sexually offending adults and juveniles be given an unequivocal message that sexually molesting children is wrong.

— The law enforcement community refocus the bulk of its activities on adult perpetrators of sex crimes against children (ie, pimps, traffickers, and customers).

— Greater federal attention be given to the role of national crime rings that include child sex among their "portfolio" of services.

— Appropriate mechanisms be found for local and state human service agencies to work more cooperatively with local, state, and federal law enforcement authorities

---

The incidence of substantiated cases of child sexual assault and child sexual abuse declined between 1993 and 2000 (Jones & Finkelhor, 2001); even so, 89 000 cases of child sexual abuse and an additional 51 100 cases of child sexual assault were substantiated to have occurred in 2000 (Sexual assault fact sheet, 2005).

in the earlier identification and apprehension of adults who commit sex crimes against children.

— Appropriate roles be found for "experiential youth" and other youthful victims of CSE to work with law enforcement to identify adult perpetrators of sex crimes against children, including adults associated with local and regional networks that recruit children into commercial pornography and prostitution.

INCREASE THE PENALTIES ASSOCIATED WITH SEXUAL CRIMES AGAINST CHILDREN

Considerable variation exists with respect to the seriousness assigned by law enforcement and, as a result, the penalties assigned to persons convicted of sex crimes against children. This is the case despite nearly a decade of national and international efforts to harmonize the legal understanding and treatment of sex crimes involving children at all levels of legal intervention. Thus, we recommend:

— Increasing uniformity across all levels of law enforcement and criminal justice concerning the nature and seriousness of crimes associated with CSE.

— Increasing uniformity across all levels of law enforcement with respect to the minimum penalties that should be associated with specific forms of CSE.

— To the fullest extent appropriate and possible, more complete integration of all federal, state, and local laws pertaining to CSE.

We further recommend:

— All sexual crimes against children involving adults be treated as felonies.

— Penalties for repeat adult offenders be severe.

— The courts and their representative agencies undertake long-term supervision of adults convicted of sex crimes against children through the use of state and nationally organized sex offender registries (SORs).

Though laden with many privacy issues, the US Supreme Court has ruled SORs constitutional; as a result, the majority of American states operate Internet-based SORs via the federally funded Jacob Wetterling Crimes Against Children and Sexually Violent Offender Registration Program. (A listing of Internet-based state SORs may be obtained from the Federal Bureau of Investigation (FBI) Web site at http://www.fbi.gov/hq/cid/cac/states.htm.) Similarly, the FBI maintains a separate national sex offender registry (NSOR) for states that are unable or unwilling to mount their own SOR (National sex offender registry, 2005). The NSOR has proven to be effective in monitoring the geographic movements of adults convicted of violent sexual crimes against children and, as such, may serve as a useful model for local and regional communities to monitor the movements of a broader range of repeat perpetrators living in their communities.

Our belief is that the adoption of these approaches to the judicial treatment of persons found guilty of CSE-related crimes is necessary to halt the epidemic of CSE and to make the treatment of CSE-related offenses more comparable to other felonies. Certainly, stronger and more consistently applied penalties for CSE-related crimes will help end the "cost/benefit" analyses engaged in by many criminals who conclude that sex crimes against children treated as misdemeanors entail high profits and lower legal risk than crimes already classified as felonies (eg, drug-related crimes, money laundering).

FULLY ENFORCE AND STRENGTHEN EXISTING NATIONAL AND STATE LAWS RELATING TO CHILD SEXUAL EXPLOITATION

A confirmed pattern of "benign neglect" exists in many communities regarding the needs of sexually exploited children and youth. This pattern is reflected in the comparatively low number of CSE cases currently being served by law enforcement and public human service agencies and in the absence of written policies and procedures for dealing with CSE cases on the part of both public and private agencies (Estes & Weiner, 2001; see the *Juvenile Arrest Rates by Offense, Sex, and Race (1980-2002)* on the National Center for Juvenile Justice Web site, http://ojjdp.ncjrs.org/ojstatbb/ crime/excel/JAR_20040801.xls, for more information). The situation is serious in cases involving runaway, homeless, and other youth who are not residents of the communities in which they are temporarily located.

We strongly recommend that the federal government provide national leadership in promoting the greatest implementation of all national, state, and local CSE laws *that already exist*, including the application of these laws in promoting the best interests of homeless and other street children and youth who are temporarily living in local communities. At a minimum, the federal government should:

— Require all federal agencies to develop strategic plans for implementing all federal laws related to the sexual exploitation of children.

— Provide financial incentives to state and local governments for implementing all laws related to CSE that currently prevail in their jurisdictions (eg, through the use of planning, coordination, and similar types of cooperation-building grants).

— Establish a system of deterrents for use with federal, state, and local government units that fail to comply with relevant laws pertaining to CSE (eg, withdrawal of funds, reassignment of responsibilities to other agencies, placing especially uncooperative agencies under court supervision).

Further, we recommend that federal statutes and laws used to adjudicate CSE-related crimes be applied in a more consistent manner. In most situations, greater consistency in the application of CSE-related laws and statutes will require clearer and more uniformly administered sentencing guidelines.

ESTABLISH A NATIONAL CHILD SEXUAL EXPLOITATION INTELLIGENCE CENTER

There is a need for full-time intelligence gathering and a strategic planning apparatus for monitoring national trends related to CSE. To that end, we recommend that a National Child Sexual Exploitation Intelligence Center (NCSEIC) be established. Though uniquely focused on issues related to CSE, the proposed goals and structure of the NCSEIC would be comparable to those of the National Drug Intelligence Center (NDIC):* (1) to support national policy makers and law enforcement decision makers with strategic domestic CSE intelligence; (2) to support national counter-CSE efforts; and (3) to conduct and report on a timely basis national, regional, and state CSE threat assessments.

In addition to other responsibilities, the functions of the NCSEIC would include:

— Efforts similar to those undertaken by Interpol (through Project INHOPE) and the European Community (through the COPINE Project) that have resulted in the creation of libraries of pornographic images with demonstrated admissibility to federal and state courts as evidence of sexual crimes against children.

— The conduct and dissemination of timely threat assessments of changing national, regional, and state trends in CSE.

— The conduct and dissemination of timely threat assessments concerning the involvement of organized criminal units in the commercial aspects of CSE.

— The promotion of continuing professional education of analysts, forensics specialists, and others needed to carry out on-going threat assessments and strategic planning on matters pertaining to CSE.

---

* *A full discussion of the mission and activities of the National Drug Intelligence Center is available from the following Web site: http://www.usdoj.gov/ndic.*

EXPAND FEDERALLY FUNDED MULTIJURISDICTIONAL TASK FORCES ON CHILD SEXUAL EXPLOITATION INTO ALL MAJOR FEDERAL AND STATE JURISDICTIONS

Federal multijurisdictional task forces (MJTFs) are emerging as powerful new mechanisms for combating serious crimes that fall within the purview of more than one federal agency (eg, drugs, money laundering, trafficking). Consisting of 2 or more federal agencies that share jurisdictional authority in a related area of criminal activity, MJTFs operate by increasing communication between agencies; promoting clearer goals; sharing intelligence, equipment, and personnel; and introducing administrative efficiencies in their cooperative undertakings. In exchange for their collaboration with one another, MJTFs receive more secure and longer-term federal funding, and they also receive technical assistance and training programs provided by experienced task force supervisors and agencies (What have we learned, 2005).

MJTFs appear to be effective in dealing more rapidly and comprehensively with federal crimes involving CSE, including pornography and trafficking in children for sexual purposes (USDOS, 2004; Whitcomb & Eastin, 1998). Among other accomplishments in combating CSE, MJTFs can:

— Sensitize local communities to the dangers of sex crimes against children.

— Promote multijurisdictional cooperation in identifying, apprehending, and prosecuting perpetrators of sex crimes against children.

— Promote new public-private partnerships in combating child pornography, the prostitution of juveniles, and trafficking in children for sexual purposes.

— Promote the strengthening of local laws designed to protect children from sexual abuse, sexual assault, and sexual exploitation.

— Serve as focal points for promoting higher levels of public and continuing professional education concerning CSE.

Given their emerging effectiveness in advancing the national agenda to combat the sexual exploitation of children, we recommend:

— Federal MJTFs on CSE be expanded into additional jurisdictions.

— MJTFs cooperate more fully with local and state law enforcement authorities to promote increasing coherence between federal, state, and local anti-CSE initiatives.

— Mechanisms be developed to further involve representatives of the private human service sector in the early identification and apprehension of adults who seek out child victims for sexual exploitation.

EXPAND FEDERALLY FUNDED INTERNET CRIMES AGAINST CHILDREN TASK FORCE PROGRAMS INTO ALL MAJOR FEDERAL AND STATE JURISDICTIONS

The federally sponsored Internet Crimes Against Children (ICAC) Task Force program has demonstrated considerable effectiveness. Since its inception in 1998, the ICAC program has contributed to the arrest of more than 1500 adults eliciting sex with children via the Internet, seized more than 5000 computers used to perpetrate such crimes, and annually reached tens of thousands of children, parents, educators, and law enforcement officials with initiatives that promote safe online procedures (USGSA, 2004). Regional ICACs work closely with the National Center for Missing & Exploited Children (NCMEC) in investigating the thousands of suspected cases of child pornography and exploitation annually reported to the NCMEC's Cyber-Tipline (USGSA, 2004). Hence, we strongly support:

— Continued use of regional ICACs to promote a safer online environment for children.

— Expansion of regional ICACs into additional federal, state, and local jurisdictions.

— Use of the ICAC Task Force program as an example of the high level of effective interagency and multijurisdictional cooperation that is possible to help reduce the risk of sexual exploitation of children.

PROMOTE EFFECTIVE PUBLIC-PRIVATE PARTNERSHIPS FOR COMBATING CHILD SEXUAL EXPLOITATION

A successful national campaign to combat CSE requires active participation and co-ordination of efforts on the part of all stakeholders committed to the prevention of CSE. Among others, these stakeholders include the following:

— Governmental agencies charged with leadership responsibility in combating CSE at the local, state, and federal levels

— Nongovernmental organizations (NGOs) and agencies that provide direct services to sexually exploited children and their families

— Associations and networks of sexually exploited children and youth

— Associations and networks of parents and guardians of sexually exploited run-away, thrownaway, homeless, and otherwise missing children

— NGOs engaged in advocacy, research, and educational activities on behalf of sexually exploited children nationally and internationally

— NGOs engaged in advocacy, research, and educational activities on behalf of adult victims of domestic violence and CSE

— Primary and secondary school educators

— Businesses that are used by abusers in the commercial sexual exploitation of children (eg, Internet Service Providers, hotel/motel chains, transportation vendors, travel agencies)

— Foundations and other public-benefit fiduciary organizations that provide financial support to programs serving sexually exploited children and their families

— Representatives of the public media (including news print, television, radio, and the film industry)

We recommend that the federal government give programmatic and fiscal leadership to:

— The development of local, state, and national councils (coalitions and task forces) of public and private stakeholders committed to the elimination of CSE.

— The development by these councils of multiyear strategic plans that include specific goals and timetables focused on combating CSE in their communities.

— The development of nationally linked coordinating mechanisms whereby local and state strategic plans for the elimination of CSE can be integrated into comprehensive national and, where appropriate, international plans of action.

ENLARGE THE NATIONAL POOL OF CHILD SEXUAL EXPLOITATION EXPERTS AND SPECIALISTS

A serious national shortage in the number and type of specialists in CSE exists. These shortages are most apparent in the forensics area and are manifest in judicial and prosecutorial agencies. An urgent need exists for more social workers, psychologists, psychiatrists, educators, physicians, lawyers, police officers, coroners, and others with special expertise in CSE. We recommend the federal government:

— Significantly expand its current programs of continuing education focused on increasing the national pool of legal, correctional, and human service professionals with specialized expertise in CSE.*

— Promote increased attention to CSE content and practices in the curricula and training programs of all professional disciplines that share responsibility for assisting sexually exploited children and their families.

— Promote increasingly higher levels of interdisciplinary education and cooperation in the field of CSE.

Health professionals (physicians, nurses, social workers, and emergency medical personnel) may often be an initial or ongoing point of contact for CSE victims and their families. Those on the front lines working in shelters and outreach sites need training, but others working in less obvious settings may encounter victims. These professionals should have the awareness, knowledge, and skills to recognize high-risk situations and screen, evaluate, and refer for the many health-related issues that need attention. The following should be provided:

— Training of first responders in recognition and intervention of CSE

— Policy statements, position papers, and standards developed by professional organizations regarding appropriate knowledge, skills, and attitudes medical professionals should have regarding CSE

— Model curricula that can be easily integrated into existing training, including the following:

— End Child Prostitution, Child Pornography and Trafficking of Children for Sexual Purposes' (ECPAT's) *The Psychosocial Rehabilitation of Children Who Have Been Commercially Sexually Exploited—A Training Guide* (Delaney & Cotterill, 2001)

— World Vision's *Crying Out: Children and Communities Speak on Abuse and Neglect* (Dorning, 2002)

— Second World Congress' East Asia and Pacific Regional Consultation's *Asia-Pacific Answers: Good Practices in Combating Commercial Sexual Exploitation of Children and Youth* (ESCAP et al, 2001)

UNDERTAKE MORE SPECIALIZED STUDIES OF PERPETRATORS AND VICTIMS OF CHILD SEXUAL EXPLOITATION

More needs to be understood about the precise nature, causes, and extent of CSE, especially that which occurs among sexually vulnerable populations of children and youth hidden from public view. Specifically, we recommend that federal priority be given to advancing research on:

— Understanding more fully those aspects of American life that appear to contribute to CSE, including changing societal values and mores, weakening family structures, the persistence of male dominance over females, and vagueness on the part of some adults concerning the right of children not to be physically, emotionally, or sexually violated.

— The development of more detailed profiles of "opportunistic" and "situational" exploiters of children for sex.

— The development of more detailed profiles of juvenile sexual offenders who exploit younger children already known to them (eg, older siblings, neighbors, children of family acquaintances).

---

* *Existing efforts include those sponsored by selected federal agencies for their own staff engaged in the investigation of CSE cases (eg, US Customs Service, US Bureau of Federal Investigation, US Postal Inspection Service) and those provided by private organizations through contractual arrangements with the Office of Juvenile Justice and Delinquency Prevention and other federal agencies, eg, the Jimmy Ryce Law Enforcement Training Center of the National Center for Missing & Exploited Children and the Fox Valley Technical College (USGSA, 2004).*

— The development of more detailed profiles of "pimps" and others (older juveniles and adults) who systematically promote the commercial sexual exploitation of juveniles.

— The development of more detailed profiles of national and international traffickers of children for sexual purposes.

— The nature and extent of CSE among children and youth who self-identify as sexual minorities (ie, gay, lesbian, bisexual, and transgender children).

— The nature and extent of CSE among girls in gangs, especially girls who are members of male-controlled gangs, ethnically organized gangs, and Native American tribal gangs.

— The nature and extent of CSE among American youth who cross international borders (especially into Mexico) in pursuit of cheaper drugs, alcohol, and sex with child nationals of those countries.

— The nature and extent of "designer sex" among middle-income and other economically well-off youth living in their own homes who engage in commercial sex to purchase more expensive clothing, jewelry, and drugs.

— The nature and extent of CSE among youth living in poverty.

— The international dimensions of CSE with a US nexus, including American youth who are trafficked outside the United States for sexual purposes and foreign children and youth who are trafficked into the United States.

— The short-term and long-term impact of sexual exploitation on children and youth as they mature into adults.

CONCLUSION

Protecting America's children from sexual exploitation is a complex and difficult responsibility. The task is more difficult given the high levels of secrecy, misinformation, and misperception that surround the involvement of children in pornography, prostitution, and even sexual trafficking, yet the problem of CSE exists and each year continues to affect hundreds of thousands of children.

Despite the difficulties involved, considerable progress has been made in combating CSE nationally and internationally. Certainly, clinicians and other practice-based professionals have been better educated to identify the warning signs associated with CSE. They understand more fully the continuum of abuse that exists between child sexual abuse, child sexual assault, and other forms of CSE. Similarly, law enforcement and human service professionals are more sensitive to the existence of child pornography and the prostitution of juveniles and are more aware of the long-term consequences of CSE on individual children, families, and society. Increasingly, people around the world have begun to understand that sexual trafficking in children and youth is a problem that afflicts impoverished nations and rich and poor countries alike.

These important advances in recognizing the existence, nature, and seriousness of CSE have contributed to a growing worldwide intolerance of the sexual victimization of children. As a result, global strategies to combat CSE have been developed, regional compacts that seek to prevent CSE have emerged, new and more comprehensive national and local laws designed to protect children from sexual victimization have been passed, and, increasingly, adults who prey on children for sex are coming under court supervision. Teachers, physicians, social workers, child advocates, and others are actively working with police, judges, and other law enforcement officials to weave a more secure safety net designed to protect children from CSE. Children themselves have joined in the effort, including "experiential youth" and other former child victims of CSE.

The editors of this publication are optimistic that, at last, nations and their leaders are prepared to confront the realities of CSE with reasonable solutions. We feel a sense of optimism that the human and fiscal resources required to implement the agreements and laws passed exist and that, in time, a growing number of political leaders and nations will join with parents, children, and child specialists in protecting children from the ravages of sexual exploitation.

REFERENCES

Delaney S, Cotterill C. *The Psychosocial Rehabilitation of Children Who Have Been Commercially Sexually Exploited: A Training Guide*. Bangkok, Thailand: ECPAT; 2001.

Dorning K. *Crying Out: Children and Communities Speak Out on Child Abuse and Neglect*. Milton Keynes, England: World Vision International; 2002.

Economic and Social Commission for Asia and the Pacific (ESCAP), End Child Prostitution, Child Pornography and Trafficking of Children for Sexual Purposes (ECPAT), United Nations Children's Fund (UNICEF), et al. *Asia-Pacific Answers: Good Practices in Combating Commercial Sexual Exploitation of Children and Youth*. Bangkok, Thailand: United Nations, ESCAP; 2001.

Estes RJ, Weiner NA. The commercial sexual exploitation of children in the US, Canada and Mexico. September 2001. Available at: http://caster.ssw.upenn.edu/~restes/CSEC.htm. Accessed January 24, 2005.

Jones L, Finkelhor D. *The Decline in Child Sexual Abuse Cases*. Washington, DC: US Dept of Justice, Office of Juvenile Justice and Prevention; 2001.

National sex offender registry. FBI Web site. Available at: http://www.fbi.gov/hq/cid/cac/registry.htm. Accessed January 17, 2005.

Sexual assault fact sheet. Crimes Against Children Research Center (CCRC) Web site. Available at: http://www.unh.edu/ccrc/factsheet/sexualassault.htm. Accessed January 24, 2005.

US Department of State (USDOS). *Trafficking in Persons Report, 2004*. Washington, DC: USDOS, Office of the Under Secretary for Global Affairs; 2004.

US General Services Administration (USGSA). *Catalogue of Federal Domestic Assistance: Missing Children's Assistance (CFDA #16.543)*. Washington, DC: Office of Justice Programs, Office of Juvenile Justice and Delinquency Prevention, US Dept of Justice; 2004.

What have we learned from evaluations of multijurisdictional task forces? Bureau of Justice Administration (BJA) Web site. Available at: http://www.bja.evaluationwebsite.org/psi_mtf/forces2.shtml. Accessed January 24, 2005.

Whitcomb D, Eastin J. *Joining Forces Against Child Sexual Exploitation: Models for a Multi-jurisdictional Team Approach*. Washington, DC: Office for Victims of Crime, US Dept of Justice; 1998.

World Health Organization (WHO). *World Report On Violence and Health*. Geneva, Switzerland: WHO; 2002. Available at: http://www.who.int/violence_injury_prevention/violence/world_report/en/. Accessed January 24, 2005.

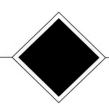

INDEX

A

C

N